PHYSIOLOGIC AND PATHOLOGIC ANGIOGENESIS - SIGNALING MECHANISMS AND TARGETED THERAPY

Edited by **Dan Simionescu**
and **Agneta Simionescu**

Physiologic and Pathologic Angiogenesis - Signaling Mechanisms and Targeted Therapy
http://dx.doi.org/10.5772/64121
Edited by Dan Simionescu and Agneta Simionescu

Contributors

Pavel Makarevich, Yelena Parfyonova, Masumi Akita, Keiko Fujita, Tomoko Takahashi, Nicolás Renna, Rodrigo Damián García, Jesica Ramirez, Roberto M. Miatello, Wiliam M. Chilian, Liya Yin, Peter Hopmann, Kathleen Graham, Bhamini Patel, Kanithra Sekaran, Mansee Desai, Lingfang Zeng, Ana Moraga, Ka Hou Lao, Tamara Franz-Odendaal, Daniel Andrews, Shruti Kumar, Susumu Minamisawa, Norika Liu, Kosuke Kaji, Hitoshi Yoshiji, Jimmy Stalin, Lucie Vivancos, Nathalie Bardin, Francoise Dignat-George, Marcel Blot-Chabaud, Marina Ziganshina, Lyubov V. Krechetova, Lyudmila V. Vanko, Zulfiya S. Khodzhaeva, Ekaterina L. Yarotskaya, Gennady T. Sukhikh, Ioana Berindan-Neagoe, Cornelia Braicu, Ciprian Tomuleasa, Diana Gulei, George Adrian Calin, Luke Brewster, Scott Robinson, Wilfred Jefferies, Singh Chaahat, Cheryl G Pfeifer, Imran Shahid, Waleed Almalki, Muhammad Hassan Hafeez, Muhammad Ahmed, Muhammed Saifullah, Mohammad Imam, Mohammed Al Rabia, Paola Guerrero, Joseph McCarty, Ivanka Dimova, Valentin Djonov, Sepehr Feizi, Lucia Napione, Maria Alvaro, Federico Bussolino, Yi Lu, Victor Gardner, Chikezie Madu, Lamia Heikal, Gordon Ferns

Published by InTech
Janeza Trdine 9, 51000 Rijeka, Croatia

Notice

Publishing Process Manager Martina Usljebrka
Technical Editor SPi Global
Cover InTech Design team

First published April, 2017
Printed in Croatia
Legal deposit, Croatia: National and University Library in Zagreb

Additional hard copies can be obtained from orders@intechopen.com

Physiologic and Pathologic Angiogenesis - Signaling Mechanisms and Targeted Therapy , Edited by Dan Simionescu and Agneta Simionescu
p. cm.
Print ISBN 978-953-51-3023-9
Online ISBN 978-953-51-3024-6

For EU product safety concerns:
IN TECH d.o.o., Prolaz Marije Krucifikse Kozulić 3, 51000 Rijeka, Croatia,
info@intechopen.com or visit our website at intechopen.com.

Meet the editor

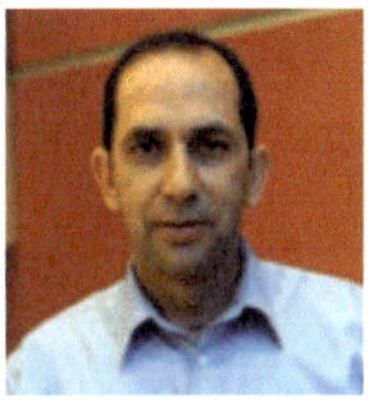

Dr. Dan Simionescu is the Harriet and Jerry Dempsey Professor of Bioengineering and Director of the Biocompatibility and Tissue Regeneration Laboratories at the Clemson University, Clemson, SC. He has published more than 80 peer-reviewed papers in highly ranked journals such as *Circulation, Cardiovascular Pathology, American Journal of Pathology, Tissue Engineering,* and *Biomaterials* and has more than 160 peer-reviewed conference proceedings presented worldwide. Dr. Simionescu's general research interests include vascular biology, pathology, and regeneration using scaffolds and stem cells. His current interest is preclinical validation of translational tissue engineering approaches and is being generously funded by the NIH and the biomedical industry for his efforts in the field of cardiovascular biology, pathology, and regenerative medicine.

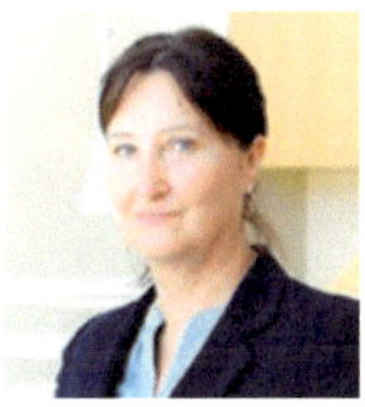

Dr. Agneta Simionescu received her PhD degree in Biochemistry/Cell Biology for the study of matrix remodeling in cardiac diseases. Agneta has research interests in translational tissue engineering, angiogenesis, remodeling, and mechanotransduction. She was the first to show that matrix metalloproteinases (MMPs) are involved in degeneration of implanted cardiovascular biomaterials and that matrix-derived degradation products (matrikines) induce pathologic osteogenic activation of cardiovascular cells. She has also shown that stabilization of biomaterials and scaffolds with mild and reversible cross-linking agents might counteract these effects. In recent years, she has developed a passion for investigating the effects of diabetes on cardiovascular tissue engineering, including diabetes-related alterations of biomaterials and scaffolds, stem cell differentiation, matrix remodeling, and microvascular network formation in vitro and in vivo models of diabetes.

Contents

Preface XI

Section 1 Signaling Mechanisms in Physiologic and Pathologic Angiogenesis 1

Chapter 1 **TGF-β Activation and Signaling in Angiogenesis 3**
Paola A. Guerrero and Joseph H. McCarty

Chapter 2 **Role of Notch, SDF-1 and Mononuclear Cells Recruitment in Angiogenesis 25**
Ivanka Dimova and Valentin Djonov

Chapter 3 **Angiogenesis Meets Skeletogenesis: The Cross-Talk between Two Dynamic Systems 47**
Tamara A. Franz-Odendaal, Daniel Andrews and Shruti Kumar

Chapter 4 **Corneal Angiogenesis: Etiologies, Complications, and Management 57**
Sepehr Feizi

Chapter 5 **Angiogenesis-Related Factors in Early Pregnancy Loss 77**
Marina M. Ziganshina, Lyubov V. Krechetova, Lyudmila V. Vanko, Zulfiya S. Khodzhaeva, Ekaterina L. Yarotskaya and Gennady T. Sukhikh

Chapter 6 **Pathogenic Angiogenic Mechanisms in Alzheimer's Disease 93**
Chaahat Singh, Cheryl G. Pfeifer and Wilfred A. Jefferies

Section 2 Angiogenesis in the Cardiovascular System 111

Chapter 7 **Hypoxia, Angiogenesis and Atherogenesis 113**
Lamia Heikal and Gordon Ferns

Chapter 8 **Coronary Collateral Growth: Clinical Perspectives and Recent Insights 133**
Bhamini Patel, Peter Hopmann, Mansee Desai, Kanithra Sekaran, Kathleen Graham, Liya Yin and William Chilian

Chapter 9 **Angiogenesis and Cardiovascular Diseases: The Emerging Role of HDACs 149**
Ana Moraga, Ka Hou Lao and Lingfang Zeng

Chapter 10 **Unique Phenotypes of Endothelial Cells in Developing Arteries: A Lesson from the Ductus Arteriosus 175**
Norika Mengchia Liu and Susumu Minamisawa

Chapter 11 **Vascular Repair and Remodeling: A Review 195**
Nicolás F. Renna, Rodrigo Garcia, Jesica Ramirez and Roberto M. Miatello

Section 3 Mechanisms of Tumor Angiogenesis 213

Chapter 12 **Tumor Angiogenesis: A Focus on the Role of Cancer Stem Cells 215**
Keiko Fujita and Masumi Akita

Chapter 13 **VEGF-Mediated Signal Transduction in Tumor Angiogenesis 227**
Lucia Napione, Maria Alvaro and Federico Bussolino

Chapter 14 **Noncoding RNAs in Lung Cancer Angiogenesis 251**
Ioana Berindan-Neagoe, Cornelia Braicu, Diana Gulei, Ciprian Tomuleasa and George Adrian Calin

Section 4 Novel Methods in Angiogenesis Research 291

Chapter 15 **Recent Advances in Angiogenesis Assessment Methods and their Clinical Applications 293**
Imran Shahid, Waleed H. AlMalki, Mohammed W. AlRabia, Muhammad Ahmed, Mohammad T. Imam, Muhammed K. Saifullah and Muhammad H. Hafeez

Chapter 16 **Novel Methods to Study Angiogenesis Using Tissue Explants 319**
Tomoko Takahashi, Keiko Fujita and Masumi Akita

Section 5 Pro-angiogenic and Anti-angiogenic Therapies 341

Chapter 17 **Therapeutic Angiogenesis: Foundations and Practical Application 343**
Pavel Igorevich Makarevich and Yelena Viktorovna Parfyonova

Chapter 18 **Platelet Lysate to Promote Angiogenic Cell Therapies 365**
Scott T. Robinson and Luke P. Brewster

Chapter 19 **Anti-VEGF Therapy in Cancer: A Double-Edged Sword 385**
Victor Gardner, Chikezie O. Madu and Yi Lu

Chapter 20 **Antiangiogenic Therapy for Hepatocellular Carcinoma 411**
Kosuke Kaji and Hitoshi Yoshiji

Chapter 21 **MCAM and its Isoforms as Novel Targets in Angiogenesis Research and Therapy 429**
Jimmy Stalin, Lucie Vivancos, Nathalie Bardin, Françoise Dignat-George and Marcel Blot-Chabaud

Preface

Welcome to the fascinating world of angiogenesis! Back by popular demand, this is the second edition of the *Vasculogenesis and Angiogenesis* Open Access book published in 2011 by InTech. The previous book comprised ten chapters of outstanding scientific content spanning the field of angiogenesis, from developmental biology to regenerative medicine. The original book elicited substantial enthusiasm, and as of January 2017, its chapters were downloaded more than 23,400 times from the InTech website.

We are now returning to the field, stronger than ever, with more than double the number of chapters and with an expanded content and focus. In order to gain an overview of the important elements in the field, we generated a "word cloud" or an objective weighted list of single-word terms gathered from all the abstracts of the current chapters. This graphical representation shown below highlights the most prominent terms, the frequency of each one being proportional to the font size. Our word cloud highlights a group of essential terms of significance to angiogenesis: factors, signaling, tumors, stem cells, blood and vascular, VEGF, endothelial cells, and therapeutic.

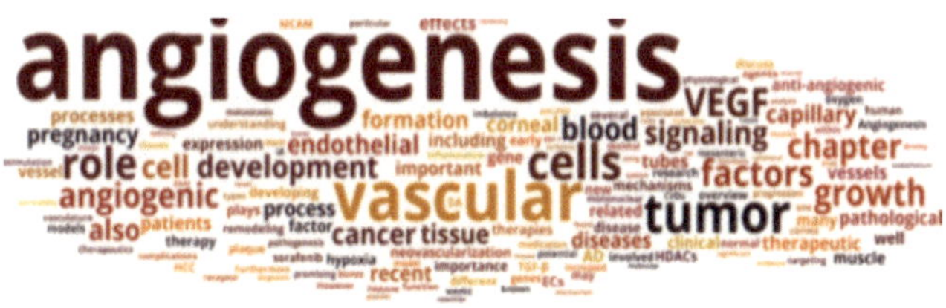

We therefore grouped the chapters into five parts. The first two parts cover cellular and molecular signaling mechanisms in physiologic and pathologic angiogenesis with application to development, the nervous system, skeletal formation, corneal angiogenesis, and the cardiovascular system. During embryonic development blood vessels form very early and aid in generation of most organs. In healthy adults, new blood vessel formation is not well represented; thus most organs appear to be "reticent" to de novo angiogenesis. Of particular note is the role of VEGF, TGF-beta, Notch, SDF-1, CXCR4, MMPs, TIMPs, histone-modifying enzymes, and other signals in angiogenesis as well as the association of imbalances in homeostasis of these factors with early loss of pregnancy, Alzheimer's disease, cardiovascular diseases, and others. Notable is also the intricate relationship between angiogenesis and endothelial cells, endothelial progenitor cells and hypoxia, and atherosclerosis and growth of coronary collaterals.

The third part grouped chapters on angiogenesis research in cancer. Starting with publication of the original hypothesis by Judah Folkman in 1971 and discovery of VEGF by Napoleone Ferrara in 1989, this topic continues to attract abundant attention and has generated many promising therapies. In addition, cancer stem cells, which can differentiate into cancer endothelial cells and influence angiogenesis, have become important targets in the fight against cancer. Since numerous experimental approaches in vitro and in vivo are being utilized in angiogenesis research, the fourth chapter was dedicated to presentation and discussion of advanced methods and models for the study of angiogenesis. Special emphasis was placed on critical analysis of pros and cons of each method, so that the reader can select adequate models for research and validation of selected targets.

Finally, in the fifth part, utilizing information from basic studies, significant focus has been placed on developing targeted therapies for either promoting or inhibiting angiogenesis. This dichotomy is quite unique to angiogenesis research and has generated a wealth of information that feeds and cross-pollinates both aspects. In scenarios where angiogenesis is desired such as ischemia relief after occlusion of blood vessels, therapies have been developed to induce new blood vessel formation using growth factor delivery and stem cell-mediated gene therapy to overexpress VEGF. Conversely, to limit tumor development, which in most cases relies on de novo vascularization, numerous treatments targeting the intentional stoppage of angiogenesis have been tested. Evidently, one major target is VEGF and its specific receptors. While initial clinical trials with anti-VEGF treatments have proven successful, we had learned throughout the years that these medications may cause significant side effects; in addition, some tumors were found to be resistant to anti-VEGF therapies. Meanwhile, additional potential targets have been identified. These include receptor tyrosine kinases, angiotensin receptors, angiotensin-converting enzymes, and cell surface receptors such as CD146, among others. Clearly there is a need for sustained research and testing of additional targets that would set the basis for effective treatment and benefit an increasing number of patients worldwide.

The purpose of this book is to highlight novel advances in the field and to incentivize scientists from a variety of fields to pursue angiogenesis as a research avenue. Blood vessel formation and maturation to capillaries, arteries, or veins is a fascinating area which can appeal to multiple scientists, students, and professors alike. Angiogenesis is relevant to medicine, engineering, pharmacology, pathology, genetics, and veterinary sciences and to the many patients suffering from blood vessel diseases and cancer, among others. We are hoping that this book will become a source of inspiration and novel ideas for all and offer this quote as a last word from Paracelsus:

“Medicine is not only a science; it is also an art. It does not consist of compounding pills and plasters; it deals with the very processes of life, which must be understood before they may be guided."

Acknowledgments

The editors would like to thank Dr. Adriana S. Bankston for helping with the angiogenesis word cloud and to acknowledge financial support from the Department of Bioengineering at the Clemson University, the Harriet and Jerry Dempsey Professorship Award, NIH grants 5P20GM103444-07 and R56HL130950-01, and grants from the Competitiveness Operational Programme 2014–2020; Tissue engineering technologies for cardiac valve regeneration, VALVE-REGEN, ID P_37_673, MySMIS code, 103431, contract 50/05.09.2016; and Targeted therapies for heart valve disease in diabetes, THERAVALDIS, ID P_37_298, MySMIS code: 104362, contract 115/13.09.2016.

Dr. Dan Simionescu and Dr. Agneta Simionescu
Clemson University, Clemson, SC, USA

Section 1

Signaling Mechanisms in Physiologic and Pathologic Angiogenesis

Chapter 1

TGF-β Activation and Signaling in Angiogenesis

Paola A. Guerrero and Joseph H. McCarty

Additional information is available at the end of the chapter

http://dx.doi.org/10.5772/66405

Abstract

The transforming growth factor-β (TGF-β) signaling pathway regulates various cellular processes during tissue and organ development and homeostasis. Deregulation of the expression and/or functions of TGF-β ligands, receptors or their intracellular signaling components leads to multiple diseases including vascular pathologies, autoimmune disorders, fibrosis and cancer. In vascular development, physiology and disease TGF-β signaling can have angiogenic and angiostatic properties, depending on expression levels and the tissue context. The objective of this chapter is to analyze the mechanisms that contribute to the activation and signaling of TGF-β in developmental, physiological and pathological angiogenesis, with a particular emphasis on the importance of TGF-β signaling in the mammalian central nervous system (CNS).

Keywords: TGF-β, vasculogenesis, angiogenesis, VEGF

1. Introduction

Discovery of TGF-βs was the result of independent efforts by several laboratories [1–4] during characterization of a secreted factor from fibroblasts transformed by the Moloney sarcoma virus (MSV). The TGF-β superfamily is now known to be composed of more than 30 chemokines such as TGF-β1-β3, activins, anti-Müllerian hormone (AMH), bone morphogenetic proteins (BMPs), growth and differentiation factors (GDFs) and NODAL that can signal via canonical and noncanonical receptors and intracellular effector proteins [5].

The best characterized member of the TGF-β family, TGF-β1, is initially produced from a single gene as a large precursor known as pre- and pro-TGF-βs which undergo two proteolytic cleavage events. The first signal peptide is cleaved in the rough endoplasmic reticulum. Furin, a proprotein convertase, subsequently cleaves the protein into two fragments [6]. The carboxy terminus corresponds to the functionally active cytokine and the large amino terminus is latency-associated protein (LAP), also referred to as the prodomain. Regardless of this processing by furin, the mature and LAP domains remain associated by noncovalent bonds to form the small latent complex (SLC). This complex subsequently covalently interacts with a second gene product, the latent TGF-β binding protein (LTBP), and is incorporated into a larger latent complex (LLC) that associates with the extracellular matrix (ECM) [6]. Three-dimensional crystal structure of porcine latent TGF-β1 shows a conformation that resembles a ring-like shape [7]. Two domains were defined in the structure: (i) an arm domain that contains an integrin-binding Arg-Gly-Asp (RGD) peptide motif and (ii) a "straitjacket" domain where the mature TGF-β is encased. At the opposite end of the arm domain, LTBP binds the prodomain forming the "ring head" [7] (**Figure 1**).

After secretion, the LLC complex interacts with various ECM proteins, such as fibronectin and fibrillin, and is maintained in an inactivated form [8]. TGF-β is activated by different mechanisms, including interactions with integrins, alterations in pH and extracellular proteases. αv integrin, which forms heterodimers with five different β integrin subunits (β1, β3, β5, β6 and β8), that bind to LAP-TGF-β1 and LAP-TGFβ-3 [9, 10]. However, only αvβ6 and αvβ8 have been shown to activate the latent TGF-β complex [11]. Activation by both αvβ6 and αvβ8 integrins requires the RGD motif in LAP. Activation by αvB6 requires an intact cytoplasmic domain [12, 13] and the presence of other ECM proteins [14]. Activation by αvβ8, however,

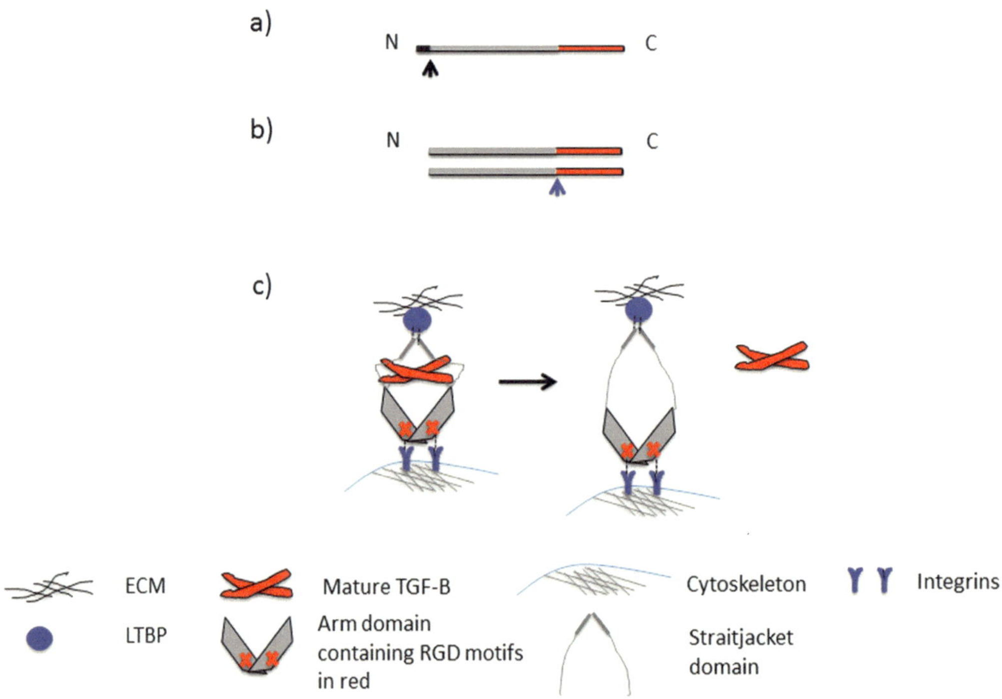

Figure 1. TGF-β processing and activation. **(a)**TGF-β precursor undergoes proteolysis at its N-terminus (black arrow head) which results in the removal of its signal peptide. **(b)**In a second proteolytic cleavage event by furin (blue arrow head), the precursor is separated into a large LAP or prodomain (gray) and the mature TGF-β (red) and **(c)**Schematic view of the closed ring structure (left) and unfastened straitjacket (right) conformation corresponding to the inactive LAP-TGF-β and mature TGF-β, respectively.

does not require the integrin cytoplasmic domain, but it is reported to require the presence of metalloproteinases (MMPs) on the cell surface or in the ECM [9]. Additionally, in T cells, αvβ6 and αvβ8 can activate LAP-TGF-β in cooperation with the glycoprotein-A repetitions predominant protein (GARP) [15, 16].

TGF-β is also activated by proteases. Aspartyl (e.g., cathepsin D) [17], cysteine (e.g., calpain) [18] and serine proteases (e.g., plasmin and kallikreins) and metalloproteases have shown to stimulate the release of chemokine from the latent complex, although most of these studies have been performed *in vitro* [19]. Moreover, TGF-β has been reported to be activated by other nonprotease mechanisms such as neuropilin1 (Nrp1), thrombospondin (TSP-1), F-spondin, pregnancy-specific beta-1-glycoprotein 1 (PSG1) and deglycosylation. Likewise, there are chemical and physical settings that activate TGF-β, for example, heat, ultraviolet radiation, physical shear, detergents and reactive oxygen species [8].

Three-dimensional structural studies of the LLC reveal that the RGD motifs are readily available for integrin engagement. Hydrophobic side chains, which have been identified near the RGD motif, likely enhance integrin binding [7]. In the presence of αvβ6, LLC can bind one or two integrin monomers. However, this binding does not induce required conformational changes to promote the complete activation of TGF-β, which is in agreement with prior mutational studies [12, 13, 20]. Furthermore, in accord with previous studies, the crystal structure of latent TGF-β predicts that pulling forces, emanating from the integrin C-terminal cytoplasmic tail that interacts with the cytoskeleton and binding RGD via the N-terminal extracellular region, are counteracted by associations with the ECM. Therefore, in the latent TGF-β, the straitjacket domain is maintained in a closed conformation until tensile forces are applied from both ends of the structure, resulting in loosening of the straitjacket domain and the release of the mature TGF-β. This study also showed that an additional feature of the prodomain is to prevent access to activating receptors [7].

2. TGF-β signaling pathways

Signaling is regulated by three major receptors: TGF-β receptor type I (TβRI), type II (TβRII) and type III (TβRIII). In general, TGF-β binds TβRIII, which facilitates its delivery to TβRII, a constitutively active kinase, leading to the subsequent phosphorylation and activation of TβRI. In humans, there are seven TβRIs, also known as activin receptor-like kinases (ALK), and five TβRIIs [5]. In most cells, ALK-5 forms a heterodimer with TβRII bound to TGF-β, which activates the ALK-5 kinase domain via phosphorylation of its GS domain. This receptor activation propagates intracellular signaling through 'canonical' effector proteins mothers against decapentaplegic homolog 2/SMAD family member 2 (Smad2) and Smad3, which are transcription factors. Once phosphorylated, these Smad proteins form a complex with Smad4 leading to nuclear translocation and initiation of genes transcription. In most normal cells, TGF-β-mediated activation of Smads leads to inhibition of cell growth. More specifically, the Smad2/3-4 complex partners with foxhead box O (FOXO) factors to activate p21Cip1 (*CDKN1A*), which inhibits cyclin-dependent kinase 1(CDK1), resulting in cell cycle arrest. Similarly, TGF-β can also activate p15Inkab (*CDKN2B*), the CDK4 inhibitor, through the SMAD2-3/4-FOXO1 axis (**Figure 2**) [5].

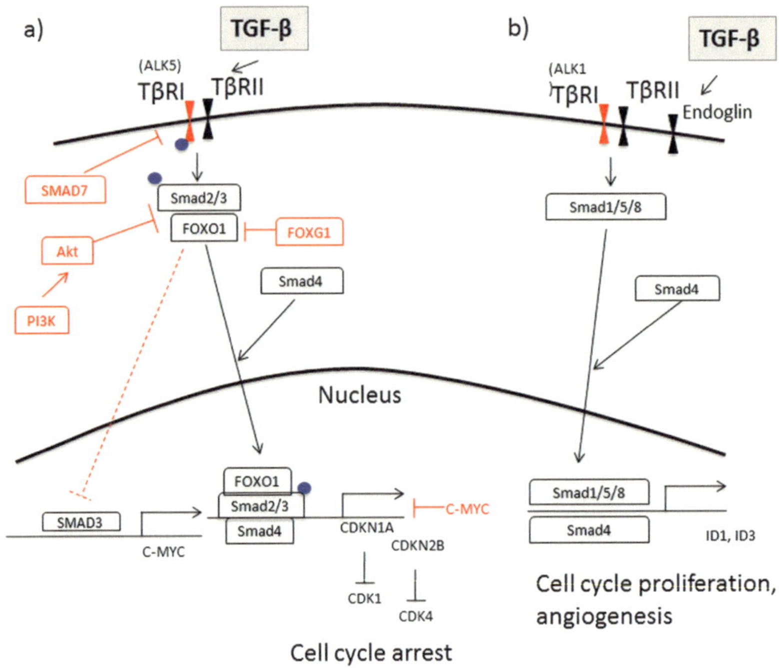

Figure 2. TGF-β canonical pathway. **(a)**In normal cells and early stages of cancer TGF-β promotes cell cycle arrest. Repressors of the pathway are shown in red. Blue dots represent protein phosphorylation and **(b)**in endothelial cells, an alternative pathway promotes cell proliferation.

Likewise, TGF-β acts as a cytostatic factor by decreasing c-Myc expression and downregulating the inhibitor of DNA-binding protein (ID) 1 and ID3 transcription factors. ID1 and ID3 are involved in differentiation, cell cycle progression and self-renewal of stem cells [21, 22]. TGF-β elicits c- Flk-1myc repression by promoting SMAD3 binding to a repressing Smad-binding element (RSBE) at the c-myc promoter [23]. c-Myc can be recruited to the promoters of *CDKN1A* and *CDKN2B* by the Myc-interacting zinc-finger (MIZ-1). This blocks CDK expression and results in apoptosis [24]. Additionally, in endothelial cells (ECs), TGF-β can target a second receptor type 1, ALK-1, which signals through Smad1/5/8 and stimulates angiogenic factors, such as interleukin 1 receptor-like 1 and ID1 (**Figure 2**) [25].

Several proteins are known to antagonize canonical TGF-β signaling. For example, (i) PI3K activates AKT which phosphorylates the SMADs-FOXO complex and inhibits its translocation to the nucleus [21], (ii) foxhead box G1 (FOXG1) inhibits the SMADs-FOXO complex [21], (iii) SMAD7 can trigger TβRI for proteosomal degradation by recruiting SMAD-specific E3 ubiquitin protein ligase (SMURF1) and SMURF2 [26], (iv) SMAD6 blocks SMAD1 through SMAD4 binding, (v) Erk proteins phosphorylate SMADs and inhibit their nuclear translocation, (vi) BAMBI, a pseudoreceptor, dimerizes with TβRI leading to its inactivation, (vii) FKBP12 binds to TβRI and impedes its phosphorylation, activation and signaling [27] and (viii) protein arginine N-methyltransferase 1 (PRMT1) methylates SMAD6 and allows BMP signaling through SMADs1/5 [28–30].

http://dx.doi.org/10.5772/66405

3. Vasculogenesis

During embryogenesis, the development of the vascular system is divided into three stages, vasculogenesis, angiogenesis and arteriogenesis. Vasculogenesis occurs in embryonic organs as well as extraembryonic tissues such as the placenta, yolk sac and allantois [31]. The earliest discernible structures in vasculogenesis, the blood islands, are formed in the mouse yolk sac by embryonic day (E) 6.5–7. This structure contains precursor cells or hemangioblasts, which differentiate to EC and hematopoietic cells [32]. At E8.5, cells located toward the periphery of the blood island, or angioblasts, differentiate into EC, while cells located toward the central region give rise to hematopoietic precursor cells. Next, lumenization takes place; tight junctions and basement membranes develop, and pericytes are recruited to blood vessels and promote maturation [33].

Several growth factors have been identified to regulate vasculogenesis, such as vascular endothelial growth factor (VEGF), fibroblast growth factor (FGF), the hedgehog family, neuropilins, integrins, fibronectin and TGF-βs. FGF-2 has been reported to participate in the generation of the angioblast in quail/chick chimeras and in vessel formation [34].

Hedgehog signaling has been shown to be crucial in the initial steps of vasculogenesis. It promotes differentiation of the primitive endoderm into both, endothelial and hematopoietic lineage [35]. For instance, blocking Indian hedgehog (Ihh) causes signaling repression from the visceral ectoderm and consequently abrogation of vasculogenesis and hematopoiesis in anterior epiblast [35]. Deletion of *Ihh* in mouse caused 50% lethality at midgestation with the remaining 50% dying at birth. Defects in blood vessel formation have been proposed as the cause for the lethality, which has been supported by experiments showing: (i) deletion of Sonic hedgehog (*Shh*) in mice resulted in a reduction in vascularization in lung [36], (ii) overexpression of *Shh* resulted in an increase in vascularization in neuroectoderm [37], (iii) depletion of *Shh* in zebrafish caused defective vasculature [38] and (iv) depletion of *Ihh* from stem cell-derived embroid bodies inhibited blood island differentiation [39].

VEGF signaling is crucial in vasculogenesis. Genetic studies have shown that deletion of *Flt-1* (VEGFR1), *Flk-1/KDR* (VEGFR2) and one or both alleles of *VEGF* cause embryonic lethality. VEGFR1 mutants exhibit aberrant central localization of the angioblasts in the blood island, instead of their normal localization toward the periphery [40]. These results implied that the growth of ECs was not inhibited in this region and led to the idea that VEGR1 hampers signaling from VEGF by ligand sequestration [33]. In addition, VEGFR2 mutants die around E9. In these embryos, both vasculogenesis and hematopoiesis do not initiate which was explained by faulty blood island in which cell migration was abrogated [41, 42]. Similarly, mutant heterozygous for VEGF die by E11 and showed impaired vasculogenesis and angiogenesis. These embryos showed severe abnormalities, such as underdeveloped brain and heart, decreased number of nucleated red blood cells in blood islands and aberrant vasculature in nervous system and placenta [43].

Neuropilins are co-receptors for VEGF receptors. Nrp1 is found in ECs of arteries, while neuropilin 2 (Nrp2) is found at the endothelium of lymphatic vessels and veins. Deletion of *Nrp1* in mice affects severely the central and peripheral nervous systems, as well as the yolk sac vasculature [44]. In contrast, depletion of *Nrp2* has no effects in the vasculature of arteries or veins, but it does affect angiogenesis of the lymphatic vasculature [45, 46]. In addition, mice harboring deletions in both neuropilins have shown obstruction in vasculogenesis in the yolk sac and in the formation of the primary vascular plexus [47].

4. Developmental angiogenesis

Angiogenesis is the formation of new blood vessels from existing vasculature. It occurs by mechanisms including sprouting angiogenesis and intussusceptive angiogenesis (**Figure 3**). Sprouting angiogenesis initiates with the selection of endothelial tip cells at the vessel wall. These cells react toward extracellular stimuli and secrete proteolytic enzymes to digest the surrounding ECM. Tip cells are connected to endothelial stalk cells to direct the vascular sprout [33, 48, 49]. Once the new tube is formed and a lumen is established, the vessel is stabilized by the recruitment of pericytes to capillaries or vascular smooth muscle cells (vSMC) to arteries and veins [6, 33], leading to re-establishment of mature blood vessels.

Intussusceptive angiogenesis, also known as splitting angiogenesis, results in the formation of intermediate intracapillary pillars. This mechanism is more efficient than sprouting angiogenesis since it does not require cell proliferation. Instead, it needs the reorganization of existing ECs. In this process, (i) ECs from opposite sides of the blood vessel make contacts, (ii) ECs from both ends reorganize and cause a splitting in the vessel wall, (iii) an interstitial pillar core is generated and (iv) myofibroblasts, pericytes and finally collagen invade the pillar and a basement membrane is formed [33, 49, 50].

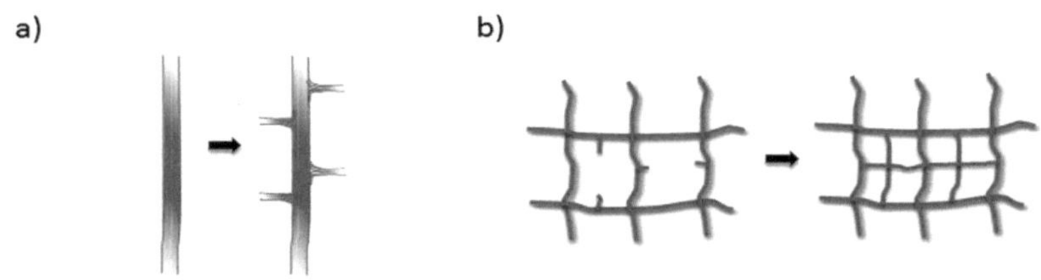

Figure 3. Mechanisms of angiogenesis. **(a)**Sprouting and **(b)**intussusceptive angiogenesis.

5. TGF-β in vasculogenesis and angiogenesis

5.1. Mutant phenotypes in mice lacking components of the TGF-B pathway

TGF-β mRNA was initially detected by PCR in preimplantation stages and in situ expression was present as early as E7.5, suggesting important roles in early development [51, 52]. In the embryo, proper TGF-β was detected in angioblast progenitors within the primitive heart mesoderm. Likewise, its expression was detected in extraembryonic tissues, including in the allantois mesoderm, and within blood islands of the yolk sac [53].

Deletion of the TGF-β1 gene in mice resulted in 50% lethality in utero, with the remaining 50% of mutant mice surviving up to three weeks postnatally. Histopathology analyses showed multifocal inflammatory cell infiltration and necrosis in several organs, especially the heart and stomach [53, 54]. It was subsequently shown that maternal contributions of *TGFB1* RNA and other genetic and epigenetic factors contributed to 50% postnatal survival [55].

The 50% of TGF-β mutants showed lethality and resorption by E10.5. Analysis of E8.5 embryos did not show significant morphological defects. However, analysis of E9.5 and E10.5 embryos resulted in a range of phenotypic defects within the yolk sac. While in some cases, vasculogenesis was delayed; in other cases, a dramatic reduction in size was observed and it was accompanied by weak and disorganized primary vessels, with some areas displaying complete vessel depletion. Analysis of the yolk sac vasculature indicated that the defects occurred during differentiation of ECs and hematopoietic cells. In contrast, the initial differentiation of mesodermal cells into ECs was not affected [52].

Genetic ablation of TβRII resulted in very similar phenotypes as in TGF-β1 mutants, with alterations in yolk sac vasculature and embryonic lethality by E10.5- E11.5 [56]. Mutants in endoglin also showed defects in vascular vessels within and outside the embryo. Embryo lethality was observed at E11.5, with mutants developing focal hemorrhage [57, 58]. Similarly, engineered mutations in mice that abrogate the expression of *ALK1, ALK5, SMAD1* or *SMAD5* resulted in defects in cardiovascular development [57, 59, 60].

5.2. Roles of TGF-β in angiogenesis

Early work to determine the roles for TGF-βs in ECs was contradictory. TGF-β signaling was initially found to inhibit cell migration and proliferation [61, 62], yet later studies indicated that it promotes cell proliferation [63–66]. The relative levels of expression of TGF-β seem to partially explain these discrepancies, with low doses promoting angiogenesis and higher levels resulting in growth inhibition of ECs and maturation of blood vessels [66, 67]. For instance, during blood vessel coverage by smooth muscle cells, TGF-β paracrine signaling from ECs to mesenchymal cells results in vascular smooth muscle cell and pericyte differentiation [6].

TGF-β also plays a role in the angiogenic process of hypoxic tissue. For instance, during infarction (stroke), neovascularization occurs primarily at the ischemic penumbra (periphery of the infarct), which correlates with high levels of both mRNA and active TGF-β protein [68]. Similarly, during organ transplant VEGF and TGF-β1, levels are increased in devascularized hypoxic tissue. TGF-β3 was also upregulated in hypoxic tissues, but to a lesser degree [69].

TGF-β regulates angiogenesis by different mechanisms; for example, it is involved in vessel proliferation and maturation by alternating two signaling cascades with opposite effects (ALK1 and ALK5). Likewise, TGF-β can promote its own expression, and it upregulates the expression of other angiogenic factors such as, platelet-derived growth factor (PDGF), interleukine-1, basic fibroblast growth factor (bFGF), tumor necrosis factor alpha and transforming growth factor alpha [70]. TGF-β can change the functions of other factors, such as VEGF, from prosurvival to pro-apoptotic [71]. Similarly, *in vitro* work has shown that in ECs TGF-β upregulates the expression of endothelin (*EDN1*), *PDGFA* and *PDGFB*, nitric oxide synthase

3 (*NOS3*), actin, alpha 2, smooth muscle, aorta (*ACTA2*), secreted protein acidic and cysteine rich (*SPARC*), *TSP-1*, fibronectin (*FN1*), collagens (*COL1A1, COL4A1,* and *COL5A1*), plasminogen activator (*PLAU*), serpin family E member 1 (*SERPINE1*) and integrins (*ITGB1, ITGB3, ITGAV, ITGA2* and *ITGA5*). It can also downregulate several genes, such as selectin-E (*SELE*), *KDR*, von Willebrand factor (*VWR*), thrombomodulin (*THBD*), monocyte chemo-attractant protein (*MCP1*), C-X-C motif chemokine ligand 1 (*CXCL1*), integrins (*ITGB1, ITGB3, ITGA5* and *ITGA6*), *TIMP1* and *PLAU* [70].

Levels of ALK1 and ALK5 determine TGF-β mitogenic or mitostatic responses in ECs. ALK5-Smad2/3 signaling stimulates transcription of ECM proteins such as fibronectin and plasminogen activator inhibitor type 1, which promote the resolution of angiogenesis by inducing vessel maturation. In contrast, signaling via the ALK1-Smad1/5/8 pathway generates anti-angiogenic responses [25, 51]. This requires a TGF-β accessory receptor, endoglin, which enhances ALK1 signaling and inhibits ALK5 cytostatic phenotype [72]. More recent work has shown that in the mouse eye retina the leucine-rich alpha-2-glycoprotein (Lrg1), which binds endoglin, promotes angiogenesis through Alk1-Smad1/5/8 in the presence of TGF-β [73].

5.2.1. TGF-β signaling in CNS development

In the mammalian CNS, neurons, astrocytes, pericytes and ECs closely interact to form a multicellular neurovascular unit [11]. During embryonic brain development, TGF-β is critical for sprouting angiogenesis of the CNS. In particular, TGF-β has been shown to work in conjunction with αv integrins to regulate paracrine signaling between neuroepithelial cells and ECs within neurovascular units. In mouse, embryos deletion of αv integrin showed vascular defects that were restricted mainly to the brain. This phenotype was recapitulated in β8 integrin mutant embryos. In contrast, deletion of β3 and β5 integrins did not cause brain vasculature abnormalities [74, 75]. Cell type-specific deletion of αv and β8 integrins in nervous system glial cells resulted in developmental intracerebral hemorrhage as well as postnatal motor dysfunction and seizures. Of note, the brain hemorrhage observed in embryos was absence in adult mice, suggesting that a compensatory mechanism that repairs hemorrhage occurs after birth [75, 76]. Interestingly, αv ablation in vascular ECs did not show a phenotype [75]. In later work, in which an outbred background was used to overcome the effects of β8−/− embryonic lethality, it was shown that adult mice lacking β8 integrin displayed neurovascular pathologies [77]. Most notably, adult β8 integrin mutants displayed a reduction in olfactory bulb size and abnormalities at the subventricular zone and rostral migratory stream. Neuroblasts generated in the subventricular zone utilize blood vessels as guides to migrate within the rostral migratory stream and differentiated to neurons within the olfactory bulbs. The size-reduced olfactory bulbs in adult β8−/− mice revealed essential roles for this integrin in promoting neuroblast migration along blood vessels. These defects correlated with a reduction in TGF-β signaling in neurospheres dissected from β8−/− mice [77].

The brain vascular defects observed in *Itgb8* null mutants are also shared by *Tgfb1* and *Tgfb3* loss of function mutants. In addition, mutating the integrin-binding RGD binding site in *Tgfb1* leads to early embryonic lethality [78]. Similarly, mice lacking both β6 and β8 integrins showed similar phenotypes as null mutants for *Tgfb1* and *Tgfb3* [78].

http://dx.doi.org/10.5772/66405

More recently, integrin β8 and Nrp1 have been shown to mediate neuroepithelial-endothelial cell interactions. β8 integrin in the neuroepithelium activates TGF-β signaling in ECs, while Nrp1 suppresses canonical TGF-β signaling, thus controlling normal sprouting angiogenesis [79]. Disruption of TGF-β signaling by targeting β8 integrin or Nrp1 results in excessive vessels sprouting and branching and formation of dysplastic glomeruloid-like vessels that are hemorrhagic [80].

The αvβ8-TGF-β connection in developmental angiogenesis in the brain also regulated neovascularization in the developing retina, where β8 integrin is expressed in astrocytes and Muller glial cells, a neuroepithelial cell type specifically found in the retina [81]. β8−/− retinas display abnormalities in the formation of the secondary vascular plexus, including impaired sprouting and formation of blood vessels with glomeruloid-like tufts. In addition, intraretinal hemorrhage was detected [81]. Furthermore, ablation of αv or β8 integrins but not of *Tgfbr2* in astrocytes resulted in defects in angiogenesis, and blocking TGF-β1 with neutralizing antibodies affected paracrine signaling to ECs [81]. This work was confirmed later in a study showing that *Tgfbr2* deletion in ECs of neonatal mice caused bleeding in the brain and vascular abnormalities, hemorrhage and deficiency in the formation of the deeper vascular network in the retina [82, 83]. Similarly, reduced Smad2 phosphorylation was observed in ECs from retina of *Tgfbr2* knockout mice [82].

6. TGF-β in pathological angiogenesis

Genetic mutations in TGF-β signaling components are associated with various human vascular pathologies. For example, mutations in the TβRIII/endoglin gene are linked to hereditary hemorrhagic telangiectasia (HHT) and Osler-Rendu-Weber syndrome. The disease is characterized, among others, by arteriovenous malformations (AVM) in the liver, brain and lung, telangiectases in skin and mucous membranes and recurrent epistaxis [84]. In trying to understand AVM, it was proposed that TGF-β paracrine signaling from ECs to vascular smooth muscle cells and/or pericytes was reduced. As a consequence, vascular smooth muscle cell differentiation was affected and this resulted in fragile, leaky blood vessels [85]. Alternatively, other suggested mechanisms underlying AVM endothelial cell apoptosis and depletion of smooth muscle cells [6]. In addition, it was discovered that brain AVM present decreased levels of integrin β8 which correlates with decreased TGF-β activation and signaling in ECs [86]. Mutations in human *ITGAV* and *ITGB8* genes also predispose some families to spontaneous brain hemorrhage [87].

In cancer, angiogenesis is not properly regulated as it occurs in developmental and physiological settings. Hypoxic conditions and proangiogenic factors released by tumor cells promote robust new blood vessel formation. The intratumoral vasculature is often disorganized and leaky with hypertension and acidosis. Similarly, tumor ECs display aneuploidy as well as centrosome and chromosomal amplifications [88]. The TGF-β pathway is affected by either mutations in the main signaling components, in particular SMADs, or by altered expression of repressive factors (e.g., FOXG1, PI3K-AKT and C-MYC) (**Figure 1**). Analysis of copy number alterations using data from The Center Genome Atlas (TCGA) and analyzed by cBioportal show that Smad2, 3 and 4 are mutated, deleted or amplified in several tumor types, but especially in pancreatic, colorectal and gastric cancers [89, 90].

During tumor growth and progression, TGF-β plays a dual role as both an angiogenic and angiostatic factor [6]. In early-stage tumors, higher TGF-β expression levels are correlative with a better prognosis. TGF-βs exert cell cycle arrest by downregulating c-Myc and Ids 1–3 in late G1 phase and by promoting the expression of cyclin-dependent protein kinase inhibitors [25]. As a proangiogenic factor, TGF-β pathway collaborates with VEGF, PDGF and bFGF in autocrine/paracrine signaling. In highly vascularized tumors, such as GBM and hepatocellular carcinoma (HCC), TGF-β levels are upregulated. In HCC cells, TGF-β induces the secretion of VEGF-A. Accordingly, inhibition of TGF-β by the TβRI/II synthetic kinase inhibitor LY2109761 showed decreased tumor size, vessel density and VEGF expression. This inhibitor also affected paracrine signaling between tumor cells and ECs. These effects on VEGF-A were dependent on SMAD2/3 expression levels [91]. Likewise, TGF-β inhibition in other cancer types such as colorectal cancer and GBM has also led to reduce intratumoral vascularization [59, 92–94]. Of note, the increase in angiogenesis caused by TGF-β in GBM was decreased by inhibition of the JNK pathway [95]. TGF-β family members also promote the secretion of MCP1 and TGF-α [96, 97], which impact inflammatory cells in the tumor microenvironment.

6.1. VEGF regulation by TGF-β

TGF-β promotes the expression of a major regulator of vasculogenesis and angiogenesis, VEGF. The VEGF family is comprised of a large group of secreted glycoproteins that interact with various cell surface receptors. VEGF-A is expressed as four different isoforms (121, 165, 189, 206 a.a.). Isoform 121 has low binding for heparan sulfate and diffuses away from its secreted location creating a chemogradient. Isoform 165 has higher affinity to heparan sulfate compared with 121, and it shows the highest mitogenic capacity among all isoforms. Finally, isoforms 189 and 206 have shown the highest binding capacity to bind heparan sulfates and are known to interact with other components of the ECM [33]. These ligands bind mainly three tyrosine kinase receptors (VEGFR) 1–3. VEGF-A has been a major therapeutic target in cancer due to its upregulation in many cancer types. Unfortunately, anti-angiogenic therapies that target VEGF-A, such as the neutralizing antibody Bevacizumab, have been unsuccessful in clinical studies where patients have shown resistance to anti-VEGF therapy. Similarly, in vitro studies performed in GBM cell lines indicated that irradiation enhances VEGF secretion [98–101].

FGF-2 induces VEGF expression in ECs via paracrine and autocrine signaling mechanisms [71]. TGF-β balances FGF-2 by suppressing the induction of plasminogen activator, a serine protease involved in the migration of cells, which is required in the formation of capillaries during angiogenesis [102]. In contrast, TGF-β induces ECs apoptosis as part of capillary remodeling and at the same time promotes ECs expression of VEGF [103]. VEGF-A is an ECs survival factor and protects ECs from apoptosis [104]. More recent work has shown that VEGF targets p38MAPK resulting in ECs survival. In contrast, in the presence of TGF-β, FGF-2 is activated, promoting VEGF upregulation, p38MAPK activation and apoptosis [71].

6.2. Upregulation of TGF-β in GBM

In GBM, an "angiogenic switch" marks the transition from low to more malignant tumors where ECs proliferate, resulting in a major increase in blood vessels. This excessive growth in vasculature was initially thought to be required for maintaining the aggressive growth rate of GBM. However, recent work suggests that these aberrant blood vessels are also required to maintain glioma stem cells (GSC), which are known to localize in close proximity to ECs in a perivascular niche. These cells secrete VEGF and express VEGFR2, and this complex is stabilized by NRP1. This axis is involved in the self-renewal, survival and tumorigenic capacity of GSCs [105]. Recent work has shown that TGF-β induces differentiation of GSCs into pericytes to support vessel formation and tumor growth [106].

TGF-β cooperates in glioma angiogenesis by enhancing the expression of FGF, VEGF, PDGF-β, and CD44. Increased expression of FGF promotes VEGF expression. High levels of TGF-β in gliomas correlate with poor prognosis, and it is known to work in conjunction with the PDGF-β to increase GSCs proliferation [107]. In vSMC, TGF-β expression increases the levels of PDGF-β, its receptor (βPDGFR) and of EGF receptor (EGFR). βPDGFR promotes VEGF expression and secretion in ECs and signals through PI3K [108].

Angiogenesis in GBM develops by two mechanisms: microvascular cell proliferation and sprouting. The origin of microvascular proliferation seems to arise from hypoxia, where cells migrate away from the hypoxic center as a result of an increase in the levels of migration-related genes. As a consequence, the center becomes necrotic and the cells surrounding it form a palisade, which secretes angiogenic factors such as VEGF. This promotes neighboring angiogenesis, known as glomeruloid-like microvascular proliferation, composed of both endothelial and smooth muscle cells. In contrast, the increase in angiogenic capillaries can be observed by staining with markers such as CD31 and Factor VIII-related antigen (**Figure 4**) [109].

TGF-β1-3 levels and endoglin-ALK1 signaling are elevated under hypoxic conditions. In addition, under hypoxia, *Snail* and *Slug* expression levels are increased. These genes are known to be involved in endothelial to mesenchymal transition and in sprouting angiogenesis and are regulated by TGF-β in ECs [110].

Integrins are important activators of the TGF-β pathway. They are important in regulating tumor angiogenesis by serving as receptors for ECM components, such as laminin, tenascin, fibronectin and collagens [111]. $\alpha v\beta 3$ is a receptor for various secreted ECM proteins, such as von Willebrand factor, TSP-1, fibrinogen, proteolyzed collagen, fibronectin and vitronectin, and it is involved in angiogenesis and vascular remodeling. For instance, $\alpha v\beta 3$ integrin associates with MMP-2 in blood vessels of melanoma tumors, and this binding facilitates collagen degradation in vitro [112]. In GBM, TGF-β enhances $\alpha v\beta 3$ integrin adhesion and expression and promotes integrin-mediated motility [111].

$\alpha v\beta 8$ is expressed in GBM cell lines and primary tumors samples. GBM cell lines overexpressing $\alpha v\beta 8$ show an increase in proliferation but when injected into the brain generate tumors with a decrease in vascularity. Silencing αv or $\beta 8$ integrin in transformed astrocytes or in human GBM cell lines leads to decreased in TGF-β signaling, resulting in increased tumor size, intratumoral hemorrhage and decreased tumor cell invasiveness [113, 114].

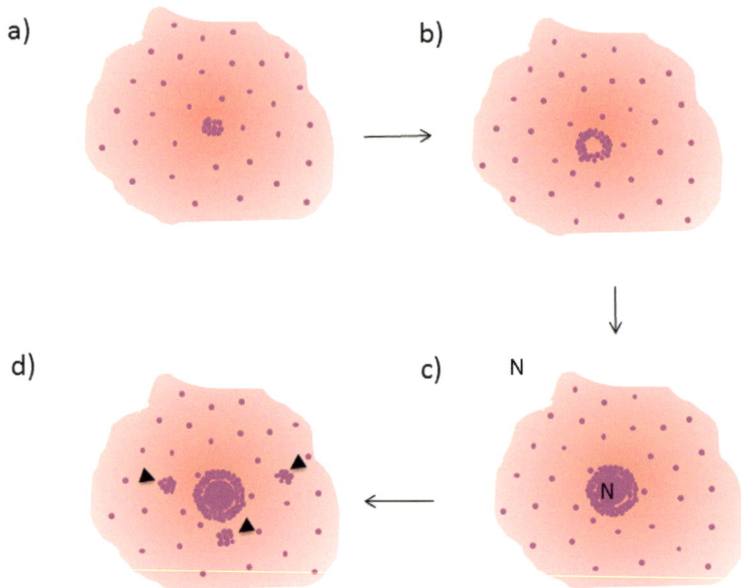

Figure 4. Microvascular proliferation. **(a)**Hypoxia center, **(b)**cell migration, **(c)**necrosis (N) and **(d)**glomeruloid microvascular proliferation (arrow heads).

In summary, TGF-β signaling is a crucial pathway in the angiogenesis of normal and tumor cells facilitating interactions between endothelial and epithelial cells. The vast majority of research has been focused on the activation of TGF-β, but more work is necessary to understand how the pathway is repressed. This could help to move forward current therapeutic attempts to target components of the TGF-β signaling pathway.

Author details

Paola A. Guerrero and Joseph H. McCarty*

*Address all correspondence to: jhmccarty@mdanderson.org

Department of Neurosurgery, University of Texas MD Anderson Cancer Center, Houston, TX, USA

References

[1] de Larco JE, Todaro GJ. Growth factors from murine sarcoma virus-transformed cells. Proceedings of the National Academy of Sciences of the United States of America. 1978;75(8):4001–5.

[2] Moses HL, Branum EL, Proper JA, Robinson RA. Transforming growth factor production by chemically transformed cells. Cancer Research. 1981;41(7):2842–8.

[3] Roberts AB, Anzano MA, Lamb LC, Smith JM, Sporn MB. New class of transforming growth factors potentiated by epidermal growth factor: isolation from non-neoplastic tissues. Proceedings of the National Academy of Sciences of the United States of America. 1981;78(9):5339–43.

[4] Moses HL, Roberts AB, Derynch R. The Discovery and Early Days of TGF-B: A Historical Perspective. Cold Spring Harbor Perspectives in Biology. 2016; 8(7): pii: a021865.

[5] Massague J. TGFbeta signalling in context. Nature Reviews Molecular Cell Biology. 2012;13(10):616–30.

[6] ten Dijke P, Arthur HM. Extracellular control of TGFbeta signalling in vascular development and disease. Nature Reviews Molecular Cell Biology. 2007;8(11):857–69.

[7] Shi M, Zhu J, Wang R, Chen X, Mi L, Walz T, et al. Latent TGF-beta structure and activation. Nature. 2011;474(7351):343–9.

[8] Robertson IB, Rifkin DB. Regulation of the bioavailability of TGF-beta and TGF-beta related proteins. Cold Spring Harbor Perspectives in Biology. 2016;8(6).pii: a021907

[9] Mu D, Cambier S, Fjellbirkeland L, Baron JL, Munger JS, Kawakatsu H, et al. The integrin alpha(v)beta8 mediates epithelial homeostasis through MT1-MMP-dependent activation of TGF-beta1. Journal of Cell Biology. 2002;157(3):493–507.

[10] Ludbrook SB, Barry ST, Delves CJ, Horgan CM. The integrin alphavbeta3 is a receptor for the latency-associated peptides of transforming growth factors beta1 and beta3. Biochemical Journal. 2003;369(Pt 2):311–8.

[11] McCarty JH. Integrin-mediated regulation of neurovascular development, physiology and disease. Cell Adhesion & Migration. 2009;3(2):211–5.

[12] Munger JS, Huang X, Kawakatsu H, Griffiths MJ, Dalton SL, Wu J, et al. The integrin alpha v beta 6 binds and activates latent TGF beta 1: a mechanism for regulating pulmonary inflammation and fibrosis. Cell. 1999;96(3):319–28.

[13] Annes JP, Chen Y, Munger JS, Rifkin DB. Integrin alphaVbeta6-mediated activation of latent TGF-beta requires the latent TGF-beta binding protein-1. Journal of Cell Biology. 2004;165(5):723–34.

[14] Fontana L, Chen Y, Prijatelj P, Sakai T, Fassler R, Sakai LY, et al. Fibronectin is required for integrin alphavbeta6-mediated activation of latent TGF-beta complexes containing LTBP-1. FASEB Journal: Official Publication of the Federation of American Societies for Experimental Biology. 2005;19(13):1798–808.

[15] Wang R, Zhu J, Dong X, Shi M, Lu C, Springer TA. GARP regulates the bioavailability and activation of TGFbeta. Molecular Biology of the Cell. 2012;23(6):1129–39.

[16] Edwards JP, Thornton AM, Shevach EM. Release of active TGF-beta1 from the latent TGF-beta1/GARP complex on T regulatory cells is mediated by integrin beta8. Journal of Immunology. 2014;193(6):2843–9.

[17] Lyons RM, Keski-Oja J, Moses HL. Proteolytic activation of latent transforming growth factor-beta from fibroblast-conditioned medium. Journal of Cell Biology. 1988;106(5):1659–65.

[18] Abe M, Oda N, Sato Y. Cell-associated activation of latent transforming growth factor-beta by calpain. Journal of Cellular Physiology. 1998;174(2):186–93.

[19] Maeda S, Dean DD, Gay I, Schwartz Z, Boyan BD. Activation of latent transforming growth factor beta1 by stromelysin 1 in extracts of growth plate chondrocyte-derived matrix vesicles. Journal of Bone and Mineral Research: The Official Journal of the American Society for Bone and Mineral Research. 2001;16(7):1281–90.

[20] Wipff PJ, Hinz B. Integrins and the activation of latent transforming growth factor beta1—an intimate relationship. European Journal of Cell Biology. 2008;87(8–9):601–15.

[21] Seoane J, Le HV, Shen L, Anderson SA, Massague J. Integration of Smad and forkhead pathways in the control of neuroepithelial and glioblastoma cell proliferation. Cell. 2004;117(2):211–23.

[22] Anido J, Saez-Borderias A, Gonzalez-Junca A, Rodon L, Folch G, Carmona MA, et al. TGF-beta receptor inhibitors target the CD44(high)/Id1(high) glioma-initiating cell population in human glioblastoma. Cancer Cell. 2010;18(6):655–68.

[23] Frederick JP, Liberati NT, Waddell DS, Shi Y, Wang XF. Transforming growth factor beta-mediated transcriptional repression of c-myc is dependent on direct binding of Smad3 to a novel repressive Smad binding element. Molecular and Cellular Biology. 2004;24(6):2546–59.

[24] Seoane J, Le HV, Massague J. Myc suppression of the p21(Cip1) Cdk inhibitor influences the outcome of the p53 response to DNA damage. Nature. 2002;419(6908):729–34.

[25] Tian M, Neil JR, Schiemann WP. Transforming growth factor-beta and the hallmarks of cancer. Cellular Signalling. 2011;23(6):951–62.

[26] Yan X, Liu Z, Chen Y. Regulation of TGF-beta signaling by Smad7. Acta Biochimica et Biophysica Sinica. 2009;41(4):263–72.

[27] Massague J, Wotton D. Transcriptional control by the TGF-beta/Smad signaling system. EMBO Journal. 2000;19(8):1745–54.

[28] Xu J, Derynck R. Does Smad6 methylation control BMP signaling in cancer? Cell Cycle. 2014;13(8):1209–10.

[29] Xu J, Wang AH, Oses-Prieto J, Makhijani K, Katsuno Y, Pei M, et al. Arginine methylation initiates BMP-induced Smad signaling. Molecular Cell. 2013;51(1):5–19.

[30] Choy L, Skillington J, Derynck R. Roles of autocrine TGF-beta receptor and Smad signaling in adipocyte differentiation. Journal of Cell Biology. 2000;149(3):667–82.

[31] Caprioli A, Minko K, Drevon C, Eichmann A, Dieterlen-Lievre F, Jaffredo T. Hemangioblast commitment in the avian allantois: cellular and molecular aspects. Developmental Biology. 2001;238(1):64–78.

[32] Choi K, Kennedy M, Kazarov A, Papadimitriou JC, Keller G. A common precursor for hematopoietic and endothelial cells. Development. 1998;125(4):725–32.

[33] Patel-Hett S, D'Amore PA. Signal transduction in vasculogenesis and developmental angiogenesis. International Journal of Developmental Biology. 2011;55(4–5):353–63.

[34] Cox CM, Poole TJ. Angioblast differentiation is influenced by the local environment: FGF-2 induces angioblasts and patterns vessel formation in the quail embryo. Developmental Dynamics: An Official Publication of the American Association of Anatomists. 2000;218(2):371–82.

[35] Dyer MA, Farrington SM, Mohn D, Munday JR, Baron MH. Indian hedgehog activates hematopoiesis and vasculogenesis and can respecify prospective neurectodermal cell fate in the mouse embryo. Development. 2001;128(10):1717–30.

[36] Pepicelli CV, Lewis PM, McMahon AP. Sonic hedgehog regulates branching morphogenesis in the mammalian lung. Current Biology: CB. 1998;8(19):1083–6.

[37] Rowitch DH, B SJ, Lee SM, Flax JD, Snyder EY, McMahon AP. Sonic hedgehog regulates proliferation and inhibits differentiation of CNS precursor cells. Journal of Neuroscience: The Official Journal of the Society for Neuroscience. 1999;19(20):8954–65.

[38] Brown LA, Rodaway AR, Schilling TF, Jowett T, Ingham PW, Patient RK, et al. Insights into early vasculogenesis revealed by expression of the ETS-domain transcription factor Fli-1 in wild-type and mutant zebrafish embryos. Mechanisms of Development. 2000;90(2):237–52.

[39] Byrd N, Becker S, Maye P, Narasimhaiah R, St-Jacques B, Zhang X, et al. Hedgehog is required for murine yolk sac angiogenesis. Development. 2002;129(2):361–72.

[40] Fong GH, Rossant J, Gertsenstein M, Breitman ML. Role of the Flt-1 receptor tyrosine kinase in regulating the assembly of vascular endothelium. Nature. 1995;376(6535):66–70.

[41] Shalaby F, Rossant J, Yamaguchi TP, Gertsenstein M, Wu XF, Breitman ML, et al. Failure of blood-island formation and vasculogenesis in Flk-1-deficient mice. Nature. 1995;376(6535):62–6.

[42] Shalaby F, Ho J, Stanford WL, Fischer KD, Schuh AC, Schwartz L, et al. A requirement for Flk1 in primitive and definitive hematopoiesis and vasculogenesis. Cell. 1997;89(6):981–90.

[43] Ferrara N, Carver-Moore K, Chen H, Dowd M, Lu L, O'Shea KS, et al. Heterozygous embryonic lethality induced by targeted inactivation of the VEGF gene. Nature. 1996;380(6573):439–42.

[44] Kawasaki T, Kitsukawa T, Bekku Y, Matsuda Y, Sanbo M, Yagi T, et al. A requirement for neuropilin-1 in embryonic vessel formation. Development. 1999;126(21):4895–902.

[45] Chen H, Bagri A, Zupicich JA, Zou Y, Stoeckli E, Pleasure SJ, et al. Neuropilin-2 regulates the development of selective cranial and sensory nerves and hippocampal mossy fiber projections. Neuron. 2000;25(1):43–56.

[46] Giger RJ, Cloutier JF, Sahay A, Prinjha RK, Levengood DV, Moore SE, et al. Neuropilin-2 is required in vivo for selective axon guidance responses to secreted semaphorins. Neuron. 2000;25(1):29–41.

[47] Takashima S, Kitakaze M, Asakura M, Asanuma H, Sanada S, Tashiro F, et al. Targeting of both mouse neuropilin-1 and neuropilin-2 genes severely impairs developmental yolk sac and embryonic angiogenesis. Proceedings of the National Academy of Sciences of the United States of America. 2002;99(6):3657–62.

[48] Adams RH, Alitalo K. Molecular regulation of angiogenesis and lymphangiogenesis. Nature Reviews Molecular Cell Biology. 2007;8(6):464–78.

[49] Ribatti D, Nico B, Crivellato E. Morphological and molecular aspects of physiological vascular morphogenesis. Angiogenesis. 2009;12(2):101–11.

[50] Adair TH, Montani JP. Angiogenesis. Integrated Systems Physiology: from Molecule to Function to Disease. San Rafael (CA) 2010.

[51] Rossant J, Howard L. Signaling pathways in vascular development. Annual Review of Cell and Developmental Biology. 2002;18:541–73.

[52] Dickson MC, Martin JS, Cousins FM, Kulkarni AB, Karlsson S, Akhurst RJ. Defective haematopoiesis and vasculogenesis in transforming growth factor-beta 1 knockout mice. Development. 1995;121(6):1845–54.

[53] Akhurst RJ, Lehnert SA, Faissner A, Duffie E. TGF beta in murine morphogenetic processes: the early embryo and cardiogenesis. Development. 1990;108(4):645–56.

[54] Shull MM, Ormsby I, Kier AB, Pawlowski S, Diebold RJ, Yin M, et al. Targeted disruption of the mouse transforming growth factor-beta 1 gene results in multifocal inflammatory disease. Nature. 1992;359(6397):693–9.

[55] Letterio JJ, Geiser AG, Kulkarni AB, Roche NS, Sporn MB, Roberts AB. Maternal rescue of transforming growth factor-beta 1 null mice. Science. 1994;264(5167):1936–8.

[56] Oshima M, Oshima H, Taketo MM. TGF-beta receptor type II deficiency results in defects of yolk sac hematopoiesis and vasculogenesis. Developmental Biology. 1996;179(1):297–302.

[57] Arthur HM, Ure J, Smith AJ, Renforth G, Wilson DI, Torsney E, et al. Endoglin, an ancillary TGFbeta receptor, is required for extraembryonic angiogenesis and plays a key role in heart development. Developmental Biology. 2000;217(1):42–53.

[58] Li DY, Sorensen LK, Brooke BS, Urness LD, Davis EC, Taylor DG, et al. Defective angiogenesis in mice lacking endoglin. Science. 1999;284(5419):1534–7.

[59] Neuzillet C, Tijeras-Raballand A, Cohen R, Cros J, Faivre S, Raymond E, et al. Targeting the TGFbeta pathway for cancer therapy. Pharmacology & Therapeutics [Internet]. 2015;147:22–31 pp. Available from: http://www.ncbi.nlm.nih.gov/pubmed/25444759.

[60] Lechleider RJ, Ryan JL, Garrett L, Eng C, Deng C, Wynshaw-Boris A, et al. Targeted mutagenesis of Smad1 reveals an essential role in chorioallantoic fusion. Developmental Biology. 2001;240(1):157–67.

[61] Baird A, Durkin T. Inhibition of endothelial cell proliferation by type beta-transforming growth factor: interactions with acidic and basic fibroblast growth factors. Biochemical and Biophysical Research Communications. 1986;138(1):476–82.

[62] Frater-Schroder M, Muller G, Birchmeier W, Bohlen P. Transforming growth factor-beta inhibits endothelial cell proliferation. Biochemical and Biophysical Research Communications. 1986;137(1):295–302.

[63] Iruela-Arispe ML, Sage EH. Endothelial cells exhibiting angiogenesis in vitro proliferate in response to TGF-beta 1. Journal of Cellular Biochemistry. 1993;52(4):414–30.

[64] Sutton AB, Canfield AE, Schor SL, Grant ME, Schor AM. The response of endothelial cells to TGF beta-1 is dependent upon cell shape, proliferative state and the nature of the substratum. Journal of Cell Science. 1991;99 (Pt 4):777–87.

[65] RayChaudhury A, D'Amore PA. Endothelial cell regulation by transforming growth factor-beta. Journal of Cellular Biochemistry. 1991;47(3):224–9.

[66] Li C, Guo B, Bernabeu C, Kumar S. Angiogenesis in breast cancer: the role of transforming growth factor beta and CD105. Microscopy Research and Technique. 2001;52(4):437–49.

[67] Hofer E, Schweighofer B. Signal transduction induced in endothelial cells by growth factor receptors involved in angiogenesis. Thrombosis and Haemostasis. 2007;97(3):355–63.

[68] Krupinski J, Kumar P, Kumar S, Kaluza J. Increased expression of TGF-beta 1 in brain tissue after ischemic stroke in humans. Stroke; A Journal of Cerebral Circulation. 1996;27(5):852–7.

[69] Dissen GA, Lara HE, Fahrenbach WH, Costa ME, Ojeda SR. Immature rat ovaries become revascularized rapidly after autotransplantation and show a gonadotropin-dependent increase in angiogenic factor gene expression. Endocrinology. 1994;134(3):1146–54.

[70] Pepper MS. Transforming growth factor-beta: vasculogenesis, angiogenesis, and vessel wall integrity. Cytokine & Growth Factor Reviews. 1997;8(1):21–43.

[71] Ferrari G, Pintucci G, Seghezzi G, Hyman K, Galloway AC, Mignatti P. VEGF, a prosurvival factor, acts in concert with TGF-beta1 to induce endothelial cell apoptosis. Proceedings of the National Academy of Sciences of the United States of America. 2006;103(46):17260–5.

[72] Lebrin F, Goumans MJ, Jonker L, Carvalho RL, Valdimarsdottir G, Thorikay M, et al. Endoglin promotes endothelial cell proliferation and TGF-beta/ALK1 signal transduction. EMBO Journal. 2004;23(20):4018–28.

[73] Wang X, Abraham S, McKenzie JA, Jeffs N, Swire M, Tripathi VB, et al. LRG1 promotes angiogenesis by modulating endothelial TGF-beta signalling. Nature. 2013;499(7458):306–11.

[74] McCarty JH, Monahan-Earley RA, Brown LF, Keller M, Gerhardt H, Rubin K, et al. Defective associations between blood vessels and brain parenchyma lead to cerebral hemorrhage in mice lacking alpha v integrins. Molecular and Cellular Biology. 2002;22(21):7667–77.

[75] McCarty JH, Lacy-Hulbert A, Charest A, Bronson RT, Crowley D, Housman D, et al. Selective ablation of alphav integrins in the central nervous system leads to cerebral hemorrhage, seizures, axonal degeneration and premature death. Development. 2005;132(1):165–76.

[76] Proctor JM, Zang K, Wang D, Wang R, Reichardt LF. Vascular development of the brain requires beta8 integrin expression in the neuroepithelium. Journal of Neuroscience: The Official Journal of the Society for Neuroscience. 2005;25(43):9940–8.

[77] Mobley AK, Tchaicha JH, Shin J, Hossain MG, McCarty JH. Beta8 integrin regulates neurogenesis and neurovascular homeostasis in the adult brain. Journal of Cell Science. 2009;122(Pt 11):1842–51.

[78] Aluwihare P, Mu Z, Zhao Z, Yu D, Weinreb PH, Horan GS, et al. Mice that lack activity of alphavbeta6- and alphavbeta8-integrins reproduce the abnormalities of Tgfb1- and Tgfb3-null mice. Journal of Cell Science. 2009;122(Pt 2):227–32.

[79] Hirota S, Clements TP, Tang LK, Morales JE, Lee HS, Oh SP, et al. Neuropilin 1 balances beta8 integrin-activated TGFbeta signaling to control sprouting angiogenesis in the brain. Development. 2015;142(24):4363–73.

[80] Glinka Y, Stoilova S, Mohammed N, Prud'homme GJ. Neuropilin-1 exerts co-receptor function for TGF-beta-1 on the membrane of cancer cells and enhances responses to both latent and active TGF-beta. Carcinogenesis. 2011;32(4):613–21.

[81] Hirota S, Liu Q, Lee HS, Hossain MG, Lacy-Hulbert A, McCarty JH. The astrocyte-expressed integrin alphavbeta8 governs blood vessel sprouting in the developing retina. Development. 2011;138(23):5157–66.

[82] Allinson KR, Lee HS, Fruttiger M, McCarty JH, Arthur HM. Endothelial expression of TGFbeta type II receptor is required to maintain vascular integrity during postnatal development of the central nervous system. PLoS One. 2012;7(6):e39336.

[83] Nguyen HL, Lee YJ, Shin J, Lee E, Park SO, McCarty JH, et al. TGF-beta signaling in endothelial cells, but not neuroepithelial cells, is essential for cerebral vascular development. Laboratory Investigation; A Journal of Technical Methods and Pathology. 2011;91(11):1554–63.

[84] Marchuk DA, Srinivasan S, Squire TL, Zawistowski JS. Vascular morphogenesis: tales of two syndromes. Human Molecular Genetics. 2003;12(Spec No 1):R97–112.

[85] Carvalho RL, Jonker L, Goumans MJ, Larsson J, Bouwman P, Karlsson S, et al. Defective paracrine signalling by TGFbeta in yolk sac vasculature of endoglin mutant mice: a paradigm for hereditary haemorrhagic telangiectasia. Development. 2004;131(24):6237–47.

[86] Su H, Kim H, Pawlikowska L, Kitamura H, Shen F, Cambier S, et al. Reduced expression of integrin alphavbeta8 is associated with brain arteriovenous malformation pathogenesis. American Journal of Pathology. 2010;176(2):1018–27.

[87] Dardiotis E, Siokas V, Zafeiridis T, Paterakis K, Tsivgoulis G, Dardioti M, et al. Integrins AV and B8 gene polymorphisms and risk for intracerebral hemorrhage in Greek and Polish populations. Neuromolecular Medicine. 2016.

[88] Chung AS, Ferrara N. Targeting the tumor microenvironment with SRC kinase inhibition. Clinical Cancer Research: An Official Journal of the American Association for Cancer Research. 2010;16(3):775–7.

[89] Cerami E, Gao J, Dogrusoz U, Gross BE, Sumer SO, Aksoy BA, et al. The cBio cancer genomics portal: an open platform for exploring multidimensional cancer genomics data. Cancer Discovery. 2012;2(5):401–4.

[90] Gao J, Aksoy BA, Dogrusoz U, Dresdner G, Gross B, Sumer SO, et al. Integrative analysis of complex cancer genomics and clinical profiles using the cBioPortal. Science Signaling. 2013;6(269):pl1.

[91] Mazzocca A, Fransvea E, Lavezzari G, Antonaci S, Giannelli G. Inhibition of transforming growth factor beta receptor I kinase blocks hepatocellular carcinoma growth through neo-angiogenesis regulation. Hepatology. 2009;50(4):1140–51.

[92] Akbari A, Amanpour S, Muhammadnejad S, Ghahremani MH, Ghaffari SH, Dehpour AR, et al. Evaluation of antitumor activity of a TGF-beta receptor I inhibitor (SD-208) on human colon adenocarcinoma. Daru: Journal of Faculty of Pharmacy, Tehran University of Medical Sciences. 2014;22:47.

[93] Zhang M, Herion TW, Timke C, Han N, Hauser K, Weber KJ, et al. Trimodal glioblastoma treatment consisting of concurrent radiotherapy, temozolomide, and the novel TGF-beta receptor I kinase inhibitor LY2109761. Neoplasia. 2011;13(6):537–49.

[94] Zhang M, Kleber S, Rohrich M, Timke C, Han N, Tuettenberg J, et al. Blockade of TGF-beta signaling by the TGFbetaR-I kinase inhibitor LY2109761 enhances radiation response and prolongs survival in glioblastoma. Cancer Research. 2011;71(23):7155–67.

[95] Yang XJ, Chen GL, Yu SC, Xu C, Xin YH, Li TT, et al. TGF-beta1 enhances tumor-induced angiogenesis via JNK pathway and macrophage infiltration in an improved zebrafish embryo/xenograft glioma model. International Immunopharmacology. 2013;15(2):191–8.

[96] Deckers MM, van Bezooijen RL, van der Horst G, Hoogendam J, van Der Bent C, Papapoulos SE, et al. Bone morphogenetic proteins stimulate angiogenesis through osteoblast-derived vascular endothelial growth factor A. Endocrinology. 2002;143(4):1545–53.

[97] Ma J, Wang Q, Fei T, Han JD, Chen YG. MCP-1 mediates TGF-beta-induced angiogenesis by stimulating vascular smooth muscle cell migration. Blood. 2007;109(3):987–94.

[98] Hovinga KE, Stalpers LJ, van Bree C, Donker M, Verhoeff JJ, Rodermond HM, et al. Radiation-enhanced vascular endothelial growth factor (VEGF) secretion in glioblastoma multiforme cell lines—a clue to radioresistance? Journal of Neuro-oncology. 2005;74(2):99–103.

[99] Lund EL, Hog A, Olsen MW, Hansen LT, Engelholm SA, Kristjansen PE. Differential regulation of VEGF, HIF1alpha and angiopoietin-1, -2 and -4 by hypoxia and ionizing radiation in human glioblastoma. International Journal of Cancer. 2004;108(6):833–8.

[100] Gupta VK, Jaskowiak NT, Beckett MA, Mauceri HJ, Grunstein J, Johnson RS, et al. Vascular endothelial growth factor enhances endothelial cell survival and tumor radioresistance. Cancer Journal. 2002;8(1):47–54.

[101] Harmey JH, Bouchier-Hayes D. Vascular endothelial growth factor (VEGF), a survival factor for tumour cells: implications for anti-angiogenic therapy. BioEssays: News and Reviews in Molecular, Cellular and Developmental Biology. 2002;24(3):280–3.

[102] Saksela O, Moscatelli D, Rifkin DB. The opposing effects of basic fibroblast growth factor and transforming growth factor beta on the regulation of plasminogen activator activity in capillary endothelial cells. Journal of Cell Biology. 1987;105(2):957–63.

[103] Pollman MJ, Naumovski L, Gibbons GH. Endothelial cell apoptosis in capillary network remodeling. Journal of Cellular Physiology. 1999;178(3):359–70.

[104] Bostrom K, Zebboudj AF, Yao Y, Lin TS, Torres A. Matrix GLA protein stimulates VEGF expression through increased transforming growth factor-beta1 activity in endothelial cells. Journal of Biological Chemistry. 2004;279(51):52904–13.

[105] Hamerlik P, Lathia JD, Rasmussen R, Wu Q, Bartkova J, Lee M, et al. Autocrine VEGF-VEGFR2-Neuropilin-1 signaling promotes glioma stem-like cell viability and tumor growth. Journal of Experimental Medicine. 2012;209(3):507–20.

[106] Cheng L, Huang Z, Zhou W, Wu Q, Donnola S, Liu JK, et al. Glioblastoma stem cells generate vascular pericytes to support vessel function and tumor growth. Cell. 2013;153(1):139–52.

[107] Bruna A, Darken RS, Rojo F, Ocana A, Penuelas S, Arias A, et al. High TGFbeta-Smad activity confers poor prognosis in glioma patients and promotes cell proliferation depending on the methylation of the PDGF-B gene. Cancer Cell. 2007;11(2):147–60.

[108] Roy LO, Poirier MB, Fortin D. Transforming growth factor-beta and its implication in the malignancy of gliomas. Targeted Oncology. 2015;10(1):1–14.

[109] Louis DN. Molecular pathology of malignant gliomas. Annual Review of Pathology. 2006;1:97–117.

[110] Doerr M, Morrison J, Bergeron L, Coomber BL, Viloria-Petit A. Differential effect of hypoxia on early endothelial-mesenchymal transition response to transforming growth beta isoforms 1 and 2. Microvascular Research. 2016;108:48–63.

[111] Platten M, Wick W, Wild-Bode C, Aulwurm S, Dichgans J, Weller M. Transforming growth factors beta(1) (TGF-beta(1)) and TGF-beta(2) promote glioma cell migration via Up-regulation of alpha(V)beta(3) integrin expression. Biochemical and Biophysical Research Communications. 2000;268(2):607–11.

[112] Brooks PC, Stromblad S, Sanders LC, von Schalscha TL, Aimes RT, Stetler-Stevenson WG, et al. Localization of matrix metalloproteinase MMP-2 to the surface of invasive cells by interaction with integrin alpha v beta 3. Cell. 1996;85(5):683–93.

[113] Tchaicha JH, Mobley AK, Hossain MG, Aldape KD, McCarty JH. A mosaic mouse model of astrocytoma identifies alphavbeta8 integrin as a negative regulator of tumor angiogenesis. Oncogene. 2010;29(31):4460–72.

[114] Tchaicha JH, Reyes SB, Shin J, Hossain MG, Lang FF, McCarty JH. Glioblastoma angiogenesis and tumor cell invasiveness are differentially regulated by beta8 integrin. Cancer Research. 2011;71(20):6371–81.

Chapter 2

Role of Notch, SDF-1 and Mononuclear Cells Recruitment in Angiogenesis

Ivanka Dimova and Valentin Djonov

Additional information is available at the end of the chapter

http://dx.doi.org/10.5772/66761

Abstract

Intussusceptive angiogenesis (IA) known also as splitting angiogenesis is a recently described mechanism of vascular growth alternative to sprouting. It plays an essential role in the vascular remodeling and adaptation of vessels during normal and pathological angiogenesis. It is an "escape" mechanism during and after irradiation and anti-VEGF therapy, both inducing angiogenic switch from sprouting to IA by formation of multiple transluminal tissue pillars. Our recently published data revealed the significant induction of IA after inhibition of Notch signaling associated with an increased capillary density by more than 50%. The induced IA was accompanied by detachment of pericytes from basement membrane, increased vessel permeability and recruitment of mononuclear cells toward the pillars; the process was dramatically enhanced after injection of bone marrow-derived mononuclear cells. The extravasation of mononuclear cells with eventual bone marrow origin was associated with upregulation of chemotaxis factors SDF-1 and CXCR4. In addition, SDF-1 expression was upregulated in the endothelium of liver sinusoids in Notch1 knockout mouse, together with vascular remodeling by intussusception. In this chapter, we discuss this important mechanism of angiogenesis, as well as the role of Notch signaling, SDF-1 signaling and mononuclear cells in the complex process of angiogenesis.

Keywords: intussusceptive angiogenesis, Notch signaling, mononuclear cells, SDF-1/CXCR4 signaling

1. Introduction: intussusceptive angiogenesis

Angiogenesis is essential for normal embryonic development and reproductive cycle and plays a key role in pathological conditions such as tumor growth and ischemic cardiovascular diseases. This is a complex process involving essential signaling pathways for instance VEGF, bFGF, and Notch, etc., in vasculature, as well as additional players such as bone marrow-derived endothelial progenitor cells. Better understanding the role of the different pathways and the crosstalk between different cells during angiogenesis is a crucial factor for developing more effective proangiogenic and antiangiogenic anticancer therapy.

Angiogenesis involves the formation of new blood vessels from a preexisting vascular plexus, and based on morphological characteristics two main distinct processes have been identified, sprouting and intussusceptive angiogenesis (IA) [1–3]. Sprouting angiogenesis has been well described since more than 150 years. Recent publications indicated that sprouting involves tip/stalk cell differentiation and crosstalk process which is tightly controlled by the VEGF and Notch/Dll4 signaling pathway [4, 5]. Intussusceptive angiogenesis (IA) is a particular form of vascular growth and remodeling in which endothelial cells make invagination intraluminally instead of extraluminally like it is in the sprouting. The cells form protrusions toward the vessel lumen resulting in the appearance of transluminal endothelial pillars–the hallmarks of intussusception. The arising pillars afterward are successively reshaped and fused and lead to "splitting" of the preexisting vessel in two segments, thus doing remodeling and organization of the vasculature. The effect is the formation of hierarchically organized vessels with supplying and draining function, pruning of arteries, and veins, and finally development of the primitive capillary plexuses into the functional vascular system. IA is a process with several consecutive steps, including intussusceptive microvascular growth, intussusceptive arborization, and intussusceptive remodeling [2, 3, 6, 7]. These processes end in the formation of mature vascular networks. In comparison to sprouting angiogenesis, intussusception is a quite fast process, enabling the vascular system to swift adaptation in unfavorable conditions. IA has been identified as the leading mode of vascular growth in animal models of liver regeneration and in alveolar angiogenesis following pneumonectomy. Intussusception appears to be predominant above sprouting in extra-embryonic vasculatures including the vitelline circulation as well [8-10]. The intensive work of our group in the past few decades clearly documented the morphological features of this specific angiogenic mode and demonstrated its definite presence during development and tumorigenesis as a complementary to sprouting vessel growth. Surprisingly, the cellular and molecular regulation of intussusception is less well known but recent evidence suggests that it might involve a component regulated by blood flow and Notch signaling [7, 9]. We provided with evidence showing that Notch regulates intussusception involving interaction with circulating mononuclear cells in developing vascular networks [11].

Intussusceptive angiogenesis (IA) is a well-documented and widely spread mode of angiogenesis, occurring during both normal development and in pathological conditions. In contrast to sprouting angiogenesis, whereby abluminal sprouts outgrow and subsequently merge with the existing capillaries, intussusceptive angiogenesis is elaborated by intraluminal growth of endothelial cell processes. The last protrude from the opposing sides of the vessel wall and form transluminal tissue pillar, representing endothelial bilayer, which is afterward perforated and stabilized from outside by collagen bindles. Repetitive formation of pillars and their subsequent fusion leads to the splitting of vessels and vascular expansion. Another way of intussusceptive angiogenesis is to increase the size of the pillar and form meshes, thus splitting the vessel. Intussusceptive angiogenesis is a process linked to both blood vessel replication and remodeling in development. It is present within the regions of increased vascular density in alveolar angiogenesis during compensatory growth after pneumonectomy in a murine model of postpneumonectomy lung growth [8]. The remodeling of the retiform meshworks in the avian lung was essentially accomplished by intussusceptive angiogenesis as well [12].

In addition to its developmental role, intussusceptive angiogenesis is well documented as a mechanism of vascular adaptation in response to different environmental stimuli. In the adult mouse retina, it was reported as a main adaptive mechanism to chronic systemic hypoxia [13]. These investigations contribute to our understanding of hypoxia-induced angiogenesis and microvascular remodeling. The process of intraluminal division participates in the inflammation-induced neovascularization associated with chemically induced murine colitis [14]. *Scanning electron microscopy* (SEM) of vascular corrosion casts demonstrated replication of the mucosal plexus without significant evidence of sprouting angiogenesis, whereas pillar formation and septation were present within days of the onset of inflammation. The authors conclude that intussusceptive angiogenesis is a fundamental mechanism of microvascular adaptation to prolonged inflammation. It is also a mechanism of compensation for vascular growth. In a capillary regression model of inflamed murine corneas, the abrupt termination of capillary sprouting is followed by an intussusceptive response [15]. The capillary repair during kidney recovery in Thy1.1 nephritis was done by intussusceptive angiogenesis [16]. Inhibitors of angiogenesis and radiation induce compensatory changes in the tumor vasculature both during and after cessation of treatment. There is a switch from sprouting to intussusceptive angiogenesis, which may be an adaptive response of tumor vasculature to cancer therapy that allows the vasculature to maintain its functional properties [17–19]. Potential candidates for molecular targeting of this angioadaptive mechanism are yet to be elucidated in order to improve the currently poor efficacy of contemporary antiangiogenic therapies. Important is the involvement of intussusceptive angiogenesis in pathological conditions. Vascular remodeling of the hepatic sinusoidal microvasculature in the course of liver nodular hyperplasia is a result of intussusceptive growth [9]. This angiogenic mode is widely involved in tumor development. By using electron and confocal microscopy, Paku et al. [20] observed intraluminal nascent pillars that contain a collagen bundle covered by endothelial cells (ECs) in the vasculature of experimental tumors. Tumor angiogenesis in liver metastasis from colon carcinoma is a controversial subject. Ceauşu et al. [21] concluded that in liver metastasis principal mechanism of neovascularization formation is based on intussusception. In metastatic tumors of the brain there was intussusceptive angiogenesis, whereby the fibrosarcoma cells were attached to the vessel, filled the developing pillars, and caused lumen splitting [22]. Branching angiogenesis was not observed either in the tumors or in control cerebral wounds. These data suggest that sprouting angiogenesis is not needed for the incipient growth of cerebral metastases and that tumor growth in this model is a result of incorporation of host vessels. Prolactin was found to directly stimulate angiogenesis in breast cancer progression, enhancing vessel density and the tortuosity of the vasculature by pillar formation, which are hallmarks of intussusceptive angiogenesis [23]. It is a preferred mode of angiogenesis in oral squamous cell carcinoma [24] and in hepatocellular carcinoma [25, 26].

Despite this variety of intussusceptive angiogenic roles, most of the current research is focused on the mechanism of sprouting angiogenesis because this mechanism was first described and most existing experimental models are related to sprouting angiogenesis. Consequently, the mechanism of intussusceptive angiogenesis is often overlooked in angiogenesis research [27]. Intussusception is an alternative to the sprouting mode of angiogenesis. The advantage of this mechanism of vascular growth is that blood vessels are generated more rapidly and the capillaries thereby formed are less leaky [1]. The regulation of intussusceptive angiogenesis is still to be elucidated. There are some hypotheses about the possible drivers of intussusception. In the sprouting type of angiogenesis related to hypoxia, there is no blood flow in the rising capillary sprout. In contrast, it has been shown that an increase of wall shear stress initiates the splitting type of angiogenesis in skeletal muscle [7]. Inflammation-associated intussusceptive angiogenesis in adult mice was associated with vessel angle remodeling and the morphometry of the vessel angles suggests the influence of blood flow on the location and orientation of remodeled vessels [28]. Regarding molecular regulation, very little is known for the molecular factors with potential significance. Application of the essential angiogenic factors VEGF and bFGF in an arteriovenous loop model demonstrated advanced neovascularization in the phase of remodeling by a higher incidence of intussusception, compared to control without these factors [29]. It was shown in Ewing sarcomas and rhabdomyosarcomas that treatment suppressing IGF-1 signaling decreases intussusceptive angiogenesis [30].

The main factors for maturation and hierarchical organization of vessels, especially arterial ones, are Notch, angiopoietin, and ephrin. In addition, it was shown that SDF-1 (CXCL12) is a crucial maturation factor in coronary arterial vasculature, since its mutants have immature capillary plexus and selective failure in arterial maturation, particularly with the onset of coronary perfusion [31].

Our preliminary results suggest that intussusception is most probably synchronized by chemokine factors since intussusceptive growth was associated with the recruitment of mononuclear cells [11]. After injection of bone marrow-derived mononuclear cells, we observed robust induction of intussusception in Notch inhibited samples. Notably, the chemotactic factors SDF-1/CXCR4 were upregulated only due to the Notch inhibition. Our hypothesis is that Notch inhibition disturbed vessel stability and led to pericyte detachment followed by extravasation of mononuclear cells due to the activation of the SDF-1/CXCR4 axis. The stromal cell-derived factor SDF-1 is binding to its receptor CXCR4 and directs migration of progenitor cells into the appropriate sites. The mononuclear cells contributed to the formation of transluminal pillars with sustained IA resulting in a dense vascular plexus.

2. Notch signaling and intussusceptive angiogenesis

The crucial role for Notch/DLL4 signaling in regulating vascular development was established based on findings from the analysis of targeted mouse and zebrafish mutants in Notch pathway components [32–35]. The common characteristics of the most of these mutants were the absence of angiogenic vascular remodeling, lack of arterial markers, and arteriovenous malformations. Mouse embryos deficient for Notch-ligand Jagged1 (Jag1), Notch1, Notch1/Notch4, or the presenilins, die between E9.5 and 10.5 and have severely disorganized vasculature [36]. Transgenic mice with inappropriate activation of Notch4 also display similar defects and die, which suggests that the appropriate Notch expression pattern (in levels, sites, and time) is critical for embryonic vascular development [37]. It was found out that Notch1, Notch2, and Notch4 are expressed predominantly in endothelial cells of aorta and arteries, whereas Notch3 was in VSMCs of arteries [38].

Recently, we have established that Notch inhibition disturbs vessel stability and induces intussusceptive neo-angiogenesis, triggering in this way the augmentation of the capillary plexus but without the accompanying vascular maturation and remodeling. It was associated with extravasation of mononuclear cells of bone marrow origin possibly by upregulation SDF-1/CXCR4 chemotactic factors.

Using the chick area vasculosa (and inhibiting Notch signaling by the γ-secretase inhibitor–GSI) and a mouse model of Notch inhibition (MxCre Notch1lox/lox mice), we have demonstrated that in already existing vascular beds disruption of Notch-signaling triggers rapid augmentation of the vasculature predominantly by intussusceptive angiogenesis [11]. The process is initiated by pericyte detachment followed by extravasation of mononuclear cells (**Figure 1**). The latter cells contributed to formation of transluminal pillars [11]. The sustained IA results in a very dense vascular plexus but without the usual concomitant vascular remodeling or maturation.

The genetic approach in mice substantiated by pharmacological studies for developing vascular networks in chicken embryo enabled us to show that Notch is critical for intussusceptive angiogenesis. In both models we demonstrated considerable changes in vascular morphogenesis, resulting in massive induction of intussusception. Inhibition of DLL4/Notch signaling by novel therapeutic antibody against DLL4, performed in a recently published study [39], was associated with threefold increase in vessel density and stimulation of vessel formation. At the same time, marked reduction in the number of smooth muscle actin (SMA)-positive mural cells was noted. Two-dimensional appearance of the blood vessels in the described phenotype highly resembles the data in our chicken and mouse models. Similar phenotypes were observed after Notch inhibition during developmental angiogenesis, in skeletal muscle and in tumor models, showing increased vessel number and increased vascular permeability [40–43]. The terminology for the resultant vascular pattern, used by authors in these studies, was "abnormal vessels" or "excessive, nonproductive angiogenesis." They focused mainly on the front of sprouting invasion after blocking Notch signaling, thus describing only newly developing, nonperfused vasculature. Along with the observed significantly increased vessel density under Notch inhibition, there was evidently demonstrated reduced mural cell coverage. The authors reported positivity for endothelial markers in the endothelial protrusions toward the vessel lumen and in the intraluminal vessel occlusions [44], but they did not attribute this phenomenon to the induced intussusceptive angiogenesis. The detailed investigation of this vascular pattern behind the sprouting mode of vessels invasion demonstrated that Notch inhibition led to IA in already perfused vascular bed and this is a complementary mechanism of angiogenesis. In fact, the authors above mentioned here nicely described the characteristic features of intussusceptive microvascular growth even though they did not use the terminology.

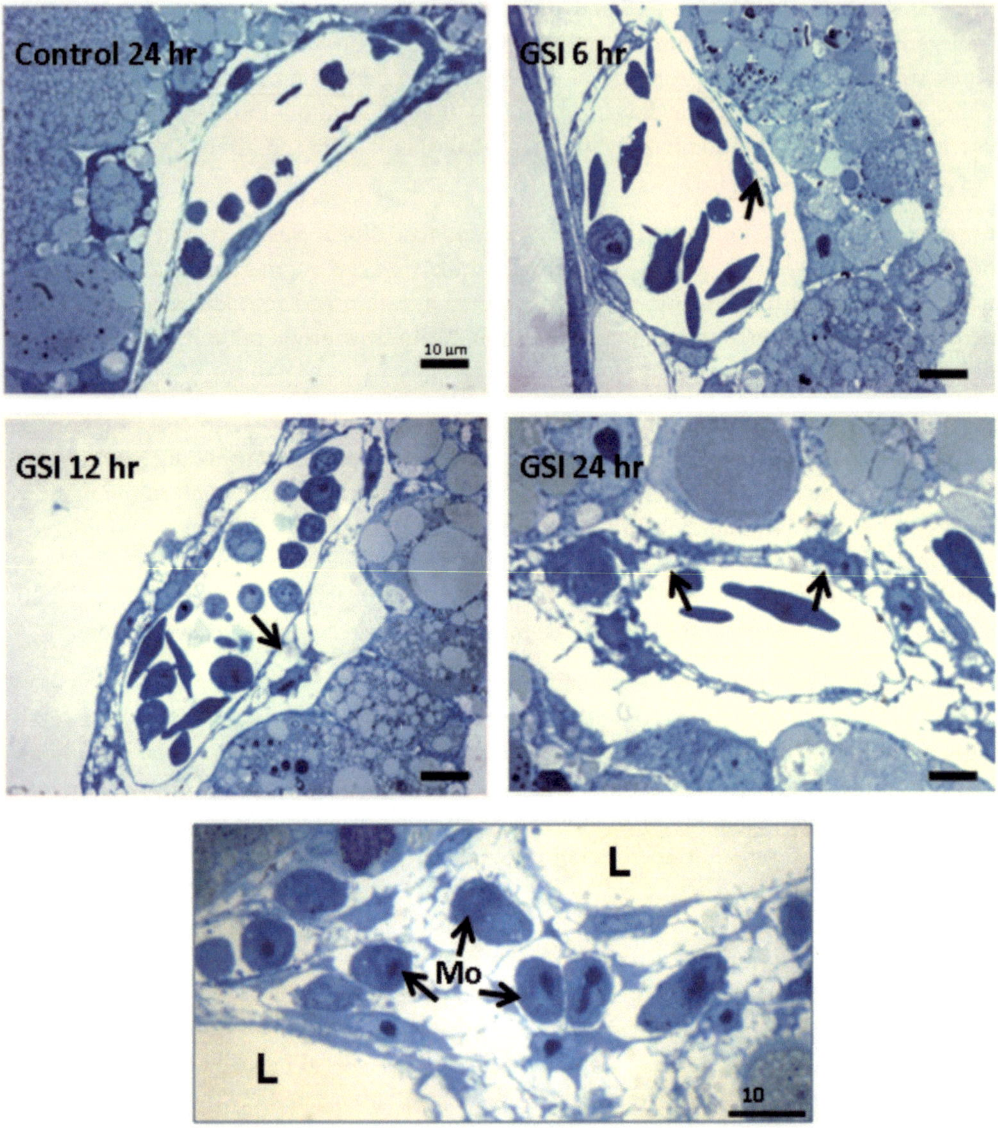

Figure 1. Inhibition of Notch signaling led to detachment of pericytes from endothelium (indicated by arrows), as it is shown at different time points after the application of GSI; it is followed by the extravasation of mononuclear cells (Mo); L–vessel lumen.

3. Role of mononuclear cells in angiogenesis

To test the role of bone marrow cells in the process of intussusception, in our previous study we isolated bone marrow mononuclear cells (BMMNC) from E14 chicken embryos and/or 4-week-old mice, labeled them with a fluorescent cell tracker (TAMRA) and injected them into the Notch inhibited (by GSI) and control samples 3 hours prior to time point 24 hours at which time the samples were visualized by FITC injection [11]. About 3–4 hours after BMMNCs injection, we observed a significant induction of intussusception in the GSI-treated area as we detected high increase in the pillar number (4.2-fold) in inhibited samples as compared to controls. Injection of BMMNCs in the area vasculosa after Notch inhibition dramatically induced increase in microvascular density by onset of IA. Microvascular area density increases significantly by 80% after injection of BMD cells in Notch-inhibited samples in comparison with injection of BMD cells in PBS. Pillar density demonstrated dramatic augmentation by 63% compared to the Notch inhibition alone and more than 400% as compared to PBS.

We have largely expanded our knowledge about the role of bone marrow-derived cells in stimulating angiogenesis after their discovery in 1997 [45] and now their capability to promote vessel formation is intensively investigated. There are large clinical perspectives for their use in many diseases, connected to angiogenesis.

With the tendency of aging, the elderly will account for a great part of population world wide. This aging will be accompanied by chronic vascular dementia, due to chronic cerebral hypoperfusion. Cellular therapy is an emerging investigational approach for cerebral ischemia. The most attractive source for such therapy is bone marrow-derived mononuclear cells (BMMNC), since they consist of different types of stem cells. Several independent studies report the significant effects of BMMNC in ischemic repair after acute and chronic ischemic disorders. The intravenous infusion of BMMNC into rat brain ischemic model reduced neurologic impairments, increased angiogenesis and cognitive function in rodent [46]. Mononuclear cells from blood have therapeutic potential as well. The neuroprotective potential of CD34+ human cord blood cells was demonstrated in regard to Parkinson's disease [47]. These cells did not differentiate into neural phenotypes, but they rather exerted their effect by stimulating the production of new neuroblasts and angiogenesis. CD34+ stem cell therapy was enrolled in 2011 for 37 patients with longstanding dilated cardiomyopathy (DCM) by cell mobilization with colony stimulating factor (G-SCF) and apheresis collection [48]. Clinical response and stem cells retention were evaluated. About half of the patients (51%) were responders to the stem cells therapy, whereby the clinical response was predefined as an increase in left ventricle ejection fraction (LVEF) of >5% in 3 months. Looking for biomarkers, which can be instrumental in prediction which patients will be responders, the authors suggested some baseline factors, positively associated with both clinical response and retention, such as G-CSF, SDF-1, LIF, MCP-1, and MCP-3. The most recent study described the significant effect of human cord blood mononuclear cells (CB-MNCs) injection for cardiac repair in ischemic heart disease, mainly by promotion of angiogenesis in the infarcted region [49].

The mechanisms of action for mononuclear cells in angiogenesis have been intensively studied. The domain comes to be multifaceted and contradictory data were sometimes arising.

First, it was proposed and evidence was provided that myeloid cells can turn into endothelial cells in hypoxic tissue demand. Asahara et al. reported that purified CD34+ hematopoietic progenitor cells in adults can differentiate *ex vivo* to an endothelial phenotype [45]. The cells were at the same time positive for VEGFR2, a specific endothelial marker and they were named endothelial progenitor cells (EPC). Thus, EPC expresses both hematopoietic stem cell and endothelial cell markers on their surface [50]. The intensive studies in the past few years allowed distinguishing subpopulations of mononuclear cells existing in the adult bone marrow and circulating in peripheral blood which support angiogenesis without incorporating permanently into the newly formed vessel–circulating angiogenic cells (CAC) [51]. Currently, bone marrow-derived (BMD) cellular populations with angiogenic properties are classified according to their phenotypic markers in the following groups: (i) EPC, which express VEGFR2, Tie2, CXCR4, CD31, CD34, CD133 (for immature progenitor cells) and they are negative for CD14; (ii) monocytes, which express CD14 and have different subclasses such as positive for Tie2, CXCR4, VEGFR2, or VEGFR1; and (iii) macrophages, mostly positive for CXCR4 and VEGFR1 [52].

Several clinical studies have shown a correlation between a high number of tumor-associated macrophages and increased microvessel density, suggesting that these cells might promote tumor angiogenesis, particularly due to production of proangiogenic and angiogenesis modulating factors [53]. A number of functional *in vitro* and *in vivo* studies demonstrate that tumors stimulate neutrophils to promote angiogenesis and immunosuppression, as well as migration, invasion, and metastasis of the tumor cells [54]. In inflammation, the SDF-1/CXCR4 signaling pathway plays an important role in the modulation of neutrophil activity, not only by promoting chemotaxis but also by suppressing cell death [55]. Although limited, there is evidence to suggest that tumor-infiltrating eosinophils can influence angiogenesis [53]. Freshly isolated human blood eosinophils or supernatants from cultured eosinophils induce endothelial cell proliferation *in vitro* and angiogenesis in the rat aortic ring assay, suggesting that eosinophils can directly influence angiogenesis. The high number of mast cells (MC) has been observed in various tumors where increased MC density positively correlates with increased microvessel density [53]. Dendritic cells (DC) promote tumor angiogenesis both by their secretion of proangiogenic cytokines (vascular endothelial growth factor (VEGF), interleukin (IL)-8, tumor necrosis factor (TNF)-alpha) and their ability to serve as a local supply of endothelial progenitors [56]. Natural killer (NK) cells control both local tumor growth and metastasis and participate in cancer elimination by inhibiting cellular proliferation and angiogenesis [57]. T helper (Th) cell-mediated immunity has traditionally been viewed as favoring tumor growth, both by promoting angiogenesis and by inhibiting cell-mediated immunity and subsequent tumor cell killing, there are also many studies demonstrating the antitumor activity of CD4+ Th2 cells, particularly in their collaboration with tumor-infiltrating eosinophils or due to direct antiangiogenic effects of IL-4 [58]. T regulatory cells (Tregs) are potent immunosuppressive cells that promote progression of cancer through their ability to limit antitumor immunity and promote angiogenesis. The accumulation of Tregs in tumors correlates with biomarkers of accelerated angiogenesis such as VEGF overexpression and increased microvessel density, providing clinical cues for an association between Tregs and angiogenesis [59].

Mononuclear cells, derived from bone marrow or umbilical cord, yielded in culture two types of cells with angiogenic properties, distinguished by morphology–late endothelial progenitor cells (EPC) and mesenchymal stem cells (MSC). Quantitative PCR analyses revealed high expression levels of Ang-1, FGF-2, SDF1α, and VEGF-A in the MSC, whereas late EPC had higher expression of PDGF-B, PlGF, KDR, CD31, VE-cadherin, and Ang-2 [60]. After transplantation of EPC and MSC in the ischemic hearts, mRNA levels of Ang-1, FGF2, SDF1α, and IGF-1 were significantly increased in tissues collected from the peri-infarct zones; notably the upregulated factors were the same in both cell types transplanted. The data demonstrate that these cells upregulate a number of paracrine factors connected to angiogenesis and cell survival during the critical period of heart repair.

Although the role of bone marrow and peripheral blood mononuclear cells in neovascularization has been convincingly shown, the question remains: how do these cells improve neovascularization? The discovery that mononuclear cells can home to sites of hypoxia and enhance neoangiogenesis has faced the possibility for using the isolated hematopoietic stem cells or EPC for therapeutic vasculogenesis [61]. Remarkably, infusion of terminally differentiated mature endothelial cells did not improve neovascularization [62, 63] suggesting that a not-yet-defined functional characteristic (e.g., chemokine or integrin receptors mediating homing) is essential for EPC-mediated vascular augmentation after ischemia [64]. Monocytic cells may play a crucial role also in collateral growth by adherence to the vascular wall during both arteriogenesis and tumor angiogenesis [53]. These data suggest that monocytic cells are necessary for arteriogenesis and possibly neovascularization. For therapeutic application, the local enhancement of monocyte recruitment might be better suited than systemic infusion of monocytic cells, which only leads to a relatively minor increase in the number of circulating monocytes. During endothelial repair after vascular injury and during tumor angiogenesis BMMNC do not seem to be involved in reendothelialization stressing rather their supportive role over trans-differentiation [65, 66].

The hypothesis for endothelial trans-differentiation of EPC and MSC was tested in the experiment with CM-Dil-labeled (red fluorescent dye) mononuclear cells and subsequent transplantation in infarcted hearts. Interestingly, both EPC and MSC were detected in the pericytic or perivascular areas with minimal and negligible endothelial trans-differentiation effects ($<1\%$). It was suggested that these cells function mainly by paracrine action and vessel stabilization in the perivascular area. The efficiency of neovascularization therefore may not solely be attributable to the incorporation of these cells in newly formed vessels, but may also be influenced by the release of proangiogenic factors in a paracrine manner [67]. It was recently shown that secreting factors from peripheral blood mononuclear cells enhance neoangiogenesis [68]. The capacity of EPC to physically contribute to vessel-like structures may contribute to their potent capacity to improve neovascularization as well [69]. Further studies are in demand to be designed to elucidate the contribution of physical incorporation, paracrine effects and possible effects on vessel remodeling and facilitating vessel branching in EPC-mediated improvement of neovascularization. Likely, paracrine effects contribute in addition to the physical incorporation of EPC into newly formed capillaries. The influence of the incorporation of a rather small number of circulating cells on remodeling and vessel maturation has to be further elucidated.

Only recently the bone marrow-derived monocytes have been related to VEGF-independent angiogenesis [70]. An open question is what drives BMD and PBM cells recruitment to the sites of angiogenesis? Ischemia is believed to upregulate VEGF or SDF-1 [71], which in turn are released to the circulation and induce mobilization of progenitor cells from the bone marrow via a MMP-9–dependent mechanism [72, 73]. Indeed, SDF-1 has been proven to stimulate recruitment of progenitor cells to the ischemic tissue [74]. SDF-1 protein levels were increased during the first day after induction of myocardial infarction [75]. Moreover, overexpression of SDF-1 augmented stem cell homing and incorporation into ischemic tissues [74, 75]. Interestingly, hematopoietic stem cells were shown to be exquisitely sensitive to SDF-1 and did not react to G-CSF or other chemokines (e.g., IL-8 and RANTES) [76]. The migratory capacity of EPC or bone marrow cells toward VEGF and SDF-1, respectively, determined the functional improvement of patients after stem cell therapy [77].

SDF-1/CXCR4 axis is crucial in the homing mechanisms of hematopoietic cells and the metastasis of solid tumors. In the past few years, numerous studies have focused on studying the role of this signaling in angiogenesis and proved its angiogenic activity in organ repair and tumor development. However, the precise mechanisms by which SDF-1 exerts its proangiogenic effects are not fully elucidated. Since it is supposed to be an angiogenic growth factor, it is a good candidate for pro- and antiangiogenic therapy. It was reported that transient disruption of the SDF-1/CXCR4 axis using CXCR4 blocking antibody blocked the recruitment of bone marrow-derived cells into the angiogenic sites of tumor tissue, and resulted in complete inhibition of accelerated tumor growth after chemotherapy in mouse [78]. SDF-1 is constitutively expressed in the bone marrow and various tissues, which enables it to regulate the trafficking, localization, and function of immature and mature leukocytes, including monocytes, neutrophils, dendritic cells, and T lymphocytes [79]. All these immune cells play an important role in tumor angiogenesis and vascularization. However, the precise role of SDF-1/CXCR4 axis on function of monocytes/macrophages, neutrophils, DC, T lymphocytes in the process of angiogenesis is still known and is worthy to be investigated.

4. SDF-1 as a key regulator of vessel development

Global mouse knockouts of SDF-1 (CXCL12) or of its receptor CXCR4 die shortly before birth with vascular deficiency in gut, kidney, and skin and with multiple hematopoietic and neural defects [80-82]. Disrupted CXCL12 signaling led to defective coronary vessel organization in mouse embryos. This signaling was connected to perfusion of the coronary arteries and respectively to embryo growth [31].

SDF-1–positive endothelium was found lining the newly formed intraluminal vessels in lobular capillary hemangiomas [83], possibly these were sites of pillar formation. Wrag et al. demonstrated that transplantation of rat bone marrow-derived progenitor cells, positive for VEGFR1, and CXCR4, in ischemic hind limbs increased capillary density by an SDF-1–dependent manner, but did not differentiate into vascular structures like endothelial cells or smooth muscle cells [84]. In our previous study, we observed upregulation of SDF-1 and CXCR4 after Notch inhibition being in association with intussusceptive angiogenesis. These chemokine factors are most probably essential for the recruitment of mononuclear cells, participating in the formation of pillars.

It is well known that blocking of SDF-1/CXCR4 axis results in prevention or delay of tumor recurrence after irradiation by inhibiting the recruitment of CD11b+ monocytes/macrophages that participate in tumor revascularization [85]. It was shown that CXCR4 is expressed on

http://dx.doi.org/10.5772/66761

eosinophils [86] and concentrations of SDF-1 correlates with eosinophil recruitment [87]. It is known that SDF-1/CXCR4 signaling has pivotal role in mast cell (MC) recruitment in tumor tissue [88] and that MC produce proangiogenic chemokines in response to SDF-1 [89]. CXCR4+ dendritic cells (DC) promote angiogenesis during embryo implantation in mice [90] and CXCR4 is known as a critical chemokine receptor for migration of plasmacytoid DC [91]. CXCR4 is expressed on both NK and NKT cells and regulates their migration in inflamed and tumor tissues in response to SDF-1 as well [92, 93]. SDF-1/CXCR4 signaling is important for migration and activation of T cells [94]. However, the role of SDF-1/CXCR4 signaling in T cell–mediated angiogenesis is unknown. B cells promote tumor progression through STAT-3 regulated angiogenesis [95] and SDF-1/CXCR4 axis is essential for B-lymphocyte production [96] and maintenance of B-cell homeostasis [97].

SDF-1 is the key regulator for homing of stem and progenitor cells to the ischemic injury and its gradient is the major determinant of these cells' recruitment. It has been shown that SDF-1 expression levels are increased in ischemic cardiomyopathy and this was accompanied by the improvement of cardiac function. In addition, SDF-1 high circulation levels were detected in patients with heart failure. Using the ELISA method, Liu et al. [98] proved significantly higher circulating SDF-1 levels in HF patients (5101 ± 1977 pg/ml) compared to controls (1879 ± 1417 pg/ml). Platelet-bound SDF-1 was correlated with acute coronary syndrome and congestive heart failure as well. It was associated with the number of circulating CD34+ progenitor cells. CD34 is coexpressed with CXCR4, which is the ultimate SDF-1 receptor, in progenitor cells, originated from bone marrow, cord blood, and fetal liver. SDF-1 levels were measured in 3359 Framingham Heart Study participants and was suggested as a biomarker of heart failure and all-cause mortality risk. In this study, CD34+ cell frequency was inversely related to SDF-1, in contrast to above-mentioned direct associations. The study has several limitations as the SDF-1 measurement at one time point. There is evidence for modulation of SDF-1 levels in humans and its effect is rather cumulative and chronic than acute.

The crucial role of SDF-1 for cardiac repair in chronic ischemic heart failure was the reason for conducting clinical trial using SDF-1 nonviral gene therapy via its endomyocardial administration [99]. This blinded placebo-controlled STOP-HF trial demonstrated improvement of clinical status based on composite endpoint of six MWD (6-min walk distance) and MLWHFQ (Minnesota Living with Heart Failure Quality of life Questionnaire). Another clinical trial–MARVEL was announced in 2015 to advance into US FDA Phase 3 clinical evaluation of regenerative/cellular therapy of chronic heart failure, planned to be combined with SDF-1.

What trigger the SDF-1 upregulation is still elusive. Some authors postulate it is induced by HIF1α in response to hypoxia. However, other mechanisms of induction are also possible such as inflammation and subsequent release of mediators like interleukin-1 or tumor necrosis factor-α into circulation. It is evident by its induction not only in ischemic, but also in nonischemic cardiomyopathy. SDF-1 circulating levels were not influenced by the local heart hypoxia, but showed positive correlation with CRP, which is a marker for inflammation.

Recently, we have demonstrated the endothelial expression of SDF-1 in liver of Notch1 knockout mouse, whereby it was associated with intussusception (**Figure 2**).

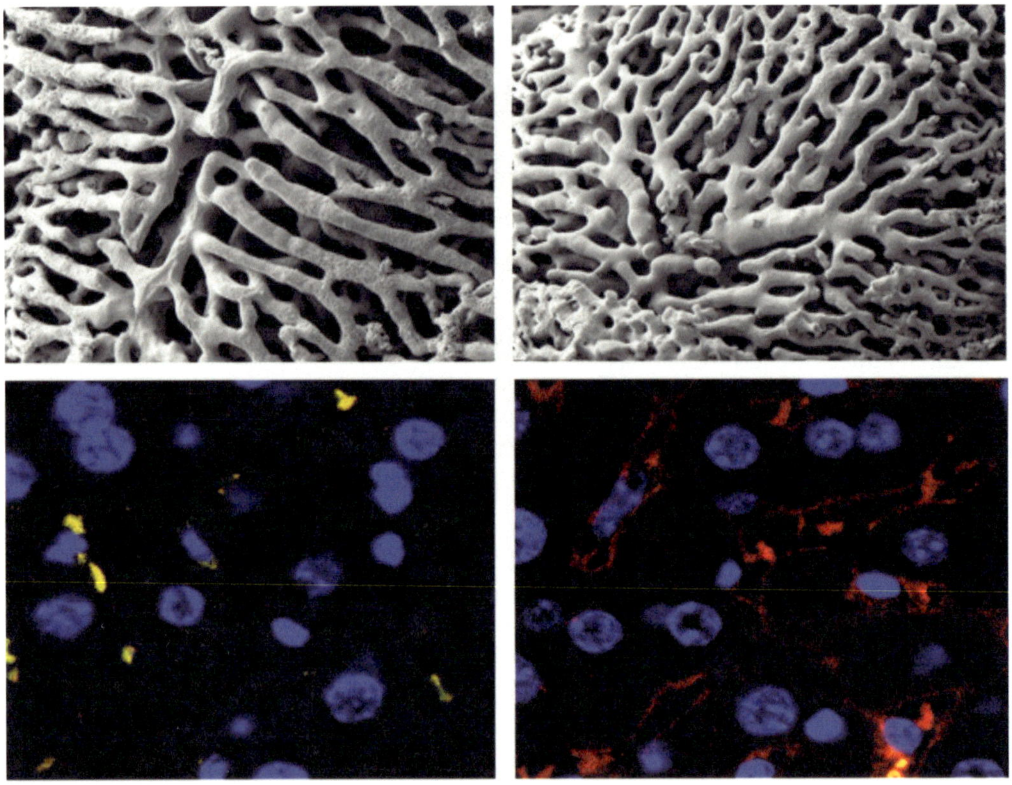

Figure 2. Vascular casts revealed predominant mode of intussusceptive angiogenesis in liver nodular regeneration after Notch1 knockout (B) compared to wild type mouse (A). Immunofluorescence for SDF-1 demonstrated strong sinusoidal positivity for this marker only in Notch1 knockout mouse (D) but not in the wild type (C).

Connecting our observations for SDF-1 positivity and mononuclear cells (MNCs) participation in intussusceptive angiogenesis, we hypothesize that both processes are involved in vessel remodeling. Using our model of chicken area vasculosa, we performed detailed ultrastructural vessel study after application of recombinant SDF-1. A specific behavior of mononuclear cells was detected during this experiment. They were involved in a step-wise process of recruitment and extravasation (**Figure 3**). We determined five distinguished states: 1, MNCs are free in the circulation; 2, MNCs are recruited to the endothelium and rolling under the blood flow; 3, MNCs are bound to the endothelium; 4, MNCs are extravasating; 5, MNCs are localized in the perivascular space.

1. MC free in circulation–nonadhesive to endothelial cells
2. MC tethered to endothelium and rolling under force of blood flow
3. MC bound to endothelium and migrating
4. Extravasation of MC from blood vessel
5. MC in perivascular space–stabilizing function

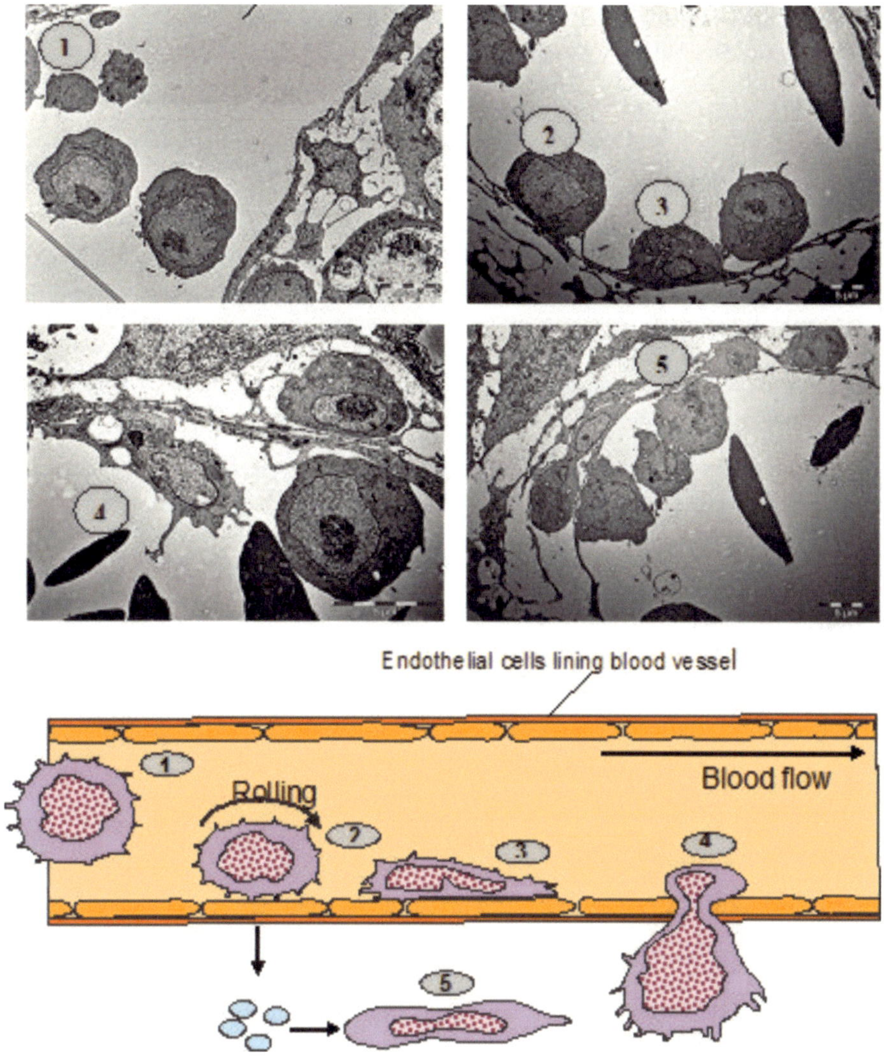

Figure 3. Transmission electron microscopy of chicken area vasculosa after the application of recombinant SDF-1 and the proposed model for mononuclear cells (MC) extravasation.

5. Summary

- Angiogenesis is a complex process involving essential signaling pathways (for instance VEGF, bFGF, Notch, etc.) in vasculature, as well as additional players such as bone marrow-derived mononuclear cells.
- Intussusceptive angiogenesis (IA) is a well-documented and widely spread mode of angiogenesis, occurring both during normal development and in pathological conditions.

- Our preliminary results suggest that IA is most probably synchronized by chemokine factors since intussusceptive growth was associated with the recruitment of mononuclear cells.
- The intensive studies in the past few years allowed distinguishing subpopulations of mononuclear cells existing in the adult bone marrow and circulating in peripheral blood which support angiogenesis.
- During endothelial repair after vascular injury and during tumor angiogenesis mononuclear cells do not seem to be involved in reendothelialization stressing rather their supportive role over trans-differentiation.
- We have demonstrated the endothelial expression of SDF-1 in liver of Notch1 knockout mouse, whereby it was associated with intussusceptive angiogenesis.
- We suggest that this chemokine factor is most probably essential for the recruitment of mononuclear cells, participating in step-wise process of extravasation and stabilizing the formation of intussusceptive pillars.

Acknowledgement

This work was supported by Contract No IZ73Z0_152454 of SNSF, Switzerland.

Author details

Ivanka Dimova[1]* and Valentin Djonov[2]

*Address all correspondence to: ivanka.i.dimova@gmail.com

1 Department of Medical genetics, Medical University Sofia, Sofia, Bulgaria

2 Institute of Anatomy, University of Bern, Bern, Switzerland

References

[1] Ribatti D, Crivellato E: "Sprouting angiogenesis", a reappraisal. Dev Biol. 2012;372(2):157–65.

[2] Djonov V, Baum O, Burri PH: Vascular remodeling by intussusceptive angiogenesis. Cell Tissue Res. 2003;314(1):107–17.

[3] Djonov V, Schmid M, Tschanz SA, Burri PH: Intussusceptive angiogenesis: its role in embryonic vascular network formation. Circ Res. 2000;86(3):286–92.

[4] Jakobsson L, Franco CA, Bentley K, Collins RT, Ponsioen B, Aspalter IM, Rosewell I, Busse M, Thurston G, Medvinsky A, Schulte-Merker S, Gerhardt H: Endothelial cells dynamically compete for the tip cell position during angiogenic sprouting. Nat Cell Biol. 2010;12(10):943–53.

[5] Blanco R, Gerhardt H: VEGF and Notch in tip and stalk cell selection. Cold Spring Harb Perspect Med. 2013 Jan 1;3(1):a006569.

[6] Makanya AN, Hlushchuk R, Djonov VG: Intussusceptive angiogenesis and its role in vascular morphogenesis, patterning, and remodeling. Angiogenesis. 2009;12(2):113–23.

[7] Styp-Rekowska B, Hlushchuk R, Pries AR, Djonov V: Intussusceptive angiogenesis: pillars against the blood flow. Acta Physiol (Oxf). 2011;202(3):213–23.

[8] Konerding MA, Gibney BC, Houdek JP, Chamoto K, Ackermann M, Lee GS, Lin M, Tsuda A, Mentzer SJ: Spatial dependence of alveolar angiogenesis in post-pneumonectomy lung growth. Angiogenesis. 2012;15(1):23–32.

[9] Dill MT, Rothweiler S, Djonov V, Hlushchuk R, Tornillo L, Terracciano L, Meili-Butz S, Radtke F, Heim MH, Semela D: Disruption of Notch1 induces vascular remodeling, intussusceptive angiogenesis, and angiosarcomas in livers of mice. Gastroenterology. 2012;142(4):967–77.

[10] Baum O, Suter F, Gerber B, Tschanz SA, Buergy R, Blank F, Hlushchuk R, Djonov V: VEGF-A promotes intussusceptive angiogenesis in the developing chicken chorioallantoic membrane. Microcirculation. 2010;17(6):447–57.

[11] Dimova I, Hlushchuk R, Makanya A, Styp-Rekowska B, Ceausu A, Flueckiger S, Lang S, Semela D, Le Noble F, Chatterjee S, Djonov V: Inhibition of Notch signaling induces extensive intussusceptive neo-angiogenesis by recruitment of mononuclear cells. Angiogenesis. 2013 Oct;16(4):921–37.

[12] Makanya AN, Hlushchuk R, Djonov V: The pulmonary blood-gas barrier in the avian embryo: inauguration, development and refinement. Respir Physiol Neurobiol. 2011 Aug 31;178(1):30–8.

[13] Taylor AC, Seltz LM, Yates PA, Peirce SM: Chronic whole-body hypoxia induces intussusceptive angiogenesis and microvascular remodeling in the mouse retina. Microvasc Res. 2010 Mar;79(2):93–101.

[14] Konerding MA, Turhan A, Ravnic DJ, Lin M, Fuchs C, Secomb TW, Tsuda A, Mentzer SJ: Inflammation-induced intussusceptive angiogenesis in murine colitis. Anat Rec (Hoboken). 2010 May;293(5):849–57.

[15] Peebo BB, Fagerholm P, Traneus-Röckert C, Lagali N: Cellular level characterization of capillary regression in inflammatory angiogenesis using an in vivo corneal model. Angiogenesis. 2011 Sep;14(3):393–405.

[16] Wnuk M, Hlushchuk R, Janot M, Tuffin G, Martiny-Baron G, Holzer P, Imbach-Weese P, Djonov V, Huynh-Do U: Podocyte EphB4 signaling helps recovery from glomerular injury. Kidney Int. 2012 Jun;81(12):1212–25.

[17] Hlushchuk R, Makanya AN, Djonov V: Escape mechanisms after antiangiogenic treatment, or why are the tumors growing again? Int J Dev Biol. 2011;55(4–5):563–67.

[18] Hlushchuk R, Riesterer O, Baum O, Wood J, Gruber G, Pruschy M, Djonov V: Tumor recovery by angiogenic switch from sprouting to intussusceptive angiogenesis after treatment with PTK787/ZK222584 or ionizing radiation. Am J Pathol. 2008 Oct;173(4):1173–85.

[19] Abdullah SE, Perez-Soler R: Mechanisms of resistance to vascular endothelial growth factor blockade. Cancer. 2012 Jul 15;118(14):3455–67.

[20] Paku S, Dezso K, Bugyik E, Tóvári J, Tímár J, Nagy P, Laszlo V, Klepetko W, Döme B: A new mechanism for pillar formation during tumor-induced intussusceptive angiogenesis: inverse sprouting. Am J Pathol. 2011 Sep;179(3):1573–85.

[21] Ceauşu RA, Cîmpean AM, Gaje P, Gurzu S, Jung I, Raica M: CD105/Ki67 double immunostaining expression in liver metastasis from colon carcinoma. Rom J Morphol Embryol. 2011;52(2):613–16.

[22] Bugyik E, Dezso K, Reiniger L, László V, Tóvári J, Tímár J, Nagy P, Klepetko W, Döme B, Paku S : Lack of angiogenesis in experimental brain metastases. J Neuropathol Exp Neurol. 2011 Nov;70(11):979–91.

[23] Reuwer AQ, Nowak-Sliwinska P, Mans LA, van der Loos CM, von der Thüsen JH, Twickler MT, Spek CA, Goffin V, Griffioen AW, Borensztajn KS: Functional consequences of prolactin signalling in endothelial cells: a potential link with angiogenesis in pathophysiology? J Cell Mol Med. 2012 Sep;16(9):2035–48.

[24] Oliveira de Oliveira LB, Faccin Bampi V, Ferreira Gomes C, Braga da Silva JL, Encarnação Fiala Rechsteiner SM: Morphological characterization of sprouting and intussusceptive angiogenesis by SEM in oral squamous cell carcinoma. Scanning. 2014 May-Jun;36(3):293-300. doi: 10.1002/sca.21104.

[25] Géraud C, Mogler C, Runge A, Evdokimov K, Lu S, Schledzewski K, Arnold B, Hämmerling G, Koch PS, Breuhahn K, Longerich T, Marx A, Weiss C, Damm F, Schmieder A, Schirmacher P, Augustin HG, Goerdt S: Endothelial transdifferentiation in hepatocellular carcinoma: loss of Stabilin-2 expression in peri-tumourous liver correlates with increased survival. Liver Int. 2013 Oct;33(9):1428–40.

[26] Piguet AC, Saar B, Hlushchuk R, St-Pierre MV, McSheehy PM, Radojevic V, Afthinos M, Terracciano L, Djonov V, Dufour JF: Everolimus augments the effects of sorafenib in a syngeneic orthotopic model of hepatocellular carcinoma. Mol Cancer Ther. 2011 Jun;10(6):1007–17.

[27] De Spiegelaere W, Casteleyn C, Van den Broeck W, Plendl J, Bahramsoltani M, Simoens P, Djonov V, Cornillie P: Intussusceptive angiogenesis: a biologically relevant form of angiogenesis. J Vasc Res. 2012;49(5):390–404.

[28] Ackermann M, Tsuda A, Secomb TW, Mentzer SJ, Konerding MA: Intussusceptive remodeling of vascular branch angles in chemically-induced murine colitis. Microvasc Res. 2013 May;87:75–82.

[29] Polykandriotis E, Arkudas A, Beier JP, Dragu A, Rath S, Pryymachuk G, Schmidt VJ, Lametschwandtner A, Horch RE, Kneser U: The impact of VEGF and bFGF on vascular stereomorphology in the context of angiogenic neo-arborisation after vascular induction. J Electron Microsc (Tokyo). 2011;60(4):267–74.

[30] Ackermann M, Morse BA, Delventhal V, Carvajal IM, Konerding MA: Anti-VEGFR2 and anti-IGF-1R-Adnectins inhibit Ewing's sarcoma A673-xenograft growth and normalize tumor vascular architecture. Angiogenesis. 2012 Dec;15(4):685–95.

[31] Cavallero S., Shen H., Yi Ch., Lien C., Ram Kumar S., Sucov H: CXCL12 signaling is essential for maturation of the ventricular coronary endothelial plexus and establishment of functional coronary circulation. Dev Cell. 2015 May 26;33(4):469–477.

[32] Kovall RA: Structures of CSL, Notch and Mastermind proteins: piecing together an active transcription complex. Curr Opin Struct Biol. 2007;17(1):117–27.

[33] Parks AL, Stout JR, Shepard SB, Klueg KM, Dos Santos AA, Parody TR, Vaskova M, Muskavitch MA: Structure-function analysis of delta trafficking, receptor binding and signalling in Drosophila. Genetics. 2006;174(4):1947–61.

[34] Seo S, Kume T: Forkhead transcription factors, Forkhead box C1 (Foxc1) and Forkhead box C2 (Foxc2), are required for the morphogenesis of the cardiac outflow tract. Dev Biol. 2006;296(2):421–36.

[35] Domenga V, Fardoux P, Lacombe P, Monet M, Maciazek J, Krebs L, Klonjkowski B, berrou E, Mericskay M, Li Z, et al: Notch3 is required for arterial identity and maturation of vascular smooth muscle cells. Genes Dev. 2004;18:2730–2735

[36] Krebs LT, et al: Notch-signalling is essential for vascular morphogenesis in mice. Genes Dev. 2000;14:1343–1352.

[37] Uyttendaele H, Ho J, Rossant J, Kitajewski J: Vascular patterning defects associated with expression of activated Notch4 in embryonic endothelium. Proc Natl Acad Sci USA. 2001;98:5643–5648.

[38] Villa N, Walker L, Lindcell CE, Gasson J, Iruela-Arispe ML, Weinmaster G: Vascular expression of Notch pathway receptors and ligands is restricted to arterial vessels. Mech Dev. 2001;108:161–164.

[39] Jenkins DW, Ross S, Veldman-Jones M, Foltz IN, Clavette BC, Manchulenko K, Eberlein C, Kendrew J, Petteruti P, Cho S, Damschroder M, Peng L, Baker D, Smith NR, Weir HM, Blakey DC, Bedian V, Barry ST: MEDI0639: a novel therapeutic antibody targeting Dll4 modulates endothelial cell function and angiogenesis in vivo. Mol Cancer Ther. 2012;11(8):1650–60.

[40] Noguera-Troise I, Daly C, Papadopoulos NJ, Coetzee S, Boland P, Gale NW, Lin HC, Yancopoulos GD, Thurston G: Blockade of Dll4 inhibits tumour growth by promoting non-productive angiogenesis. Novartis Found Symp. 2007;283:106–20.

[41] Ridgway J, Zhang G, Wu Y, Stawicki S, Liang WC, Chanthery Y, Kowalski J, Watts RJ, Callahan C, Kasman I, Singh M, Chien M, Tan C, Hongo JA, de SF, Plowman G, Yan M: Inhibition of Dll4 signalling inhibits tumour growth by deregulating angiogenesis. Nature. 2006;444(7122):1083–87.

[42] Thurston G, Noguera-Troise I, Yancopoulos GD: The Delta paradox: DLL4 blockade leads to more tumour vessels but less tumour growth. Nat Rev Cancer. 2007;7(5):327–31.

[43] Al Haj ZA, Oikawa A, Bazan-Peregrino M, Meloni M, Emanueli C, Madeddu P: Inhibition of delta-like-4-mediated signaling impairs reparative angiogenesis after ischemia. Circ Res. 2010;107(2):283–93.

[44] Kalen M, Heikura T, Karvinen H, Nitzsche A, Weber H, Esser N, Yla-Herttuala S, Hellstrom M: Gamma-secretase inhibitor treatment promotes VEGF-A-driven blood vessel growth and vascular leakage but disrupts neovascular perfusion. PLoS One. 2011;6(4):e18709.

[45] Asahara T, Murohara T, Sullivan A, Silver M, van der Zee R, Li T, Witzenbichler B, Schatteman G, Isner JM: Isolation of putative progenitor endothelial cells for angiogenesis. Science. 1997 Feb 14;275(5302):964–67.

[46] Wang J, Fu X, Yu L, Li N, Wang M, Liu X, Zhang D, Han W, Zhou C, Wang J: Preconditioning with VEGF enhances angiogenic and neuroprotective effects of bone marrow mononuclear cell transplantation in a rat model of chronic cerebral hypoperfusion. Mol Neurobiol. 2016 Nov;53(9):6057–6068.

[47] Corenblum MJ, Flores AJ, Badowski M, Harris DT, Madhavan L: Systemic human CD34(+) cells populate the brain and activate host mechanisms to counteract nigrostriatal degeneration. Regen Med. 2015;10(5):563–77.

[48] Haddad F, Sever M, Poglajen G, Lezaic L, Yang P, Maecker H, Davis M, Kuznetsova T, Wu JC, Vrtovec B: Immunologic network and response to intramyocardial CD34+ stem cell therapy in patients with dilated cardiomyopathy. J Card Fail. 2015 Jul;21(7):572–82.

[49] Chang MY, Huang TT, Chen CH, Cheng B, Hwang SM, Hsieh PC: Injection of human cord blood cells with hyaluronan improves postinfarction cardiac repair in pigs. Stem Cells Transl Med. 2016 Jan;5(1):56–66.

[50] Zhao YH, Yuan B, Chen J, Feng DH, Zhao B, Qin C, Chen YF: Endothelial progenitor cells: therapeutic perspective for ischemic stroke. CNS Neurosci Ther. 2013 Feb;19(2):67–75.

[51] Fang S, Salven P: Stem cells in tumor angiogenesis. J Mol Cell Cardiol. 2011 Feb;50(2):290–95.

[52] Favre J, Terborg N, Horrevoets AJ: The diverse identity of angiogenic monocytes. Eur J Clin Invest. 2013 Jan;43(1):100–7.

[53] Murdoch C, Muthana M, Coffelt SB, Lewis CE: The role of myeloid cells in the promotion of tumour angiogenesis. Nat Rev Cancer. 2008 Aug;8(8):618–31.

[54] Dumitru CA, Lang S, Brandau S: Modulation of neutrophil granulocytes in the tumor microenvironment: mechanisms and consequences for tumor progression. Semin Cancer Biol. 2013 Jun;23(3):141–48.

[55] Yamada M, Kubo H, Kobayashi S, Ishizawa K, He M, Suzuki T, Fujino N, Kunishima H, Hatta M, Nishimaki K, Aoyagi T, Tokuda K, Kitagawa M, Yano H, Tamamura H, Fujii N, Kaku M: The increase in surface CXCR4 expression on lung extravascular neutrophils and its effects onneutrophils during endotoxin-induced lung injury. Cell Mol Immunol. 2011 Jul;8(4):305–14.

[56] Strioga M, Schijns V, Powell DJ Jr, Pasukoniene V, Dobrovolskiene N, Michalek J: Dendritic cells and their role in tumor immunosurveillance. Innate Immun. 2013 Feb;19(1):98–111.

[57] Levy EM, Roberti MP, Mordoh J: Natural killer cells in human cancer: from biological functions to clinical applications. J Biomed Biotechnol. 2011;2011:676198.

[58] Ellyard JI, Simson L, Parish CR: Th2-mediated anti-tumour immunity: friend or foe? Tissue Antigens. 2007 Jul;70(1):1–11.

[59] Facciabene A, Motz GT, Coukos G: T-regulatory cells: key players in tumor immune escape and angiogenesis. Cancer Res. 2012 May 1;72(9):2162–71.

[60] Kim SW, Jin HL, Kang SM, Kim S, Yoo KJ, Jang Y, Kim HO, Yoon YS: Therapeutic effects of late outgrowth endothelial progenitor cells or mesenchymal stem cells derived from human umbilical cord blood on infarct repair. Int J Cardiol. 2016 Jan 15;203:498–507.

[61] Wara AK, Croce K, Foo S, Sun X, Icli B, Tesmenitsky Y, Esen F, Rosenzweig A, Feinberg MW: Bone marrow-derived CMPs and GMPs represent highly functional proangiogenic cells: implications for ischemic cardiovascular disease. Blood. 2011 Dec 8;118(24):6461–64.

[62] Kocher AA, Schuster MD, Szabolcs MJ, Takuma S, Burkhoff D, Wang J, Homma S, Edwards NM, Itescu S: Neovascularization of ischemic myocardium by human bone-marrow-derived angioblasts prevents cardiomyocyte apoptosis, reduces remodeling and improves cardiac function. Nat Med. 2001 Apr;7(4):430–36.

[63] Hur J, Yoon CH, Kim HS, Choi JH, Kang HJ, Hwang KK, Oh BH, Lee MM, Park YB: Characterization of two types of endothelial progenitor cells and their different contributions to neovasculogenesis. Arterioscler Thromb Vasc Biol. 2004 Feb;24(2):288–93.

[64] Cochain C, Rodero MP, Vilar J, Récalde A, Richart AL, Loinard C, Zouggari Y, Guérin C, Duriez M, Combadière B, Poupel L, Lévy BI, Mallat Z, Combadière C, Silvestre JS: Regulation of monocyte subset systemic levels by distinct chemokine receptors controls post-ischaemic neovascularization. Cardiovasc Res. 2010 Oct 1;88(1):186–95.

[65] Dudley AC, Udagawa T, Melero-Martin JM, Shih SC, Curatolo A, Moses MA, Klagsbrun M: Bone marrow is a reservoir for proangiogenic myelomonocytic cells but not endothelial cells in spontaneous tumors. Blood. 2010 Oct 28;116(17):3367–71.

[66] Hagensen MK, Raarup MK, Mortensen MB, Thim T, Nyengaard JR, Falk E, Bentzon JF: Circulating endothelial progenitor cells do not contribute to regeneration of endothelium after murine arterial injury. Cardiovasc Res. 2012 Feb 1;93(2):223–31.

[67] Ribatti D, Crivellato E: Immune cells and angiogenesis. J Cell Mol Med. 2009 Sep;13(9A):2822–33.

[68] Mildner M, Hacker S, Haider T, Gschwandtner M, Werba G, Barresi C, Zimmermann M, Golabi B, Tschachler E, Ankersmit HJ: Secretome of peripheral blood mononuclear cells enhances wound healing. PLoS One. 2013;8(3):e60103.

[69] Urbich C, Heeschen C, Aicher A, Dernbach E, Zeiher AM, Dimmeler S: Relevance of monocytic features for neovascularization capacity of circulating endothelial progenitor cells. Circulation. 2003 Nov 18;108(20):2511–16.

[70] Botta C, Barbieri V, Ciliberto D, Rossi A, Rocco D, Addeo R, Staropoli N, Pastina P, Marvaso G, Martellucci I, Guglielmo A, Pirtoli L, Sperlongano P, Gridelli C, Caraglia M, Tassone P, Tagliaferri P, Correale P: Systemic inflammatory status at baseline predicts bevacizumab benefit in advanced non-small cell lung cancer patients. Cancer Biol Ther. 2013 Jun;14(6):469–75.

[71] Lee SH, Wolf PL, Escudero R, Deutsch R, Jamieson SW, Thistlethwaite PA: Early expression of angiogenesis factors in acute myocardial ischemia and infarction. N Engl J Med. 2000 Mar 2;342(9):626–33.

[72] Heissig B, Hattori K, Dias S, Friedrich M, Ferris B, Hackett NR, Crystal RG, Besmer P, Lyden D, Moore MA, Werb Z, Rafii S: Recruitment of stem and progenitor cells from the bone marrow niche requires MMP-9 mediated release of kit-ligand. Cell. 2002 May 31;109(5):625–37.

[73] Shintani S, Murohara T, Ikeda H, Ueno T, Honma T, Katoh A, Sasaki K, Shimada T, Oike Y, Imaizumi T: Mobilization of endothelial progenitor cells in patients with acute myocardial infarction. Circulation. 2001 Jun 12;103(23):2776–79.

[74] Yamaguchi J, Kusano KF, Masuo O, Kawamoto A, Silver M, Murasawa S, Bosch-Marce M, Masuda H, Losordo DW, Isner JM, Asahara T: Stromal cell-derived factor-1 effects on ex vivo expanded endothelial progenitor cell recruitment for ischemic neovascularization. Circulation. 2003 Mar 11;107(9):1322–28.

[75] Askari AT, Unzek S, Popovic ZB, Goldman CK, Forudi F, Kiedrowski M, Rovner A, Ellis SG, Thomas JD, DiCorleto PE, Topol EJ, Penn MS: Effect of stromal-cell-derived factor 1 on stem-cell homing and tissue regeneration in ischaemic cardiomyopathy. Lancet. 2003 Aug 30;362(9385):697–703.

[76] Wright DE, Bowman EP, Wagers AJ, Butcher EC, Weissman IL: Hematopoietic stem cells are uniquely selective in their migratory response to chemokines. J Exp Med. 2002 May 6;195(9):1145–54.

[77] Britten MB, Abolmaali ND, Assmus B, Lehmann R, Honold J, Schmitt J, Vogl TJ, Martin H, Schächinger V, Dimmeler S, Zeiher AM: Infarct remodeling after intracoronary progenitor cell treatment in patients with acute myocardial infarction (TOPCARE-AMI): mechanistic insights from serial contrast-enhanced magnetic resonance imaging. Circulation. 2003 Nov 4;108(18):2212–28.

[78] Murakami J, Li TS, Ueda K, Tanaka T, Hamano K: Inhibition of accelerated tumor growth by blocking the recruitment of mobilized endothelial progenitor cells after chemotherapy. Int J Cancer. 2009;124(7):1685–1692.

[79] Karin N: The multiple faces of CXCL12 (SDF-1alpha) in the regulation of immunity during health and disease. J Leukoc Biol. 2010 Sep;88(3):463–73.

[80] Ma Q, Jones D, Borghesani PR, Segal RA, Nagasawa T, Kishimoto T, Bronson RT, Springer TA: Impaired B-lymphopoiesis, myelopoiesis, and derailed cerebellar neuron migration in CXCR4- and SDF-1-deficient mice. Proc Natl Acad Sci U S A. 1998 Aug 4;95(16):9448–53.

[81] Nagasawa T, Hirota S, Tachibana K, Takakura N, Nishikawa S, Kitamura Y, Yoshida N, Kikutani H, Kishimoto T: Defects of B-cell lymphopoiesis and bone-marrow myelopoiesis in mice lacking the CXC chemokine PBSF/SDF-Nature. 1996 Aug 15;382(6592):635–38.

[82] Tachibana K, Hirota S, Iizasa H, Yoshida H, Kawabata K, Kataoka Y, Kitamura Y, Matsushima K, Yoshida N, Nishikawa S, Kishimoto T, Nagasawa T: The chemokine receptor CXCR4 is essential for vascularization of the gastrointestinal tract. Nature. 1998 Jun 11;393(6685):591–94.

[83] Morrow D, Cullen JP, Cahill PA, Redmond EM: Cyclic strain regulates the Notch/CBF-1 signaling pathway in endothelial cells: role in angiogenic activity. Arterioscler Thromb Vasc Biol. 2007;27(6):1289–96.

[84] Williams CK, Segarra M, Sierra ML, Sainson RC, Tosato G, Harris AL: Regulation of CXCR4 by the Notch ligand delta-like 4 in endothelial cells. Cancer Res. 2008;68(6):1889–95.

[85] Tseng D, Vasquez-Medrano DA, Brown JM: Targeting SDF-1/CXCR4 to inhibit tumour vasculature for treatment of glioblastomas. Br J Cancer. 2011 Jun 7;104(12):1805–9.

[86] Dulkys Y, Buschermöhle T, Escher SE, Kapp A, Elsner J: T-helper 2 cytokines attenuate senescent eosinophil activation by the CXCR4 ligand stromal-derived factor-1alpha (CXCL12). Clin Exp Allergy. 2004 Oct;34(10):1610–20.

[87] Negrete-García MC, Velazquez JR, Popoca-Coyotl A, Montes-Vizuet AR, Juárez-Carvajal E, Teran LM: Chemokine (C-X-C motif) ligand 12/stromal cell-derived factor-1 is associated with leukocyte recruitment in asthma. Chest. 2010 Jul;138(1):100–doi: 10.1378/chest.09-Epub 2010 Mar 18.

[88] Põlajeva J1, Sjösten AM, Lager N, Kastemar M, Waern I, Alafuzoff I, Smits A, Westermark B, Pejler G, Uhrbom L, Tchougounova E: Mast cell accumulation in glioblastoma with a potential role for stem cell factor and chemokine CXCLPLoS One. 2011;6(9):edoi: 10.1371/journal.pone.0025222.

[89] Lin TJ, Issekutz TB, Marshall JS: SDF-1 induces IL-8 production and transendothelial migration of human cord blood-derived mast cells. Int Arch Allergy Immunol. 2001 Jan–Mar;124(1–3):142–45.

[90] Barrientos G, Tirado-González I, Freitag N, Kobelt P, Moschansky P, Klapp BF, Thijssen VL, Blois SM: CXCR4(+) dendritic cells promote angiogenesis during embryo implantation in mice. Angiogenesis. 2013 Apr;16(2):417–27.

[91] Umemoto E1, Otani K, Ikeno T, Verjan Garcia N, Hayasaka H, Bai Z, Jang MH, Tanaka T, Nagasawa T, Ueda K, Miyasaka M: Constitutive plasmacytoid dendritic cell migration

to the splenic white pulp is cooperatively regulated by CCR7- and CXCR4-mediated signaling. J Immunol. 2012 Jul 1;189(1):191–doi: 10.4049/jimmunol.1200802.

[92] Robertson MJ: Role of chemokines in the biology of natural killer cells. J Leukoc Biol. 2002 Feb;71(2):173–83.

[93] Lindau D, Gielen P, Kroesen M, Wesseling P, Adema GJ: The immunosuppressive tumour network: myeloid-derived suppressor cells, regulatory T cells and natural killer T cells. Immunology. 2013 Feb;138(2):105–15.

[94] Patrussi L1, Baldari CT: Intracellular mediators of CXCR4-dependent signaling in T cells. Immunol Lett. 2008 Jan 29;115(2):75–82.

[95] Yang C1, Lee H, Pal S, Jove V, Deng J, Zhang W, Hoon DS, Wakabayashi M, Forman S, Yu H: B cells promote tumor progression via STAT3 regulated-angiogenesis. PLoS One. 2013 May 29;8(5):edoi: 10.1371/journal.pone.0064159.

[96] Nagasawa T: A chemokine, SDF-1/PBSF, and its receptor, CXC chemokine receptor 4, as mediators of hematopoiesis. Int J Hematol. 2000 Dec;72(4):408–11.

[97] Mountz JD, Wang JH, Xie S, Hsu HC: Cytokine regulation of B-cell migratory behavior favors formation of germinal centers in autoimmune disease. Discov Med. 2011 Jan;11(56):76–85.

[98] Liu K, Yang S, Hou M, Chen T, Liu J, Yu B: Increase of circulating stromal cell-derived factor-1 in heart failure patients. Herz. 2015 Mar;40(Suppl 1):70–doi: 10.1007/s00059-014-4169-z.

[99] Chung ES, Miller L, Patel AN, et al: Changes in ventricular remodelling and clinical status during the year following a single administration of stromal cell-derived factor-1 non-viral gene therapy in chronic ischaemic heart failure patients: the STOP-HF randomized Phase II trial. European Heart Journal. 2015;36(33):2228–doi:10.1093/eurheartj/ehv254.

Chapter 3

Angiogenesis Meets Skeletogenesis: The Cross-Talk between Two Dynamic Systems

Tamara A. Franz-Odendaal, Daniel Andrews and
Shruti Kumar

Additional information is available at the end of the chapter

http://dx.doi.org/10.5772/66497

Abstract

In this chapter, we describe the complex relationship between angiogenesis and skeletogenesis. While much is known about the interactions of these two dynamic systems for bones that ossify via a cartilage template, comparatively little is known about directly ossifying bones. Most of the bones of the head develop from osteogenic condensations and undergo intramembranous (direct) ossification during development. Our understanding of the relationship between osteogenic cell condensations (in particular) and angiogenesis is currently inadequate and prevents a comprehensive understanding of vertebrate head development. This chapter highlights our understanding of both direct and indirectly ossifying bones shedding light on where there are important gaps in our understanding.

Keywords: avascular, skeletogenic condensation, osteoblasts, chondrocytes, cell culture, VEGF, HIF

1. Introduction

The coordinated development of tissues is critical for proper development. Bone is a highly vascularized tissue that also houses the hematopoetic cell niche, which provides a lifelong supply of blood cells (in humans and most other vertebrates). In this chapter, we will explore the role angiogenesis plays during the development of bones. Bones that ossify endochondrally (from cartilage) versus bones that ossify intramembranously (without cartilage) have different relationships with vasculature and hence with the process of angiogenesis. These bones start development by forming a skeletogenic condensation, however, the molecular signals within these condensations differ [1]. We begin with a discussion of bones that develop from a cartilage precursor (endochondral ossification) since more is known about this process than about directly ossifying bones (intramembranous ossification). We also discuss data from cell culture and bone grafts that shed light on the cross talk between these two dynamic processes, angiogenesis and skeletogenesis. Some pathological implications are also included.

2. Bones that ossify via endochondral ossification

2.1. Angiogenesis during formation of the cartilage template

Endochondrally ossifying bones are bones that form via a cartilage template. The process of endochondral ossification begins with stem cells originating from the mesenchyme in the future area of bone development. These stem cells aggregate to form a chondrogenic condensation. Once this cell aggregation reaches a critical size, cells begin to differentiate into chondrocytes (chondroblasts) that will then secrete extracellular matrix (ECM), collagen type II. This matrix matures into the cartilage template that will eventually ossify (e.g., long bones). Cartilage itself is avascular when first deposited, however, differentiated chondrocytes secrete anti-angiogenic factors (inhibitors) to maintain the avascular nature of the cartilage. These early chondrocytes are typically referred to as pre-hypertrophic chondrocytes. As these chondrocytes mature, they gradually become hypertrophic and begin to secrete a number of pro-angiogenic factors. Vascular endothelial-derived growth factor (VEGF), a protein which is important for angiogenesis and the subsequent ossification of the cartilage, is a key angiogenic factor during bone development. Hypoxia-inducible factor is one of the key upstream regulators of VEGF, and changes in the level of HIF can alter the level of VEGF thus dramatically changing bone mass (discussed later).

During the maturation of hypertrophic chondrocytes, these cells release VEGF into the extracellular matrix and into the area surrounding the perichondrium layer of the cartilage. The hypertrophic chondrocytes also secrete fibroblast growth factor (FGF), bone morphogenetic protein (BMP) and connective tissue growth factor (CTGF) [2, 3]. With the arrival of these factors to the site of bone formation, angiogenesis in the bone can now occur. There is a complex cross talk between bone-forming cells (osteoblasts), the angiogenic factors present, and the invading vasculature. These growth factors, in particular VEGF, recruit osteo/chondro-clasts, osteoprogenitors and other bone precursors to the area in order to initiate the primary ossification center, the first site of bone formation within the cartilage template [2, 4].

Osteoclasts are bone matrix resorbing cells, and once recruited, they secrete multiple factors that contribute to the initiation of vascularization, including the release of more VEGF and FGFs [2, 5]. Among these factors are matrix metalloproteinases (MMPs) and hypoxia-inducible factors (HIFs) which, along with VEGF, are other key proteins important in the development of vasculature in bone. The MMPs break down the ECM and release matrix-bound VEGF that allows for the resorption of cartilage so that osteoblasts can infiltrate and deposit bone. MMPs, primarily MMP9 and MMP13, also function to recruit osteoclasts and osteoprogenitors, further aiding in the subsequent deposition of bone [2, 4]. The matrix-bound VEGF that is released is a key player in the formation of bone vasculature. HIFs regulate VEGF

http://dx.doi.org/10.5772/66497

expression in bone, which has an effect on angiogenesis [2]. Thus VEGF, MMPs and HIFs play a central role in angiogenesis during endochondral ossification.

2.2. Vascular invasion of the cartilage

Vascular invasion of the cartilage template is the first major step in angiogenesis in the developing bone. The vasculature from the perichondrium penetrates the previously avascular cartilage and begins to invade the rest of the cartilage. Vascular invasion is coupled to a number of events in the cartilage, the degradation of the extracellular matrix by MMPs, which releases matrix-bound VEGF and favors the invasion of the cartilage, as well as apoptosis of the hypertrophic chondrocytes which were responsible for secreting many of the growth factors that resulted in the invasion [2, 4, 6]. As vasculature penetrates the cartilage and the hypertrophic chondrocytes undergo apoptosis, they are promptly replaced by osteoblasts in the resulting bone cavity (i.e., by the osteoblasts previously recruited by factors such as VEGF). These osteoblasts then secrete collagen type I to initiate ossification to form the bone matrix in the primary ossification center. The same growth factors in and around the growth plate of the bone will allow the vasculature to continue its invasion of the bone to the secondary ossification centers located at either ends of the long bone, in the same way that the primary ossification centers were formed [2].

Angiogenesis during endochondral ossification is heavily dependent on the cellular components of the skeleton, namely osteoblasts and chondrocytes. Without these cells, the valuable pro-angiogenic factors would not be properly secreted and will not be able to induce vascular invasion. However, the reverse is also true. In order for bone to continue to form properly, efficient and effective vascular invasion is required. The vasculature that invades cartilage likely also carries required factors for bone growth; the vascular epithelium is thought to carry osteoprogenitors, more VEGF, FGFs and other factors which assist with the resorption of the surrounding cartilage and the ossification of bone [6]. Without vasculature invading the cartilage, bone formation is impaired. A study on mouse long bones showed that expression of SOX9 can block the expression of VEGFA, which results in impaired vascular invasion, and as a result, the bones do not ossify [7]. (SOX9 is a key marker of chondrogenic condensations [1].) VEGF also plays a role in the ongoing maintenance of bone vasculature endogenous VEGF was shown to enhance vascularization of bone and subsequently allows more rapid healing of injured bones, indicating the role of vascularization in the formation and turnover of endochondral bone [6].

Along with VEGF, another key factor in the invasion of vasculature into bone is hypoxia. The lack of oxygen will result in the release of hypoxia-inducible factors (HIFs) which regulate the production of the extracellular matrix and VEGF expression. The matrix binds VEGF triggering vascular invasion. The HIFs expressed by osteoblasts support both the proper vascularization of bone as well as the proper functioning of osteoblasts. Increased expression of HIFs results in more vascularization and thicker bones, whereas deletion of HIFs (and the resulting reduced expression of VEGF) results in less vascularization and thinner bones [2]. Thus, VEGFs and HIFs are two major factors that couple angiogenesis to endochondral bone formation [2, 6].

Thus in summary, endochondral ossification is dependent on the interaction between pro-angiogenic factors acting on bone-forming cells (**Figure 1**), and endochondral ossification is impaired in the absence of these factors.

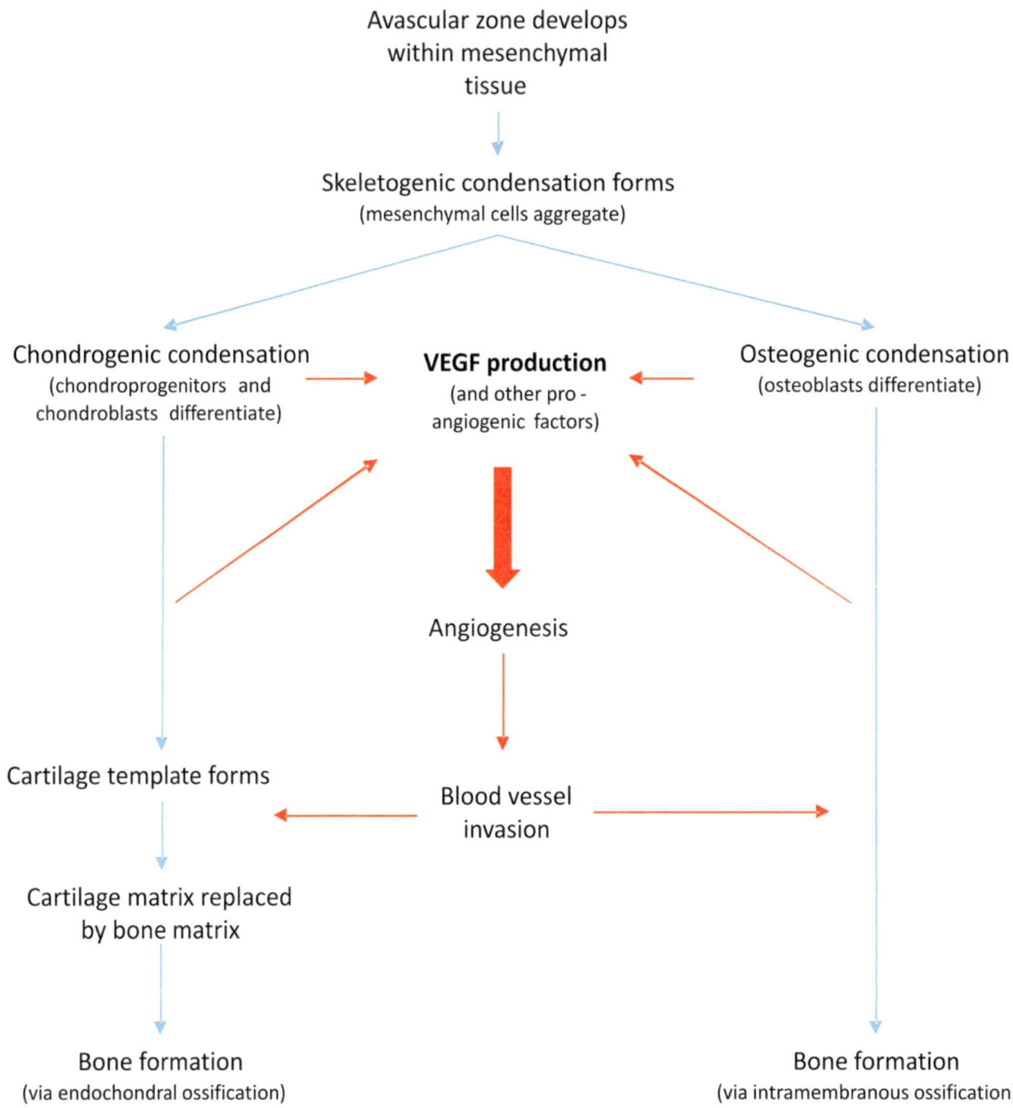

Figure 1. Schematic showing the complex cross talk between angiogenesis and skeletogenesis. Mesenchymal cells aggregate in an avascular (hypoxic) zone to form skeletogenic condensations. Differences in the molecular characteristics of these cells determine the fate of the condensation. Cells within this condensation produce VEGF and other pro-angiogenic factors, and this induces angiogenesis. Left side: Cells within the chondrogenic condensation continue to produce these angiogenic factors, and ultimately, the condensation differentiates into a cartilage template, which is still avascular. Following angiogenesis surrounding this template, blood vessels invade the cartilage perichondrium layer, and this triggers osteoblast differentiation, cartilage matrix degradation, bone matrix production and the further release of more pro-angiogenic factors. Ossification begins in the diaphysis (shaft) of long bones and spreads to the epiphyses (ends of the bone). Right side: As cells within the skeletogenic condensation differentiate, they continue to produce angiogenic factors. These factors induce angiogenesis and subsequent blood vessel invasion into the outer edges of the condensation. As more cells within the condensation differentiate, the wave of bone matrix deposition and blood vessel invasion spreads outwards.

3. Bones that ossify via intramembranous ossification

3.1. Directly ossifying bones

Intramembranously ossifying bones form without a cartilage template. Motile mesenchymal cells fated to differentiate into osteoblasts aggregate to from skeletogenic condensations at the site of the future bone. As these osteogenic aggregations enlarge and reach a critical size, the central cells begin to differentiate into osteoblasts, lose their mobility and deposit bone matrix. This process results in osteoblasts becoming embedded or trapped in bone matrix, forcing them to differentiate into osteocytes [8]. The majority of the craniofacial skeleton forms via intramembranous ossification [9]. A common example is the skull vault (the calvariae). Less common examples are the scleral ossicles (in reptiles), parts of the clavicles and scapula (in mammals), the cleithra and opercula (in fish) and sesamoid bones (e.g., the patella in humans) [9]. Although vascularization has been extensively studied in endochondral ossification as discussed above, comparatively little research has been conducted to understand the relationship between angiogenesis and intramembranous ossification.

3.2. Angiogenesis during formation of the initial phase of directly ossifying bones

The most studied intramembranous bones are the calvariae (or skull vault). Cells in the osteogenic condensations proliferate resulting in growth of the condensations until a critical size is reached. Ossification begins at the center of the condensation and expanding outwards toward the apex of the head [10]. Once this has occurred, cells at the osteogenic front proliferate, and the bones grow toward one another [11]. Areas that ossified first form a trabecular bone structure that later becomes woven bone [10]. Interestingly, the frontal and parietal bones in humans each develop two condensations, each with their own ossification centers; these centers then fuse as ossification progresses [12].

There is a significant difference in the gene expression patterns in prechondrogenic and preosteogenic condensations [1]. Avascularity within condensations may be necessary for the formation of the condensations themselves and/or to provide positional cues [10, 13]. Indeed, in scleral ossicles, an avascular zone develops surrounding the condensation [14, 15]. Manipulating the size of this avascular zone has a direct effect on subsequent bone development [15]. Although not much is known about the process of vascularization during intramembranous ossification, it is thought that similar to endochondral bones, hypoxic conditions are important to induce angiogenesis. Avascular zones likely surround all preosteogenic condensations in mammals and avians, however, the mechanism by which these zones are established is not known [10]. Percival and colleagues [10] postulate that this avascularity may be important for condensation growth, and subsequent intramembranous ossification (as in the case for prechondrogenic condensations of endochondrally ossifying bones, **Figure 1**).

A single study describes in detail, the association of angiogenesis and intramembranous bones [16]. This study of the development of the chick frontal bone showed that small capillaries invade the thin avascular layer of loose mesenchymal cells of the condensation prior to invading the condensation at/near the site of initial ossification [16]. This association between vascular invasion and ossification continues and cascades as the bone expands in all directions. As the bone mineralizes in the wake of this vascular invasion front, the internal and external vasculature is remodeled.

Based on studies of endochondral ossification and distraction osteogenesis, Percival and colleagues [10] recently developed a model of angiogenesis during intramembranous ossification. They propose that prior to the onset of mineralization, small capillaries begin to invade the surrounding avascular loose mesenchymal tissue due to the presence of pro-angiogenic factors. At around the time of mineralization onset, these capillaries invade the osteogenic condensations and branch outwards from the ossification center (**Figure 1**). These capillaries branch toward regions of pro-angiogenic factor expression and thus support the proliferating mesenchymal cells of the condensation. Mineralization thus first occurs at sites closest to the capillaries and then at sites progressively further away. Once the osteogenic condensation stops expanding, the capillaries along with the mineralization front continue to moves toward the presumptive sutures (i.e., the edges of the future bone), thus allowing continued calvarial growth.

Interestingly, while osteoblasts in endochondrally ossifying bones express both HIF1α and HIF2α, only HIF2α is detected in the osteoblasts of directly ossifying bones (i.e., those that undergo intramembranous ossification) [17]. This altered expression pattern of the HIFα subunits could suggest that alternative regulatory pathways trigger angiogenesis in these distinct types of ossification [17]. Percival and Richtsmeier [10] provide a comprehensive list of hypotheses relating to intramembranous osteogenesis and angiogenesis that require testing. The cross talk between these two dynamic processes is summarized in **Figure 1**.

4. Insights from cell culture and bone graft studies

VEGF is a chemoattractant for primary osteoblasts and mesenchymal progenitor cells [18] and can directly promote differentiation of primary human osteoblasts in culture in a dose-dependent manner [19]. Osteoblasts and mesenchymal stem cells are the two cell types most often used in bone tissue engineering. Interestingly, the type of cell used can influence the mode of ossification that occurs and the organization of blood vessels [20]. Implantation of osteoblasts leads to the formation of fibrous tissue and disorganized blood vessels. The osteoblasts become trapped in the secreted bone matrix (i.e., intramembranous ossification occurs). In contrast, implantation of stem cells leads to the formation of cartilaginous tissue (i.e., endochondral ossification) and well-organized blood vessels.

Basic fibroblast growth factor (bFGF) is another important pro-angiogenic factor. When bone mesenchymal stem cells were transfected with bFGF and then implanted into rats with calvarial defects, an increase in vascularization and osteogenesis was observed [21]. Similarly, the addition of sonic hedgehog (Shh) in engineered bone grafts *in vitro* also promotes vascularization of the grafts [22]. Shh is expressed during fracture healing and neovascularization after trauma and has been used *in vitro* to promote the organization of blood vessels in artificial tissue grafts similarly to VEGF [22, 23]. Furthermore, when these grafts were implanted subcutaneously in mice, there was increased bone formation of both directly and indirectly ossifying bone types [22]. For large defects, supplementing the graft with platelet-rich plasma results in increased bone formation [24].

5. Pathological implications

The role of growth factors like VEGF, FGF, CTGFs and others in both bone growth and angiogenesis has been demonstrated in a number of recent studies investigating the growth and healing of bones. For example, $FGF9^{+/-}$ mice exhibit a reduction in the healing of bones accompanied by a lack of VEGF expression in the area of injury, suggesting that FGF9 is required for angiogenesis and for healing long bones [25]. Hypomorphic $VEGF^{120/120}$ mice have reduced mineralization of the calvarial bones and consequently reduced bone thickness. This has been attributed to a reduction and delay in vascular invasion [26]. Additionally, conditional deletion of VEGFA in mice cranial neural crest cells causes cleft palate with reduced ossification of the mandibular bone due to reduced endothelial cell proliferation and decreased angiogenesis [27]. Mice with a VEGF-deficient osteoblastic lineage exhibit age-dependent loss of bone mass and increased bone marrow fat, similar to the changes associated with osteoporosis in humans [28].

6. Conclusions and summary

VEGF mediates angiogenesis, chondrocyte differentiation, osteoblast differentiation and osteoclast recruitment [29], and thus, its role during osteogenesis is complex ([10], **Figure 1**). Yang et al. [30] provide a useful tabulation of the effects of VEGF on intramembranous and endochondral ossification. Importantly, this chapter highlights that the relationship between angiogenesis and intramembranous ossification is not well understood. For example, only one study describes the detailed relationship between these two dynamic systems [16], and a very recent study provides a model of this process [10]. This model should be examined in several directly ossifying bones in the skeleton in order to confirm whether all directly ossifying bones follow the model or whether subtle differences exist depending perhaps on the location of the bone or the origin of the bone cells. This lack of a fundamental understanding about the developmental interactions between angiogenesis and skeletogenic condensations (particularly with respect to directly ossifying bones) contributes to our inadequate understanding of skull formation [10].

It should be noted that bones that ossify from the perichondrium of a cartilage template can be considered endochondral or intramembranous (since the perichondrium is a membrane of the cartilage). An example is Meckel's cartilage. The relationship between angiogenesis and bones that develop via the perichondrium has not been studied.

Acknowledgements

The authors acknowledge funding from the Natural Sciences and Engineering Research Council of Canada. We also acknowledge M. Bhade who collated literature for this book chapter.

Author details

Tamara A. Franz-Odendaal[1,2]*, Daniel Andrews[1] and Shruti Kumar[1,2]

*Address all correspondence to: tamara.franz-odendaal@msvu.ca

1 Mount Saint Vincent University, Nova Scotia, Canada

2 Saint Mary's University, Nova Scotia, Canada

References

[1] Eames BF, Helms JA: Conserved molecular program regulating cranial and appendicular skeletogenesis. Developmental Dynamics. 2004;231:4–13.

[2] Silvaraj KK, Adams RH: Blood vessel formation and function in bone. Development. 2016;513:2706–2715. doi:10.1242/dev.136861

[3] Liu ES, Raimann A, Chae BT, Martins JS, Baccarini M, Demay MB: C-Raf promotes angiogenesis during normal growth plate maturation. Development. 2016;143:348–355. doi:10.1242/dev.127142

[4] Ortega N, Wang K, Ferrara N, Werb Z, Vu TH: Complementary interplay between matrix metalloproteinase-9, vascular endothelial growth factor and osteoclast function drives endochondral bone formation. Disease Models and Mechanisms. 2010;3:224–235. doi:10.1242/dmm004226

[5] Berendsen AD, Olsen BR: How vascular endothelial growth factor-A (VEGF) regulated differentiation of mesenchymal stem cells. Journal of Histochemistry & Cytochemistry. 2014;62:103–108. doi:10.1369/0022155413516347

[6] Maes C: Role and regulation of vascularization processes in endochondral bones. Calcified Tissue International. 2013;92:307–323. doi:10.1007/s00223-012-9689-z

[7] Hattori T, Muller C, Gebhard S, Bauer E, Pausch F, Schlund B, Bosl MR, Hess A, Surmann-Schmitt C, von der Mark H, de Crombrugghe B, von der Mark K: SOX9 is a major negative regulator of cartilage vascularization, bone marrow formation and endochondral ossification. Development. 2010;137:901–911. doi:10.1242/dev.045203

[8] Franz-Odendaal TA, Hall BK, Witten PE: Buried alive: how osteoblasts become osteocytes. Developmental Dynamics. 2006;235:176–190.

[9] Franz-Odendaal, TA: Induction and patterning of intramembranous bone. (Special Issue – Signaling Mechanisms in Development) Frontiers in Biosciences. 2011;16: 2734–2746.

[10] Percival CJ, Richtsmeier JT: Angiogenesis and intramembranous osteogenesis. Developmental Dynamics. 2013;242(8):909–22.

[11] Rice R, Rice DP, Olsen BR, Thesleff I: Progression of calvarial bone development requires Foxc1 regulation of Msx2 and Alx4. Developmental Biology. 2003;262(1):75–87.

[12] Lemier RJ: Embryology of the skull. In Craniosynostosis: Diagnosis, Evaluation and Management. Cohen MM Jr. ed. Raven Press, New York, Chapter 5; 1986.

[13] Yin M, Pacifici M: Vascular regression is required for mesenchymal condensation and chondrogenesis in the developing limb. Devlopmental Dynamics. 2001;222:5–533.

[14] Jourdeuil K, Franz-Odendaal TA: Vasculogenesis and the induction of skeletogenic condensations in the avian eye. The Anatomical Record. 2012;285:691–698.

[15] Jabalee J, Franz-Odendaal TA: Vascular endothelial growth factor signaling regulates angiogenesis and osteogenesis during the development of scleral ossicles. Developmental Biology 2015:406:52–62.

[16] Thompson TJ, Owens PD, Wilson DJ: Intramembranous osteogenesis and angiogenesis in the chick embryo. Journal of Anatomy. 1989;166:55–65.

[17] De Spiegelaere W, Cornillie P, Casteleyn C, Burvenich C, Van Den Broeck W: Detection of hypoxia inducible factors and angiogenic growth factors during foetal endochondral and intramembranous ossification. Anatomia, Histologia, Embryologia. 2010;39(4):376–384.

[18] Fiedler J, Leucht F, Waltenberger J. et al.: VEGF-A and PIGF-1 stimulate chemotactic migration of human mesenchymal progenitor cells. Biochemical and Biophysical Research Communications. 2005;334(2):561–568.

[19] Street J, Bao M, deGuzman L. et al.: Vascular endothelial growth factor stimulates bone repair by promoting angiogenesis and bone turnover. Proceedings of the National Academy of Sciences of the United States of America. 2002;99(15):9656–9661.

[20] Tortelli F, Tasso R, Loiacono F, Cancedda R: The development of tissue-engineered bone of different origin through endochondral and intramembranous ossification following the implantation of mesenchymal stem cells and osteoblasts in a murine model. Biomaterials. 2010;31(2):242–249.

[21] Qu D, Li J, Li Y, Gao Y, Zuo Y, Hsu Y, Hu J: Angiogenesis and osteogenesis enhanced by bFGF ex vivo gene therapy for bone tissue engineering in reconstruction of calvarial defects. Journal of Biomedical Materials Research Part A. 2011;96(3):543–551.

[22] Rivron NC, Raiss CC, Liu J, Nandakumar A, Sticht C, Gretz N, Truckenmüller R, Rouwkema J, van Blitterswijk CA: Sonic Hedgehog-activated engineered blood ves-

sels enhance bone tissue formation. Proceedings of the National Academy of Sciences. 2012;109(12):4413–4418.

[23] Correia C, Grayson WL, Park M, Hutton D, Zhou B, Guo XE, Niklason L, Sousa RA, Reis RL, Vunjak-Novakovic G: In vitro model of vascularized bone: synergizing vascular development and osteogenesis. PLoS One. 2011;6(12):e28352.

[24] Dong Z, Li B, Liu B, Bai S, Li G, Ding A, Zhao J, Liu Y: Platelet-rich plasma promotes angiogenesis of prefabricated vascularized bone graft. Journal of Oral and Maxillofacial Surgery. 2012;70(9):2191–2197.

[25] Behr B, Leucht P, Longaker MT, Quarto N: *Fgf-9* is required for angiogenesis and osteogenesis in long bone repair. PNAS. 2010;107:11853–11858. doi:10.1073/pnas.100331710.

[26] Zelzer E, McLean W, Ng YS, Fukai N, Reginato AM, Lovejoy S, D'Amore PA, Olsen BR: Skeletal defects in VEGF120/120 mice reveal multiple roles for VEGF in skeletogenesis. Development. 2002;129(8):1893–1904.

[27] Hill C, Jacobs B, Kennedy L, Rohde S, Zhou B, Baldwin S, Goudy S: Cranial neural crest deletion of VEGFa causes cleft palate with aberrant vascular and bone development. Cell and Tissue Research. 2015;361(3):711–722.

[28] Lui Y, Olsen BR: Distinct VEGF functions during bone development and homeostasis. Archivum Immunologiae et Therapiae Experimentalis. 2014;62:363–368.

[29] Zelzer E, Olsen BR: Multiple roles of vascular endothelial growth factor (VEGF) in skeletal development, growth, and repair. Current Topics in Developmental Biology. 2004;65:169–187.

[30] Yang Y, Tan Y, Wong R, Wenden A, Zhang L, Rabie ABM: The role of vascular endothelial growth factor in ossification. International Journal of Oral Science. 2012;4:64–68. doi:10.1038/ijos.2012.33

Chapter 4

Corneal Angiogenesis: Etiologies, Complications, and Management

Sepehr Feizi

Additional information is available at the end of the chapter

http://dx.doi.org/10.5772/66713

Abstract

A large subset of corneal pathologies involves the formation of new blood vessels, leading to compromised visual acuity. Additionally, neovascularization of the cornea worsens the prognosis of subsequent penetrating keratoplasty, keeping the patient in a vicious circle of poor prognosis. Ocular angiogenesis results from the upregulation of proangiogenic and downregulation of antiangiogenic factors. There is a tremendous need for developing effective measures to prevent and/or treat corneal neovascularization. Topical steroid medication, cautery, argon and yellow dye laser, and fine needle diathermy have all been advocated with varying degrees of success. The process of corneal neovascularization is primarily mediated by the vascular endothelial growth factor family of proteins, and current therapies are aimed at disrupting the various steps in this pathway. This article aims to review the clinical causes and presentations of corneal neovascularization caused by different etiologies. Moreover, this chapter reviews different complications caused by corneal neovascularization and summarizes the most relevant treatments available so far.

Keywords: cornea, angiogenesis, etiologies, complications, management

1. Introduction

A normal cornea is necessary to protect the eye against structural damage to the deeper ocular components as well as to provide a proper anterior refractive surface. Optimal vision and corneal clarity entail an avascular cornea, and maintaining the stromal avascularity is an important feature of the corneal pathophysiology. Corneal vascularization, which is a sign of corneal disease processes than a diagnosis, results from an imbalance between angiogenic and antiangiogenic factors [1]. The angiogenic factors stimulate the proliferation and migration of vascular endothelial cells, resulting in the formation of a capillary tube [2, 3]. Corneal neovascularization is part of the natural healing processes, which are triggered by exposure of the cornea to trauma or pathogens, and is not necessarily 'harmful.' In the long-term and under certain circumstances, however, corneal neovascularization can surpass a threshold, invading the cornea, reducing visual acuity, and, in case of lamellar keratoplasty or penetrating keratoplasty, endangering corneal graft survival [4–7]. These complications have prompted clinicians to devise means to shut vessels. Topical steroid medication, cautery, argon and yellow dye laser, and fine needle diathermy (FND) have all been advocated with varying degrees of success. The advent of anti-vascular endothelial growth factor (VEGF) antibodies has resulted in a surge of interest in using these agents to treat corneal neovascularization. These approaches, however, have a limited clinical efficacy and can result in a multitude of undesirable complications. This chapter aims to review the causes, pathogenesis, and clinical presentations of corneal neovascularization caused by different etiologies, such as contact lens–induced keratitis, corneal ulcers, and herpes simplex stromal keratitis. Moreover, it reviews different complications caused by corneal neovascularization and summarizes the most relevant treatments available so far.

2. Etiologies

Corneal vascularization occurs as a nonspecific response to different clinical insults. Diseases associated with corneal neovascularization include corneal graft rejection, inflammatory disorders, chemical burns, contact lens–related hypoxia, stromal ulceration, infectious keratitis, limbal stem cell deficiency, and congenital disease (**Table 1**) [8–10].

Categories	Cause
Infectious keratitis	Parasitic
	Viral
	Bacterial
	Fungal
Hypoxia	Contact lens wearing
Conjunctival/corneal degeneration	Pterygium
Inflammatory disorder	Stevens-Johnson syndrome
	Mucous membrane pemphigoid
	Corneal graft rejection
	Rosacea
	Atopic conjunctivitis
Ocular surface neoplasia	Conjunctival or corneal intraepithelial neoplasia
	Conjunctival or corneal squamous cell carcinoma
	Papilloma
Loss of limbal barrier function	Congenital (e.g., aniridia)
	Thermal burn, chemical burn, or other injury

Table 1. Causes of corneal neovascularization.

Hypoxia related to contact lens wear is a common cause where corneal neovascularization is usually superficial and involves only the corneal periphery [11, 12]. However, if contact lens wear is not discontinued, deep stromal and central corneal invasion can take place.

Infections can result in corneal neovascularization with the patterns of response being different. Herpes simplex virus (HSV) keratitis is likely to cause extensive vascularization and lipid keratopathy, while, in Acanthamoeba keratitis, vascularization tends to develop late in the course of the disease (**Figure 1**). The continued presence of HSV-DNA and HSV-immune complexes

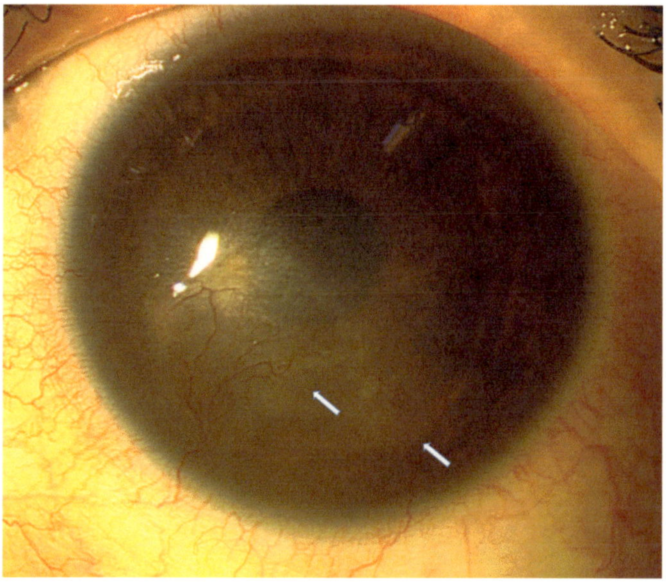

Figure 1. Acanthamoeba keratitis. Corneal opacity and vascularization (arrows) developed four months after corneal ulcer caused by Acanthamoeba in a contact lens wearer.

contributes to inflammation and angiogenesis in HSV stromal keratitis through increased levels of matrix metalloproteinase (MMP)-9 and vascular endothelial growth factor (VEGF) [13, 14]. There is a close link between extent (i.e., superficial or stromal) and location (i.e., central or peripheral) of infections, and the location and extent of corneal neovascularization.

Limbal stem cell deficiency (LSCD) occurs in a variety of ocular pathologies both congenital (e.g., aniridia) and acquired (e.g., contact lens use, drugs, chemical burns, etc.), which lead to partial or total loss of limbal stem cells [15, 16]. Chemical (acidic and alkaline) substances can penetrate and damage the cornea and anterior chamber, with alkali burns being more severe [17]. Conjunctivalization of the cornea with massive neovascularization may develop, leading to severe reductions in corneal clarity and visual acuity through the pannus formation on the cornea and an unstable and irregular epithelium [17, 18]. Deep vascularization may develop in the late healing phase following severe chemical burns (**Figure 2**).

Degenerative conditions such as pterygium are associated with corneal neovascularization that usually is accompanied with a fibrovascular pannus located on, rather than in, the corneal stroma. Long-standing irritation of the ocular surface such as in vernal keratoconjunctivitis can lead to aggressive corneal neovascularization (**Figure 3**).

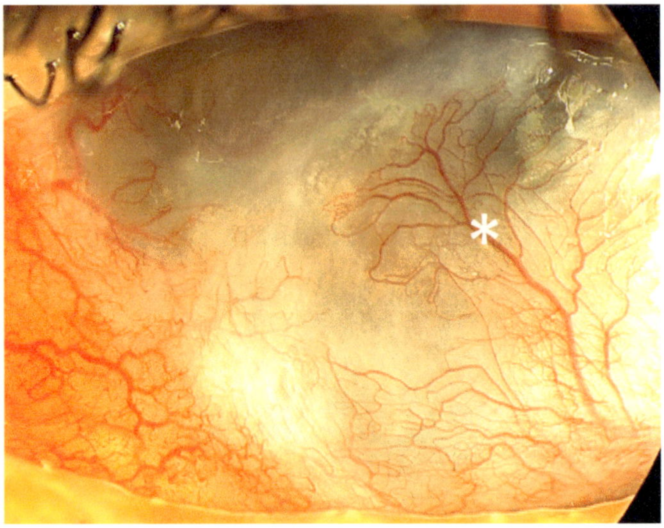

Figure 2. Limbal stem cell deficiency after alkali burn. The Figure demonstrates invasion of conjunctival vessels into the cornea (conjunctivalization) along with corneal stromal opacification and vascularization (asterisk).

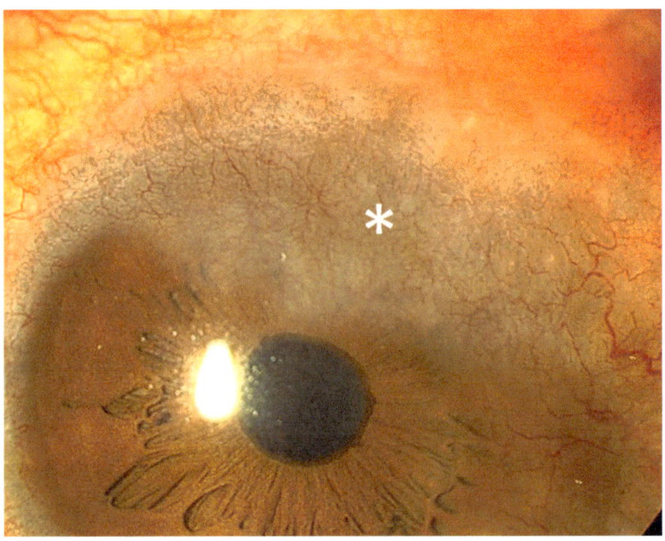

Figure 3. Corneal vascularization (asterisk) in a patient with vernal keratoconjunctivitis.

Ocular surface neoplasia, including papilloma and conjunctival/corneal intraepithelial neoplasia, can cause corneal neovascularization as part of the tumor angiogenic response. Initially, the vessels can be limited to the tumor but eventually invade the entire cornea. Other specific etiologies of corneal neovascularization include persistent corneal edema as in chronic hydrops of keratoconus and bullous keratopathy as well as corneal allograft rejection. Less common causes of corneal neovascularization are corneal foreign bodies and exposure to chemical toxins including mustard gas, radiation, or sun [19–21]. Intrastromal corneal ring implants, loose sutures, suture knots, and broken sutures seem to provide a stimulus for corneal vascularization

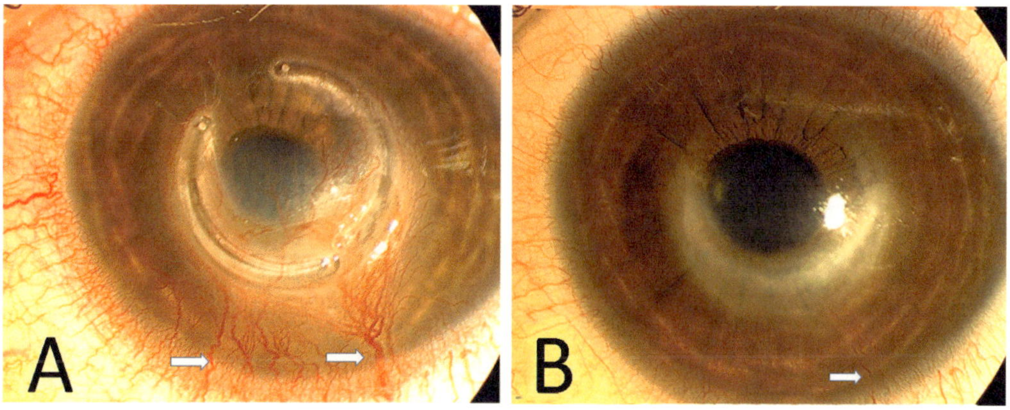

Figure 4. Intrastromal corneal ring segment implants complicated by corneal neovascularization. (A) Active young vessels (arrows) emanating from the limbus invade to the site of segment implantation. (B) The vessels have regressed after intrastromal corneal ring segment implants were removed. Partially regressed vessels are present in the inferior cornea (arrow).

(**Figure 4**). The mucus that collects around loose and broken sutures can trap polymorphonuclear cells and microbes inciting localized inflammation/infection, thus attracting vessels.

3. Pathogenesis

The upstream molecular pathway mechanisms resulting in corneal neovascularization differ in the different underlying pathologies. Nonetheless, core molecular pathways governing the processes of corneal hemangiogenesis seem to be shared among various conditions leading to the active stage of corneal neovascularization. The normally avascular cornea may vascularize in circumstances in which a disequilibrium between angiogenic and antiangiogenic stimuli results in a surplus of proangiogenic factors, such as VEGF, basic fibroblast growth factor (bFGF), interleukin-1 (IL-1), and MMP, and a deficiency in antiangiogenic agents, such as endostatin, angiostatin, and pigment epithelium-derived factor (PEDF) [22].

The so-called VEGF family consists of VEGF-A, VEGF-B, VEGF-C, VEGF-D, and placental growth factor [23]. VEGF-A is the most important member of this family, especially relating to pathologic hemangiogenesis through VEGF receptor (VEGFR)-2. VEGF-C and VEGF-D can stimulate lymphangiogenesis through VEGFR-2 and VEGFR-3, respectively [24, 25]. Macrophages, activated by injury or inflammation, can also produce VEGF-A, VEGF-C, and VEGF-D in corneal stroma [26]. VEGF-A sustains various steps of hemangiogenesis including vascular endothelial cell proliferation and migration, capillary lumen formation, and proteolytic activity [1]. The importance of VEGF-A in corneal neovascularization was exhibited experimentally on animal studies by inhibiting angiogenesis following stromal application of an anti-VEGF-A antibody [27].

Platelet-derived growth factors (PDGFs) are involved in cell division, growth, tissue remodeling, and angiogenesis. Receptors, such as PDGFR-a and PDGFR-b, and ligands, such as PDGF-A and PDGF-B, can be found in cornea and are associated with corneal neovascularization [28, 29]. Improved understanding of the molecular mechanisms of vascularization has enabled identification of specific factors that suppress angiogenesis to maintain the avascularity of the cornea. Because several molecules are involved in corneal neovascularization, a multipronged approach is desirable.

4. Clinical presentations

Corneal neovascularization which arises from the limbus, conjunctiva, and iris can lead to a reduction in the clarity of the cornea and visual acuity because of edema, scarring, intracorneal lipid and protein deposition, and persistent inflammation. Additionally, there is a robust association between the presence of corneal neovascularization and corneal graft rejection with the risk increasing as more quadrants are affected by vessels (**Figure 5**) [4–7]. The presence of corneal neovascularization can also cause intraoperative bleeding, which can be associated with hyphema.

Abnormal vessels may invade the cornea at different planes depending on the location and nature of the inflammatory stimulus. Corneal neovascularization has three clinical patterns, based on the depth of involvement. The first type, superficial vascularization, results from ocular surface disease (**Figure 6**). The second type is stromal vessels, which results from alkaline injury or stromal keratitis (**Figure 7**). The third is deep vessels overlying Descemet's membrane, which can be associated with interstitial keratitis or HSV keratitis, or after deep anterior lamellar keratoplasty (**Figure 8**) [1, 8, 9, 22]. Mixed patterns are often observed clini-

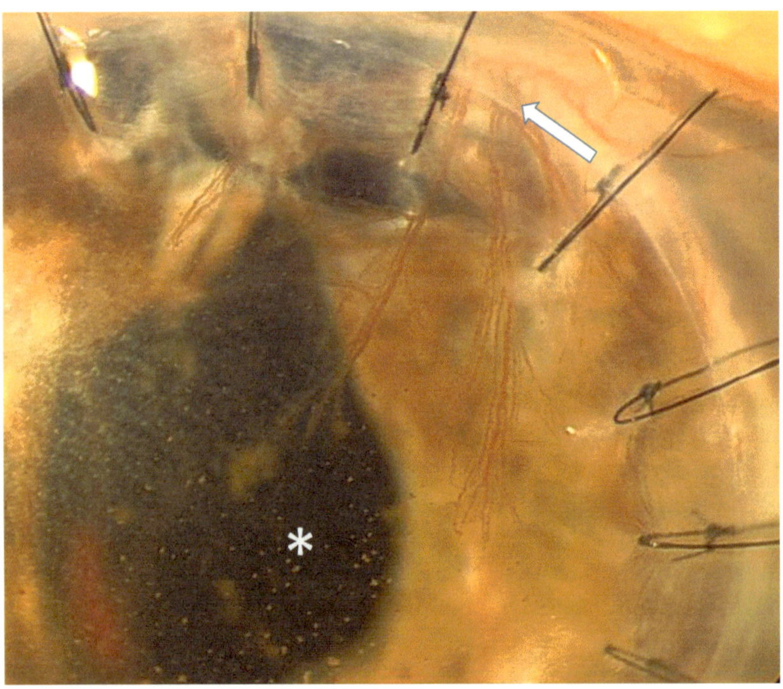

Figure 5. Endothelial corneal graft rejection in a high-risk graft. Active old corneal vessels (arrow) arising from the limbus sharply dip into a deep suture track and continue to the graft in an eye that underwent penetrating keratoplasty. The presence of keratic precipitates (asterisk) indicates an episode of endothelial graft rejection.

http://dx.doi.org/10.5772/66713

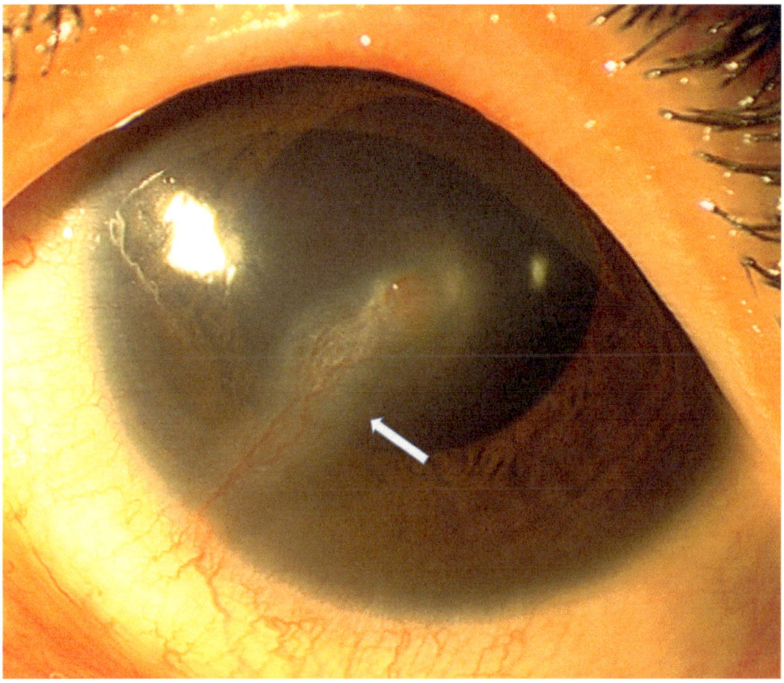

Figure 6. Phlyctenular keratitis. Superficial corneal vascularization (arrow) is evident in an eye with severe blepharitis. Adjacent stroma shows edema and infiltration.

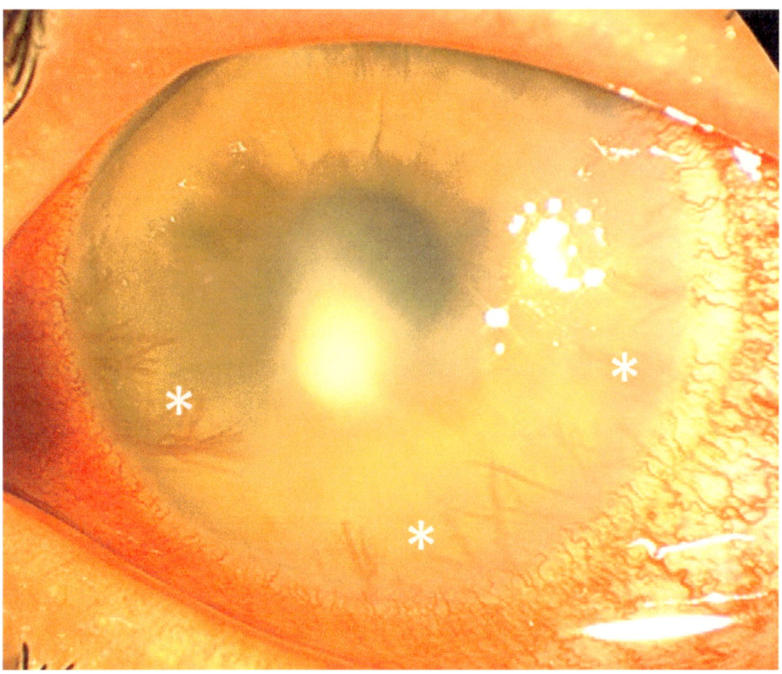

Figure 7. Deep stromal vascularization in an eye with recurrent herpes simplex stromal keratitis. Active young, bright red, brush-like vessels (asterisks) invade in to the corneal stroma.

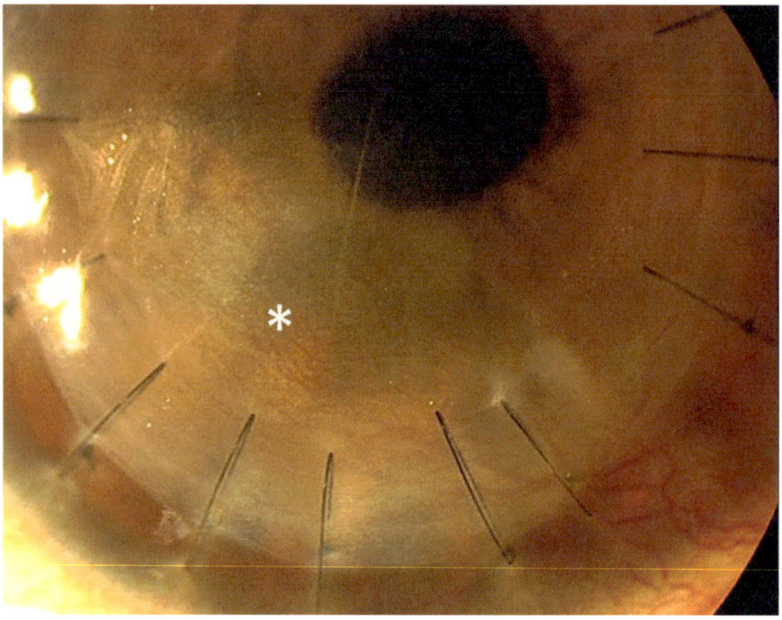

Figure 8. Partially regressed vessels with lipid keratopathy (asterisk) at the donor-recipient interface in a patient who underwent deep anterior lamellar keratoplasty (DALK). Vessels arising from the limbus sharply dip into a deep suture track and continue to the deep lamellar plane created by the DALK procedure, before fanning out. The vessels are dull red with a slow circulation, and some parts of the complex are less visible or have undergone attrition.

cally. The level of vascularization is chiefly related to the level of pathology rather than to the etiology. Superficial corneal pathology results in superficial vascularization, and deep pathology results in deep vessels. Often when the disease process extends through the thickness of the cornea, superficial and deep vessels are seen in the same cornea.

A detailed clinical evaluation of corneal neovascularization, including extension (the number of quadrants involved) and depth, is crucial for treatment planning. In addition to the extent and level of corneal vascularization, the state of vessel activity is also important [30]. Clinically, corneal vascularization can be classified as active young, active old, mature, partially regressed, and regressed. This often corresponds with the stage of activity or chronicity of the disease. Active young vessels are freshly formed vessels that are full of blood, appear bright red in color, have minimal surrounding fibrous tissue sheathing, and are actively progressing in the cornea with a well-defined arborizing network of fine (capillary) vessels (**Figures 4A** and **7**). The corneal stroma surrounding the vessels shows signs of leakage and edema. Active old vessels appear less bright and maintain a brisk circulation (**Figure 5**). This represents the stage when the vessels have reached and surrounded or covered the offending lesion in the cornea. Their progression ceases but consolidation continues. Mature vessels are relatively large vessels, with minimal arborization and regressed or absent capillary networks, seen to persist in scar tissue or in the corneal stroma after the corneal pathology has healed. These vessels contain blood and maintain a circulation (**Figure 9**). Partially regressed vessels are seen when the corneal pathology has abated in response to therapy or the arrival

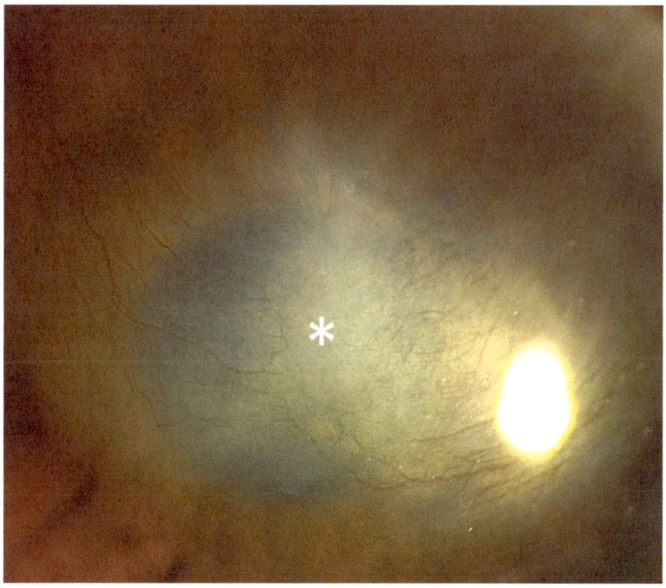

Figure 9. Mature vessels in the corneal stroma after the improvement of corneal ulcer (asterisk). The vessels are relatively large, with minimal arborization and regressed or absent capillary networks. These vessels which persist in scar tissue contain blood and maintain a circulation.

of corneal vessels. The circulation in the vascular complex is relatively slow, the vessels are less engorged, and some parts of the complex have become less visible or undergo attrition (**Figures 4B** and **8**). Regressed (ghost) vessels present as fine white lines mirroring the morphology of the original vessels. These do not have an active circulation, and the cornea where they are located is not edematous. Although clinically undetectable, lymphangiogenesis almost always accompanies hemangiogenesis in the cornea [31].

5. Paraclinical evaluation of corneal vascularization

Accurate evaluation and documentation of corneal neovascularization are essential to monitor the effect of any treatment modality employed. Case note entries can be used to assess the extent of corneal vascularization, and the depth of penetration and the centripetal progression of vessels, which allows a semiquantitative measurement of corneal neovascularization. It is neither time efficient nor practical, however, to manually trace the corneal vessels in each follow-up examination. Furthermore, the reproducibility is questionable, and the opportunity for variability and human error is very high.

The need to measure corneal neovascularization motivated researchers to explore measurement tools. An ideal measurement tool should allow rapid, reproducible, accurate, and objective measurement of corneal neovascularization. Digitized photographs with good contrast can be analyzed, based on the grayscale values, to evaluate the progression of vascularization [32]. Corneal vessels can be quantified on the basis of contrast enhancement, density threshold identification for the blood vessels, and pixel measurement [33]. A more novel automatic approach on the basis of gray filter sampling and threshold analyses of digital photographs using an image analysis software has also been investigated [34, 35]. Despite the recent progress in the graphic editing software, automated methods have some limitations. First, the optimization and validation of any automated quantitative tool are questionable [36–38]. Second, it does not allow sufficient appreciation of details on vessel extent, localization, leakage, origin, and differentiation of the afferent and efferent systems. This information is of importance for guidance of clinical judgment and treatment [39].

Corneal angiography, using fluorescein and indocyanine green, provides excellent details of the neovascular complexes, thus enabling an enhanced clinical assessment and decision-making even in patients with complex corneal neovascularization [39]. The required technological equipment for corneal angiography is readily available in most ophthalmologic centers, as angiography is widely used to diagnose vascular disorders of the retina of various origin. It is a relatively inexpensive and safe diagnostic intervention, and serious adverse events like anaphylaxis to the intravenous dye are extremely rare [40, 41].

Fluorescein angiography gives an indication of the vessel maturity and leakage activity, whereas indocyanine green angiography allows better depiction of capillaries and deeper corneal neovascularization, particularly in the presence of vessel obscuration because of corneal haze and scarring [39]. It is possible to calculate the area of corneal neovascularization, the time to first detection of fluorescein dye leakage, corneal neovascular vessel diameter, and vascular tortuosity and activity. These parameters reliably quantify changes in corneal neovascularization over time [39]. Therefore, it allows monitoring of the natural course and treatment success [42].

6. Treatments

The treatment for corneal neovascularization aims at the occlusion of afferent corneal blood vessels to reduce exudative lipid keratopathy, and stromal edema and inflammation or as a preoperative conditioning intervention before keratoplasty to increase chances of graft survival [17, 43]. Current treatments for corneal neovascularization consist of topical nonsteroid anti-inflammatory and corticosteroid medications [44], photodynamic therapy [45], laser photocoagulation [46, 47], fine needle diathermy [48], and limbal, conjunctival, and amniotic membrane transplantation (AMT) [49]. More recently, manipulation of VEGF activity and manipulation of proangiogenic mediators like interleukin have been under investigation [50, 51]. Unfortunately, all of these approaches have a limited clinical efficacy, especially when the vessels are large because large vessels are difficult to occlude and easily recanalized. In addition, a multitude of undesirable side effects can occur after the treatment of corneal neovascularization. The following section reviews the available treatment approaches for corneal neovascularization and their limitations.

6.1. Corticosteroid therapy

Inflammation is a potent driver for corneal neovascularization. When inflammation settles, spontaneous regression of corneal neovascularization can occur and lead to gradual resolution of lipid keratopathy if present. Topical and periocular steroids have been popular and can effectively reduce inflammation and consequently corneal neovascularization in various disease conditions. However, the risks of superinfection, glaucoma, and cataract associated with the long-term use of corticosteroids have been a limiting factor [44]. Additionally, steroids have only limited antiangiogenic effects [52]. Cyclosporine A and nonsteroidal anti-inflammatory agents were reported to be largely ineffective in controlling or limiting corneal angiogenesis [53].

6.2. Laser photocoagulation

Photocoagulation of vessels has been shown to be an effective method to obliterate corneal vascularization [46, 47]. The argon laser [46] and the 577 nm yellow dye lasers [47] have been used effectively for treating vascularization in lipid keratopathy and graft rejection. Laser obliteration of corneal efferent vessels is comparatively easy as they are wider and have a relatively slower blood flow. Conversely, the afferent vessels are narrower and deeper, have a rapid blood flow, and are more difficult to obliterate. Consequently, reopening of the afferent vessels takes place in a high proportion of patients. In such cases, the procedure can be repeated more than once. Laser photocoagulation may not be effective in cases with extensive corneal neovascularization [46]. Other drawbacks include damage to iris and accidental suture lysis, which has a significant implication for grafts with running sutures. Furthermore, the expense of this equipment and the lack of availability in most centers make the treatment inaccessible to most surgeons.

6.3. Fine needle diathermy

Fine needle diathermy (FND) is an inexpensive and useful procedure that can serve as an adjunct or alternative to laser photocoagulation for the management of established corneal vessels. FND is simple and inexpensive and can be performed under topical anesthesia by any ophthalmologist. It can be applied at any depth to obliterate both afferent and efferent vessels with equal efficacy. However, it may have to be repeated to obtain the desired result [48]. Corneal microperforation is a potentially serious adverse event that can occur during passage of the needle. This is particularly so when the vascularized cornea is thin [48]. Other adverse events, such as striae, whitening, and intracorneal hemorrhages, are reversible [48]. Transient opacification of the cornea is observed in the stroma immediately surrounding the needle in all patients and persists for 24–48 h, with complete resolution. Intracorneal hemorrhage occurring intraoperatively or immediately postoperatively is the commonest adverse event. Though dramatic in appearance, intracorneal hemorrhages all resolve over a week or two. Sometimes, crystalline deposits can develop in the site of hemorrhage [48].

6.4. Corneal anti-angiogenesis target therapies

The advent of anti-VEGF agents has introduced a new dimension to the management of corneal vessels [54]. Active young vessels which usually indicate an underlying ongoing pathology continuing to induce further vascularization are probably best treated with anti-VEGF drops or subconjunctival injections. There is a growing list of therapeutic agents that target corneal angiogenesis (**Table 2**). Currently, only limited experience using anti-VEGFs on the cornea and only in an off-label setting is available [54].

Targets	Mechanisms	Therapeutics
Vascular endothelial growth factor	Anti–VEGF-A antibodies	Bevacizumab
		Ranibizumab
	Soluble or modified VEGF receptors	VEGFR-2-Fc
		sVEGFR-3 overexpression gene therapy
		VEGFR-1 morpholino
		Recombinant dimeric
		sVEGFR-1 overexpression gene therapy
		VEGFR intraceptor gene therapy (Flt23k, Flt24k)
		Aflibercept/VEGF-Trap(R1R2)
	VEGF-A aptamer	Pegaptanib
Pigment epithelium-derived factor	PEDF direct effect	PEDF
		PEDF gene therapy
		PEDF-derived peptide
Angiostatin	Angiostatin direct effect	Angiostatin pump
Platelet-derived growth factor	Multitargeted receptor tyrosine kinase inhibitor	Sunitinib
	PDGF receptor inhibitor	AG 1296
12-Hydroxyeicosatrienoic acid	siRNA for cytochrome P450 mono-oxygenase	CYP4B1 siRNA gene therapy
Hypoxia-inducible factors	shRNA for hypoxia-inducible factors	HIF-1a shRNA gene therapy (HIF-1a RNAi-A)
Decorin	Decorin direct effect	Decorin gene therapy
Vascular adhesion protein	VAP-1/SSAO inhibitor	U-V002
		LJP1207
Cannabinoid receptor CB1	CB1 antagonist	Rimonabant
Vasohibin-1	Vasohibin-1 directly effect	Vasohibin-1 gene therapy

HIF-1a: hypoxia-inducible factor 1a, CYP: cytochrome P450 mono-oxygenase, PDGF: platelet-derived growth factor, SSAO: semicarbazide-sensitive amine oxidase, PEDF: pigment epithelium-derived factor, VAP-1: vascular adhesive protein-1, sVEGFR: soluble form of vascular endothelial growth factor receptor, VEGF: vascular endothelial growth factor, VEGFR: vascular endothelial growth factor receptor.

Table 2. Corneal antiangiogenesis target therapies.

6.4.1. Anti-VEGF antibody

Inhibition of VEGF activity by a specific neutralizing anti-VEGF antibody is one possible strategy for treating corneal angiogenesis. VEGF inhibitors such as pegaptanib sodium (Macugen™, OSI/Eyetech), off-label bevacizumab (Avastin™, Genentech), and ranibizumab (Lucentis™, Genentech) are currently used for the treatment of different retinal pathologies including wet-type age-related macular degeneration [55]. Both animal models and clinical trials have demonstrated that these agents are effective in reducing corneal neovascularization. Both ranibizumab and bevacizumab use the same mechanisms and nonspecifically inhibit the VEGF-A isoforms [56]. Nevertheless, differently from ranibizumab and bevacizumab, pegaptanib specifically binds to VEGF-A165 and does not inhibit all of the VEGF isoforms. Subconjunctival ranibizumab, pegaptanib sodium, and bevacizumab are effective with no epitheliopathy in reducing corneal angiogenesis. Repeated subconjunctival injections with higher doses and concentrations and combination therapy with other antiangiogenic agents may be valid options to improve the effectiveness of treatments [57].

Treating corneal new vessel with the anti-VEGF antibody has some limitations. In contrast to superficial and active vascularization, in which clear regression is observed, anti-VEGF agents have a lower effect on deep vascularization. The effect of the anti-VEGF antibodies depends on the time of the treatment after the onset of neovascularization. In contrast to newly formed vessels, stable vessels are less affected by VEGF blockade [58]. The vessels mature in chronic neovascularization, and pericytes are recruited to the area around the region of corneal neovascularization [59]. Such coverage may reduce the influence of anti-VEGF agents on the regression of newly formed immature vessels. Anti-VEGF therapy is only a symptomatic treatment of corneal neovascularization that does not cure the underlying pathology, making it necessary to repeat the treatment to maintain its positive effect over a span of time [27].

Bevacizumab, which is FDA approved for intravenous administration in the treatment of various cancers, is a full-length, humanized murine monoclonal antibody with a molecular weight of 149 kD. Bevacizumab recognizes all isoforms of VEGF and is in widespread use, off-label, as an intravitreal injection to treat different retinal diseases [60]. Additionally, studies have demonstrated that topical, subconjunctival, and intraocular application of bevacizumab can partially reduce corneal angiogenesis and inflammatory response, resulting in an increase in corneal transparency [61, 62]. Bevacizumab can inhibit macrophage migration to the corneal stroma in early but not late treatment. Macrophages are known to trigger neovascularization in ischemic or inflamed corneas [63]. There is a concern about the interference of the topical form but not subconjunctival form of bevacizumab with nerve regeneration and delayed wound healing [54, 64, 65].

Ranibizumab, which has VEGF-binding characteristics similar to bevacizumab, is a recombinant humanized monoclonal antibody fragment that binds and inhibits all VEGF-A isoforms. Bevacizumab and ranibizumab are related to each other, but ranibizumab is the Fab fragment from the same antibody used to create bevacizumab. Therefore, ranibizumab has a molecular weight of 48 kD, making it approximately one-third the size of bevacizumab and theoretically allowing a better corneal penetration. In addition, it has been affinity matured to optimize the VEGF-A binding potential. These characteristics may enable ranibizumab to reduce corneal angiogenesis more effectively than bevacizumab [66]. Subconjunctival ranibizumab significantly reduces VEGF levels not only in the bulbar conjunctiva and cornea but also in the iris and aqueous humor [67]. Clinically, stable corneal neovascularization can be effectively treated by topical ranibizumab 1% as evidenced by a significant reduction in vessel caliber and neovascular area with no significant change in invasion area. These findings suggest that the main outcome of ranibizumab treatment for stable corneal neovascularization is to induce the narrowing of vessels more than a reduction in their length.

6.4.2. *Pigment epithelium-derived factor*

PEDF is a glycoprotein with neurotrophic, antitumorigenic, and antiangiogenic functions. PEDF can inhibit FGF, VEGF, and interlukin-8 (IL-8/CXCL8)-mediated angiogenesis by inducing the cells' apoptosis and reducing endothelial cell migration simultaneously [68, 69]. It is also found to play an important role in the antiangiogenic effect of AMT [70]. Topical PEDF or PEDF-derived (P5-2 and P5-3) peptides can downregulate VEGF expression and inhibit corneal neovascularization in a chemical-induced corneal model [71].

6.4.3. *Tyrosine kinase inhibitors*

Anti-VEGF antibodies block the effect of VEGF before it attaches to the endothelial receptors. Tyrosine kinase with immunoglobulin and epidermal growth factor homology domain 2 (TIE2) that is predominantly or exclusively expressed in endothelial cells is an important regulator of angiogenesis. Tyrosine kinase inhibitors inhibit the activity of VEGF by blocking tyrosine kinase in the intracellular part of the VEGF cell membrane receptor. This may offer a different opportunity for the management of the angiogenesis process in corneal diseases. Regorafenib is a multikinase inhibitor that targets various kinases, including PDGF β, VEGFR1, VEGFR2, and VEGFR3, mutant oncogenic kinases, TIE2, and the FGF receptor, which are involved in neovascularization. The inhibitory effects of topical regorafenib are comparable to those of topical bevacizumab and dexamethasone [72]. Sunitinib is a multitargeted receptor tyrosine kinase inhibitor that blocks both VEGF and PDGF. Topically administered sunitinib can reduce corneal neovascularization more effectively than bevacizumab [73].

Trastuzumab is a monoclonal antibody that interferes with the HER2/ neu receptor. Lapatinib is a dual tyrosine kinase inhibitor, which interrupts the epidermal growth factor receptor (EGFR) and HER2/ neu pathways. Lapatinib used in the form of lapatinib ditosylate is an orally active drug for solid tumors such as breast cancer. In recent studies, both substances were compared for the treatment of experimental corneal angiogenesis. The results suggested that systemically administered lapatinib is more effective than systemically administered trastuzumab in preventing corneal angiogenesis [74].

7. Conclusion

Corneal neovascularization is a common clinical feature in different corneal diseases including ocular traumatic or chemical injury, autoimmune diseases, chronic contact lens wear, infectious keratitis, and keratoplasties. Although corneal neovascularization can serve a beneficial role in arresting stromal melts, wound healing, and the clearing of infections, its disadvantages are numerous and it frequently results in edema, tissue scarring, persistent inflammation, and lipid deposition that may significantly reduce vision. Furthermore, it plays a major role in corneal graft rejection by breaching corneal immune privilege. VEGF, which plays a crucial role in angiogenesis and the pathologic neovascularization associated with a variety of eye diseases, is the most important target for antiangiogenic therapies. Experience indicates that anti-VEGFs are effective in occluding actively growing corneal neovascularization but not established vessels. Surgical procedures, including laser photocoagulation or fine needle diathermy, are useful particularly to obliterate large, established corneal vessels.

Author details

Sepehr Feizi

Address all correspondence to: sepehrfeizi@yahoo.com

Ophthalmic Research Center and Department of Ophthalmology, Labbafinejad Medical Center, Shahid Beheshti University of Medical Sciences, Tehran, Iran

References

[1] Chang JH, Gabison EE, Kato T, Azar DT. Corneal neovascularization. Curr Opin Ophthalmol 2001;12(4):242–249.

[2] Strömblad S, Cheresh DA. Integrins, angiogenesis and vascular cell survival. Chem Biol 1996;3(11):881–885.

[3] Lee HS, Chung SK. The effect of subconjunctival suramin on corneal neovascularization in rabbits. Cornea 2010;29(1):86–92.

[4] Bachmann B, Taylor RS, Cursiefen C. Corneal neovascularization as a risk factor for graft failure and rejection after keratoplasty: an evidence-based meta-analysis. Ophthalmology 2010;117(7):1300–1305.

[5] Huang PT. Penetrating keratoplasty in infants and children. J AAPOS 2007;11(1):5–6.

[6] Panda A, Vanathi M, Kumar A, Dash Y, Priya S. Corneal graft rejection. Surv Ophthalmol 2007;52(4):375–396.

[7] Sellami D, Abid S, Bouaouaja G, Ben Amor S, Kammoun B, Masmoudi M, Dabbeche K, Boumoud H, Ben Zina Z, Feki J. Epidemiology and risk factors for corneal graft rejection. Transplant Proc 2007;39(8):2609–2611.

[8] Menzel-Severing J. Emerging techniques to treat corneal neovascularisation. Eye (Lond) 2012;26(1):2–12.

[9] Tshionyi M, Shay E, Lunde E, Lin A, Han KY, Jain S, Chang JH, Azar DT. Hemangiogenesis and lymphangiogenesis in corneal pathology. Cornea 2012;31(1):74–80.

[10] Beebe DC. Maintaining transparency: a review of the developmental physiology and pathophysiology of two avascular tissues. Semin Cell Dev Biol 2008;19(2):125–133.

[11] Madigan MC, Penfold PL, Holden BA, Billson FA. Ultrastructural features of contact lens-induced deep corneal neovascularization and associated stromal leukocytes. Cornea 1990;9(2):144–1451.

[12] Wong AL, Weissman BA, Mondino BJ. Bilateral corneal neovascularization and opacification associated with unmonitored contact lens wear. Am J Ophthalmol 2003;136(5):957–958.

[13] Remeijer L, Duan R, van Dun JM, Wefers Bettink MA, Osterhaus AD, Verjans GM. Prevalence and clinical consequences of herpes simplex virus type 1 DNA in human cornea tissues. J Infect Dis 2009;200(1):11–19.

[14] Hayashi K, Hooper LC, Detrick B, Hooks JJ. HSV immune complex (HSV-IgG: IC) and HSV-DNA elicit the production of angiogenic factor VEGF and MMP-9. Arch Virol 2009;154(2):219–226.

[15] Dua HS, Azuara-Blanco A. Limbal stem cells of the corneal epithelium. Surv Ophthalmol 2000;44(5):415–425.

[16] Kokotas H, Petersen MB. Clinical and molecular aspects of aniridia. Clin Genet 2010;77(5):409–420.

[17] Lee P, Wang CC, Adamis AP. Ocular neovascularization: an epidemiologic review. Surv Ophthalmol 1998;43(3):245–269.

[18] Mochimaru H, Usui T, Yaguchi T, Nagahama Y, Hasegawa G, Usui Y, Shimmura S, Tsubota K, Amano S, Kawakami Y, Ishida S. Suppression of alkali burn-induced corneal neovascularization by dendritic cell vaccination targeting VEGF receptor 2. Invest Ophthalmol Vis Sci 2008;49(5):2172–2177.

[19] Applegate LA, Ley RD. DNA damage is involved in the induction of opacification and neovascularization of the cornea by ultraviolet radiation. Exp Eye Res 1991;52(4):493–497.

[20] Cogan DG. Corneal vascularization. Invest Ophthalmol Vis Sci 1962;1:253–261.

[21] Javadi MA, Jafarinasab MR, Feizi S, Karimian F, Negahban K. Management of mustard gas-induced limbal stem cell deficiency and keratitis. Ophthalmology 2011;118(7):1272–1281.

[22] Chang JH, Garg NK, Lunde E, Han KY, Jain S, Azar DT. Corneal neovascularization: an anti-VEGF therapy review. Surv Ophthalmol 2012;57(5):415–429.

[23] Neufeld G, Cohen T, Gengrinovitch S, Poltorak Z. Vascular endothelial growth factor (VEGF) and its receptors. FASEB J 1999;13(1):9–22.

[24] Goldman J, Rutkowski JM, Shields JD, Pasquier MC, Cui Y, Schmökel HG, Willey S, Hicklin DJ, Pytowski B, Swartz MA. Cooperative and redundant roles of VEGFR-2 and VEGFR-3 signaling in adult lymphangiogenesis. FASEB J 2007;21(4):1003–1012.

[25] Shibuya M. Vascular endothelial growth factor (VEGF) and its receptor (VEGFR) signaling in angiogenesis: a crucial target for anti- and pro-angiogenic therapies. Genes Cancer 2011;2(12):1097–1105.

[26] Cursiefen C, Chen L, Borges LP, Jackson D, Cao J, Radziejewski C, D'Amore PA, Dana MR, Wiegand SJ, Streilein JW. VEGF-A stimulates lymphangiogenesis and hemangiogenesis in inflammatory neovascularization via macrophage recruitment. J Clin Invest 2004;113(7):1040–1050.

[27] Krizova D, Vokrojova M, Liehneova K, Studeny P. Treatment of corneal neovascularization using Anti-VEGF bevacizumab. J Ophthalmol. 2014;2014:178132. doi:10.1155/2014/178132.

[28] Kim WJ, Mohan RR, Mohan RR, Wilson SE. Effect of PDGF, IL-1alpha, and BMP2/4 on corneal fibroblast chemotaxis: expression of the platelet-derived growth factor system in the cornea. Invest Ophthalmol Vis Sci 1999;40(7):1364–1372.

[29] Hoppenreijs VP, Pels E, Vrensen GF, Felten PC, Treffers WF. Platelet-derived growth factor: receptor expression in corneas and effects on corneal cells. Invest Ophthalmol Vis Sci 1993;34(3):637–649.

[30] Pillai CT, Dua HS, Hossain P. Fine needle diathermy occlusion of corneal vessels. Invest Ophthalmol Vis Sci 2000;41(8):2148–2153.

[31] Cursiefen C, Chen L, Dana MR, Streilein JW. Corneal lymphangiogenesis: evidence, mechanisms, and implications for corneal transplant immunology. Cornea 2003;22(3):273–281.

[32] Proia AD, Chandler DB, Haynes WL, Smith CF, Suvarnamani C, Erkel FH, Klintworth GK. Quantitation of corneal neovascularization using computerized image analysis. Lab Invest 1988;58(4):473–479.

[33] Conrad TJ, Chandler DB, Corless JM, Klintworth GK. In vivo measurement of corneal angiogenesis with video data acquisition and computerized image analysis. Lab Invest 1994;70(3):426–434.

[34] Bock F, König Y, Kruse F, Baier M, Cursiefen C. Bevacizumab (Avastin) eye drops inhibit corneal neovascularization. Graefes Arch Clin Exp Ophthalmol 2008;246(2):281–284.

[35] Cursiefen C, Bock F, Horn FK, Kruse FE, Seitz B, Borderie V, Früh B, Thiel MA, Wilhelm F, Geudelin B, Descohand I, Steuhl KP, Hahn A, Meller D. GS-101 antisense oligonucleotide eye drops inhibit corneal neovascularization: interim results of a randomized phase II trial. Ophthalmology 2009;116(9):1630–1637.

[36] Wu PC, Liu CC, Chen CH, Kou HK, Shen SC, Lu CY, Chou WY, Sung MT, Yang LC. Inhibition of experimental angiogenesis of cornea by somatostatin. Graefes Arch Clin Exp Ophthalmol 2003;241(1):63–69.

[37] You IC, Kang IS, Lee SH, Yoon KC. Therapeutic effect of subconjunctival injection of bevacizumab in the treatment of corneal neovascularization. Acta Ophthalmol 2009;87(6):653–658.

[38] Jhanji V, Liu H, Law K, Lee VY, Huang SF, Pang CP, Yam GH. Isoliquiritigenin from licorice root suppressed neovascularisation in experimental ocular angiogenesis models. Br J Ophthalmol 2011;95(9):1309–1315.

[39] Kirwan RP, Zheng Y, Tey A, Anijeet D, Sueke H, Kaye SB. Quantifying changes in corneal neovascularization using fluorescein and indocyanine green angiography. Am J Ophthalmol 2012;154(5):850–858.

[40] Kwan AS, Barry C, McAllister IL, Constable I. Fluorescein angiography and adverse drug reactions revisited: the Lions Eye experience. Clin Experiment Ophthalmol 2006;34(1):33–38.

[41] Hope-Ross M, Yannuzzi LA, Gragoudas ES, Guyer DR, Slakter JS, Sorenson JA, Krupsky S, Orlock DA, Puliafito CA. Adverse reactions due to indocyanine green. Ophthalmology 1994;101(3):529–533.

[42] Steger B, Romano V, Kaye SB. Corneal indocyanine green angiography to guide medical and surgical management of corneal neovascularization. Cornea 2016;35(1):41–45.

[43] Romano V, Spiteri N, Kaye SB. Angiographic-guided treatment of corneal neovascularization. JAMA Ophthalmol 2015;133(3):e143544.

[44] Al-Torbak A, Al-Amri A, Wagoner MD. Deep corneal neovascularization after implantation with intrastromal corneal ring segments. Am J Ophthalmol 2005;140(5):926–927.

[45] Brooks BJ, Ambati BK, Marcus DM, Ratanasit A. Photodynamic therapy for corneal neovascularisation and lipid degeneration. Br J Ophthalmol 2004;88(6):840.

[46] Baer JC, Foster CS. Corneal laser photocoagulation for treatment of neovascularization. Efficacy of 577 nm yellow dye laser. Ophthalmology 1992;99(2):173–179.

[47] L'sEsperance FA Jr. Clinical photocoagulation with organic dye laser. A preliminary communication. Arch Ophthalmol 1985;103(9):1312–1316.

[48] Faraj LA, Elalfy MS, Said DG, Dua HS. Fine needle diathermy occlusion of corneal vessels. Br J Ophthalmol 2014;98(9):1287–1290.

[49] Liang L, Li W, Ling S, Sheha H, Qiu W, Li C, Liu Z. Amniotic membrane extraction solution for ocular chemical burns. Clin Exp Ophthalmol 2009;37(9):855–863.

[50] Oliveira HB, Sakimoto T, Javier JA, Azar DT, Wiegand SJ, Jain S, Chang JH. VEGF Trap(R1R2) suppresses experimental corneal angiogenesis. Eur J Ophthalmol 2010;20(1):48–54.

[51] Hos D1, Bock F, Dietrich T, Onderka J, Kruse FE, Thierauch KH, Cursiefen C. Inflammatory corneal (lymph) angiogenesis is blocked by VEGFR-tyrosine kinase inhibitor ZK 261991, resulting in improved graft survival after corneal transplantation. Invest Ophthalmol Vis Sci 2008;49(5):1836–1842.

[52] Cursiefen C, Wenkel H, Martus P, Langenbucher A, Nguyen NX, Seitz B, Küchle M, Naumann GO. Impact of short-term versus long-term topical steroids on corneal neovascularization after non-high-risk keratoplasty. Graefes Arch Clin Exp Ophthalmol 2001;239(7):514–521.

[53] Ey RC, Hughes WF, Bloome MA, Tallman CB. Prevention of corneal vascularization. Am J Ophthalmol 1968;66(6):1118–1131.

[54] Dastjerdi MH, Al-Arfaj KM, Nallasamy N, Hamrah P, Jurkunas UV, Pineda R 2nd, Pavan-Langston D, Dana R. Topical bevacizumab in the treatment of corneal neovascularization: results of a prospective, open-label, noncomparative study. Arch Ophthalmol 2009;127(4):381–389.

[55] Heier JS, Antoszyk AN, Pavan PR, Leff SR, Rosenfeld PJ, Ciulla TA, Dreyer RF, Gentile RC, Sy JP, Hantsbarger G, Shams N. Ranibizumab for treatment of neovascular age-related macular degeneration: a phase I/ II multicenter, controlled, multidose study. Ophthalmology 2006;113(4):633.e1–4.

[56] Bhisitkul RB. Vascular endothelial growth factor biology: clinical implications for ocular treatments. Br J Ophthalmol 2006;90(12):1542–1547.

[57] Akar EE, Oner V, Küçükerdönmez C, Aydın Akova Y. Comparison of subconjunctivally injected bevacizumab, ranibizumab, and pegaptanib for inhibition of corneal neovascularization in a rat model. Int J Ophthalmol 2013;6(2):136–140.

[58] Ferrari G, Dastjerdi MH, Okanobo A, Cheng SF, Amparo F, Nallasamy N, Dana R. Topical ranibizumab as a treatment of corneal neovascularization. Cornea 2013;32(7):992–997.

[59] Cursiefen C, Hofmann-Rummelt C, Küchle M, Schlötzer-Schrehardt U. Pericyte recruitment in human corneal angiogenesis: an ultrastructural study with clinicopathological correlation. Br J Ophthalmol 2003;87(1):101–106.

[60] Keating AM, Jacobs DS. Anti-VEGF treatment of corneal neovascularization. Ocul Surf 2011;9(4):227–237.

[61] Avisar I, Weinberger D, Kremer I. Effect of subconjunctival and intraocular bevacizumab injections on corneal neovascularization in a mouse model. Curr Eye Res 2010;35(2):108–115.

[62] Lee SH, Leem HS, Jeong SM, Lee K. Bevacizumab accelerates corneal wound healing by inhibiting TGF-beta2 expression in alkali-burned mouse cornea. BMB Rep 2009;42(12):800–805.

[63] Chen WL, Chen YM, Chu HS, Lin CT, Chow LP, Chen CT, Hu FR. Mechanisms controlling the effects of bevacizumab (avastin) on the inhibition of early but not late formed corneal neovascularization. PLoS One 2014;9(4):e94205. doi:10.1371/journal.pone.0094205.

[64] Kim TI, Chung JL, Hong JP, Min K, Seo KY, Kim EK. Bevacizumab application delays epithelial healing in rabbit cornea. Invest Ophthalmol Vis Sci 2009;50(10):4653–4659.

[65] Koenig Y, Bock F, Horn F, Kruse F, Straub K, Cursiefen C. Short- and long-term safety profile and efficacy of topical bevacizumab (Avastin) eye drops against corneal neovascularization. Graefes Arch Clin Exp Ophthalmol 2009;247(10):1375–1382.

[66] Stevenson W, Cheng SF, Dastjerdi MH, Ferrari G, Dana R. Corneal neovascularization and the utility of topical VEGF inhibition: ranibizumab (Lucentis) vs bevacizumab (Avastin). Ocul Surf 2012;10(2):67–83.

[67] Liarakos VS, Papaconstantinou D, Vergados I, Douvali M, Theodossiadis PG. The effect of subconjunctival ranibizumab on corneal and anterior segment neovascularization: study on an animal model. Eur J Ophthalmol 2014;24(3):299–308.

[68] Duh EJ, Yang HS, Suzuma I, Miyagi M, Youngman E, Mori K, Katai M, Yan L, Suzuma K, West K, Davarya S, Tong P, Gehlbach P, Pearlman J, Crabb JW, Aiello LP, Campochiaro PA, Zack DJ. Pigment epithelium-derived factor suppresses ischemia-induced retinal neovascularization and VEGF-induced migration and growth. Invest Ophthalmol Vis Sci 2002;43(3):821–829.

[69] Mori K, Gehlbach P, Ando A, McVey D, Wei L, Campochiaro PA. Regression of ocular neovascularization in response to increased expression of pigment epithelium-derived factor. Invest Ophthalmol Vis Sci 2002;43(7):2428–2434.

[70] Shao C, Sima J, Zhang SX, Jin J, Reinach P, Wang Z, Ma JX. Suppression of corneal neovascularization by PEDF release from human amniotic membranes. Invest Ophthalmol Vis Sci 2004;45(6):1758–1762.

[71] Jin J, Ma JX, Guan M, Yao K. Inhibition of chemical cautery-induced corneal neovascularization by topical pigment epithelium-derived factor eyedrops. Cornea 2010;29(9):1055–1061.

[72] Onder HI, Erdurmus M, Bucak YY, Simavli H, Oktay M, Kukner AS. Inhibitory effects of regorafenib, a multiple tyrosine kinase inhibitor, on corneal neovascularization. Int J Ophthalmol 2014;7(2):220–225.

[73] Pérez-Santonja JJ1, Campos-Mollo E, Lledó-Riquelme M, Javaloy J, Alió JL. Inhibition of corneal neovascularization by topical bevacizumab (Anti-VEGF) and sunitinib (Anti-VEGF and Anti-PDGF) in an animal model. Am J Ophthalmol 2010;150(4):519–528.

[74] Kaya MK, Demir T, Bulut H, Akpolat N, Turgut B. Effects of lapatinib and trastuzumab on vascular endothelial growth factor in experimental corneal neovascularization. Clin Exp Ophthalmol 2015;43(5):449–457.

Chapter 5

Angiogenesis-Related Factors in Early Pregnancy Loss

Marina M. Ziganshina, Lyubov V. Krechetova,

Lyudmila V. Vanko, Zulfiya S. Khodzhaeva,

Ekaterina L. Yarotskaya and Gennady T. Sukhikh

Additional information is available at the end of the chapter

http://dx.doi.org/10.5772/66410

Abstract

The habitual loss of early pregnancy is one of the major problems of obstetrics nowadays, provided that the cause of more than 50% of all early pregnancy losses is unknown. Adequate angiogenesis is one of the main indicators of proper formation of placental system, making the basis of fetal life support. The objective description of angiogenesis in physiological development of pregnancy and in pathological conditions is complicated by the difficulties in obtaining and characterizing placental tissue in early pregnancy. Thus, angiogenesis-related factors are promising indicators to characterize angiogenesis in pregnancy. This chapter draws attention to alteration in angiogenesis-related factors in peripheral blood of patients with habitual early pregnancy losses. Investigation of factors (vascular endothelial growth factor (VEGF), sFlt-1, sKDR, metalloproteinase (MMP)-2, MMP-9, tissue inhibitor (TIMP)-1, TIMP-2 and placental growth factor (PLGF)), which specifically and nonspecifically regulate angiogenesis in pregnancy, was performed in the most significant terms for placentogenesis: 6 weeks, 7–8 weeks and 11–14 weeks of pregnancy. It was found that in a missed abortion there was a significant imbalance of angiogenesis-related factors compared with normal pregnancy. These results reflect a disturbance of angiogenesis in a missed abortion and point to the importance of the studied factors in the pathogenesis of early pregnancy losses.

Keywords: Angiogenesis, angiogenic factors, pregnancy, angiogenesis inhibitors, matrix metalloproteinases, pro- and antiangiogenic factors ratio, VEGF/VEGF-R1, VEGF/VEGF-R2, MMP-9/TIMP-1

1. Introduction

Adequate formation of uteroplacental and fetal placental blood flow is the determining factor of physiological pregnancy and fetal development. Successful uterine-placental vascular morphogenesis and embryonic morphogenesis of fetal blood system are the basis of these processes. There are two stages of vascular morphogenesis: vasculogenesis—primary formation and development of blood vessels *de novo* from committed mesodermal cells—and angiogenesis—formation of new blood vessels from existing vascular structures, which reflect the formation of vascular system of a fetus and placenta during pregnancy [1–4].

"Early pregnancy" period includes several time intervals when the most significant for angiogenesis events occur, determining further course and outcome of pregnancy. During gestation up to 6 weeks, the primary fetal circulatory system and placental bed with the development of villi are formed, and extensive vascularization of placental villous tree occurs. The 6–8th weeks of pregnancy are marked by the start of transition to the placental circulation, as well as by the most expressed invasion of extravillous trophoblast into maternal spiral arteries (first wave of trophoblast invasion). The period of 11–13 weeks is considered to be borderline and is characterized by the completion of embryogenesis, the starting period of fetal development, fading of the first wave of trophoblast invasion and further increase in the volume of uteroplacental blood flow [4–8].

During trophoblast invasion into endometrium, interactions with components of the extracellular matrix, which is mediated by cell adhesion molecules, occur. Proteinases participate in the degradation of extracellular matrix and cell migration deep into the myometrium through the uterine spiral arteries. Cytotrophoblast cells change their phenotype from epithelial to endothelial, producing a large number of soluble factors contributing to the development of the vasculature [9, 10].

Growth factors play the key role in vessels formation. They serve as cell mitogens, as attractants in the formation of vascular architectonics, and most important, as morphogens. The main regulators of angiogenesis are members of the family of vascular endothelial growth factor (VEGF). In addition to direct activators of angiogenesis, there is a large group of factors, whose effect on angiogenesis is nonspecific. It includes matrix metalloproteinases (MMPs) and their tissue inhibitors (TIMPs) [11–14].

Decidual NK-cells in early pregnancy, at the stage preceding the invasion of trophoblast into the maternal arteries, produce VEGF, placental growth factor (PLGF) and matrix metalloproteinases (MMPs), in particular MMP-2 and MMP-9 [15–17]. These MMPs are collagenases of IV type which specifically hydrolyze the collagen of basement membranes and thereby facilitate cell invasion through the basement membranes and stimulate angiogenesis [18–21]. Decidual NK-cells are the main source of MMP-2 and TIMP-2 from the group of tissue inhibitors of matrix metalloproteinases (TIMPs) [22–24].

Trophoblast also produces factors regulating processes of vessels formation. Particularly, MMP-9, TIMP-1, TIMP-2 and TIMP-3 are produced by the cells of extravillous trophoblast. Villous cytotrophoblast cells and invasive endovascular trophoblast produce MMP-2 which is considered a key regulator of cell invasion in early gestation (up to 8 weeks), according to some authors [17, 19].

Production of anti-angiogenic factors is an integral part of the normal angiogenesis. As a result of the molecular dialog during vascularization, production of inhibitors serves as a hamper for excessive trophoblast invasion, as well as an obstacle for the further development of the vascular bed and for vascularization of pathologically changed tissue sites. Angiogenic factors are specifically expressed in endothelium and in the placenta during pregnancy. These include receptors VEGF-R1 (Flt-1), VEGF-R2 (Flk-1, KDR) and VEGF-R3 (Flt-4). Soluble forms of these receptors are able to bind growth factors in circulation, slowing or blocking angiogenesis [25].

Humoral factors involved in vascular formation processes are more accessible for research in maternal circulation, and change of their content in mother's blood reflects changes in the content of these factors in the fetal blood circulation and tissues. In this regard, a complex study of angiogenesis-related factors and their ratios is crucial for understanding and predicting vascular morphogenesis disorders during pregnancy.

2. Characteristics of the groups and study design

The prospective study included 66 patients with early stage pregnancy.

The control group consisted of 20 patients with normal pregnancy. All the patients had one or two previous pregnancies uneventfully completed at term.

The main subgroup A consisted of 16 patients with the history of miscarriage and current threatening miscarriage. All patients from the main subgroup A gave live births at term. The main subgroup B included 30 patients whose pregnancy ended as «missed abortion».

In patients of the control group and of the main subgroup A, the study of angiogenesis-related factors in peripheral blood samples was performed within 6 weeks, at 7–8 weeks and at 11–14 weeks of pregnancy. In the main subgroup B, the investigation was conducted at the time of diagnosis of «missed abortion» (8 patients were examined before 6 weeks, 14 patients—at 7-8 weeks and 8 patients—at 11-14 weeks).

The criteria for inclusion into the main groups were as follows: history of two and more early pregnancy losses, no childbirth in current marriage, singleton natural pregnancy.

Exclusion criteria were endometriosis, POS, uterine fibroids, induced pregnancy and/or extragenital conditions (diabetes mellitus, psoriasis and systemic autoimmune diseases, and malignancies), FV L and FII G20210A gene mutations, and activation of bacterial viral infections. Groups were matched for the patient's age.

Diagnosis of recurrent miscarriage was established according to the International Classification of Diseases 10th Edition (ICD-10-CM). Pregnancy was diagnosed based on the ultrasonography study and HCG.

The samples of peripheral blood for investigation of angiogenesis-related factors were obtained from the cubital vein not later than 5 days after ultrasonic detection of cessation of pregnancy development in the patients of the main subgroup B in case of intact chorion (absence of retroplacental and/or retro amniotic hematomas, vaginal tract bleedings). Prior to investigation, the serum was stored at the temperature of «-80°C».

3. Methods

Determination of serum levels of VEGF, VEGF-R1 (sFlt-1), VEGF-R2 (sKDR), MMP-2, MMP-9, TIMP-1, TIMP-2 and PLGF was performed by enzyme-linked immunosorbent assay (ELISA) using standard test systems: Bender MedSystems GmbH (Austria) and R&D Systems (USA). The optical density was measured using the plate reader BioTek (USA) at the wavelength of 450 nm. Construction of the calibration curve and calculation of the concentrations of VEGF, sFlt-1, sKDR, MMP-2, MMP-9, TIMP-1, TIMP-2 and PLGF were performed by linear regression equation in logarithmic coordinates.

The statistical processing was carried out using statistical analysis package for Microsoft Office Excel 2007 and software package Statistica for Windows 7.0, Statsoft Inc. (USA). Control of the normality of obtained parameters in studied groups was performed with Shapiro-Wilk W test. The significance of differences of mean values of the measured parameters was evaluated using unpaired t-test with different dispersions. Differences were considered significant at a significance level $p < 0.05$.

4. Results

Results of the study of angiogenesis-related factors are presented in **Tables 1** and **2**.

4.1. Time course of angiogenesis-related factors in patients with normal pregnancy

It was found that VEGF had the maximum concentration in blood at terms up to 6 weeks of gestation: Contents of this factor was significantly higher (more than 10 times) compared with further points of study. Concentration of PLGF at terms up to 6 weeks and at 7–8 weeks remained unchanged but increased more than two times by 11–14 weeks; this is consistent with the published data [24]. This trend in changing of VEGF and PLGF during early pregnancy probably provides pro-angiogenic effect because under the decrease in VEGF, PLGF is able to synergistically enhance angiogenesis promoted by VEGF [26].

Level of sVEGF-R1 was minimal at the starting point of the study but significantly increased reaching maximum values at 11-14 weeks. In contrast, the concentration of sVEGF-R2 was decreased only at 7-8 weeks of pregnancy. It is known that VEGF interacts with receptors VEGF-R1 and VEGF-R2, while VEGF-R1 is the only receptor for PLGF [27]. These factors compete for binding with VEGF-R1. Under increased secretion of VEGF and PLGF, this leads to exhaustion of VEGF-R1 and predominance of VEGF-R2 in circulation. PLGF is also supposed to be able to replace VEGF in the VEGF/VEGF-R1 complex, activating the

http://dx.doi.org/10.5772/66410

Factor (u.m.)	Groups	Factor's values in terms of study		
		Up to 6 weeks	7–8 weeks	11–14 weeks
VEGF (pg/ml)	Control	100.5 ± 24.5	5.5 ± 1.3#	8.9 ± 3.2#
	Main subgroup A	202.7 ± 82.3	5.9 ± 0.9#	4.2 ± 1.2#
	Main subgroup B	49.6 ± 28.6	4.7 ± 1.9	3.2 ± 0.4
VEGF-R1 (ng/ml)	Control	0.4 ± 0.1	1.1 ± 0.2#	1.7 ± 0.4#
	Main subgroup A	0.9 ± 0.1*	1.4 ± 0.1*#	1.7 ± 0.1#•
	Main subgroup B	0.4 ± 0.1**	5.8 ± 2.6*#	0.5 ± 0.2*,**•
VEGF-R2 (ng/ml)	Control	9.4 ± 1.9	4.9 ± 0.6#	9.3 ± 1.5•
	Main subgroup A	8.4 ± 1.9	10.6 ± 0.4*	10.5 ± 0.6
	Main subgroup B	12.5 ± 2.0	11.6 ± 1.5*	12.5 ± 2.0
PLGF (pg/ml)	Control	12.2 ± 1.4	13.2 ± 2.5	28.9 ± 4.1#•
	Main subgroup A	7.5 ± 0.6*	9.9 ± 0.8#	22.5 ± 2.5#•
	Main subgroup B	8.5 ± 0.7*	9.5 ± 2.0	8.8 ± 2.4*,**

*Comparison with the control group;
**comparison with the main subgroup A;
#the differences within one group in comparison with the data obtained before 6 weeks.
•the differences within one group in comparison with data obtained at 7-8 weeks (# < 0.05).

Table 1. Blood levels of pro- and antiangiogenic factors of the first trimester of pregnancy.

Factor (u.m.)	Groups	Factor's values in terms of study		
		up to 6 weeks	7–8 weeks	11–14 weeks
MMP-2 (ng/ml)	Control	330.6 ± 31.1	331.8 ± 13.2	364.2 ± 30.9
	Main subgroup A	415.3 ± 21.9*	411.1 ± 30.0*	392.6 ± 34.8
	Main subgroup B	526.8 ± 16.0*,**	378.7 ± 33.7#	271.8 ± 21.9*, **#•
MMP-9 (ng/ml)	Control	556.5 ± 71.4	379.6 ± 50.1#	558.8 ± 92.8
	Main subgroup A	537.2 ± 78.6	500.1 ± 51.1	578.9 ± 109.0
	Main subgroup B	296.1 ± 132.6	403.6 ± 79.3	278.0 ± 67.7*,**
TIMP-1 (ng/ml)	Control	435.6 ± 31.0	357.5 ± 26.1#	388.5 ± 23.9
	Main subgroup A	440.3 ± 62.1	458.8 ± 34.1*	344.0 ± 42.3•
	Main subgroup B	321.4 ± 27.9*	403.9 ± 48.9	342.0 ± 27.4
TIMP-2 (ng/ml)	Control	22.6 ± 2.1	19.4 ± 1.5	21.0 ± 1.5
	Main subgroup A	23.3 ± 2.4	21.2 ± 2.6	29.4 ± 4.1*
	Main subgroup B	30.4 ± 1.4*,**	25.3 ± 3.0*	18.1 ± 1.3**#•

*Comparison with the control group;
**comparison with the main subgroup A;
#the differences within one group in comparison with the data obtained before 6 weeks.
•the differences within one group in comparison with data obtained at 7-8 weeks ($p < 0.05$).

Table 2. Blood levels of matrix metalloproteinases and their tissue inhibitors in the first trimester of pregnancy.

expression of VEGF-R2 [28]. According to the published data, VEGF-R2 is a key receptor in angiogenesis [29] although its affinity to VEGF is quite lower than VEGF-R1 [30].

It is known that normally pro-angiogenic molecules are less than their inhibitors; nevertheless, intensive vascularization of placenta and of fetal developing organs occurs in pregnancy. This situation can be described as "pro-angiogenic state." However, it is quite difficult to quantify it, as the described models of angiogenic factors-receptor interactions do not give guide on the factor/inhibitor ratio, allowing to specify the pro-angiogenic state or block of angiogenesis [26, 31]. Therefore, trends observed in normal pregnancy may serve as references for challenging cases.

Blood levels of MMP-2 and TIMP-2 vary insignificantly in the studied terms of normal pregnancy. Significant decrease in MMP-9 and TIMP-1 concentration was found at 7–8 weeks compared with the terms before 6 weeks of pregnancy.

Normally, MMPs blood level is insignificant. Soluble forms of MMPs are present in blood as inactive proenzymes and transfer into active forms after propeptide cleavage under the impact of activation factors including inhibitors. Constant concentrations in the system "protease-antiprotease" (MMP-2/TIMP-2) may indicate extracellular matrix remodeling and vascular morphogenesis which intensively go at these terms; degradation of interstitial collagens and basement membrane collagens under the participation of these factors is obvious.

4.2. Time course of angiogenesis-related factors in patients of the main subgroup A

Blood levels of PLGF and sVEGF-R1 in patients of main subgroup A significantly increased with gestational age. In contrast, concentration of VEGF was maximum at the starting point of the study but significantly decreased (more than 30 times) by 7-8 weeks and then remained at the same level till 11–14 weeks of gestation.

Lack of significant differences in dynamics of MMP-2, MMP-9, TIMP-2 and sVEGF-R2 was observed during entire pregnancy. Concentration of TIMP-1 significantly decreased by 11–14 weeks.

Thus, in the main subgroup A, we found significant fluctuations of certain soluble factors. For several factors (VEGF, PLGF, MMP-2, TIMP-2), trends of this levels alterations at the same study points coincided with those observed during normal pregnancy; there was no statistically significant differences between the groups and the most studied terms. At the same time, for sVEGF-R1, sVEGF-R2, MMP-9 and TIMP-1, the trends were significantly different from the control group. However, these differences do not seem sufficient to cause dramatic consequences in pregnancy. Probably for successful outcome of pregnancy, a balanced production of VEGF and PLGF, key angiogenic factors for pregnancy [14, 24, 32], is necessary, as well as the balance between MMP-2 and TIMP-2, because MMP-2 is the key regulator of trophoblast invasion [17, 19] especially in early pregnancy.

4.3. Angiogenesis-related factors in the main subgroup B

4.3.1. Blood levels of angiogenesis-related factors in patients with missed abortion before 6 weeks of gestation

Missed abortion before 6 weeks was characterized by significant differences of the levels of angiogenesis-related factors: sVEGF-R1, PLGF, MMP-2, TIMP-1 and TIMP-2. Thus, with missed abortion, the level of PLGF was lower than in the control group; however, there was no significant difference with the main subgroup A. Blood level of sVEGF-R1 did not differ from the values of the control group. However, comparison with the main subgroup A showed that in complicated pregnancy which further accomplished with childbirth, level of sVEGF-R1 was higher than in missed abortion. These results may indicate the existence of subtle mechanisms of regulation in the system "ligand/receptor," where the most important aspect is not a certain level of material content of the molecule, but the impacts of the factors on each other.

The concentrations of MMP-2 in the main subgroups A and B were significantly higher than in the control group. The maximum level of MMP-2 in blood was detected in missed abortion. TIMP-1 and TIMP-2 levels in the control group and main subgroup A differed insignificantly; in the main subgroup B, the level of TIMP-1 was significantly lower and the level of TIMP-2 was significantly higher at these terms.

Thus, more distinct differences specific for missed abortion were found in the group of factors "protease-antiprotease." The content of the factors in the system MMP-2–TIMP-2 at this term is, probably, critical for pregnancy. It is known that MMP-2 and TIMP-2 are most important at early terms of gestation during trophoblast invasion into maternal tissues [19]. Constant expression of MMP-2 and TIMP-2 was detected in apical layer of the syncytiotrophoblast and decidual NK-cells [19]. The published data suggest a possibility of syncytium activation by MMP-2, and the participation of this molecule in the processing of paracrine factors synthesized by these cells [19, 21]. There is a probability of change in the balance of production of biologically active molecules determining the development of pregnancy, due to the excessive production of MMP-2 or TIMP-2.

Pregnancy-initiated angiogenesis is closely associated with tissue remodeling and vascularization. Changes occurring in the endometrium decidualization include as follows: infiltration of tissues by immune cells (uNK-cells and macrophages), extracellular matrix remodeling with cell invasion through the matrix and membrane, and lysis of muscle-elastic tissue elements. In this period, the most important processes are formation of the placental bed and vascularization of the villi [6, 8, 10]. It is known that embryos which stopped to develop at 3–5 weeks had vascular villi, large hydropic dystrophy of the villous stroma and no embryonic blood vessels [33–35]. The disbalance of angiogenic factors, causing autocrine and paracrine effects to each other and to the cells, leads to microenvironment that is not compatible with the development of pregnancy. Excessive protease activity under these conditions may also reflect degenerative processes in the uterus before abortion.

4.3.2. Blood levels of angiogenesis-related factors in patients with missed abortion at 7–8 weeks

Pathological changes specific for missed abortion at 7–8 weeks were reflected by the significant increase in VEGF-R1, VEGF-R2 and TIMP-2 levels compared with the control group.

The interval of 7–8 weeks of gestation is marked by the first wave of trophoblast invasion into the mother's arteries and the start of uteroplacental blood flow. Extravillous trophoblast has a high invasive potential and expresses VEGF, PLGF and VEGF-R1 [36]. The receptor VEGF-R2 is expressed by the cells of fetoplacental complex [36, 37]. It should be noted that the level of VEGF-R1 is five times higher and VEGF-R2 more than two times differ from these factor levels in the control group. According to the published data, soluble forms of VEGF-R1 and VEGF-R2 are able to block angiogenesis and adversely affect the migration and proliferation of endothelial cells [27, 38, 39]. However, comparison with the main subgroup A did not show any significant differences in the studied period. Therefore, excessive levels of soluble forms of VEGF-R1 and VEGF-R2 in maternal circulation are not the main cause of this pathology at this term. It is known that adequate angiogenesis of villous tree and chorionic villi are critical stage and condition for further development of the placenta and fetus [1–4]. Inadequate start of restriction of uterine arteries at these terms initiates a chain of troubles in the system mother-placenta-fetus.

The key process of pregnancy is cytotrophoblast invasion into uterine arteries. At the same time, there is arteriolar lumen expansion under the impact of metalloproteinases. Excess of tissue inhibitors at 7–8 weeks, probably, leads to incomplete trophoblast invasion and insufficient lumen expansion which under the increased secretion of VEGF-R1 and VEGF-R2 can result in vasospasm and enhanced vascular permeability-specific manifestations of increased contents of these factors [36, 40] which adversely affect the embryo development.

4.3.3. Blood levels of angiogenesis-related factors in patients with missed abortion at 11–14 weeks of pregnancy

Missed abortion detected at of 11–14 weeks was characterized by a significant decrease in sVEGF-R1, PLGF, MMP-2 and MMP-9 compared with the control group and main subgroup A. Level of TIMP-2 was significantly lower than in the main subgroup A, but close to the control group.

The end of the first trimester of pregnancy is marked by the start of the fetal period of intrauterine human development, fading of the first wave of trophoblast invasion and preparation for a second wave at 16-18 weeks of pregnancy. Significant decrease in soluble forms of VEGF-R1 and PLGF in the main subgroup B could evidence the role of these factors in the pathologic processes leading to pregnancy loss. PLGF is the main regulatory factor in the first trimester of physiological pregnancy [2, 24] that acts as paracrine regulator of decidual angiogenesis and autocrine regulator of trophoblast function [24]. The synergy of effects of PLGF and VEGF on angiogenesis manifests with the morphogenesis of more mature and stable vasculature [24, 27]. Its effect is more significant in angiogenesis than in vasculogenesis [2]. Besides inhibition of angiogenesis, soluble form of the receptor VEGF-R1 also provides "support," and thus, the effect depends on the factor blood level. Probably in this situation, levels of sVEGF-R1 and PLGF are insufficient for adequate angiogenesis.

4.4. Ratio of angiogenesis-related factors

Dynamic balance in the system ligand/receptor provides a state of the system which empowers the implementation of its function, if this system tends towards the harmonic balance. The equilibrium point in such systems is always moving, because ligand/receptor pairs, being complex systems, are influenced by a variety of factors. In terms of the dynamic balance theory, ligand's positions in this study were occupied by the factors which specifically and nonspecifically affect angiogenesis, while the receptor's positions were occupied by its inhibitors. Studied ligands and receptors have multiple substrate specificity, but because their activity is affected by other factors that are present in the bloodstream and were not included in this study, investigation of ligand/receptor pairs in terms of classical concepts is difficult. Moreover, current models describing interactions of VEGF family members with the receptors [26] as well as of the matrix metalloproteinase family members with the inhibitors [31] do not provide quantitative binding characteristics of the system receptor/ligand for these molecules. The situation is complicated by the different levels of expression of these factors by various cell types. Therefore, the use of any index or ratio characterizing the dynamic situation in the selected time interval as a pro-angiogenic or nonproangiogenic state does not seem possible. To describe such situations, "surrogate" indexes characterizing the ligand/receptor ratio may be most appropriate to define any process, particularly angiogenesis. Such ratios are used to calculate the risk of development of pregnancy complications, such as preeclampsia [41–44].

Changes of the ligand/receptor pair ratio (VEGF/VEGF-R1, VEGF/VEGF-R2, PLGF/VEGF-R1, MMP-9/TIMP-1, MMP-2/TIMP-2) in the studied groups are presented in **Figure 1**.

4.4.1. VEGF/VEGF-R1 and VEGF/VEGF-R2 ratios

VEGF/VEGF-R1 ratio (**Figure 1A**) in the control group before 6 weeks was significantly higher than in the main subgroups A and B (0.562; 0.178 and 0.0312, respectively). In the control group, we observed significant differences between the terms before 6 weeks of gestation and other terms. Interestingly, the pattern of the VEGF/VEGF-R1 ratio change in the main subgroup A had tendencies similar to the control group. In the main subgroup B, the values of ligand/receptor pairs were significantly low, except for the last study term (0.0086) compared with the control group (0.006) and the main subgroup A (0.0024).

VEGF/VEGF-R2 ratio changed in a similar way (**Figure 1B**). Before 6 weeks of pregnancy, the significant changes were noted only in the main subgroup B (0.0023), compared with the control group (0.020) and the main subgroup A (0.011).

Tendencies of changes of VEGF/VEGF-R2 were similar in the control and the main subgroup A, demonstrating at the same time significant differences at 7-8 weeks. The main subgroup B was characterized by minimal values of the ratio which significantly differed in terms before 6 and 7–8 weeks compared with the other groups, but do not change within group in all terms of pregnancy.

It is known that realization of different mechanisms of angiogenesis depends on the type of receptor interacting with VEGF. Activation of VEGF-R2 leads to stimulation of angiogenesis

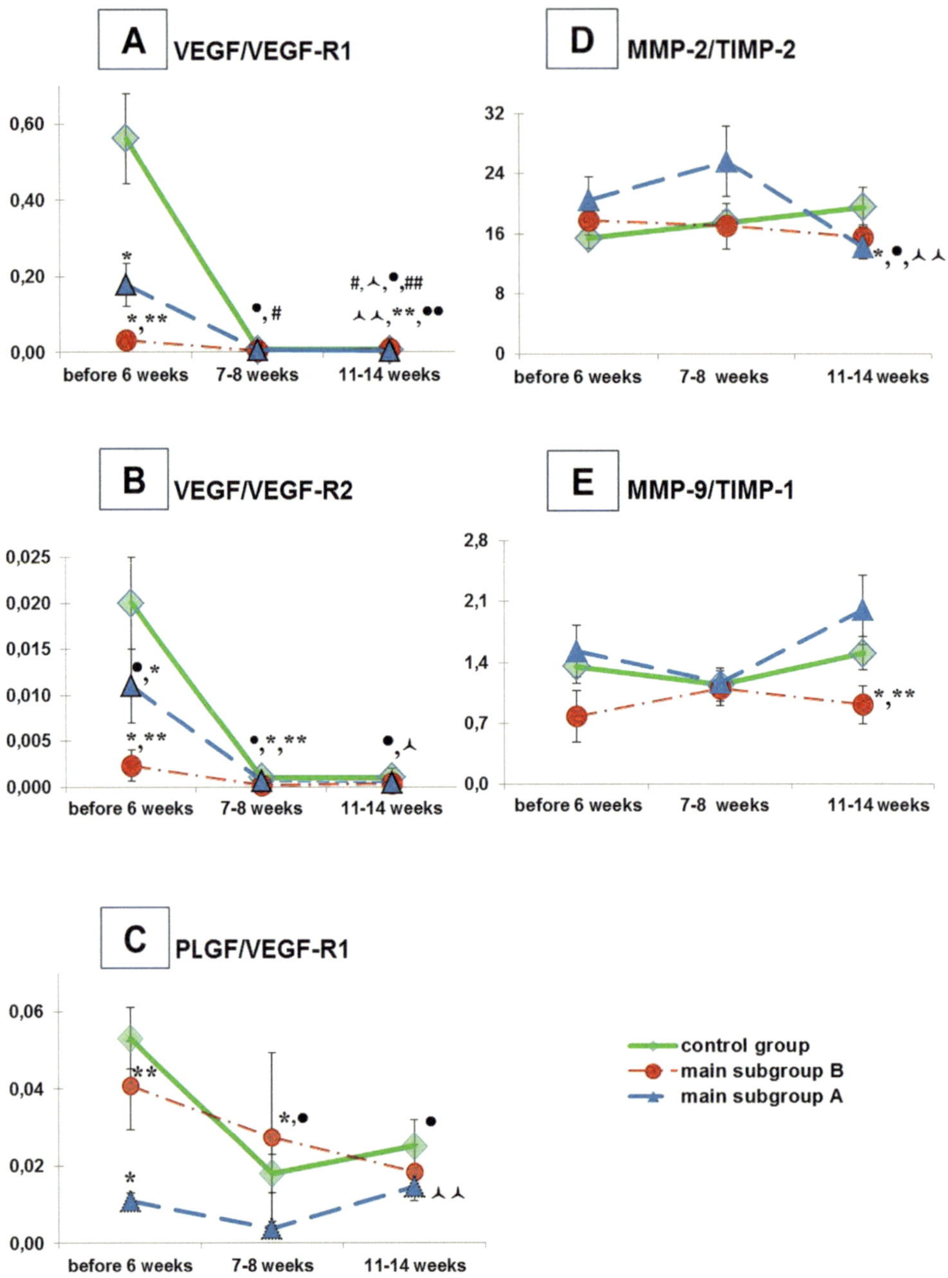

Figure 1. Factor/receptor (A, B, C) and factor/inhibitor (D, E) ratio in the blood of women at early terms of pregnancy. *Significant difference from the control group; **significant difference from the main subgroup A; •significant differences inside the control group in comparison with terms before 6 weeks; ••significant difference inside the control group in comparison with terms 7-8 weeks; #significant difference inside the main subgroup A in comparison with terms before 6 weeks; ##significant difference inside the main subgroup A in comparison with terms 7–8 weeks; ⅄significant difference inside the main subgroup B in comparison with terms before 6 weeks; ⅄⅄significant difference inside the main subgroup B in comparison with terms 7–8 weeks ($p < 0.05$).

by triggering proliferation, migration, differentiation and inhibition of apoptosis of endothelial cells. Activated VEGF-R1 receptor stimulates intercellular interactions, branching of vascular network and regulates the trophoblast invasion into the spiral arteries [27]. Use of blocking antibodies for VEGF-R2 causes reduction in decidual angiogenesis and pregnancy loss in mice, while use of antibodies of similar effect for VEGF-R1 does not cause such effects [37]. In other studies, the lack of VEGF-R1 in experimental animals led to overdevelopment of disorganized vessels and clusters of endothelial cells, and the absence of VEGF-R2—to reduction in development of vasculature [2]. It has been demonstrated that interaction of VEGF/VEGF-R2 regulates the development of fetoplacental complex [27] and acts as a paracrine system in the processes of formation of primitive embryo vascular network [24, 29]. On the contrary, the formation of an active complex VEGF/VEGF-R1 mostly affects the processes of differentiation and migration of trophoblast and also regulates invasion [27].

4.4.2. PLGF/VEGF-R1 ratio

PLGF factor affects endothelium through specific binding with the receptor VEGF-R1 (**Figure 1C**). According to the published data, PLGF more impacts the processes of angiogenesis, than vasculogenesis; however, PLGF and VEGF-R1 also affect the mobilization of mesenchymal progenitors of endothelial cells, which are involved in vasculogenesis [2]. PLGF enhances angiogenesis acting synergistically with VEGF, and it is also able to replace VEGF in the complex with VEGF/VEGF-R1 releasing it for VEGF-R2 activation. It is also known that PLGF is a paracrine regulator of decidual angiogenesis and autocrine regulator of trophoblast's functions in differentiation and invasion [24] and also the main regulating factor in normal pregnancy in the first trimester [2, 24].

The ratio of PLGF/VEGF-R1 for each group of pregnant women had its own tendencies. There were significant differences between the main subgroup A and control group before 6 and at 7–8 weeks. However, there was notable misbalance of factors in ligand/receptor pair PLGF/VEGF-R1 manifesting with significant deviations from the average value of the factors ratio at 7-8 weeks of pregnancy in the main subgroup B. Moreover, low ratio values were noted in the ligand/receptor pair of the main subgroup A at all studied points. The reduced value of this ratio in the main subgroup A may be due to the changes in the dynamic system PLGF/VEGF-R1 (both toward the increase in sVEGF-R1 and toward the decrease in PLGF). Obtained ratio values for the given ligand/receptor pair for all groups at early terms of pregnancy may evidence the acceptable fluctuations of the values of the factors in this pair, which are nonsignificant for the development of pregnancy.

4.4.3. MMP-9/TIMP-1 and MMP-2/TIMP-2 ratio

Analysis of the obtained results showed no significant differences of ratios of free forms of MMPs and tissue inhibitors TIMPs (MMPs/TIMPs) between the groups at the most studied terms of pregnancy (**Figure 1D, E**). Significant differences were shown for the MMP-9/TIMP-1 ratio at 11-14 weeks for the main subgroup B (0.91) and the control group (1.48). The significant decrease in this ratio in the main subgroup B may evidence degradation processes and autolysis in missed abortion. The character of changes of the ligand/receptor ratio within studied groups confirms some stable dynamic equilibrium of the factors concentrations. Probably, nonspecific effects of the factors in the studied ligand/receptor pairs on angiogenesis processes are of somewhat conservative nature comprising prevention of excessive protease activity, and sufficient for an adequate angiogenesis at the studied terms of pregnancy. However, use of these ratios is not informative to characterize the pathologic processes at studied terms in patients of these groups, excluding the ratio MMP-9/TIMP-1 at 11-14 weeks of pregnancy. The observed reduction in MMP-9/TIMP-1 at 11-14 weeks may serve as an alert of the development of critical events.

5. Conclusions

This study revealed the features of humoral systems regulating angiogenesis during physiological pregnancy and in patients with successful and unsuccessful perinatal outcomes. We found that deviations in the peripheral blood contents of angiogenesis-related factors: VEGF-R1, VEGF-R2, MMP-9 and TIMP-1 in patients with the history of missed abortion do not reflect critical for angiogenesis events in the first trimester of pregnancy. However, a significant disbalance of soluble factors, regulating angiogenesis, detected in patients with missed abortion shows that matrix metalloproteinases and their tissue inhibitors play the leading role in pregnancy losses before 6 and 7–8 weeks. Analysis of ligand/receptor ratios complements the obtained results, as we have found a significant decrease in the VEGF/VEGF-R1 and VEGF/VEGF-R2 ratios before 6 weeks of pregnancy despite the fact that there were no significant differences between individual molecules forming these pairs. The nature of VEGF/VEGF-R1 and VEGF/VEGF-R2 ratios alterations within the groups at the studied terms suggests the presence of a single mechanism that regulates interactions between VEGF and its receptors VEGF-R1 and VEGF-R2. In patients with pregnancy losses at 11-14 weeks, we found low concentrations of PLGF and sVEGF-R1 and also of MMP-2 and MMP-9, and reduction in MMP-2/TIMP-2 ratio, which are probably insufficient for an adequate angiogenesis at this term. Since an adequate angiogenesis is the determining factor for the development of pregnancy, early identification of criteria alerting about a trouble in fetoplacental system will also have diagnostic and prognostic value. Detection of the markers is especially important in cases of habitual pregnancy loss of unknown origin, because the disturbance of angiogenesis may be one of the causes of missed abortion. Taking into account difficulties with obtaining placental tissue at the studied terms of pregnancy, the angiogenesis-related factors may serve as unbiased indicators of placental angiogenesis. The obtained results allow to presume various mechanisms of pregnancy pathology at early terms and to demonstrate the possibility of using the analysis of ligand/receptor pairs to characterize the angiogenesis processes in early pregnancy.

Acknowledgements

The authors express their deep appreciation and gratitude to employee of Department of Perinatal Pathology, Kulikova G.V and the Department of Library and Information Resources and Telemedicine, A.L. Komarovsky, V.I. Kulakov Research Center for Obstetrics, Gynecology and Perinatology of the Russian Ministry of Health, for his help in preparing this manuscript.

Author details

Marina M. Ziganshina*, Lyubov V. Krechetova, Lyudmila V. Vanko, Zulfiya S. Khodzhaeva, Ekaterina L. Yarotskaya and Gennady T. Sukhikh

*Address all correspondence to: mmz@mail.ru

Federal State Budget Institution "The Research Center for Obstetrics, Gynecology and Perinatology" of the Ministry of Healthcare of the Russian Federation, Moscow, Russia

References

[1] Demir R, Seval Y, Huppertz B. Vasculogenesis and angiogenesis in the early human placenta. Acta Histochem. 2007;109(4):257–65. doi:10.1016/j.acthis.2007.02.008

[2] Burton GI, Charnock-Jones DS, Jauniaux E. Regulation of vascular growth and function in the human placenta. Reproduction. 2009;138(6):895–902. doi:10.1530/REP-09-0092

[3] Zygmunt M, Herr F, Münstedt K, Lang U, Liang OD. Angiogenesis and vasculogenesis in pregnancy. Eur J Obstet Gynecol Reprod Biol. 2003;110(Suppl 1):S10–8. doi:10.1016/S0301-2115(03)00168-4

[4] Milovanov AP, Kirichenko AK. Molecular mechanisms of regulation of cytotrophoblastic invasion in uteroplacental region. Arkh Patol. 2001;63(5):3–8.

[5] Mihu CM, Susman S, Rus Ciucă D, Mihu D, Costin N. Aspects of placental morphogenesis and angiogenesis. Rom J Morphol Embryol. 2009;50(4):549–57. http://www.rjme.ro/RJME/resources/files/500409549557.pdf

[6] Kingdom J, Huppertz B, Seaward G, Kaufmann P. Development of the placental villous tree and its consequences for fetal growth. Eur J Obstet Gynecol Reprod Biol. 2000;92(1):35–43. doi:10.1016/S0301-2115(00)00423-1

[7] James JL, Carter AM, Chamley LW. Human placentation from nidation to 5 weeks of gestation. Part I: What do we know about formative placental development following implantation? Placenta. 2012;33(5):327–34. doi:10.1016/j.placenta.2012.01.020.

[8] Benirschke K, Burton GJ, Bergen RN. Pathology of the human placenta. 6th ed., Springer, NewYork, 2012.

[9] Kaufmann P, Black S, Huppertz B. Endovascular trophoblast invasion: implications for the pathogenesis of intrauterine growth retardation and preeclampsia. Biol Reprod. 2003;69(1):1–7. doi:10.1095/biolreprod.102.014977

[10] Pollheimer J, Knöfler M. The role of the invasive, placental trophoblast in human pregnancy. Wien Med Wochenschr. 2012;162(9–10):187–90. doi:10.1007/s10354-012-0071-6

[11] Raza SL, Cornelius LA. Matrix metalloproteinases: pro- and anti-angiogenic activities. J Investig Dermatol Symp Proc. 2000;5(1):47–54. doi:10.1046/j.1087-0024.2000.00004.x

[12] Rundhaug JE. Matrix metalloproteinases and angiogenesis. J Cell Mol Med. 2005;9(2):267–85. doi:10.1111/j.1582-4934.2005.tb00355.x

[13] Vrachnis N, Kalampokas E, Sifakis S, Vitoratos N, Kalampokas T, Botsis D, Iliodromiti Z. Placental growth factor (PlGF): a key to optimizing fetal growth. J Matern Fetal Neonatal Med. 2013;26(10):995–1002. doi:10.3109/14767058.2013.766694

[14] Andraweera PH, Dekker GA, Roberts CT. The vascular endothelial growth factor family in adverse pregnancy outcomes. Hum Reprod Update. 2012;18(4):436–57. doi:10.1093/humupd/dms011

[15] Lash GE, Schiessi B, Kirkley M, Innes BA, Cooper A, Searle RF et al. Expression of angiogenic growth factors by uterine natural killer cells during early pregnancy. J Leukoc Biol. 2006;80:572–580. doi:10.1189/jlb.0406250

[16] Quenby S, Nik H, Innes B, Lash G, Turner M, Drury J, Bulmer J. Uterine natural killer cells and angiogenesis in recurrent reproductive failure. Hum Reprod. 2009;24:45–54. doi:10.1093/humrep/den348

[17] Naruse K, Lash GE, Innes B, Otun HA, Searle RF, Robson SC, Bulmer JN. Localization of matrix metalloproteinase (MMP)-2, MMP-9 and tissue inhibitors for MMPs (TIMPs) in uterine natural killer cells in early human pregnancy. Hum Reprod. 2008;1:1–9. doi:10.1093/humrep/den408

[18] Anacker J, Feix S, Kapp M, et al. Expression pattern of matrix metalloprotenases (MMPs) in human deciduas during pregnancy. J Reprod Immunol. 2010;86:79–111.

[19] Bai SX, Wang YL, Qin L, Xiao ZJ, Herva R, Piao YS. Dynamic expression of matrix metalloproteinases (MMP-2,-9 and -14) and the tissue inhibitors of MMPs (TIMP-1,-2 and -3) at the implantation site during tubal pregnancy. Reproduction. 2005;129:103–113. doi:10.1530/rep.1.00283

[20] Cockle J, Gopichandran N, Walker J, Levene MI, Orsi NM. Matrix metalloproteinases and their tissue inhibitors in preterm perinatal complications. Reprod Sci. 2007;14:629–645. doi:10.1177/1933719107304563

[21] Smith SD, Dunk CE, Aplin J, Harris LK, Jones RL. Evidence for immune cell involvement in decidual spiral arteriole remodeling in early human pregnancy. Am J Pathol. 2009;174:1959–1971. doi:10.2353/ajpath.2009.080995

[22] Forbes K, Westwood M. Maternal growth factor regulation of human placental development and fetal growth. J Endocrinol. 2010;207:1–16. doi:10.1677/JOE-10-0174

[23] Florio P, Gabbanini M, Borges LE, Bonaccorsi L, Pinzauti S, Reis FM et al. Activins and related proteins in the establishment of pregnancy. Reprod Sci. 2010;17:320–330. doi:10.1177/1933719109353205

[24] Plaisier M, Dennert I, Rost E, Koolwijk P, van Hinsbergh VW, Helmerhorst FM. Decidual vascularization and the expression of angiogenic growth factors and proteases in first trimester spontaneous abortions. Hum Reprod. 2009;24:185–197. doi:10.1093/humrep/den296

[25] Sugimoto H, Hamano Y, Charytan D, Cosgrove D, Kieran M, Sudhakar A, Kalluri R. Neutralization of circulating vascular endothelial growth factor (VEGF) by anti-VEGF antibodies and soluble VEGF receptor 1 (sFlt-1) induced proteinuria. J Biol Chem. 2003;278:12605–12608. doi:10.1074/jbc.C300012200

[26] Gabhann FM, Popel AS. Model of competitive binding of vascular endothelial growth factor and placental growth factor to VEGF receptors on endothelial cells. Am J Physiol Heart Circ Physiol. 2004;286:H153–H164. doi:10.1152/ajpheart.00254.2003

[27] Wulff C, Weigand M, Kreienberg R, Fraser HM. Angiogenesis during primate placentation in health and disease. Reproduction. 2003;126:569–577. doi:10.1530/rep.0.1260569

[28] Dewerchin M, Carmeliet P. PlGF: a multitasking cytokine with disease-restricted activity. Cold Spring Harb Perspect Med. 2012;2(8). pii: a011056. doi:10.1101/cshperspect.a011056

[29] Plaisier M, Streefland E, Koolwijk P, van Hinsbergh VW, Helmerhorst FM, Erwich JJ. Angiogenic growth factors and their receptors in first-trimester human decidua of pregnancies further complicated by preeclampsia or fetal growth restriction. Reprod Sci. 2008;15:720–726. doi:10.1177/1933719108317300

[30] Molskness TA, Stouffer RL, Burry KA, Gorrill MJ, Lee DM, Patton PE. Circulating levels of free and total vascular endothelial growth factor (VEGF)-A, soluble VEGF recepror-1 and -2, and angiogenin during ovarian stimulation in non-human primates and women. Hum Reprod. 2004;19:822–830. doi:10.1093/humrep/deh132

[31] Olson MW, Gervasi DC, Mobashery S, Fridman R. Kinetic analysis of the binding of human matrix metalloproteinase-2 and -9 to tissue inhibitor of metalloproteinase (TIMP-1) and (TIMP-2). J Biol Chem. 1997;272:29975–29983. doi:10.1074/jbc.272.47.29975

[32] Kalkunte SS, Mselle NF, Norris WE, Wira CR, Sentman CL, Sharma S. Vascular endothelial growth factor C facilitates immune tolerance and endovascular activity of human uterine NK cells at the maternal-fetal interface. J Immunol. 2009;182:4085–4092. doi:10.4049/jimmunol.0803769

[33] Cherstvoi ED, Kirillova IA, Kravtsova GI, Laziuk GI. The prospective directions of research in teratology. Arkh Patol. 1990;52(4):3–9.

[34] Laziuk GI. Human Teratology. A Guide for Physicians. (in Russian) 1991. 480p.

[35] Carmeliet P, Ferreira V, Breier G, Pollefeyt S, Kieckens L, Gertsenstein M, et al. Abnormal blood vessel development and lethality in embryos lacking a single VEGF allele. Nature. 1996;380(6573):435–9. doi:10.1038/380435a0

[36] Wang A, Rana S, Karumanchi SA. Preeclampsia: the role of angiogenic factors in its pathogenesis. Physiology. 2009;24:147–158. doi:10.1152/physiol.00043.2008

[37] Douglas NC, Tang H, Gomez R, Pytowski B, Hicklin DJ, Sauer CM et al. Vascular endothelial growth factor receptor 2 (VEGF-2) functions to promote uterine decidual angiogenesis during early pregnancy in the mouse. Endocrinology. 2009;150:3845–3854. doi:10.1210/en.2008-1207

[38] Lorquet S, Berndt S, Blacher S, Pequeux C. Implication of VEGF receptor soluble forms, sVEGFR-1 and sVEGFR-2, in pathological angiogenesis. Abstracts of the 23rd Annual Meeting of the ESHRE1-4; July 2007; Lyon, France, pp.1174–1175.

[39] Wathen KA, Tuutti E, Stenman UH, Alfthan H, Halmesmäki E, Finne P, Ylikorkala O, Vuorela P. Maternal serum-soluble vascular endothelial growth factor receptor-1 in early pregnancy ending in preeclampsia or intrauterine growth retardation. J Clin Endocrinol Metab. 2006;91:180–184. doi:10.1210/jc.2005-1076

[40] Bates DO. Vascular endothelial growth factors and vascular permeability. Cardiovasc Res. 2010;87:262–271. doi:10.1093/cvr/cvq105

[41] Erez O, Romero R, Espinoza J, Fu W, Todem D, Kusanovic JP, et al. The change in concentrations of angiogenic and anti-angiogenic factors in maternal plasma between the first and second trimesters in risk assessment for the subsequent development of preeclampsia and small-for-gestation age. J Matern Fetal Neonatal Med. 2008;21:279–287. doi:10.1080/14767050802034545

[42] Verlohren S, Galindo A, Schlembach D, Zeisler H, Herraiz I, Moertl MG, et al. An automated method for determination of the sFlt-1/PLGF ratio in the assessment of preeclampsia. Am J Obstet Gynecol. 2010;202:161. e1-161.e11. doi:10.1016/j.ajog.2009.09.016

[43] Schoofs K, Grittner U, Engels T, Pape J, Denk B, Henrich W, Verlohren S. The importance of repeated measurements of the sFlt-1/PlGF ratio for the prediction of preeclampsia and intrauterine growth restriction. J Perinat Med. 2014;42(1):61–8. doi:10.1515/jpm-2013-0074

[44] Herraiz I, Simón E, Gómez-Arriaga PI, Martínez-Moratalla JM, García-Burguillo A, Jiménez EA, Galindo A. Angiogenesis-related biomarkers (sFlt-1/PLGF) in the prediction and diagnosis of placental dysfunction: an approach for clinical integration. Int J Mol Sci. 2015;16(8):19009–26. doi:10.3390/ijms160819009

Chapter 6

Pathogenic Angiogenic Mechanisms in Alzheimer's Disease

Chaahat Singh, Cheryl G. Pfeifer and
Wilfred A. Jefferies

Additional information is available at the end of the chapter

http://dx.doi.org/10.5772/66403

Abstract

Vascular dysfunction is a crucial pathological hallmark of Alzheimer's disease (AD). Studies have reported that beta amyloid (Aβ) causes increased blood vessel growth in the brains of AD mouse models, a phenomenon that is also seen in AD patients. This has given way to an alternative angiogenesis hypothesis according to which, increased leakiness in the blood vessels disrupts the blood-brain barrier (BBB) and allows unwanted blood products to enter the brain causing progression of disease pathology, promoting amyloid clumping and aggregation along with impaired cerebral blood flow. Furthermore, the expression of melanotransferrin in AD model and patients may contribute to angiogenesis. The objective of this chapter is to attempt to establish a link between the vascular damage and AD pathology. Curbing the vascular changes and resulting damage seen in the brains of AD model mice and improving their cognition by treating with FDA-approved anti-angiogenic drugs may expedite the translational potential of this research into clinical trials in human patients. This direction into targeting angiogenesis will facilitate new preventive and therapeutic interventions for AD and related vascular diseases.

Keywords: Alzheimer's disease, amyloid beta, blood-brain barrier, angiogenesis

1. Introduction: history of vascular dysfunction in Alzheimer's disease

Alzheimer's disease (AD) presents itself as a progressive neurological disorder, which is the major cause of dementia leading to death in the elderly. It affects thinking, orientation and memory, causing impairment in cognition, social behaviour and motivation [1]. Approximately 47.5 million people worldwide have dementia, of which the most common contributor is AD with 60–70% [1]. In 2010, the total global societal costs were estimated to be US $604 billion corresponding to 1.0% of the worldwide gross domestic product [1].

In 1906, Dr. Alois Alzheimer [2] noted two microscopic neuropathological findings, which were further characterized and eventually established as the hallmarks of AD: senile neuritic plaques, which are aggregates that are primarily composed of beta-amyloid (Aβ) peptides; [3, 4] and neurofibrillary tangles, which are primarily composed of intra-neuronal hyperphosphorylated tau aggregates [5]. Aβ, a 4 kDa peptide, is a proteolytic cleavage product of the amyloid precursor protein (APP) by the action of α and γ secretase enzymes [6, 7]. Mutations either in the *APP* gene or in the secretase enzyme complex lead to a β secretase cleavage, forming a pathogenic Aβ species (Aβ1-42). These Aβ molecules aggregate to form oligomers, which multimerize into protofibrils, followed by the formation of dense core amyloid plaques [8–10].

1.1. Initial clinical observations linking AD and vascular disease

Post-mortem analysis has established that 50–84% of the brains of persons, who die aged 80–90+ years, show appreciable cerebrovascular lesions and although there is a debate around their impact on AD pathology, it is suggested that the independent dementia caused by vascular and AD-type pathologies may have additive or synergistic effect on cognitive impairment [11]. Vascular pathologies that have been seen in the aged human brain include: cerebral amyloid angiopathy (CAA), cerebral atherosclerosis, small vessel disease in most cases caused by hypertensive vasculopathy or microvascular degeneration, blood-brain barrier (BBB) dysfunction causing white matter lesions, microinfarctions, lacunar infarcts and microbleeds [11]. Studies in post-mortem of human brains also found evidence of increased angiogenesis in the hippocampus, midfrontal cortex, substantia nigra pars compacta, and locus coeruleus of AD brains compared to control brains suggesting that vascular dysfunction is an inherent part of AD pathology [12, 13].

1.2. Genetic risk factors linking AD and vascular disease

Epidemiological studies have identified risk factors for AD that are similar to those for cardiovascular disease (CVD) [14] such as hypertension during midlife, diabetes mellitus, smoking, apolipoprotein E (APOE) 4 isoforms, hypercholesterolemia, homocysteinemia and, in particular, age [1]. Familial AD is caused most commonly by presenilin 1 (*PSEN1*) or presenilin 2 (*PSEN2*) mutations. It is also seen that the presenilins are expressed in the heart and are critical to cardiac development. The work by Li *et al.* indicated that *PSEN1* and *PSEN2* mutations are associated with dilated cardiomyopathy (DCM) and heart failure and implicate novel mechanisms of myocardial disease [15]. Amyloid is a known vasculotrope and an

http://dx.doi.org/10.5772/66403

increased amyloid aggregation in AD brains is seen to be in interaction with the angiogenic and CAA positive vessels [14]. Apolipoprotein 3 (APOE3) is responsible for normal lipid metabolism; however, the APOE4 isoforms is strongly associated with the late onset of AD [13]. Carriers of this isoform show a decreased cerebral blood flow and have also been linked to disorders associated with elevated cholesterol levels or lipid derangements (*i.e.* hyperlipoproteinemia type III, coronary heart disease, strokes, peripheral artery disease and diabetes mellitus) [15]. These overlapping genetic risk factors might give us a direction for understanding the mechanisms of the disease-related pathways.

1.3. Factors linked to AD and increased angiogenesis: melanotransferrin (p97), VEGF, transglutaminases (factor XIIIa and tTG)

Melanotransferrin (also known as p97 or melanoma tumour antigen) is a member of the transferrin family and is responsible for the cellular uptake of iron. P97 was shown to be present in the capillary endothelium in a normal brain, in contrast to the brain from patients with AD, where it is found to be localized in microglia cells, associated with senile plaques [16, 17]. Serum normally contains very low levels of p97; however, it is reported to increase by five- and six-fold in patients with AD [18, 19]. From this observation, it was proposed that serum p97 could be a potential biochemical marker for this disease. It was further demonstrated that melanotransferrin exerts an angiogenic response quantitatively similar to that elicited by fibroblast growth factor 2 [20], and hypervascularity has been shown to be a feature in the brains of AD patients [12]. Overexpression of vascular endothelial growth factor (VEGF) receptor 2 was observed in newly formed vessels, suggesting that the angiogenic activity of melanotransferrin may depend on activation of endogenous VEGF [20]. VEGF is the major player in pathological/dysfunctional blood vessel formation. It is shown that VEGF is highly up-regulated in AD brains via the inflammatory pathway and also that VEGF co-aggregates with Aβ in AD brains [13]. The role of transglutaminases in AD is highly debated; however, it is shown that the activity of these enzymes might contribute to both angiogenesis and in the formation of protein aggregates in the AD brain [21, 22].

2. Alzheimer's disease and the blood-brain barrier pathogenesis: angiogenesis and inflammation

A physical seal is present between the vasculature in the brain and the central nervous system that restricts fluid and entrained molecules from being transported into the brain from the systemic circulation [13, 23]. Dysfunction of the BBB was originally seen in animal models of AD [24] and was later established as a prominent, but unexplained clinical feature of AD in patients [23]. Though it is unknown where the BBB dysfunction stems from, it is, however, argued that Aβ may be directly involved in this process [25, 26]. Leakiness of the BBB has been demonstrated in a number of AD transgenic animal models that have overexpression of *APP*, including the Tg2576, which manifests a form of early-onset AD [24, 25]. Studies show that BBB integrity is compromised in this mouse model as early as 4 months of age, much before the onset of other disease pathology, such as the consolidated amyloid plaques [24, 27]. Hence, the mechanism leading to the BBB disruption is a potential target for AD therapy.

2.1. Tight junction disruption in mouse models

The brain has a unique structure termed as the blood-brain barrier (BBB), which is a specialized physical seal that precludes the transport of various, large and/or hydrophilic, peripheral blood molecules from entering the brain parenchyma [13, 25]. This restricted exchange protects the brain from indiscriminate exposure to peptides, macromolecules and potentially toxic molecules [13, 25]. The integrity of the BBB is maintained by inter-endothelial complexes called tight junctions (TJ), in the brain capillaries, that are composed of a variety of plasma membrane spanning proteins (occludin), scaffold proteins (zonula occludens protein-1; ZO-1) and the actin cytoskeleton [12, 13, 25]. The peripheral membrane protein, ZO-1, localizes along blood vessels in the brain parenchyma and along with claudins and occludin ensures the intactness and permeability of the BBB [26, 28]. A second barrier is presented by the basal lamina, composed of type IV collagen, fibronectin and heparan sulphate along with other molecules, which operates as a molecular weight filter [26]. Lastly, there are cells that interact to protect the BBB, known as the neurovascular unit (NVU). This is composed of neurons, cerebral endothelial cells, basal lamina, astrocytic foot processes (containing proteases and neurotransmitters) and perivascular macrophages called pericytes [26].

Since the BBB plays crucial role in maintaining central nervous system (CNS) homeostasis, its dysfunction proves deleterious for the smooth working of the brain. The BBB dysfunction includes: (1) BBB disruption, resulting in the discharge of potentially neurotoxic circulating substances into the CNS; (2) transporter dysfunction, which consequently creates deficiency of nutrient supply and amplify toxic substances in the CNS; and (3) altered protein expression and NVU cell secretions, potentially resulting in inflammatory activation, oxidative stress and neuronal damage [28]. The three effects stated above have been reported in AD patients, although the scope of this chapter pertains only to BBB disruption.

The compromised integrity of the BBB has been indicated by increased CSF/serum albumin ratios seen in AD patients [28]. Albumin is a macromolecule that is unable to cross an intact BBB [27, 28]. Histological studies have also revealed the presence of albumin staining around microvessels that shows co-localization of amyloid plaques and angiopathy [12, 13, 26]. It is suggested that this staining is a result of an affinity of extravasated albumin for amyloid [28].

Prothrombin is seen at elevated levels particularly around the microvessels in the brains of AD patients [29]. Highest levels of the protein were observed in people scoring higher in the Braak staging [30, 31].

The increased vesicularization of brain endothelial cells damages the BBB by altering the tight junction function. This is consistent with increased transcytotic disruption of the BBB initiated by the release of inflammatory cytokines that are angiogenic triggers, promoting paracellular leakage [28].

http://dx.doi.org/10.5772/66403

2.2. CBF impairment: a road to hypervascularity in mouse models and humans

Vascular dysfunction is a crucial pathological hallmark of AD [12, 32]. The two key precursors to neurodegenerative changes and Aβ deposition in AD are the BBB breakdown [12, 32] and cerebral blood flow (CBF) impairment [33]. Various studies with the help of a non-invasive imaging technique (arterial spin labelling MRI) have shown that AD is associated with a global, as well as a regional CBF impairment, also known as cerebral hypoperfusion [34]. While AD patients exhibit a global decrease in blood flow (averaged 40%), compared to healthy controls, the CBF reduction is seen only in specific regions that are usually implicated in the disease state [14, 34]. It is, however, argued whether a diminished blood flow in AD is a cause or consequence of the disease.

Hypoperfusion is associated with both structural and functional changes in the brain and hence plays a pivotal role in influencing the permeability of the BBB [34]. Severe reductions in CBF have been seen in the elderly at a high risk for cognitive decline and AD [34]. Individuals that are carriers of the major AD risk allele, (APOE4), have a more impacted regional deteriorated CBF than non-carriers of the allele [35, 36]. AD-related vascular pathology impairs cerebral autoregulation and causes cerebrovascular insufficiency [37]. This impaired CBF and compromised BBB result in the accumulation of potentially neurotoxic molecules (*e.g.* increased Aβ concentration) in the brain along with the entry of unwanted blood products via peripheral circulation [38, 39]. Data obtained from structural MRI scans show atrophy in different regions of the brain, and an overall change in cortical thickness is observed due to hypoperfusion in AD patients [34]. The thickness of the cortex is an important predictive measure of evolution to AD for subjects with mild cognitive impairment [34]. Carriers of the APOE4 allele, a demographic reported to have glucose hypo-metabolism, demonstrate hastened cortical thinning in areas most vulnerable to aging (medial prefrontal and peri-central cortices) as well as in areas associated with AD and amyloid-aggregation (*e.g.* occipito-temporal, basal temporal cortices and hippocampus) [34]. Ageing is the leading risk factor for the development of late-onset AD. Aberrations in vascular ultrastructure, vascular reactivity, resting cerebral blood flow and oxygen metabolism are all associated with age and act as a catalyst for cerebrovascular diseases and subsequent cognitive deficits [40]. To cope with the decrease in blood flow, the brain has evolved a compensatory mechanism whereby it increases the formation of blood vessels resulting in hypervascularity, a phenomenon which is seen not only in mouse models [40–43] but also in post-mortem samples of AD patients [43].

2.3. Involvement of angiogenesis and not apoptosis

The 'vascular hypothesis' as stated currently, defends that the vascular damage is a consequence of diminished blood perfusion of the brain, leading to hypoperfusion/hypoxia causing the BBB dysfunction [44]. A subsequent amalgamation of accumulated Aβ, neuro-inflammation, and the eventual disintegration of the neurovascular unit is seen, culminating in vascular death [13, 25, 45]. In a state of hypoperfusion, the hypoxia-inducible factors initiate angiogenesis (the formation of blood vessels) through the up-regulation of pro-angiogenic factors [25]. The main player in this blood vessel formation is VEGF, which induces differentiation and proliferation of endothelial cells from its progenitors, the hemangioblast and the angioblast

[46]. This forms an inefficiently differentiated primitive vascular plexus (vasculogenesis) [47]. The vascular plexus undergoes remodelling, that is triggered by the angiopoietin-1 (Ang-1), into a hierarchically structured mature vascular system established through endothelial cell sprouting, trimming differentiation and pericyte recruitment (normal angiogenesis) [48]. In contrast to these events in AD, it is observed that, a downstream cell signalling molecule to VEGF, angiopoietin-2 (Ang-2), destabilizes the vessel wall of mature vessels [32, 49–51]. The quiescent endothelial cells become sensitive to VEGF (and other angiogenic factors), proliferate indiscriminately, migrate to form new vessels that are not able to mature and eventually lead to the establishment of a leaky network of blood vessels [32]. This phenomenon is termed as pathological angiogenesis, which is a common occurrence seen during the evolution of tumours. In accordance with the current version of the 'vascular hypothesis', the BBB disruption is due to vascular cell death caused by apoptosis and angiogenesis would only be required to ensure tissue regeneration and likely be limited to replacing the damaged tissues and ensuring oxygenation of brain tissues [12, 13]. However, this role of apoptosis in BBB dysfunction is highly debated. Recent studies have shown that endothelial cell proliferation, during pathological angiogenesis, results in hypervascularity [12]. As a compensatory mechanism to the decreased blood flow caused by the leaky blood vessel network, vascular remodelling and structural changes take place in the physical arrangement of the tight junction proteins, resulting in compromised BBB integrity [12, 52]. The work of Biron *et al.* characterized the relationship between amyloidogenesis and BBB integrity, through changes in the TJ morphology in the Tg2576 AD mouse. They reported that the Tg2576 AD mice exhibit no apparent vascular apoptosis but have significant TJ disruption, which was seen directly linked to pathological angiogenesis, resulting in a significant increase in vascular density in AD brain [12]. Hence, it can be said that these data support the model that TJ disruption results from increased vascular permeability that takes place during extreme neovascularization in AD.

2.4. Angiogenesis: inflammation and vascular activation

Increasing evidence suggest that the vascular perturbation appears as a common feature in AD pathology as its hallmarks: amyloid plaques and neurofibrillary tangles. Over the years, emphasis has still been given to the accumulation of Aβ in AD, which, as a result of its impaired clearance from the brain, is thought to be responsible for the onset of cognitive decline [39, 53–55]. Paradoxical to this hypothesis, aggregated Aβ can be extensively present in the human brain in the absence of AD symptoms [56–58]. Although Aβ plays a crucial role in AD, it is neither necessary nor by itself sufficient to cause full AD pathology [27]. The alternate idea is that the mere production of Aβ (amyloidogenesis), promotes extensive pathological angiogenesis, leading to the redistribution of TJs, which then causes disruption to the BBB integrity, thereby increasing vascular permeability, subsequent hypervascularization and eventual AD pathology. This alternate 'vascular hypothesis' stems from a body of data that now establishes hypervascularization as a mechanistic explanation for amyloid-associated TJ pathology [12]. It provides new modalities for therapeutic intervention that target the restoration of the BBB by modulating angiogenesis, thereby possibly preventing AD onset and potentially repairing damage in the AD brain. A second study by Biron *et al.* demonstrated that immunization with Aβ peptides neutralized the amyloid trigger that causes pathological angiogenesis and thereby reverses hypervascularity in Tg2576 AD mice [59]. The Aβ plaques were seen to be dissolved, solubilized Aβ removed from the brain parenchyma along perivascular drainage routes, which resulted in a decrease in the hypervascularity [59]. This supports a vascular angiogenesis model for AD pathophysiology and provides the first evidence that modulating angiogenesis repairs damage in the AD brain.

Pathological angiogenesis and hypervascularization in an AD brain occurs in response to impaired cerebral perfusion (oligaemia) and inflammatory response to vascular injury [60]. We have already discussed the impaired perfusion in Section 2.2. In this section, we will look at the inflammatory activation of angiogenesis. Morphological and biochemical evidences present themselves in the form of regionally increased capillary density, unresolved vascular sprouting, glomeruloid vascular structure formation, and up-regulated expression of angiogenic factors: VEGF, transforming growth factor β (TGF β) and tumour necrosis factor α (TNF α) [60]. In AD, inflammatory pathways, when stimulated, cause the release of angiogenic cytokines such as thrombin and VEGF, contributing to pathological angiogenesis [60]. It is hypothesized that a thrombogenic region develops in the endothelial cells of the vessel wall, leading to intra-vascular accumulation of thrombin. This thrombin activates the vascular endothelial cells to secrete amyloid precursor protein via a receptor-mediated protein kinase C-dependent pathway [60]. Progressive deposition of amyloid precursor protein leads to accumulation of the Aβ plaques, which generates more reactive oxygen species and induces further endothelial damage in a cycle of neurotoxic insult. This establishes a cycle of neurotoxicity and death, instituted by the discharge of thrombin following Aβ-induced neuroinflammatory responses [60]. Other studies further support the interaction of Aβ with thrombin and fibrin throughout the clotting cascade, to increase neurovascular damage and neuroinflammation [61–63]. Astrocytes, cultured *in vitro* and stimulated with Aβ, showed a release of neuroinflammatory cytokines that resulted in the increased expression of VEGF [49, 50]. Other pro-inflammatory cytokines, such as interleukin-1β are increased during AD and known to induce VEGF and growth of new blood vessels [52, 64].

Consequential evidence is present implicating Aβ as a vasculotrope, modulating blood vessel density and vascular remodelling through angiogenic mechanisms. Brain microvessels have been shown to be closely associated with Aβ plaques with the aid of ultrastructural studies. It was observed that that AD brain capillaries contained pre-amyloid deposits [60]. Aβ stimulates angiogenesis in a highly conserved manner, which is speculated to be mediated through γ-secretase activity and Notch signalling [60, 65]. The *in vitro* studies of human umbilical vein endothelial cells (hUVEC), exposed directly to Aβ1-40 and Aβ1-42, show an angiogenic effect on the hUVEC, which exhibited an increase in the number of tip cells and branching [60].

The indication for Aβ-related angiogenesis has been extended *in vivo* as well, which can be observed with the chick embryo chorioallantoic membrane assay [65]. Aβ1-40 and Aβ1-42 stimulated embryos illustrated escalated vascular growth [65]. *In vivo* studies, using various APP mutant AD mouse models that have an overproduction of Aβ, show modifications in brain vasculature compared to the wild-type animals [12, 25]. APP23 AD model mice exhibit significant blood flow alterations correlated with structural modifications of blood vessels [51].

A study using three-dimensional architectural analysis [51], revealed significant changes to be accelerated only in the amyloid positive vessels [64]. Interestingly, brain homogenates taken from Aβ-overexpressing AD model mice, demonstrated an increase in the formation of new vessels in an *in vivo* angiogenesis assay [52]. This increase in vessels was blocked on exposure to a VEGF antagonist [52]. The vascular changes observed in these mice may be thought to be due to unrelated, 'off-target' effects of the APP mutation. However, the fact that the vascular changes observed in transgenic mice correlate well with vascular disturbances reported in human AD brains, it is safe to say that angiogenesis plays a crucial role in the establishment of AD pathology.

Post-mortem studies of human brains also show evidence of increased angiogenesis in the hippocampus, mid-frontal cortex, substantia nigra pars compacta, and locus coeruleus of AD brains compared to healthy individuals [43]. Further analysis found no correlation between the number of microglia (activation of apoptosis) and angiogenesis or microglia with vessel density, suggesting that it may be the presence of Aβ that is initiating angiogenesis (and not activation of apoptosis) and subsequently causing BBB dysfunction [66, 67].

It is seen that there are additional proteins at the BBB, which act to regulate brain Aβ levels and the disruption of which takes the brain towards up-regulated angiogenesis. The receptor for advanced glycation products (RAGE), a multi-ligand receptor, regulates the entry of peripheral Aβ to the brain [67–69]. Its expression is up-regulated by binding with ligands including Aβ and pro-inflammatory cytokine-like mediators [67]. This facilitates the entry of Aβ into the cerebral neurons, microglia and vasculature [69]. *In vitro* studies have also implicated RAGE in the vascular pathogenesis of AD, by suppressing the CBF, leading to hypoperfusion [67, 70].

3. Haemostatic mechanisms in relation to angiogenesis in AD

Maintenance of the fluidity of blood and limiting its loss upon blood vessel endothelium injury is a crucial physiological process known as haemostasis [71]. Haemostasis is possible due to the existence of a delicate balance between pro-coagulation and anti-coagulation along with numerous pathways and feedback loops [71, 72]. Haemostasis has three distinct phases—where the primary haemostasis is involved in adhering platelets to site of injury, forming a 'haemostatic or platelet plug' [71]; secondary haemostasis—which involves the activation of coagulation cascade, culminating in a fibrin clot; the last stage—which is fibrinolysis, or the dissolution of the clot [71]. Accompanied with vascular dysfunction, an altered haemostatic scenario is increasingly implicated in AD. Majority of the research, barring a few, support an association of pro-coagulation mechanism in AD. The proteins like transglutaminases are core components of the coagulation system that could be used as therapeutics to resolve the altered haemostasis in AD.

3.1. The involvement of haemostatic factors in angiogenesis: transglutaminases (factor XIIIa and tTG)

Transglutaminases (TG) are a family of enzymes, which catalyse irreversible post-translational modifications of proteins [22, 73]. Yamada *et al.* put forward the suggestion that TG activity might contribute to the formation of protein aggregates in AD brain [21]. Though this idea is debated, tau proteins have been shown to be in support of this hypothesis by being an appropriate *in vitro* substrate of TGs [22]. Studies also show that transglutaminase-catalysed cross-links, co-localize with pathological lesions in AD brain. More recently, amyloid β-protein oligomerization and aggregation, at physiologic levels *in vitro,* have seen to be induced by the activity of TGs [22]. By these molecular mechanisms, TGs could contribute to AD symptoms and progression. Though the studies mentioned above support the involvement of TG in neurodegeneration, they fail to indicate whether aberrant TG activity, *per se,* directly determines the disease's progression [22].

Factor XIII (FXIII), a plasma TG, besides clot stabilization, plays an important role in wound healing and embryo implantation—a process that involves angiogenesis [74]. Haemostasis and angiogenesis are inter-related as can be seen by the haemostatic proteins assisting the spatial localization and stabilization of endothelial cells, which is succeeded by growth and repair of damaged vessels [74]. Post clot stabilization, the coagulation and fibrinolytic proteins regulate angiogenesis [74]. Thrombin-activated FXIII promotes endothelial cell migration, proliferation and inhibits apoptosis [74]. It is known to bind endothelial cell integrin $\alpha v\beta 3$. This binding enhances the integrin's interaction with VEGFR2, which then activates downstream, the Erk and Akt, thus augmenting cell proliferation [74]. This body of data suggests that there is an altered state of haemostasis that could contribute to AD pathology through angiogenesis.

4. Therapeutic modalities in treating pathogenic angiogenesis in AD

Angiogenesis, as stated by the studies mentioned in this chapter, can be viewed as that stage in AD pathology where all the different pathways (hypoperfusion, BBB dysfunction, inflammation) merge, leading to the AD pathology. Observations showing increased cerebrovascular permeability prior to the appearance of the hallmarks of AD, sprout a novel paradigm for integrating vascular remodelling (angiogenesis) with the pathophysiology of the disease. Targeting this integral step in the pathophysiology of AD and developing a novel therapeutic intervention using anti-angiogenic drugs can help to alleviate the global societal burden of AD.

4.1. Anti-angiogenics: small molecule tyrosine kinase inhibitors

Anti-angiogenics, including small molecule tyrosine kinase inhibitors have been tested and approved as anti-cancer therapeutics and have shown to maintain normal vascular [75–77]. Sunitinib is a broad spectrum tyrosine kinase inhibitor. This is known to inhibit the phosphorylation of multiple receptor tyrosine kinases and is a potent inhibitor of VEGF as well as platelet-derived growth factor (PDGF-β). Currently, it is in use for gastrointestinal stromal tumours, renal cell cancer and pancreatic cancer. Sunitinib was shown to decrease the amyloid burden and reverse cognitive decline in AD model mice, suggesting that if we target angiogenesis, we can revert the increase in the accumulation of Aβ and abate the cognitive decline associated with AD [76].

4.2. Biologics and small molecule VEGFR inhibitors

We now know that VEGF is the prime and central component of pathological blood vessel formation. There are biologics and small molecules that specifically target the ligand or its receptor. This specific-targeted therapy could prove more efficient and less deleterious due to avoidance of unwanted 'off target' effects. A potential therapeutic is Bexarotene, a retinoid X receptor agonist, is shown to facilitate Aβ clearance via activation of apolipoprotein (APOE) expression and promoting microglial phagocytosis [78]. Bexarotene counteracts VEGF-mediated angiogenesis by decreasing blood vessel density and reversing cognitive deficits in AD mice [78].

These are examples of some of the therapeutic routes that could target angiogenesis; however, understanding the molecular mechanism behind angiogenesis causing eventual AD pathology is of utmost importance in order to look for safe and effective novel therapeutics for AD and other vascular diseases.

5. Concluding remarks

As the Western world ages, AD represents an ailment that will place a significant burden on all the aspects of society. This burden, primarily placed on family caregivers, has been estimated to cost billions in lost productivity and healthcare costs (both direct and indirect). Currently, there is a lack of understanding regarding the cause(s) of the disease that translates into a lack of viable treatments or cures. Over the years, limited progress has been made with regards to the clinical translation of the popular amyloid hypothesis for treating AD and hence new thinking towards AD pathogenesis is required. Vascular risk factors and neurovascular dysfunction associated with hypotension, hypertension, cholesterol levels, type II diabetes mellitus, smoking, oxidative stress and iron overload have been found to play integral roles in the pathogenesis of stroke and AD. Observations showing increased cerebrovascular permeability prior to the appearance of the hallmarks of AD, sprout a novel paradigm for integrating vascular remodelling (angiogenesis) with the pathophysiology of the disease. Taking this into account, research focused on understanding the molecular mechanism behind the pathophysiology of angiogenesis leading to AD pathology will mediate in developing novel therapeutic interventions targeting this pathological blood vessel formation help to alleviate the global societal burden of AD.

Author details

Chaahat Singh[1,3], Cheryl G. Pfeifer[1] and Wilfred A. Jefferies[1,2,3,4,5,6*]

*Address all correspondence to: wilf@msl.ubc.ca

1 The Michael Smith Laboratories, University of British Columbia, Vancouver, Canada

2 Department of Microbiology & Immunology, University of British Columbia, Vancouver, Canada

3 Department of Medical Genetics, University of British Columbia, Vancouver, Canada

4 Department of Zoology, University of British Columbia, Vancouver, Canada

5 Centre for Blood Research, University of British Columbia, Vancouver, Canada

6 Djavad Mowafaghian Centre for Brain Health, University of British Columbia, Vancouver, Canada

References

[1] WHO: Dementia—Fact sheet. April 2016. http://www.who.int/mediacentre/factsheets/fs362/en/

[2] Alzheimer A: About a peculiar disease of the cerebral cortex. By Alois Alzheimer, 1907 (Translated by L. Jarvik and H. Greenson). Alzheimer Dis Assoc Disord 1987, 1:3–8.

[3] Glenner GG, Wong CW: Alzheimer's disease: initial report of the purification and characterization of a novel cerebrovascular amyloid protein. Biochem Biophys Res Commun 1984, 120:885–90.

[4] Glenner GG, Wong CW: Alzheimer's disease: initial report of the purification and characterization of a novel cerebrovascular amyloid protein. Biochem Biophys Res Commun 2012, 425:534–9.

[5] Gorevic PD, Goni F, Pons-Estel B, Alvarez F, Peress NS, Frangione B: Isolation and partial characterization of neurofibrillary tangles and amyloid plaque core in Alzheimer's disease: immunohistological studies. J Neuropathol Exp Neurol 1986, 45:647–64.

[6] Hardy JA, Higgins GA: Alzheimer's disease: the amyloid cascade hypothesis. Science 1992, 256:184–5.

[7] Thinakaran G, Koo EH: Amyloid precursor protein trafficking, processing, and function. J Biol Chem 2008, 283:29615–9.

[8] Citron M, Oltersdorf T, Haass C, McConlogue L, Hung AY, Seubert P, Vigo-Pelfrey C, Lieberburg I, Selkoe DJ: Mutation of the beta-amyloid precursor protein in familial Alzheimer's disease increases beta-protein production. Nature 1992, 360:672–4.

[9] Haass C, Lemere CA, Capell A, Citron M, Seubert P, Schenk D, Lannfelt L, Selkoe DJ: The Swedish mutation causes early-onset Alzheimer's disease by beta-secretase cleavage within the secretory pathway. Nat Med 1995, 1:1291–6.

[10] Haass C, De Strooper B: The presenilins in Alzheimer's disease—proteolysis holds the key. Science 1999, 286:916–9.

[11] Attems J, Jellinger KA: The overlap between vascular disease and Alzheimer's disease —lessons from pathology. BMC Med 2014, 12:206.

[12] Biron KE, Dickstein DL, Gopaul R, Jefferies WA: Amyloid triggers extensive cerebral angiogenesis causing blood brain barrier permeability and hypervascularity in Alzheimer's disease. PLoS One 2011, 6:e23789.

[13] Jefferies WA, Price KA, Biron KE, Fenninger F, Pfeifer CG, Dickstein DL: Adjusting the compass: new insights into the role of angiogenesis in Alzheimer's disease. Alzheimers Res Ther 2013, 5:64.

[14] Claassen JA, Zhang R: Cerebral autoregulation in Alzheimer's disease. J Cereb Blood Flow Metab 2011, 31:1572–7.

[15] Li D, Parks SB, Kushner JD, Nauman D, Burgess D, Ludwigsen S, Partain J, Nixon RR, Allen CN, Irwin RP, Jakobs PM, Litt M, Hershberger RE: Mutations of presenilin genes in dilated cardiomyopathy and heart failure. Am J Hum Genet 2006, 79:1030–9.

[16] Jefferies WA, Food MR, Gabathuler R, Rothenberger S, Yamada T, Yasuhara O, McGeer PL: Reactive microglia specifically associated with amyloid plaques in Alzheimer's disease brain tissue express melanotransferrin. Brain Res 1996, 712:122–6.

[17] Yamada T, Tsujioka Y, Taguchi J, Takahashi M, Tsuboi Y, Moroo I, Yang J, Jefferies WA: Melanotransferrin is produced by senile plaque-associated reactive microglia in Alzheimer's disease. Brain Res 1999, 845:1–5.

[18] Feldman H, Gabathuler R, Kennard M, Nurminen J, Levy D, Foti S, Foti D, Beattie BL, Jefferies WA: Serum p97 levels as an aid to identifying Alzheimer's disease. J Alzheimers Dis 2001, 3:507–16.

[19] Kennard ML, Feldman H, Yamada T, Jefferies WA: Serum levels of the iron binding protein p97 are elevated in Alzheimer's disease. Nat Med 1996, 2:1230–5.

[20] Sala R, Jefferies WA, Walker B, Yang J, Tiong J, Law S, Carlevaro MF, Di Marco E, Vacca A, Cancedda R: The human melanoma associated protein melanotransferrin promotes endothelial cell migration and angiogenesis in vivo. Eur J Cell Biol 2002, 81:599–607.

[21] Yamada T, Yoshiyama Y, Kawaguchi N, Ichinose A, Iwaki T, Hirose S, Jefferies W: Possible roles of transglutaminases in Alzheimer's disease. Dementia Geriatr Cogn Disorder 1998, 9:103–10.

[22] Martin A, De Vivo G, Gentile V: Possible role of the transglutaminases in the pathogenesis of Alzheimer's disease and other neurodegenerative diseases. Int J Alzheimers Dis 2011, 2011:865432.

[23] Rosenberg GA: Blood-brain barrier permeability in aging and Alzheimer's disease. J Prev Alzheimers Dis 2014, 1:138–9.

[24] Ujiie M, Dickstein D, Carlow D, Jefferies WA: Blood-brain barrier permeability precedes senile plaque formation in an Alzheimer disease model. Microcirculation 2003, 10:463–70.

[25] Kook SY, Seok Hong H, Moon M, Mook-Jung I: Disruption of blood-brain barrier in Alzheimer disease pathogenesis. Tissue Barriers 2013, 1:e23993.

[26] Erickson MA, Banks WA: Blood-brain barrier dysfunction as a cause and consequence of Alzheimer's disease. J Cereb Blood Flow Metab 2013, 33:1500–13.

[27] Vagnucci AH, Jr., Li WW: Alzheimer's disease and angiogenesis. Lancet 2003, 361:605–8.

[28] Banks WA, Gray AM, Erickson MA, Salameh TS, Damodarasamy M, Sheibani N, Meabon JS, Wing EE, Morofuji Y, Cook DG, Reed MJ: Lipopolysaccharide-induced blood-brain barrier disruption: roles of cyclooxygenase, oxidative stress, neuroinflammation, and elements of the neurovascular unit. J Neuroinflamm 2015, 12:223.

[29] Arai T, Miklossy J, Klegeris A, Guo JP, McGeer PL: Thrombin and prothrombin are expressed by neurons and glial cells and accumulate in neurofibrillary tangles in Alzheimer disease brain. J Neuropathol Exp Neurol 2006, 65:19–25.

[30] Zipser BD, Johanson CE, Gonzalez L, Berzin TM, Tavares R, Hulette CM, Vitek MP, Hovanesian V, Stopa EG: Microvascular injury and blood-brain barrier leakage in Alzheimer's disease. Neurobiol Aging 2007, 28:977–86.

[31] Lewczuk P, Wiltfang J, Lange M, Jahn H, Reiber H, Ehrenreich H: Prothrombin concentration in the cerebrospinal fluid is not altered in Alzheimer's disease. Neurochem Res 1999, 24:1531–4.

[32] Desai BS, Schneider JA, Li JL, Carvey PM, Hendey B: Evidence of angiogenic vessels in Alzheimer's disease. J Neural Transm 2009, 116:587–97.

[33] Austin BP, Nair VA, Meier TB, Xu G, Rowley HA, Carlsson CM, Johnson SC, Prabhakaran V: Effects of hypoperfusion in Alzheimer's disease. J Alzheimers Dis 2011, 26 Suppl 3:123–33.

[34] Thomas T, Miners S, Love S: Post-mortem assessment of hypoperfusion of cerebral cortex in Alzheimer's disease and vascular dementia. Brain 2015, 138:1059–69.

[35] Olichney JM, Hansen LA, Galasko D, Saitoh T, Hofstetter CR, Katzman R, Thal LJ: The apolipoprotein E epsilon 4 allele is associated with increased neuritic plaques and

cerebral amyloid angiopathy in Alzheimer's disease and Lewy body variant. Neurology 1996, 47:190–6.

[36] Verghese PB, Castellano JM, Holtzman DM: Apolipoprotein E in Alzheimer's disease and other neurological disorders. Lancet Neurol 2011, 10:241–52.

[37] Zlokovic BV: The blood-brain barrier in health and chronic neurodegenerative disorders. Neuron 2008, 57:178–201.

[38] D'Esposito M, Jagust W, Gazzaley A: Methodological and conceptual issues in the study of the aging brain: Oxford University Press, Oxford, UK, 2009.

[39] Selkoe DJ: Toward a comprehensive theory for Alzheimer's disease. Hypothesis: Alzheimer's disease is caused by the cerebral accumulation and cytotoxicity of amyloid beta-protein. Ann N Y Acad Sci 2000, 924:17–25.

[40] Kara F, Dongen ES, Schliebs R, Buchem MA, Groot HJ, Alia A: Monitoring blood flow alterations in the Tg2576 mouse model of Alzheimer's disease by *in vivo* magnetic resonance angiography at 17.6 T. Neuroimage 2012, 60:958–66.

[41] Beckmann N, Schuler A, Mueggler T, Meyer EP, Wiederhold KH, Staufenbiel M, Krucker T: Age-dependent cerebrovascular abnormalities and blood flow disturbances in APP23 mice modeling Alzheimer's disease. J Neurosci 2003, 23:8453–9.

[42] Thal DR, Capetillo-Zarate E, Larionov S, Staufenbiel M, Zurbruegg S, Beckmann N: Capillary cerebral amyloid angiopathy is associated with vessel occlusion and cerebral blood flow disturbances. Neurobiol Aging 2009, 30:1936–48.

[43] Pfeifer LA, White LR, Ross GW, Petrovitch H, Launer LJ: Cerebral amyloid angiopathy and cognitive function: the HAAS autopsy study. Neurology 2002, 58:1629–34.

[44] de la Torre JC, Mussivand T: Can disturbed brain microcirculation cause Alzheimer's disease? Neurol Res 1993, 15:146–53.

[45] de la Torre JC: How do heart disease and stroke become risk factors for Alzheimer's disease? Neurol Res 2006, 28:637–44.

[46] Rose JA, Erzurum S, Asosingh K: Biology and flow cytometry of proangiogenic hematopoietic progenitors cells. Cytometry A 2015, 87:5–19.

[47] Patan S: Vasculogenesis and angiogenesis. Cancer Treat Res 2004, 117:3–32.

[48] Herbert SP, Stainier DY: Molecular control of endothelial cell behaviour during blood vessel morphogenesis. Nat Rev Mol Cell Biol 2011, 12:551–64.

[49] Chiarini A, Whitfield J, Bonafini C, Chakravarthy B, Armato U, Dal Pra I: Amyloid-beta (25–35), an amyloid-beta (1–42) surrogate, and proinflammatory cytokines stimulate VEGF-A secretion by cultured, early passage, normoxic adult human cerebral astrocytes. J Alzheimers Dis 2010, 21:915–26.

[50] Pogue AI, Lukiw WJ: Angiogenic signaling in Alzheimer's disease. Neuroreport 2004, 15:1507–10.

[51] Meyer EP, Ulmann-Schuler A, Staufenbiel M, Krucker T: Altered morphology and 3D architecture of brain vasculature in a mouse model for Alzheimer's disease. Proc Natl Acad Sci U S A 2008, 105:3587–92.

[52] Schultheiss C, Blechert B, Gaertner FC, Drecoll E, Mueller J, Weber GF, Drzezga A, Essler M: *In vivo* characterization of endothelial cell activation in a transgenic mouse model of Alzheimer's disease. Angiogenesis 2006, 9:59–65.

[53] Selkoe DJ: The cell biology of beta-amyloid precursor protein and presenilin in Alzheimer's disease. Trends Cell Biol 1998, 8:447–53.

[54] Selkoe DJ: Translating cell biology into therapeutic advances in Alzheimer's disease. Nature 1999, 399:A23–31.

[55] de la Torre JC: Alzheimer's disease: how does it start? J Alzheimers Dis 2002, 4:497–512.

[56] Mielke R, Schroder R, Fink GR, Kessler J, Herholz K, Heiss WD: Regional cerebral glucose metabolism and postmortem pathology in Alzheimer's disease. Acta Neuropathol 1996, 91:174–9.

[57] Davis DG, Schmitt FA, Wekstein DR, Markesbery WR: Alzheimer neuropathologic alterations in aged cognitively normal subjects. J Neuropathol Exp Neurol 1999, 58:376–88.

[58] Morris GP, Clark IA, Vissel B: Inconsistencies and controversies surrounding the amyloid hypothesis of Alzheimer's disease. Acta Neuropathol Commun 2014, 2:135.

[59] Biron KE, Dickstein DL, Gopaul R, Fenninger F, Jefferies WA: Cessation of neoangiogenesis in Alzheimer's disease follows amyloid-beta immunization. Sci Rep 2013, 3:1354.

[60] Cortes-Canteli M, Paul J, Norris EH, Bronstein R, Ahn HJ, Zamolodchikov D, Bhuvanendran S, Fenz KM, Strickland S: Fibrinogen and beta-amyloid association alters thrombosis and fibrinolysis: a possible contributing factor to Alzheimer's disease. Neuron 2010, 66:695–709.

[61] Zamolodchikov D, Strickland S: Abeta delays fibrin clot lysis by altering fibrin structure and attenuating plasminogen binding to fibrin. Blood 2012, 119:3342–51.

[62] Paul J, Strickland S, Melchor JP: Fibrin deposition accelerates neurovascular damage and neuroinflammation in mouse models of Alzheimer's disease. J Exp Med 2007, 204:1999–2008.

[63] Fioravanzo L, Venturini M, Di Liddo R, Marchi F, Grandi C, Parnigotto PP, Folin M: Involvement of rat hippocampal astrocytes in beta-amyloid-induced angiogenesis and neuroinflammation. Curr Alzheimer Res 2010, 7:591–601.

[64] Boulton ME, Cai J, Grant MB: gamma-Secretase: a multifaceted regulator of angiogenesis. J Cell Mol Med 2008, 12:781–95.

[65] Boscolo E, Folin M, Nico B, Grandi C, Mangieri D, Longo V, Scienza R, Zampieri P, Conconi MT, Parnigotto PP, Ribatti D: Beta amyloid angiogenic activity *in vitro* and *in vivo*. Int J Mol Med 2007, 19:581–7.

[66] Johnston H, Boutin H, Allan SM: Assessing the contribution of inflammation in models of Alzheimer's disease. Biochem Soc Trans 2011, 39:886–90.

[67] Yan SD, Chen X, Fu J, Chen M, Zhu H, Roher A, Slattery T, Zhao L, Nagashima M, Morser J, Migheli A, Nawroth P, Stern D, Schmidt AM: RAGE and amyloid-beta peptide neurotoxicity in Alzheimer's disease. Nature 1996, 382:685–91.

[68] Mackic JB, Stins M, McComb JG, Calero M, Ghiso J, Kim KS, Yan SD, Stern D, Schmidt AM, Frangione B, Zlokovic BV: Human blood-brain barrier receptors for Alzheimer's amyloid-beta 1–40. Asymmetrical binding, endocytosis, and transcytosis at the apical side of brain microvascular endothelial cell monolayer. J Clin Invest 1998, 102:734–43.

[69] Stern D, Yan SD, Yan SF, Schmidt AM: Receptor for advanced glycation endproducts: a multiligand receptor magnifying cell stress in diverse pathologic settings. Adv Drug Deliv Rev 2002, 54:1615–25.

[70] Deane R, Du Yan S, Submamaryan RK, LaRue B, Jovanovic S, Hogg E, Welch D, Manness L, Lin C, Yu J, Zhu H, Ghiso J, Frangione B, Stern A, Schmidt AM, Armstrong DL, Arnold B, Liliensiek B, Nawroth P, Hofman F, Kindy M, Stern D, Zlokovic B: RAGE mediates amyloid-beta peptide transport across the blood-brain barrier and accumulation in brain. Nat Med 2003, 9:907–13.

[71] McMichael M: New models of hemostasis. Top Companion Anim Med 2012, 27:40–5.

[72] Versteeg HH, Heemskerk JW, Levi M, Reitsma PH: New fundamentals in hemostasis. Physiol Rev 2013, 93:327–58.

[73] Martin A, Giuliano A, Collaro D, De Vivo G, Sedia C, Serretiello E, Gentile V: Possible involvement of transglutaminase-catalyzed reactions in the physiopathology of neurodegenerative diseases. Amino Acids 2013, 44:111–8.

[74] Inbal A, Dardik R: Role of coagulation factor XIII (FXIII) in angiogenesis and tissue repair. Pathophysiol Haemost Thromb 2006, 35:162–5.

[75] Powles T, Chowdhury S, Jones R, Mantle M, Nathan P, Bex A, Lim L, Hutson T: Sunitinib and other targeted therapies for renal cell carcinoma. Br J Cancer 2011, 104:741–5.

[76] Grammas P, Martinez J, Sanchez A, Yin X, Riley J, Gay D, Desobry K, Tripathy D, Luo J, Evola M, Young A: A new paradigm for the treatment of Alzheimer's disease: targeting vascular activation. J Alzheimers Dis 2014, 40:619–30.

[77] Barrascout E, Medioni J, Scotte F, Ayllon J, Mejean A, Cuenod CA, Tartour E, Elaidi R, Oudard S: Angiogenesis inhibition: review of the activity of sorafenib, sunitinib and bevacizumab. Bull Cancer 2010, 97:29–43.

[78] Tousi B: The emerging role of bexarotene in the treatment of Alzheimer's disease: current evidence. Neuropsychiatr Dis Treat 2015, 11:311–5.

Section 2

Angiogenesis in the Cardiovascular System

Chapter 7

Hypoxia, Angiogenesis and Atherogenesis

Lamia Heikal and Gordon Ferns

Additional information is available at the end of the chapter

http://dx.doi.org/10.5772/66714

Abstract

The balance between vascular oxygen supply and metabolic demand for oxygen within the vasculature is tightly regulated. An imbalance leads to hypoxia and a consequential cascade of cellular signals that attempt to offset the effects of hypoxia. Hypoxia is invariably associated with atherosclerosis, wound repair, inflammation and vascular disease. There is now substantial evidence that hypoxia plays an essential role in angiogenesis as well as plaque angiogenesis. It controls the metabolism, and responses of many of the cell types found within the developing plaque and whether the plaque will evolve into a stable or unstable phenotype. Hypoxia is characterized in molecular terms by the stabilization of hypoxia-inducible factor (HIF)-1α, a subunit of the heterodimeric nuclear transcriptional factor HIF-1 and a master regulator of oxygen homeostasis. The expression of HIF-1 is localized to perivascular tissues, inflammatory macrophages and smooth muscle cells where it regulates several genes that are important to vascular function including vascular endothelial growth factor, nitric oxide synthase, endothelin-1 and erythropoietin. This chapter summarizes the effects of hypoxia on the functions of cells involved in angiogenesis as well as atherogenesis (plaque angiogenesis) and the evidence for its potential importance from experimental models and clinical studies.

Keywords: hypoxia, HIF-1, proliferation, atherosclerosis, plaque formation, blood vessel

1. Introduction

The circulatory system develops early in mammalian embryogenesis. An oxygen supply is essential for normal tissue function, development and homeostasis. The vascular network within the cardiovascular system is essential for the delivery of oxygen, nutrients and other molecules to the tissues of the body [1]. Oxygen availability serves as an important regulator of the cardiovascular system. Oxygen balance may be perturbed if there is reduced oxygen diffusion, or increased oxygen consumption that may be a consequence of rapid cellular division during embryonic development, by tumour growth, or by vasculature dysfunction due to vessel occlusion or rupture [2].

Hypoxia is defined by a reduced oxygen tension relative to those normally extant within a particular tissue. It has multiple impacts on the vascular system and cell function [3]. The effects of moderate hypoxia (3–5% O_2) are usually reversible and are usually accompanied by adaptive physiological responses in the cells. A lower oxygen tension (0–1% O_2) contributes to the pathophysiology of tumour progression and cell apoptosis [4] and is a feature of conditions that include cancer, ischemic heart disease, peripheral artery disease, wound healing and neovascular retinopathy. Hypoxia promotes vessel growth by stimulating an upregulation of multiple proangiogenic pathways that mediate key aspects of endothelial, stromal and vascular support cell biology. The role of hypoxia in human disease is now becoming increasingly clear [5] including the association between hypoxia and endothelial dysfunction that affects several cellular processes and signal transduction.

Hypoxia can occur in several ways: (1) hypoxic hypoxia is caused by an insufficient oxygen concentration in the air in the lungs, which may occur during sleep apnea, when the diffusion of oxygen to the blood is reduced, or at high altitude; (2) hypoxemic hypoxia occurs when the blood has reduced transport capacity as seen in carbon monoxide poisoning when haemoglobin cannot carry oxygen at its normal concentrations; (3) stagnant hypoxia results when the cardiac output does not match the demands of the body and the flow is not sufficient to deliver enough oxygenated blood to the tissue and (4) histotoxic hypoxia occurs when cells cannot utilize the available oxygen, for example following cyanide poisoning when oxygen cannot be used to produce ATP as the mitochondrial electron transport is inhibited.

Chronic tissue hypoxia (an oxygen tension of 2–3% for a prolonged period of time) may cause uncontrolled proliferation of cells. When physiological oxygen concentrations are restored, the increased blood flow supplies excessive oxygen; this may then lead to increased free-radical generation, tissue damage and concomitant activation of stress-response genes; a condition known as 'reoxygenation injury'. In these circumstances, normal cells/tissues may not survive; but tumour cells are still able to proliferate despite the hypoxic milieu, as they have developed genetic and adaptive changes leading to resistance to hypoxia [6].

Hypoxia plays important roles in normal human physiology and development. For example, it is integral to normal embryonic development. Whatever the cause, or the severity of hypoxia, it leads to an induction of adaptive responses within the endothelial and vascular smooth muscle cells through the activation of genes that participate in angiogenesis, cell proliferation/survival and in glucose and iron metabolism [7].

In healthy vascular tissue, vascular smooth muscle cells (SMCs) and endothelial cells (ECs) proliferate at very low levels. However, SMCs and ECs can be stimulated to re-enter the cell cycle in response to several physiological and pathological stimuli. Hypoxia is considered an important stimulus of SMC and EC proliferation and is found in atherosclerotic lesions and rapidly growing tumours [4].

The proliferation of ECs is pivotal to the formation of new micro-vessels and is important during organ development in embryogenesis and tumour growth, and also contributes to diabetic retinopathy, psoriasis, rheumatoid arthritis and atherosclerosis. Abnormal SMC proliferation contributes to atherosclerosis, intimal hyperplasia after angioplasty and graft atherosclerosis after coronary transplantation [8, 9].

2. Consequences of hypoxia

Most cells are able to survive under hypoxic conditions through the transcriptional activation of a series of genes. The oxygen-sensitive transcriptional activator, hypoxia-inducible factor-1 (HIF-1) is the key transcriptional mediator of the hypoxic response and master regulator of O_2 homeostasis. It orchestrates the profound changes in cellular transcription that accompanies hypoxia by controlling the expression of numerous angiogenic, metabolic and cell cycle genes. Accordingly, the HIF pathway is currently viewed as a master regulator of angiogenesis [5].

HIF-1 is normally only found in hypoxic cells. It is a heterodimer that is composed of an O_2-regulated HIF-1α subunit and a constitutively expressed HIF-1β subunit [10]. In the α-subunit, there is an oxygen-dependent degradation (ODD) domain, where the 4-hydroxyproline formation is catalysed by proline-hydroxylase-2 (PHD-2). This leads to its ubiquitination by the von Hippel-Lindau E3 ubiquitin ligase (VHL) and subsequent proteasomal degradation under normoxic cellular conditions. This prevents the formation of a functional HIF dimer [11]. Since PHDs require oxygen for their catalytic activity, and function as cellular oxygen sensors, HIF degradation only occurs under normoxic conditions. Factor inhibiting HIF-1 (FIH) protein, which hydroxylates HIF-1, also contributes to HIF-1 inactivation in normoxic conditions, and thereby prevents the interaction of this subunit with the two transcriptional co-activators of HIF-1: p300 and CREB-binding protein (CBP) which are essential for HIF-1 transcription. Expression and stabilization of the HIF-1 complex is also regulated through feedback inhibition, as PHD-2 itself is activated by HIF-1 [12].

Under hypoxic conditions, HIF-1 protein is stable and active as the hydroxylase, VHL proteins, and FIH are all inhibited by a lack of oxygen. HIF-1 is then able to interact with its co-activators and can dimerize with its constitutively expressed β-subunit [12]. Once stabilized, the HIF-1 protein can bind to the regulatory regions of its target genes, inducing their expression; these target genes include VEGF (vascular endothelial growth factor) [13], erythropoietin [14] and nitric oxide synthase (NOS) [15, 16] and other proangiogenic factors such as PlGF (placental growth factor), or angiopoietins [12] (**Figure 1**).

It has been proposed that the induction of a pseudo-hypoxic response by inhibiting HIF prolyl 4-hydroxylases may provide a novel therapeutic target in the treatment of hypoxia-associated diseases [17].

Several small molecules, such as dimethyloxalyl glycine [18], Roxadustat (FG-4592) [19] and ZYAN1 [20], have been developed to inhibit prolyl hydroxylase domain-containing (PHD) enzymes, and cause HIF activation [21]. These agents have been applied to the treatment of renal anaemia in which there is a deficiency of erythropoietin [22, 23]. The administration of

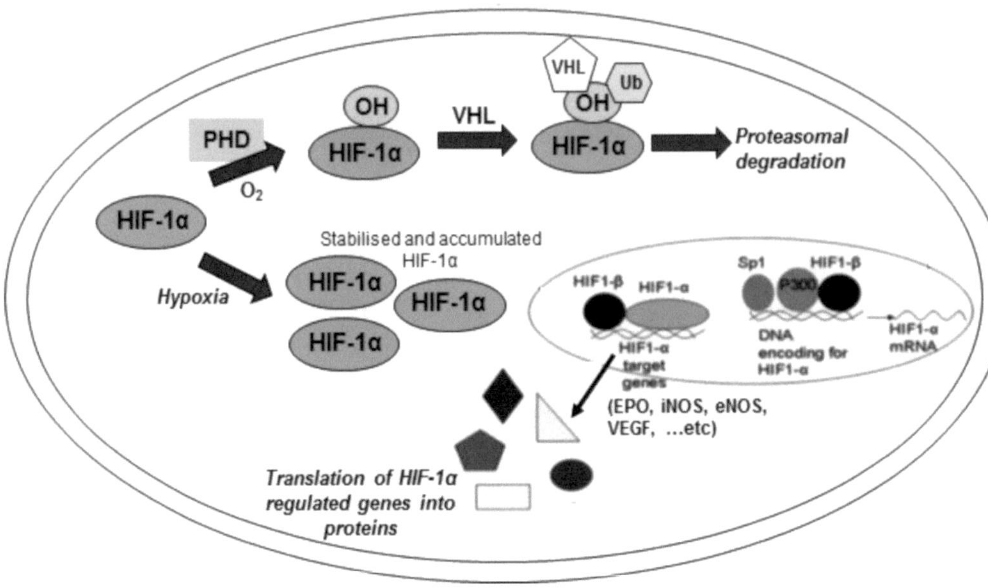

Figure 1. Regulation of the hypoxia-inducible transcription factor (HIF-1α) pathway. Under normal oxygen tensions (normoxia), prolyl hydroxylase (PHD) enzymes, von Hippel-Lindau protein (pVHL), the ubiquitin ligase complex (Ub) and factor inhibiting HIF-1 (FIH) are active leading to HIF-1α proteasomal degradation. Under hypoxic conditions, PHD, pVHL and Ub are not active leading to its cytoplasmic accumulation of HIF-1α. The HIF-1α gene is transcribed in the nucleus with the help of specificity protein (Sp) 1, P300, and HIF-1β leading to transcription of HIF target genes such as EPO, NOS and VEGF.

these compounds is associated with an improved iron profile and an increase of endogenous erythropoietin production to near the physiological range. The clinical trials currently underway aim to address whether PHD enzyme inhibitors will improve clinical end-points, including cardiovascular events [24]. PHD inhibitors have been reported to reduce blood pressure [22] and plasma cholesterol concentrations [19]. Hence, there is a good reason to believe that some PHD inhibitors will reduce cardiovascular endpoints in patients with renal disease. Whether they will benefit a broader category of patients with high risk of cardiovascular disease is difficult to predict.

Hydroxylase activity can be also rescued by mutating specific regions, or by adding cobalt ions to the cell, the latter of which presumably compete for iron-binding sites. Some hydroxylases in the prolyl family can be selectively inhibited by Adriamycin *in vitro*. Cobalt (II) and nickel (II) ions increase HIF-1 activity in cells, presumably because these ions displace iron from the active sites of 2-oxo-glutarate (2OG) hydroxylases [12].

It has been shown that HIF-1α can be regulated by non-hypoxic stimuli such as lipopolysaccharides (LPS), thrombin and angiotensin II (Ang II) [25]. Hormones such as angiotensin II and platelet-derived growth factor stimulate the HIF pathway by increasing HIF-1α protein levels through production of reactive oxygen species (ROS) within the cell. Although the exact mechanism for this is unclear, it appears to be entirely distinct from the hypoxia pathways.

Thrombin and other growth factors appear to increase angiogenesis through HIF-1α protein agonist mechanisms. Insulin similarly activates HIF-1α through the action of multiple protein kinases necessary for expression and function. p53 is responsible for promoting ubiquitination of HIF-1α, and may be an another possible target for enhancing HIF-1. Homozygous deletion of the p53 gene has been found to cause HIF-1 activation [26]. Gene therapy may eventually be used to increase HIF-1 levels and relieve complications of ischemia. For example, delivery of a stabilized, recombinant form of HIF-1α through adeno-associated virus (AAV) in order to overexpress HIF-1 has been shown to result in significantly increased capillary density in skeletal muscle [27]. While gene therapy approaches aimed at the process and effects of angiogenesis continue to be developed and studied, higher levels of success in preclinical trials currently are being sought before clinical applications are pursued. Amongst the remaining obstacles in using gene therapy for this purpose is the effective mode of delivery [12]. Inhibition of PHD2 using siRNA has been shown to decrease cardiac infarction size in murine models [28, 29].

In addition to HIF-1α, there are two other members of HIF superfamily that have been described: HIF-2 and HIF-3 [30]. Both are important regulators of the hypoxia response with similar actions as HIF-1 [31] and lead to the transcriptional activation of target genes in hypoxia [32]. However, Eubank et al demonstrated opposing roles for the HIFs in tumour angiogenesis, with HIF-1 exhibiting proangiogenic properties that act through its effects on VEGF secretion, whereas HIF-2 exhibits anti-angiogenic activity by inducing the production of the endogenous angiogenesis inhibitor, sVEGFR-1 [33]. HIF-3α has complementary functions, rather than redundant to HIF-1α induction in protection against hypoxic damage in alveolar epithelial cells in protection against hypoxic damage in alveolar epithelial cells [34].

Although the oxygen-sensing mechanism involving oxygen-dependent hydroxylation of the HIF-α subunits is probably a universal mechanism in cells, and has been highly conserved during evolution, additional regulatory steps appear to determine which of the alternative subunits is induced [34]. One of the best studied hypoxic responses that will be discussed in this chapter is the induction of angiogenic factors and growth factors, which lead to the formation and growth of new blood vessels.

3. Hypoxia and angiogenesis

Blood vessels formation occurs through two basic mechanisms: (1) vasculogenesis represents de novo formation of blood vessels, and is derived from endothelial progenitors and (2) angiogenesis and arteriogenesis (formation of blood vessels from pre-existing blood vessels).

Angiogenesis is a tightly regulated multi-step process that begins when cells within a tissue respond to hypoxia. When tissues grow beyond the physiological oxygen diffusion limit, the relative hypoxia triggers expansion of vascular beds by inducing angiogenic factors in the cells of the vascular beds, which are physiologically oxygenated by simple diffusion of oxygen. Angiogenesis may be a physiological process, as in the case in embryonic development, wound healing or vessel penetration into avascular regions. It may also be pathological, for example when it occurs during the formation of solid tumours, eye disease, chronic inflammatory disorders such as rheumatoid arthritis, psoriasis and periodontitis and atherosclerosis.

The regulation of angiogenesis (whether in physiological or pathological cases) by hypoxia is an important component of homeostatic mechanisms that link vascular oxygen supply to metabolic demand. An understanding of the processes involved in angiogenic, the role of the interacting proteins involved, and how all this is regulated by hypoxia through an ever-expanding number of pathways in multiple cell types may lead to the identification of novel therapies and modalities for ischemic vascular diseases as well as diseases characterized by excessive angiogenesis, such as rheumatoid arthritis, psoriasis, tumours, ischemic brain and heart attack [5, 6].

Angiogenesis in hypoxia is regulated by several pro- and anti-angiogenic factors [1]. HIF-1 has been established as the major inducer of angiogenesis [35]. It regulates the transcription of VEGF, a major regulator of angiogenesis which promotes endothelial cell migration towards the hypoxic area. During hypoxia, HIF-1 binds to the regulatory region of the VEGF gene, inducing its transcription and initiating its expression. VEGF is then secreted and binds to cognate receptor tyrosine kinases (VEGFR1 and VEGFR2) located on the surface of vascular endothelial cells triggering a cascade of intracellular signalling pathways that initiate angiogenesis [10]. These endothelial cells are recruited to form new blood vessels which ultimately supply the given area with oxygenated blood [12]. Interestingly, recent studies have shown that hypoxia influences additional aspects of angiogenesis, including vessel patterning, maturation and function [5].

Other factors such as angiopoietin-2/angiopoietin-1 [36, 37], angiopoietin receptor (Tie2) [38], platelet-derived growth factor (PDGF) [39], basic fibroblast growth factor (bFGF) [40] and monocyte chemoattractant protein 1 (MCP-1) [41] have also been reported to be responsible not only for increasing vascular permeability, endothelial sprouting, maintenance, differentiation and remodelling but also cell proliferation, migration, enhancement of endothelial assembly and lumen formation (**Figure 2**). In hypoxia, angiogenesis is also modulated by several factors that are secreted by leucocytes, which produce a high abundance of angiogenic factors, various interleukins such as TGF-β1 and MCP-1 and proteinases [42]. Thus, hypoxia provides an important environmental stimulus not only for angiogenesis but also for related phenomena in the hypoxic or surrounding area, suggesting that hypoxia is more than simply a regulator of angiogenesis [6].

Angiogenesis may be detrimental when it is excessive. Therefore, angiogenic factors must be highly active but also be tightly regulated. Angiogenesis that is associated with pathological consequences may exhibit differences in the responsible molecular pathways in comparison to physiological angiogenesis. Mutations in oncogenes and tumour suppressor genes and disruptions in growth factor activity play an important role in tumour angiogenesis. The activation of the most prominent proangiogenic factor VEGF might be due to physiological stimuli such as hypoxia or inflammation or due to oncogene activation and tumour suppression function loss. Physiological angiogenesis that occurs during embryonic development or wound healing seems to be dependent on VEGF signalling, whereas tumour angiogenesis adopts

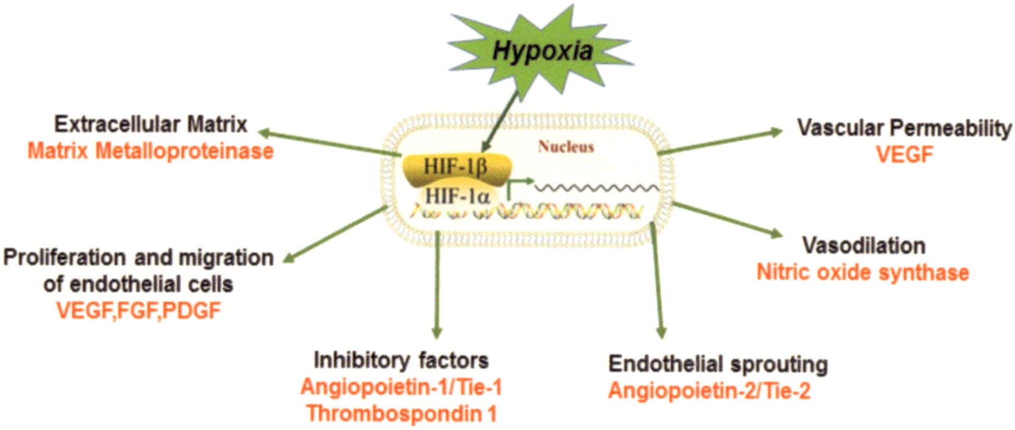

Figure 2. HIF-1α regulates factors involved in developmental and pathological angiogenesis. HIF-1α directly regulates genes involved in steps such as vasodilation, increased vascular permeability, extracellular matrix remodelling and proliferation.

the ability to shift its dependence from VEGF to other proangiogenic pathways, for example, through the recruitment of myeloid cells and the upregulation of alternative vascular growth factors (PlGF and FGF) [1].

The identification of alternative ways of inhibiting tumour growth by disrupting the growth-triggering mechanisms of increasing vascular supply through angiogenesis will depend on the understanding of how tumour cells develop their own vasculature. Other cofactors are essential to ensure maximum efficiency of the transcriptional machinery related to changes in oxygen availability within cells/tissues, and the roles of different HIFs in eliciting hypoxic responses seem to be more divergent as originally assumed. Chen et al. have shown new regulatory interactions of HIF-related mechanisms involving the interactions of basic HIFs, HIF-1α and HIF-2α with their regulatory binding proteins, histone deacetylase 7 (HDAC7) and translation initiation factor 6 (Int6), respectively [6]. Int6 induces HIF- 2 degradation. In addition, silencing of *Int6* produces a potent, physiological induction of angiogenesis that may be useful in the treatment of diseases related to insufficient blood supply. The newly discovered binding proteins-HDAC7 for HIF-1 and Int6 for HIF-2 support the assumption that the 2 HIF isoforms play distinct roles in eliciting hypoxia-related responses. HIF-2 may be considered as one of the master switches for inducing angiogenic factors at least in some cell types [6].

The hypoxia/reoxygenation cycle leads to the formation of reactive oxygen species (ROS) that may subsequently regulate HIF-1 but in a rather complex manner. It has been suggested that ROS promote angiogenesis, either directly through stimulation of HIF-1 genes that are involved in stimulating angiogenesis, such as NOS and NADPH oxidase orthrough the generation of active oxidation products, including lipid peroxides. ROS are associated with the development of several chronic diseases that include atherosclerosis, type 2 diabetes mellitus, and cancer [43]. Although ROS have damaging effects on tissues, causing cell death at high concentrations, lesser degrees of oxidative stress may play a positive role during angiogenesis, or other pathophysiological processes. Angiogenesis induced by oxidative stress involves vascular endothelial growth factor (VEGF) signalling, although VEGF-independent pathways have also been identified [44].

The clinical importance of this biological process has become increasingly apparent over the last decade, and angiogenesis now represents a major focus for novel therapeutic approaches to the prevention and treatment of multiple diseases, most notably ischemic cardiovascular disease and cancer [10].

4. Atherosclerosis and plaque angiogenesis

Considering the important contributions of HIF-1 in angiogenesis, it may also be a promising target for treating ischaemic disease [1] and pressure-overload heart failure [45].

Atherosclerosis causes clinical disease through the occlusion of the arteries as a result of excessive build-up of plaque within the artery wall resulting from the accumulation of cholesterol, fatty material and extracellular matrix. This causes obstruction in the blood flow to the myocardium (coronary heart disease), brain (ischemic stroke) or lower extremities (peripheral vascular). The most common of these manifestations is coronary heart disease that includes stable angina pectoris and the acute coronary syndromes [46].

Coronary heart disease (CHD) is a major cause of mortality globally (1 in every 6 deaths annually). An estimated £2bn per annum is used to treat CHD and its co-morbidities [47]. Arterial injury plays a key role in the initiation and progression of CHD [48]. Treatments for CHD range from lifestyle changes and non-invasive medical therapies to pharmacological therapies and open surgical interventions. Despite the widespread use of drugs such as statins, there remains a significant proportion of individuals for whom response to therapy is sub-optimal, and who develop atherosclerosis [49, 50].

Atherosclerosis is a lipoprotein-driven disease affecting medium and large arteries that leads to plaque formation at specific sites of the arterial tree through intimal inflammation, necrosis, fibrosis and calcification. It is a chronic inflammatory process that involves increased oxidative stress, endothelial damage, and smooth muscle cell proliferation and migration. It is associated with several established risk factors, including hypertension, hyperglycaemia, ageing and dyslipidaemia [51]. It is important to control the factors involved in the progression of atherosclerosis because advanced atherosclerotic lesions are prone to rupture, leading to disability or death. Plaque at risk of rupture has been a major focus of research [52]. There is an emerging need for new therapies to stabilize atherosclerotic lesions. Further understanding of the effects of hypoxia in atherosclerotic lesions could indicate potential therapeutic targets [53, 54]. The presence of hypoxia in human carotid atherosclerotic lesions correlates with angiogenesis. Hypoxia plays a key role in the progression and development of advanced lesions by promoting lipid accumulation, increased inflammation, ATP depletion and angiogenesis. A recent study has convincingly demonstrated the presence of hypoxia in macrophage-rich regions of advanced human carotid atherosclerotic lesions [53].

http://dx.doi.org/10.5772/66714

4.1. Evidence for hypoxia within atherosclerotic plaque

Hypoxia in atherosclerotic plaques is now widely recognized, because of the use of specific probes in imaging studies [4]. Imaging plaque hypoxia could provide a means of assessing putative culprit lesions that are at risk of rupture, and are consequentially liable to adverse outcomes.

Hypoxia has been consistently found in atherosclerotic plaques *in vivo* in humans and animal models using different biomarkers [55]. The immunologically identifiable hypoxia marker, 7-(4″-(2-nitroimidazole-1-yl)-butyl)-theophylline (NITP), has been used to assess hypoxia in three murine models *in vivo*. NITP can bind to cells under low-oxygen conditions [56, 57].

Other non-invasive imaging techniques have also been applied, which directly target plaque hypoxia, and these techniques are now being further validated in human studies. The metabolic marker F-fluorodeoxyglucose (FDG) has been used to detect human atherosclerosis *in vivo* and may also serve as an indirect marker of plaque hypoxia as the enhanced glucose uptake in anaerobic metabolism results in an increased uptake of the labelled FDG [58]. F-18-fluoromisonidazole positron emission tomographic (PET) has been used for the *in vivo* assessment of hypoxia in advanced aortic atherosclerosis in rabbits where hypoxia has been found to be predominantly confined to the macrophage-rich regions within the atheromatous core, whereas the macrophages close to the lumen were hypoxia negative [47]. This was then related to hypoxia assessed by *ex vivo* tissue staining using pimonidazole, and immuno-staining for macrophages (RAM-11), new vessels (CD31) and hypoxia-inducible factor-1 α. ^{18}F-fluoromisonidazole (^{18}F-FMISO), a cell permeable 2-nitroimidazole derivative that is reduced i*n vivo* by nitroreductases, regardless of the intracellular oxygen concentration, has been one of the leading radiotracers for imaging hypoxia [47]. In human studies, this imaging approach has been coupled with quantitative polymerase chain reaction (qPCR) and immune-staining of plaques tissues recovered by carotid endarterectomy to determine the gene expression of HIF-1α and cluster of differentiation 68 (CD68, a marker of inflammation). HIF-1α and CD68 expression were both found to be significantly correlated with F-FDG-uptake, indicating an association between the presence of hypoxia, inflammation and increased glucose metabolism *in vivo* [59].

Imaging plaque biomarkers such as CRP, interleukins 6, 10 and 18, soluble CD40 ligand, P- and E-selectin, NT-proBNP, fibrinogen and cystatin C show great potential in the prediction and improvement for vascular patients [60].

4.2. The development of a hypoxic environment within the atherosclerotic plaque

Hypoxia has been identified as a potential factor in the formation of vulnerable plaque, and it is clear that decreased oxygen plays a role in the development of plaque angiogenesis leading to plaque destabilization [61]. There have been a number of hypotheses of atherogenesis (plaque angiogenesis) proposing that an imbalance between the demand for and supply of oxygen in the arterial wall is a key factor in the development of atherosclerosis [2, 62].

During atherogenesis, the intima (the innermost layer of the artery wall) may thicken by the accumulation of cells and matrix, and the diffusion of oxygen can then become impaired. The vasa vasorum, forming the network of small blood vessels, are vulnerable to hypoxia especially at the site of arterial branching as they are end arteries and the blood flow is reduced in this region. It has been hypothesized that hypoxia within the vasa vasorum is due to reduced blood flow and consequent endothelial dysfunction, local inflammation and permeation of large particles such as microbes, LDL-lipoprotein and fatty acids which are transformed by macrophages into foam cells [63, 64], which may be an initiating factor in atherosclerosis [65]. Therefore, the micro-environment within the atherosclerotic plaque is thought to be an important determinant of whether a plaque progresses, and the likelihood of clinical complications. Recent reports provide substantial evidence that there are regions within the plaque in which hypoxia can be identified [46].

In addition to being a marker of hypoxia, HIF-1α may directly enhance atherogenesis through several mechanisms, including smooth muscle cell proliferation and migration, new vessel formation (angiogenesis) and altered lipid metabolism [66]. The effects of HIF-1α on macrophage biology and subsequent promotion of atherogenesis has been studied in mice. HIF-1α expression in macrophages affects their intrinsic inflammatory profile and promotes the development of atherosclerosis [67]. Hence, HIF-1α may play a key role in the progression of atherosclerosis by initiating and promoting the formation of foam cells, endothelial cell dysfunction, apoptosis, increasing inflammation and angiogenesis [68].

It has been also proposed that the state of hypoxia, present in the atherosclerotic plaques of mice deficient in apolipoprotein E (ApoE$^{-/-}$ mice), may promote lipid synthesis, and reduce cholesterol efflux through the ATP-binding cassette transporter (ABCA1) pathway: processes that are known to be mediated by HIF-1α [55]. Hypoxia has also been reported to increase the formation of lipid droplets in macrophages to promote the secretion of inflammatory mediators, and atherosclerotic lesion progression by exacerbating ATP depletion and lactate accumulation in this model of atherosclerosis [53].

Several HIF-responsive genes have been found to be upregulated in atherosclerosis, such as VEGF, endothelin-1 and matrix-metalloproteinase-2 [69]. Hypoxia has the potential to fundamentally change the function, metabolism and responses of many of the cell types found within the developing atherosclerotic plaque, and this may in turn determine whether the plaque evolves into a stable or unstable phenotype. It is likely that this is mediated through effects on angiogenesis, extracellular matrix elaboration and lipoprotein metabolism. The hypoxic milieu in the atherosclerotic plaque may therefore also have implications for the putative therapeutic interventions for atherosclerosis. However, most *in vitro* studies have been conducted under normoxic conditions. The effects observed under these conditions may not accurately reflect those extant within the plaque [69].

The role of HIF-1 in atherosclerosis is not univocal. Silencing of HIF-1α in macrophages reduces proinflammatory factors and increases macrophage apoptosis. Hyperlipidaemia impairs angiogenesis in an HIF-1b and nuclear factor (NF)-κB-dependent manner. Specific knockdown of HIF-1α in endothelial cells reduces atherosclerosis through reduced monocyte recruitment [26], whereas knockdown in antigen-presenting cells results in aggravation of atherosclerosis through T-cell polarization [70]. There is another non-lipid-driven mechanism by which alternative macrophages present in human atherosclerosis M(Hb) promote plaque neoangiogenesis and microvessel incompetence throughan HIF-1α/VEGF-A-dependent pathway [71].

HIF-1α has also been also implicated in the pathogenesis of in-stent restenosis following coronary revascularisation, stroke, peripheral artery disease, aortic aneurysm formation and pulmonary artery hypertension [72], and also appears to be involved in the calcification of blood vessels, which often accompanies atherosclerosis [73]. Despite being an intracellular transcription factor, HIF-1 could be possible released into the circulation from damaged cells, similar to other transcriptional factors such as NF-κB and p53 [73-75].

4.3. Other atherogenic mechanisms of hypoxia

Although plaque angiogenesis is a physiological response that facilitates the increased oxygen demand in the plaque, it can have adverse effects by facilitating intra-plaque haemorrhage (IPH) and the influx of inflammatory mediators. IPH as a result of immature plaque neovessels is associated with subsequent ischemic events. Inflammatory cell, endothelial cell and pericyte interactions can provide insight into the biological mechanisms of plaque angiogenesis [70].

The recruitment of T lymphocytes and proliferation and migration of smooth muscle and endothelial cells are essential for atherosclerotic plaque formation and development. During this process, a number of pro-inflammatory factors and cytokines, leukotrienes and chemokines are increased in expression, especially in lipid-loaded foam cells, such as IL8, tumour necrosis factor α (TNFα), interleukin (IL)-1,vascular cell adhesion molecule 1 (VCAM-1) and 15-lipoxygenase-2 (15-LOX-2). Moreover, macrophages are trapped in hypoxic areas of the lesion; however, the exact mechanisms have yet to be determined.

The majority of inflammatory cells contributing to early atherosclerosis probably enter the artery wall from the lumen [76, 77]. However, the vasa vasorum and associated microvessels may provide an alternate route by which leucocytes can enter the vascular wall [78]. As atherosclerosis progresses, angiogenic factors within the micro-environment of the plaque may stimulate new vessel formation. This combination of delicate new vessel network and inflammatory cells, that elaborate proteolytic enzymes, may contribute to intra-plaque haemorrhage and subsequent plaque rupture [79]. The involvement of vasa vasorum and intimal hyperplasia in the pathophysiology of atherosclerosis is supported by several experimental animal studies [80, 81].

Hypoxia may also induce macrophage migration inhibitory factor (MIF). MIF plays a critical role in the progression of atherosclerosis by several different mechanisms. These include the MIF-triggered arrest and chemotaxis of monocytes and T cells through its receptors CXCR2/4. Further, *in vivo* studies have shown that the blockade of MIF in mice with advanced atherosclerosis leads to plaque regression and reduced monocyte and T-cell content. Additionally, the neuronal signalling molecule Netrin-1 was recently shown to play an important role in macrophage retention in atherosclerotic plaques. Notably, netrin-1 expression has been shown to be regulated by hypoxia, but this may be tissue or disease specific [55].

Atherosclerotic lesion formation is associated with vessel wall thickening resulting in regional limited oxygen exchange. Vascular cells respond to hypoxic conditions with changes in cell metabolism, angiogenesis, apoptosis and inflammatory responses comparable to cells in tumours. Local hypoxic regions and hypoxic cells have been identified in human atherosclerotic lesions and in experimental models. Increased oxygen consumption by cells with a high metabolic activity, such as macrophages, further depletes the oxygen availability, creating a hypoxic environment in the atherosclerotic lesion. In macrophages, hypoxia not only affects the metabolism and lipid uptake but also results in an increased inflammatory response characterized by increased IL-1β and caspase-1 activation. Hypoxia also augments the thrombogenic potential of atherosclerotic plaques through upregulation of tissue factor.

The identification of specific inflammatory markers pertaining to the arterial wall in atherosclerosis may be useful for both diagnosis and treatment. These include macrophage inhibiting factor (MIF), leucocytes and P-selectin. Purinergic signalling is involved in the control of vascular tone and remodelling. Endothelial cells release purines and pyrimidines in response to changes in blood flow (evoking shear stress) and hypoxia. They then act on P2Y, P2X and P1 receptors on endothelial cells leading to release of EDRF mediated by nitric oxide and prostaglandins and EDHF, resulting in vasodilatation. The therapeutic potential of purinergic compounds for the treatment of vascular diseases, including hypertension, ischaemia, atherosclerosis, migraine and coronary artery and diabetic vascular disease as well as vasospasm is discussed [82]. Modern therapeutic modalities involving endothelial progenitor cells therapy, angiotensin II type-2 (AT2R) and ATP-activated purinergic receptor therapy are notable to mention. Future drugs may be designed to target three signalling mechanisms of AT2R which are (a) activation of protein phosphatases resulting in protein dephosphorylation, (b) activation of bradykinin/nitric oxide/cyclic guanosine 3″,5″-monophosphate pathway by vasodilation and (c) stimulation of phospholipase A(2) and release of arachidonic acid. Drugs may also be designed to act on ATP-activated purinergic receptor channel type P2X7 molecules which acts on cardiovascular system. Better understanding of the vascular inflammatory processes and the cells involved in the formation of plaques may prove to be beneficial for future diagnosis, clinical treatment and planning innovative novel anti-atherosclerotic drugs [83].

Systemic hypoxia that is, for example, associated with obstructive sleep apnoea (OSA) also promotes atherosclerosis. The processes by which it may do this include effects on lipid metabolism and efflux, inflammation, altered macrophage polarization and glucose metabolism [84].

5. Conclusion

Hypoxia is involved in several pathophysiological processes, including embryogenesis, angiogenesis and atherogenesis. HIF-1 appears to be an important mediator controlling cellular response to hypoxia. It also appears to be related to atherosclerotic progression and rupture. A better understanding of the mechanism involved in these processes may provide some novel therapeutic approaches to the treatment of cardiovascular disease.

Author details

Lamia Heikal * and Gordon Ferns

*Address all correspondence to: l.heikal@bsms.ac.uk

Brighton and Sussex Medical School, University of Sussex, Brighton, United Kingdom

References

[1] Zimna A and Kurpisz M. Hypoxia-inducible factor-1 in physiological and pathophysiological angiogenesis: applications and therapies. BioMed Research International. 2015;**2015**:13DOI: 10.1155/2015/549412

[2] Bjornheden T, Levin M, Evaldsson M and Wiklund O. Evidence of hypoxic areas within the arterial wall in vivo. Arteriosclerosis, Thrombosis and Vascular Biology. 1999;**19** (4):870-6 (4PT).

[3] Michiels C, Deleener F, Arnould T, Dieu M and Remacle J. Hypoxia stimulates human endothelial cells to release smooth muscle cell mitogens–role of prostaglandins and BFGF. Experimental Cell Research. 1994;**213**(1):43–54. DOI: 10.1006/excr.1994.1171

[4] Humar R, Kiefer FN, Berns H, Resink TJ and Battegay EJ. Hypoxia enhances vascular cell proliferation and angiogenesis in vitro via rapamycin (mTOR) -dependent signaling. The FASEB Journal. 2002;**16**(8):771–780. DOI: 10.1096/fj.01-0658com

[5] Krock BL, Skuli N and Simon MC. Hypoxia-induced angiogenesis: good and evil. Genes & Cancer. 2011;**2**(12):1117–33. DOI: 10.1177/1947601911423654

[6] Chen L, Endler A and Shibasaki F. Hypoxia and angiogenesis: regulation of hypoxia-inducible factors via novel binding factors. Experimental and Molecular Medicine. 2009;**41**:849–857.

[7] Chan CK and Vanhoutte PM. Hypoxia, vascular smooth muscles and endothelium. Acta Pharmaceutica Sinica B. 2013;**3**(1):1–7. DOI: 10.1016/j.apsb.2012.12.007

[8] Singh RB, Mengi SA, Xu Y-J, Arneja AS and Dhalla NS. Pathogenesis of atherosclerosis: a multifactorial process. Experimental & Clinical Cardiology. 2002;**7**(1):40–53.

[9] Cines DB, Pollak ES, Buck CA, et al.. Endothelial cells in physiology and in the pathophysiology of vascular disorders. Blood. 1998;**91**(10):3527–3561.

[10] Semenza GL. Regulation of hypoxia-induced angiogenesis: a chaperone escorts VEGF to the dance. The Journal of Clinical Investigation. 2014;**108**(1):39–40. DOI: 10.1172/JCI13374

[11] Goggins BJ, Chaney C, Radford-Smith GL, Horvat JC and Keely S. Hypoxia and integrin-mediated epithelial restitution during mucosal inflammation. Frontiers in Immunology. 2013;**4**DOI: 10.3389/fimmu.2013.00272

[12] Ziello JE, Jovin IS and Huang Y. Hypoxia-inducible factor (HIF)-1 regulatory pathway and its potential for therapeutic intervention in malignancy and ischemia. The Yale Journal of Biology and Medicine. 2007;**80**(2):51–60.

[13] Ahluwalia A and Tarnawski AS. Critical role of hypoxia sensor HIF-1 alpha in VEGF gene activation. Implications for angiogenesis and tissue injury healing. Current Medicinal Chemistry. 2012;**19**(1):90–97.

[14] Fandrey J. Oxygen-dependent and tissue-specific regulation of erythropoietin gene expression. American Journal of Physiology–Regulatory, Integrative and Comparative Physiology. 2004;**286**(6):R977–R988. DOI: 10.1152/ajpregu.00577.2003

[15] Heikal L, Ghezzi P, Mengozzi M, Stelmaszczuk B, Feelisch M and Ferns GAA. Erythropoietin and a nonerythropoietic peptide analog promote aortic endothelial cell repair under hypoxic conditions: role of nitric oxide. Hypoxia. 2016;**4**:121–133.

[16] Heikal L, Ghezzi P, Mengozzi M and Ferns G. Low oxygen tension primes aortic endothelial cells to the reparative effect of tissue-protective cytokines. Molecular Medicine. 2015;**21**:709–716. DOI: 10.2119/molmed.2015.00162

[17] Myllyharju J. Prolyl 4-hydroxylases, master regulators of the hypoxia response. Acta Physiologica. 2013;**208**(2):148–165. DOI: 10.1111/apha.12096

[18] Milkiewicz M, Pugh CW and Egginton S. Inhibition of endogenous HIF inactivation induces angiogenesis in ischaemic skeletal muscles of mice. The Journal of Physiology. 2004;**560**(1):21–26. DOI: 10.1113/jphysiol.2004.069757

[19] Provenzano R, Besarab A, Sun CH, et al. Oral hypoxia-inducible factor prolyl hydroxylase inhibitor roxadustat (FG-4592) for the treatment of anemia in patients with CKD. Clinical Journal of the American Society of Nephrology. 2016;**11**(6):982–991. DOI: 10.2215/cjn.06890615

[20] Jain MR, Joharapurkar AA, Pandya V, et al. Pharmacological characterization of ZYAN1, a novel prolyl hydroxylase inhibitor for the treatment of anemia. Drug Research. 2016;**66**(2):107–112. DOI: 10.1055/s-0035-1554630

[21] Beuck S, Schaenzer W and Thevis M. Hypoxia-inducible factor stabilizers and other small-molecule erythropoiesis-stimulating agents in current and preventive doping analysis. Drug Testing and Analysis. 2012;**4**(11):830–845. DOI: 10.1002/dta.390

[22] Yousaf F and Spinowitz B. Hypoxia-inducible factor stabilizers: a new avenue for reducing BP while helping hemoglobin?. Current Hypertension Reports. 2016;**18**(3)DOI: 10.1007/s11906-016-0629-6

[23] Forristal CE, Winkler IG, Nowlan B, Barbier V, Walkinshaw G and Levesque JP.. Pharmacologic stabilization of HIF-1α increases hematopoietic stem cell quiescence in vivo and accelerates blood recovery after severe irradiation. Blood. 2013;**121**(5):759–769. DOI: 10.1182/blood-2012-02-408419

[24] Maxwell PH and Eckardt KU. HIF prolyl hydroxylase inhibitors for the treatment of renal anaemia and beyond. Nature Reviews in Nephrology. 2016;**12**(3):157–168. DOI: 10.1038/nrneph.2015.193

[25] Kuschel A, Simon P and Tug S. Functional regulation of HIF-1a under normoxi-auis there more than post-translational regulation?. Journal of Cellular Physiology. 2012;**227**(2):514–524. DOI: 10.1002/jcp.22798

[26] Pajusola K, Kunnapuu J, Vuorikoski S, et al. Stabilized HIF-1 alpha is superior to VEGF for angiogenesis in skeletal muscle via adeno-associated virus gene transfer. Faseb Journal. 2005;**19**(8):1365. DOI: 10.1096/fj.05-3720fje

[27] Tsurumi Y, Takeshita S, Chen DF, et al. Direct intramuscular gene transfer of naked DNA encoding vascular endothelial growth factor augments collateral development and tissue perfusion. Circulation. 1996;**94**(12):3281–3290.

[28] Eckle T, Köhler D, Lehmann R, El Kasmi KC and Eltzschig HK. Hypoxia-inducible factor-1 is central to cardioprotection. A New Paradigm for Ischemic Preconditioning. 2008;**118**(2):166–175. DOI: 10.1161/circulationaha.107.758516

[29] Tekin D, Dursun AD and Xi L. Hypoxia inducible factor 1 (HIF-1) and cardioprotection. Acta Pharmacologica Sinica. 2010;**31**(9):1085–1094. DOI: 10.1038/aps.2010.132

[30] Zhao J, Du F, Shen G, Zheng F and Xu B. The role of hypoxia-inducible factor-2 in digestive system cancers. Cell Death Disease. 2015;**6**:e1600. DOI: 10.1038/cddis.2014.565

[31] Agnieszka L, Alicja J and Jozef D. HIF-1 and HIF-2 transcription factors - similar but not identical. Molecules and Cells. 2010;**29**(5):435–442.

[32] Carroll VA and Ashcroft M. Role of hypoxia-inducible factor (HIF)-1 alpha-versus HIF-2 alpha in the regulation of HIF target genes in response to hypoxia, insulin-like growth factor-1, or loss of von Hippel-Lindau function: implications for targeting the HIF pathway. Cancer Research. 2006;**66**(12):6264–6270. DOI: 10.1158/0008-5472.can-05-2519

[33] Eubank TD, Roda JM, Liu HW, O'Neil T and Marsh CB. Opposing roles for HIF-1 alpha and HIF-2 alpha in the regulation of angiogenesis by mononuclear phagocytes. Blood. 2011;**117**(1):323–332. DOI: 10.1182/blood-2010-01-261792

[34] Li QF, Wang XR, Yang YW and Lin H. Hypoxia upregulates hypoxia inducible factor (HIF)-3 alpha expression in lung epithelial cells: characterization and comparison with HIF-1 alpha. Cell Research. 2006;**16**(6):548–558. DOI: 10.1038/sj.cr.7310072

[35] Pugh CW and Ratcliffe PJ. Regulation of angiogenesis by hypoxia: role of the HIF system. Nature Medicine. 2003;**9**(6):677–684.

[36] Graham CH, Fitzpatrick TE and McCrae KR. Hypoxia stimulates urokinase receptor expression through a heme protein-dependent pathway. Blood. 1998;**91**(9):3300–3307.

[37] Phelan MW, Forman LW, Perrine SP and Faller DV. Hypoxia increases thrombospondin-1 transcript and protein in cultured endothelial cells. Journal of Laboratory and Clinical Medicine. 1998;**132**(6):519–529. DOI: 10.1016/s0022-2143(98)90131-7

[38] Kuwabara K, Ogawa S, Matsumoto M, et al. Hypoxia-mediated induction of acidic/basic fibroblast growth factor and platelet derived growth factor in mononuclear phagocytes stimulates growth of hypoxic endothelial cells. Proceedings of the National Academy of Sciences of the United States of America. 1995;**92**(10):4606–4610. DOI: 10.1073/pnas.92.10.4606

[39] Wykoff CC, Pugh CW, Maxwell PH, Harris AL and Ratcliffe PJ. Identification of novel hypoxia dependent and independent target genes of the von Hippel-Lindau (VHL) tumour suppressor by mRNA differential expression profiling. Oncogene. 2000;**19**(54):6297–6305. DOI: 10.1038/sj.onc.1204012

[40] Sakuda H, Nakashima Y, Kuriyama S and Sueishi K. Media conditioned by smooth muscle cells cultured in a variety of hypoxic environments stimulates in vitro angiogenesis-a relationship to transforming growth factor-beta-1. American Journal of Pathology. 1992;**141**(6):1507–1516.

[41] Phillips PG, Birnby LM and Narendran A. Hypoxia induces capillary network formation in cultured bovine pulmonary microvessel endothelial cells. American Journal of Physiology-Lung Cellular and Molecular Physiology. 1995;**268**(5):L789–L800.

[42] Norrby K. Mast cells and angiogenesis. Apmis. 2002;**110**(5):355–371. DOI: 10.1034/j.1600-0463.2002.100501.x

[43] Goerlach A, Dimova EY, Petry A, et al. Reactive oxygen species, nutrition, hypoxia and diseases: Problems solved?. Redox Biology. 2015;**6**:372–385. DOI: 10.1016/j.redox.2015.08.016

[44] Kim YW and Byzova TV.. Oxidative stress in angiogenesis and vascular disease. Blood. 2014;**123**(5):625–631. DOI: 10.1182/blood-2013-09-512749

[45] Semenza G L. Hypoxia-inducible factor 1 and cardiovascular disease. Annual Review of Physiology. 2014;**76**:39–56. DOI: 10.1146/annurev-physiol-021113-170322

[46] Lahoz C and Mostaza JM. Atherosclerosis as a systemic disease. Revista Espanola De Cardiologia. 2007;**60**(2):184–195. DOI: 10.1157/13099465

[47] Mateo J, Izquierdo-Garcia D, Badimon JJ, Fayad ZA and Fuster V. Noninvasive assessment of hypoxia in rabbit advanced atherosclerosis using (18)F-fluoromisonidazole PET imaging. Circulation. Cardiovascular imaging. 2014;**7**(2):312–320. DOI: 10.1161/CIRCIMAGING.113.001084

[48] Varani J and Ward PA. Mechanisms of endothelial cell injury in acute inflammation. Shock. 1994;**2**(5):311–319.

[49] Andrade PJ, Medeiros MM, Andrade AT, Lima AA. Coronary angioplasty versus CABG: review of randomised trials. Arquivos Brasileiros De Cardiologia. 2011;**97**(3):E60–E69.

[50] Solomon AJ, Gersh BJ. Management of chronic stable angina: medical therapy, percutaneous transluminal coronary angioplasty and coronary artery bypass graft surgery-Lessons from randomized trials. Annals of Internal Medicine. 1998;**128**(3):216–223.

[51] Xiao W, Jia Z, Zhang Q, Wei C, Wang H and Wu Y. Inflammation and oxidative stress, rather than hypoxia, are predominant factors promoting angiogenesis in the initial phases of atherosclerosis. Molecular Medical Report. 2015;**12**(3):3315–3322. DOI: 10.3892/mmr.2015.3800

[52] Nie XY, Randolph GJ, Elvington A, et al. Imaging of hypoxia in mouse atherosclerotic plaques with Cu-64-ATSM. Nuclear Medicine and Biology. 2016;**43**(9):534–542. DOI: 10.1016/j.nucmedbio.2016.05.011

[53] Hulten LM and Levin M. The role of hypoxia in atherosclerosis. Current Opinion in Lipidology. 2009;**20**(5):409–414. DOI: 10.1097/MOL.0b013e3283307be8

[54] Van der Veken B, De Meyer GRY and Martinet W. Intraplaque neovascularization as a novel therapeutic target in advanced atherosclerosis. Expert Opinion on Therapeutic Targets. 2016;**20**(10):1247–1257. DOI: 10.1080/14728222.2016.1186650

[55] Parathath S, Yang Y, Mick S and Fisher EA. Hypoxia in murine atherosclerotic plaques and its adverse effects on macrophages. Trends in Cardiovascular Medicine. 2013;**23**(3):80–84. DOI: 10.1016/j.tcm.2012.09.004

[56] Bjornheden T, Evaldsson M and Wiklund O. A method for the assessment of hypoxia in the arterial wall, with potential application in vivo. Arteriosclerosis, Thrombosis and Vascular Biology. 1996;**16**(1):178–185.

[57] Webster L, Hodgkiss RJ and Wilson GD. Cell cycle distribution of hypoxia and progression of hypoxic tumour cells in vivo. British Journal of Cancer. 1998;**77**(2):227–234.

[58] Buscombe JR. Exploring the nature of atheroma and cardiovascular inflammation in vivo using positron emission tomography (PET). British Journal of Radiology. 2015;**88**(1053) DOI: 10.1259/bjr.20140648

[59] Pedersen SF, Grabe M, Hag AMF, Hojgaard L, Sillesen H and Kjar A. (18)F-FDG imaging of human atherosclerotic carotid plaques reflects gene expression of the key hypoxia marker HIF-1alpha. American Journal of Nuclear Medicine and Molecular Imaging. 2013;**3**(5):384–92.

[60] van Lammeren GW, Moll FL, Borst GJD, de Kleijn DPV, de Vries JPPM and Pasterkamp G.. Atherosclerotic plaque biomarkers: beyond the horizon of the vulnerable plaque. Current Cardiology Reviews. 2011;**7**(1):22–27. DOI: 10.2174/157340311795677680

[61] Sluimer JC and Daemen MJ. Novel concepts in atherogenesis: angiogenesis and hypoxia in atherosclerosis. Journal of Pathology. 2009;**218**(1):7–29. DOI: 10.1002/path.2518

[62] Gainer JL. Hypoxia and atherosclerosis. Re-evaluation of the old hypothesis. Atherosclerosis. 1987;**68**(3):263–266. DOI: 10.1016/0021-9150(87)90206-1

[63] Jarvilehto M and Tuohimaa P. Vasa vasorum hypoxia: initiation of atherosclerosis. Medical Hypotheses. 2009;**73**(1):40–41. DOI: 10.1016/j.mehy.2008.11.046

[64] Barger AC, Beeuwkes R, Lainey LL and Silverman KJ. Hypothesis-vasa vasorum and neovascularisation of human coronary arteries- a possible role in the path-physiology of atherosclerosis. New England Journal of Medicine. 1984;**310**(3):175–177. DOI: 10.1056/nejm198401193100307

[65] Ferns G and Heikal L. Atherogenesis and hypoxia. Angiology. 2016; August 27:1-22. DOI: 10.1177/0003319716662423

[66] Lim CS, Kiriakidis S, Sandison A, Paleolog EM and Davies AH. Hypoxia-inducible factor pathway and diseases of the vascular wall. Journal of Vascular Surgery. 2013;**58**(1):219–230. DOI: 10.1016/j.jvs.2013.02.240

[67] Aarup A, Pedersen TX, Junker N, et al. Hypoxia-inducible factor-1α expression in macrophages promotes development of atherosclerosis. Arteriosclerosis, Thrombosis, and Vascular Biology. 2016; 36:1782-1790;DOI: 10.1161/atvbaha.116.307830

[68] Gao L, Chen Q, Zhou X and Fan L. The role of hypoxia-inducible factor 1 in atherosclerosis. Journal of Clinical Pathology. 2012;**65**(10):872–876. DOI: 10.1136/jclinpath-2012-200828

[69] Sluimer JC, Gasc J-M, van Wanroij JL, et al. Hypoxia, hypoxia-inducible transcription factor, and macrophages in human atherosclerotic plaques are correlated with intraplaque angiogenesis. Journal of the American College of Cardiology. 2008;**51**(13):1258–1265. DOI: 10.1016/j.jacc.2007.12.025

[70] de Vries MR and Quax PHA. Plaque angiogenesis and its relation to inflammation and atherosclerotic plaque destabilisation. Current Opinion in Lipidology. 2016;**27**(5):499–506.

[71] Finn AV, Akahori H, Guo L, et al. Alternative macrophages promote intraplaque angiogenesis and vascular permeability in human atherosclerosis. Journal of the American College of Cardiology. 2016;**67**(13):2241–2241.

[72] Kasivisvanathan V, Shalhoub J, Lim CS, Shepherd AC, Thapar A and Davies AH. Hypoxia-inducible factor-1 in arterial disease: a putative therapeutic target. Current Vascular Pharmacology. 2011;**9**(3):333–349.

[73] Li G, Lu W-h, Ai R, Yang J-h, Chen F and Tang Z. The relationship between serum hypoxia-inducible factor 1 alpha and coronary artery calcification in asymptomatic type 2 diabetic patients. Cardiovascular Diabetology. 2014;**13**DOI: 10.1186/1475-2840-13-52

[74] Ismail S, Mayah W, Battia HE, et al. Plasma nuclear factor kappa B and serum peroxiredoxin 3 in early diagnosis of hepatocellular carcinoma. Asian Pacific Journal of Cancer Prevention: APJCP. 2015;**16**(4):1657–63.

[75] Attallah AM, Abdel-Aziz MM, El-Sayed AM and Tabll AA. Detection of serum p53 protein in patients with different gastrointestinal cancers. Cancer Detection and Prevention. 2003;**27**(2):127–131. DOI: http://dx.doi.org/10.1016/S0361-090X(03)00024-2

[76] Faggiotto A, Ross R and Harker L. Studies of hypercholesterolemia in the non-human primate. 1. Changes that lead to fatty streak formation. Arteriosclerosis. 1984;**4**(4):323–340.

[77] Ross R. Mechanisms of disease - atherosclerosis - an inflammatory disease. New England Journal of Medicine. 1999;**340**(2):115–126.

[78] Rademakers T, Douma K, Hackeng TM, et al. Plaque-associated vasa vasorum in aged apolipoprotein E-deficient mice exhibit proatherogenic functional features In Vivo. Arteriosclerosis, Thrombosis and Vascular Biology. 2013;**33**(2):249–256. DOI: 10.1161/atvbaha.112.300087

[79] Moreno PR, Purushothaman KR, Zias E, Sanz J and Fuster V. Neovascularization in human atherosclerosis. Current Molecular Medicine. 2006;**6**(5):457–477. DOI: 10.2174/156652406778018635

[80] Barker SGE, Talbert A, Cottam S, Baskerville PA and Martin JF. Arterial intimal hyperplasia after occlusion of the adventitial vasa vasorum in the pig. Arteriosclerosis and Thrombosis. 1993;**13**(1):70–77.

[81] Khurana R, Zhuang Z, Bhardwaj S, et al. Angiogenesis-dependent and independent phases of intimal hyperplasia. Circulation. 2004;**110**(16):2436–2443. DOI: 10.1161/01.cir.0000145138.25577.f1

[82] Burnstock G. Purinergic signalling and endothelium. Current Vascular Pharmacology. 2016;**14**(2):130–145. DOI: 10.2174/1570161114666151202204948

[83] Thent ZC, Chakraborty C, Mahakkanukrauh P, Kosai N, Rajan R and S D. The molecular concept of atheromatous plaques. Current Drug Target. 2016; 17: 1–9.

[84] Marsch E, Sluimer JC and Daemen MJAP. Hypoxia in atherosclerosis and inflammation. Current Opinion in Lipidology. 2013;**24**(5):393–400. DOI: 10.1097/MOL.0b013e32836484a4

Chapter 8

Coronary Collateral Growth: Clinical Perspectives and Recent Insights

Bhamini Patel, Peter Hopmann, Mansee Desai,
Kanithra Sekaran, Kathleen Graham, Liya Yin and
William Chilian

Additional information is available at the end of the chapter

http://dx.doi.org/10.5772/67164

Abstract

This chapter summarizes recent research on the coronary collateral circulation. The chapter is focused on clinical perspectives and importance of a well-developed coronary collateral circulation, the mechanisms of growth induced by chemical factors and a role for stem cells in the process. Some discussion is devoted to the role of shear stress and mechanical signaling, but because this topic has been reviewed so extensively in the recent past, there is only small mention of its role in the growth of the coronary collateral circulation.

Keywords: arteriogenesis, coronary collateral, ischemic heart disease

1. Introduction

Although arteriogenesis has been studied for approximately a hundred years, there are still fundamental unanswered questions about the causes of collateral vessel growth, and whether different factors control growth at varying points in the maturation process. One line of investigation, spurred by the myriad contributions of Schaper and his colleagues have focused on mechanical shear stress being the main factor that stimulates collateral growth [1–4]. Although this hypothesis is well-founded on a large body of experimental data, it does not explain other observations that show collateral growth in the absence of altered shear stress [5, 6]. Accordingly investigators have proposed that ischemia (via cytokine, chemokine, and growth factor expression), and the consequential inflammation, is the cause of collateral growth, but assessing it has proven to be difficult due to the unclear lines between ischemic regions, normal circulation, and collateral growth. The hypotheses regarding the causative factor(s) for collateral growth are not mutually exclusive as there are likely many mechanisms that are the principal driver, which vary at various points of the process. For example, even if one maintains that ischemia is the initiating mechanism for collateral growth, it is likely that other stimuli continue the growth of the vessel after the ischemic stimulus has waned. To provide perspective for this chapter, we refer to **Figure 1**, which summarizes four factors that exert important effects in this adaptive process. The bulk of this chapter will focus on the collateral growth from a clinical perspective, the role of stem cells, and chemical factors involved in this process. We will not extensively review the role that shear stress in coronary collateral growth as this has been reviewed ample times in the past. We also will not review the genetic aspects because the bulk of this information has been derived from studies of collateral growth in vascular beds other than the heart, e.g., skeletal muscle and brain [7, 8], although there is some preliminary information about genetic links to collateral growth in patients [9]. **Figure 1** also shows the anatomical structure of a collateral; namely, an arterial-arterial anastomosis that connect large coronary perfusion territories. Collateral growth, also known as arteriogenesis, in the heart involves the abluminal expansion of a preexisting arterial-arterial anastomosis [10]. The degree of expansion is profound—the caliber of collateral vessels can increase over an order of magnitude [10]. This degree of expansion would greatly reduce vascular resistance of these vessels, thereby increasing flow in the area of risk. This increase in flow is the reason why the collateral circulation exerts beneficial effects through the reduction in infarct size (following a coronary occlusive event) and reduction in the incidence of sudden cardiac death.

We also would like to point out an obvious distinction between the growth of collateral vessels (arteriogenesis) and angiogenesis. These processes are often confused as the same, but

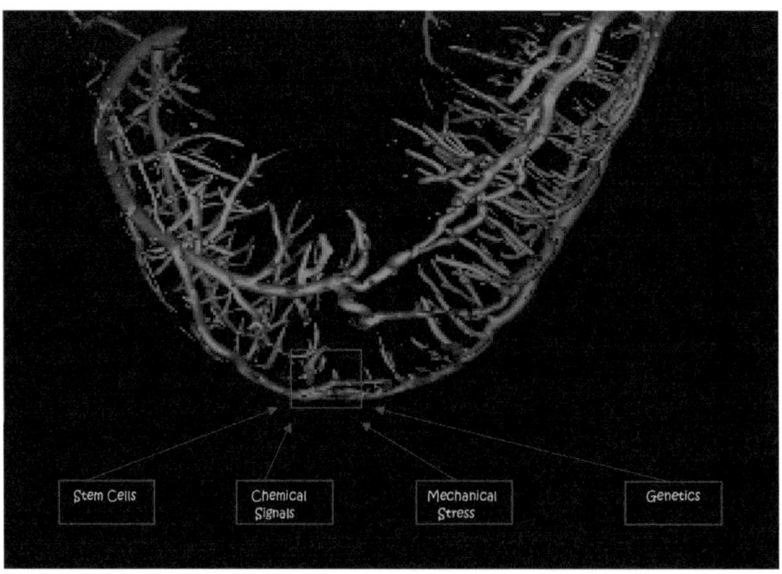

Figure 1. An image of the human coronary circulation depicting large collateral vessels that connect perfusion territories of major arteries and some factors that regulate their development.

http://dx.doi.org/10.5772/67164

they are distinct and have distinguishing characteristics. In *A Brief Etymology of the Collateral Circulation*, Faber et al. describe angiogenesis as the formation of capillaries from preexisting capillaries [11]. In contrast to angiogenesis, arteriogenesis is more the remodeling of preexisting vessels through the "anatomic increase in lumen area and wall thickness." The causes of arteriogenesis are more physical, specially, mechanical shear stress and ischemic conditions, while angiogenesis is caused by chemical conditions such as hypoxia [11].

2. Clinical perspective

Heart disease is extremely prevalent in the United States, where it accounts for every one in four deaths and almost 735,000 Americans suffer a heart attack each year (Centers for Disease Control, USA). However, there are numerous differences between these individuals in terms of response to treatment, future adverse events, and long-term survival rates. One explanation for these differences involves the presence of good collateral growth in certain individuals. A 5-year study called Osaka Acute Coronary Insufficiency Study (OACIS) assessed both acute and long-term survival in patients and came to three important conclusions: (1) patients with a Rentrop collateral score (RCS) of one or two showed the most promising 5-year survival rates, (2) RCS of three was associated with a worse 5-year survival rate, (3) RCS of three was associated with the best survival rates in a specific subgroup of patients with single vessel disease without previous myocardial infarction (MI) [12]. These first two conclusions can be explained due to the fact a higher baseline RCS can be indicative of a worse background of clinical characteristics such as previous MI or angina pectoris resulting in increased mortality rates, whereas an RCS of one or two was developed in the acute setting negating any adverse effects of chronic ischemia [12]. The third conclusion states RCS of three is more beneficial in the setting of single vessel occlusion and without previous MI, which would liken it to individuals who have RCS of one or two, but without any previous adverse events. In this subgroup, patients are having increased collateral flow, but without the chronic angina pectoris or previous MI improving survival rates [12]. This information leads to an important conclusion where the increased number of collaterals does not equate to decreased mortality rates, but rather is dependent upon a multitude of factors.

2.1. Methods

The literature is replete with the salubrious effects of a well-developed coronary collateral circulation and the potential benefit of a therapeutic process aimed at stimulating coronary collateral growth [13–19]. One patient study focused on coronary collateral growth in patients that had stable coronary artery disease. Specifically, the Möbius-Winkler et al. study looked at the impact of exercise on coronary collateral growth [20]. The patients were put into groups of usual care, moderate intensity exercise, and high-intensity exercise. The main findings of this study were that moderate and high-intensity exercise increased the coronary collateral blood flow. Scientists in this study postulated the cause of the coronary collateral growth. They questioned whether ischemia triggers collateral growth, since a percutaneous coronary intervention was performed before the study began; however, there is a large body of literature suggesting the PCI procedures may not completely resolve myocardial ischemia. The authors further speculated that the cause could be this increased blood flow and could have been from either increasing work done by preexisting blood vessels or an "improvement in endothelial function of small intramyocardial vessels." There was a CFI increase of 39% in the group of patients that did high-intensity exercise and a 41% CFI increase in the group that did moderate intensity exercise, which emphasized that exercise increased the coronary collateral blood flow in patients with coronary artery disease [20].

There has been much discussion for stimulating arteriogenesis in patients in order to give them proper blood perfusion to ischemic areas. Collaterals have been found to give patients many benefits over individuals who do not have collaterals, with a long-term mortality reduction, reduced myocardial infarct size, a greater postinfarction ejection fraction, and a reduced risk for rupture of the papillary muscle, myocardial free wall, or interventricular septum [21]. A reduction in infarct size was noted by the decreased peak creatinine levels as the number of collaterals increased depicting a cardioprotective effect [12]. Additionally, specific benefits have been noted between the presence of collaterals and sudden cardiac death and myocardial infarction.

There are three prevalent assessment methods of collateral growth circulation: the Rentrop score, collateral flow index (CFI), and intracoronary electrocardiogram. The Rentrop score can be most easily assessed when using coronary angiography as a visual assessment method. Circulation is then categorized into four different grades: Grade 0, Grade 1, Grade 2, and Grade 3. These categories range from no filling of the coronary collaterals to complete filling of collaterals, respectively. Although successful, the Rentrop method has some limitations due to being easily influenced by blood pressure changes and the force of injections during imaging procedures. Currently, the method considered to be the most accurate is the collateral flow index measurement. This method centers around utilizing a Doppler sensor tipped guide wire to quantify flow velocity in an occluded vessel compared with a normal vessel. Briefly mentioned was the intracoronary electrocardiogram, which is regarded as "simpler, cheaper, and very accurate" [22].

2.2. Benefits of coronary collaterals

Although many in the preclinical models have been employed in the study of coronary collateral growth, there is a relative paucity of clinical studies that have attempted to elucidate mechanisms of growth. One of the first studies done was in 1971 and was published in the *New England Journal of Medicine* [23]. This study only had three successful trials that demonstrated collaterals alleviating cardiovascular mortality. The inconsistency, according to Meier et al., could be rooted in the method by which they measured coronary collateral growth. The 1971 study "qualified" collaterals visually using coronary angiography, but Meier et al. postulates that had a better measurement method such as CFI been used, results could have been more promising [22].

One successful clinical study was performed by Seiler et al., which found that there is a direct correlation between collateral function and atherosclerotic lesions [24]. Patients with chronic total coronary occlusions had higher CFI values than those patients who did not have this condition. A CFI shift was quantified that patients with coronary occlusions had a CFI of 0.365 ± 0.190 versus 0.180 ± 0.105 of that of patients without occlusions. This study directly demonstrated that "collateral function is a direct indicator of CAD severity." The clinical importance of these findings suggests that human coronary collaterals can act as a "marker of poor outcome" in diseases such as acute coronary syndromes.

Sudden cardiac death (SCD) has several causes including electrical instability of the heart, specifically QRS complex variabilities can be used as markers for SCD and at times even trigger SCD [25]. The Oregon Sudden Unexpected Death Study (Ore-SUDS) has shown that prolongation of the QRS complex is associated with a large increase of SCD due to both known and unknown causes; therefore, methods to reduce this adverse event in the presence of myocardial ischemia can reduce mortality [26]. Additionally, fragmented QRS (fQRS), which are various RSR patterns in two continuous leads, have a well-established relationship with cardiac fibrosis caused by previous myocardial infarction or ischemia [27]. fQRS patterns have also been associated with increased morbidity and mortality, SCD, and repeat cardiovascular (CV) events and were found more often in individuals with poor collateral growth [27]. The presence of a well-developed collateral network has been shown to reduce QRS prolongation in left coronary artery occlusion and occurrence of fQRS in patients with chronic total occlusion [25, 27]. With this information, it can be concluded that with an increased number of coronary collaterals, patients can avoid QRS complex abnormalities thereby decreasing the chances of sudden cardiac death.

Additionally, the presence of collaterals has shown an increased time from symptom-onset-to-perfusion (>6 hours in good collateral versus poor collateral). This enables patients to increase the amount of time before onset of detrimental cardiac damage [28]. During an acute MI, the presence of a well-developed collateral circulation was seen in infarcted tissue that did not undergo cell necrosis, proving that increased collaterals will increase the chances of myocardial viability [29–31].

Overall, the presence of a well-developed collateral circulation in conjunction with healthy baseline characteristics (absence of repeat MI or angina pectoris) will be protective in patients who may suffer SCD, MI, or bouts of ischemia. Working to induce this collateral growth in patients both mechanically and chemically will prove to be very beneficial in decreasing mortality rates of patients with heart disease and perhaps ameliorate the possibility of recurrent cardiac events.

3. Mechanical factors involved in coronary collateral growth

The precise stimulation of arteriogenesis is yet to be found; however, both mechanical and chemical influences are required to induce the formation of collaterals in the heart. Mechanical shear stress occurs due to increased pressure gradients that form when an occlusion is present [32]. A stenotic artery will increase the pressure prior to the occlusion while decreasing the pressure distal to the occlusion. The increased pressure above the occlusion will cause an increase in blood flow into capillary beds prior to the occlusion increasing the shear stress [32]. The increased movement of blood into pre-existing collaterals and the resultant increased shear stress leads to several changes in the capillary endothelium. The first of which includes an increase in MCP-1 that serves to attract more monocytes to the proliferative site in order to transform them into the subsequent macrophages. The macrophages play a vital role in releasing cytokines and growth factors required for arteriogenesis. TNF-α, released by macrophages, helps form the inflammatory environment required for the growth of collaterals [33]. Another major factor includes basic fibroblast growth factor (bFGF), which helps with the actual development of collaterals [32]. A more in depth analysis on chemical inducers will be discussed later on in this chapter.

Although mechanical shear stress is thought to be a major contributor to arteriogenesis, it cannot be the sole solution due to the inability of fluid shear stress to completely replace the conducting artery. Fluid shear stress (FSS) has been found to only reach 35–40% of the maximal conductance possessed by the original stenotic artery [34]. An explanation for this phenomenon can be found in the relationships: FSS and blood flow velocity and FSS and cube of the vessel radius. FSS and blood flow velocity have a proportional relationship, while FSS is inversely related to the cube of the vessel radius [34]. The increase in blood flow velocity in the pre-existing collaterals leads to an increase in FSS. Since the shear stress causes growth in the collaterals (meaning an increase in the vessel radius), the FSS begins to decline preventing full recovery of the stenotic artery [34]. This indicates the need for both mechanical and chemical effectors for the production of proper coronary collaterals.

4. Chemical factors involved in coronary collateral growth

In addition to mechanical mechanisms of arteriogenesis, there are several chemical mediators involved in regulation of the process. Many of these chemical factors modulate the functions of the various cell types involved in arteriogenesis, including induction of cell proliferation, chemotaxis, and cellular remodeling. In this section, we will outline the various chemical mediators that are currently known to play a role in arteriogenesis.

4.1. Vascular endothelial growth factor (VEGF)

Vascular endothelial growth factor (VEGF) is known to play a major role in development of new vasculature. Under hypoxic conditions, VEGF production and release stimulates new capillary formation (angiogenesis) via endothelial cell sprouting, proliferation, and migration [35]. Alternatively, under different conditions, it can instead stimulate growth of new arteries, formation of collateral vessels, and modulation of lumen expansion—these actions are collectively referred to as arteriogenesis [35].

In VEGF signaling, there are three primary cell-surface receptors to which it binds: two tyrosine kinase receptors VEGFR-1 and VEGFR-2 and a nonkinase receptor neuropilin-1 (NRP-1) [35–37]. There are multiple isoforms of VEGF, with VEGF-A playing the major role in endothelial cell function via binding to VEGFR-2 [35]. VEGFR-2 is also involved in signaling pathways that lead to arteriogenesis via stimulation of proliferation, migration, survival, and lumenization of endothelial cells [35].

The first of these signaling cascades is activation of phosphatidylinositol 3-kinase (PI3K)/Akt that inhibits apoptosis in endothelial cells thus promoting cell survival [35]. The cascade is initiated by binding of VEGF-A to VEGFR-2 (Flk-1), which initiates receptor internalization via clathrin-coated pits followed by receptor autophosphorylation [35]. Active VEGFR-2 then phosphorylates PI3K, which goes on to phosphorylate the serine/threonine kinase Akt, which will go on to phosphorylate targets to inhibit apoptosis [38].

The second signal cascade is phosphorylation of profilin-1, indirectly via Src/FAK as well as directly via VEGFR-2, which stimulates migration of endothelial cells [35, 37]. Like the previous mechanism, this cascade is initiated by binding of VEGF-A to VEGFR-2. Activated VEGFR-2 then goes on to phosphorylate profilin-1 as well as Src kinase, which also phosphorylates profilin-1 [37]. Phosphorylated profilin-1 then goes on to catalyze the exchange of ADP for ATP on G-actin that stimulates polymerization of actin and resultant remodeling of the endothelial cell cytoskeleton [37]. This remodeling results in formation of actin-rich filopodia extending in the direction of the concentration gradient of VEGF, thus stimulating endothelial cell migration [37].

The third signal cascade is activation of the Raf-MEK-ERK signal cascade, which stimulates proliferation of endothelial cells, network formation, and increase in lumen size via phosphorylation of ERK1/2 [35]. While the exact mechanism of ERK1/2 action on cell proliferation and motility is not yet well understood, it has been suggested that a major component of this signaling cascade is downregulation of Rho-Kinase activity [39].

Finally, it is important to note that VEGF has been shown to be a critical factor in the process of coronary collateral growth. In a study of collateral growth following myocardial infarction in rats, it was observed that when the endogenous functions of VEGF were blocked by anti-VEGF neutralizing antibody, the result was a complete lack of collateral growth and subsequently no increase in coronary flow in the anti-VEGF group [40]. Additionally, upon treatment with dipyridamole (a potent vasodilator), it was observed that the increased coronary flow seen in the control group was in fact due to collateral growth, as there was no observed increase in coronary flow in the anti-VEGF group after the dipyridamole [40]. This study solidifies the importance of VEGF in the process of angiogenesis, particularly as it relates to coronary collateral growth.

4.2. bFGF and PDGF

In addition to VEGF, other growth factors are known to play a role in arteriogenesis—notably basic fibroblast growth factor (bFGF) and platelet-derived growth factor (PDGF) [41]. Basic FGF and PDGF are known to induce mitosis in both endothelial and smooth muscle cells and also exert other mitogenic effects such as promoting cell migration and differentiation [41, 42]. Basic FGF stimulates these mitogenic effects via binding to FGF receptors (FGFRs) expressed on cell surfaces [43]. These FGFRs are a part of the tyrosine kinase receptor family, and following binding of bFGF dimerize are autophosphorylated to become activated [43]. Activated FGFRs, notably FGFR-2 (FGFR-1 is thought to be a regulator of bFGF concentration available to bind FGFR-2), then continue the signal cascade by activation of cytoplasmic mitogen-activated protein kinase (MAPK), which then is translocated to the nucleus to initiate transcription promoting the aforementioned mitogenic effects [43]. PDGF, on the other hand, is known to activate multiple other downstream targets including PI3K, phospholipase C (PLC), as well as MAPK to mediate its mitogenic effects [44].

4.3. MCP-1 and macrophages

In addition to endothelial cells, macrophages are also heavily involved in arteriogenesis, but in order to do so must be directed to the correct location [36]. The primary molecule that has been studied as part of this mechanism is monocyte chemotactic protein 1 (MCP-1) [36]. Secretion of MCP-1 is initiated by activation of endothelial cell MAP-kinase-protein-kinase-2 (MK2) by elevation of fluid shear stress [45]. Released MCP-1 subsequently activates monocyte MK2, initiating migration to the correct location [45]. In the last step of the cycle, release of inflammatory cytokines by recruited monocytes cause increased secretion of MCP-1 from the endothelium, resulting in further monocyte recruitment [45]. Of similarly significant importance to MCP-1 are two adhesive molecules, intracellular adhesion molecule-1 (ICAM-1), and vascular cell adhesion molecule-1 (VCAM-1), which serve to bind the surface of migrating monocytes allowing them to roll along the luminal surface of the vasculature [36].

Once the macrophages have reached their destination, the correct phenotype must be expressed to stimulate new vessel growth [36]. There are two primary phenotypes of monocyte macrophages: M1 macrophages that secrete inflammatory molecules and help fight pathogens and M2 macrophages that play a role in vascular growth and wound healing [36]. These two phenotypes are induced by different cytokines, with interferon-γ causing a shift toward the M1 phenotype, while IL-4, IL-13, and several other factors such as IL-10 and IL-33 causing M2 differentiation. In histological analysis of hypoxia-induced arteriogenesis, the number of M2 macrophages was shown to increase indicating their essential role in development of new vasculature [36].

4.4. NO and eNOS

Nitric oxide (NO) is a potent vasodilator that is produced via the activity of endothelial nitric oxide synthase (eNOS). eNOS has been shown to function in stimulating production of new vasculature, and its expression is also known to be upregulated in response to elevated fluid shear stresses—a principal mechanical stimulus of arteriogenesis [46]. While the exact effects of NO and eNOS on arteriogenesis are still controversial, it has been shown that one contribution of elevated NO due to increased expression of eNOS is a reduction of vascular endothelial cadherin (VE-cadherin), resulting in increased vascular permeability and indirect promotion of macrophage invasion [46]. Additionally, eNOS activity and pharmacological inhibition of eNOS were shown to play a role in mediating vascular remodeling during collateral growth [47, 48].

4.5. Catestatin

Catestatin is a neuroendocrine peptide derived from a specific cleavage of the larger protein human chromogranin A (CgA) [49]. It functions in many different processes within the body including secretion of histamine from mast cells, defense against microbes, vasodilation, and attraction of monocytes. It has also been observed that catestatin acts in a pro-angiogenic capacity, involved in inducing proliferation and migration of endothelial cells

http://dx.doi.org/10.5772/67164

as well as formation of capillary tubes [49, 50]. This is accomplished through stimulating release of bFGF, which in turn will activate MAPK via binding to FGFR-1 as previously discussed [49, 50]. It has also been shown that catestatin activates other signal cascades such as PI3K/Akt, serving an anti-apoptotic role to promote cell survival [50]. Finally, catestatin influences effects in both endothelial progenitor cells (EPCs) and vascular smooth muscle cells (VSMCs) in addition to its direct effects on endothelial cells, inducing chemotaxis to incorporate these cell types into formation of new vasculature [50].

4.6. Neuregulins

Neuregulins (NRG) are another class of molecules produced by endothelial cells. These growth factor ligands bind to erbB receptors expressed on the surface of endothelial cells—this action has been shown to induce angiogenesis [51]. NRG involvement in angiogenesis and arteriogenesis is tied to regulation of $\alpha_v\beta_3$ integrin, thus playing a role in cell migration, proliferation, and differentiation mechanisms as shown in a NRG-erbB knockout mouse model. The mechanism by which this occurs involves another proangiogenic protein, Cyr61, the expression of which is upregulated by NRG-erbB signaling, in addition to mediation via induction of VEGF release and subsequent activation of the ERK signaling cascade [51]. ErbB receptors have also been found to be expressed on EPCs, playing a role in increasing cell survival, and on certain types of VSMCs, though the role NRG-erbB signaling plays here is not well known [51].

4.7. Early growth response 1 (Egr-1)

Early growth response 1 (Egr-1) is a transcription factor of the zinc-finger family that has been shown to be upregulated during arteriogenesis [52]. It plays a major role in modulating the levels of other growth factors that are involved in the process of collateral growth, including playing a role in the recruitment and proliferation of leukocytes [52, 53]. Specific genes that are upregulated by Egr-1 include PDGF and transforming growth factor β (TGF-β), which then indirectly upregulates other factors involved in collateral growth such as VEGF and metalloproteinases [53]. Interestingly, despite the fact that most of these factors have been primarily shown to affect angiogenesis, it has been observed that Egr-1 primarily affects the growth of arterioles rather than capillaries, indicating its primary role in regulation of arteriogenesis [53].

Much like the other factors mentioned here, Egr-1 production is stimulated primarily by elevations in fluid shear stress, in this case by activating the Egr-1 gene promoter [54]. It has been suggested that this is mediated by the Ras-MEK-ERK1/2 signal cascade in which shear stress leads to activation of MEK1, which proceeds to activate ERK1/2 of the MAPK family, and finally ERK1/2 activate the protein Elk-1 that induces transcription of Egr-1 [54]. Interestingly, this pathway can be activated by very low levels of shear stress due to the sensitivity of ERK1/2 [54].

There are many varying chemical mediators of arteriogenesis, many of which share similar signaling pathways leading to their involvement. While some of these mediators have been studied extensively and are relatively well understood, there are others whose mechanisms have not yet been elucidated and require more investigation. There are likely even more chemical mediators involved that have not yet been studied. Going forward, more research will be extremely valuable in understanding the overall chemical mechanism behind collateral vessel growth and how to apply this knowledge to a clinical setting.

5. Role of Stem Cells in Coronary Collateral Growth

In addition to the aforementioned chemical mediators that mitigate the consequences of vascular occlusive diseases by stimulating collateral growth, in recent years, stem cell-based therapy has been implicated as a possible avenue for vascular regeneration. Stem cells have the unique potential of developing into many different cell types in the body. Under certain physiologic and experimental conditions, they can be manipulated to grow into specific tissues and organ cells with exclusive functionality. This revolutionary discovery for stem cells has demonstrated a clinical potential to create new networks of blood-perfused vessels and treat human patients with cardiovascular and vascular diseases [55]. The current theory is that stem cells may release a series of angiogenic factors, such as VEGF and bFGF, which mobilize vascular endothelial cells through a paracrine effect [56]. In this section, we will summarize the current state of regenerative approaches using stem cells to stimulate coronary collateral growth.

A 2012 study programmed endothelial cells to develop into induced vascular progenitor cells (iVPCs) and assessed their ability to induce coronary collateral growth in a rat model in efforts to increase blood flow to the collateral-dependent region of risk [57]. iVPCs are also known to be less tumorigenic compared with induced pluripotent cells (iPSCs) and are more likely to commit to a line of vascular differentiation (they will not turn into cardiomyocytes) [57]. When the iVPCs were transplanted into myocardium, they formed blood vessels and improved blood flow markedly better than did natural endothelial cells, mesenchymal stem cells, or iPSCs [57]. However, while results showed that partial programming of the endothelial cells was promising enough to sprout new blood vessels in the myocardium, one big challenge persists: how to maintain the partial programmed state of the cells until they get to their intended destination [57].

In addition, current literature posits that bone marrow-derived stem cells and endothelial progenitor cells in arteriogenesis do not physically deposit onto the walls of newly generated arteries but rather play the role of supporting cells [58]. The therapeutic induction of collateral growth from already established arteries improves any blood flow deficiencies caused by blockage in major arteries. Transplanted bone marrow-derived cells act as "cytokine factors" and secrete specific growth factors that mediate their effects through paracrine activity [59]. As Dr. Matthias Heil of the Netherlands puts it, "bone marrow stem cells provide the software and not the hardware in vascular growth" [59]. His group's study on the hindlimb ischemic model with mice revealed that GFP-tagged bone marrow was not localized to endothelial and smooth cell markers, but around burgeoning collaterals that were secreting chemokines and growth factors [59]. Hence, therapeutic arteriogenesis functions to boost the body's natural angiogenic ability by stimulating the release of pro-angiogenic factors rather than actually providing the buildings block for a new artery. A caveat to this is if the processes in the heart are different from those in the peripheral circulation.

While there is a continued debate on whether bone marrow-derived multipotent stromal cells (MSCs) exert their effect via transdifferentiation or through paracrine activity, there is unequivocal evidence showing that MSCs must first travel to ischemic tissue to achieve a therapeutic benefit [60]. MSCs localize to injured tissues by adhering to endothelial cells and migrating across the cell wall. Homing of MSCs to injured tissues is optimized by an expression of ligands on endothelial cells [60]. A 2009 study showed the importance of epidermal growth factor (EGF) and heparin-binding epidermal growth factor-like growth factor (HB-EGF) in inducing increased expression of these ligands [60]. Specifically, phosphorylation of the EGF-R leads to higher expression of ligands, VCAM-1, and ICAM-1 that enhanced MSC adherence and ultimately stimulated coronary collateral growth in rats that had undergone repetitive instances of myocardial ischemia [60]. Coronary collateral growth was assessed with the ratio of collateral dependent flow (CZ) to normal zone flow (NZ). Exposure of both MSCs and coronary endothelial cells (CECs) to a 100 ng/mL dose of EGF for 16 hours maximally increased expression of adhesion molecules compared with samples untreated with EGF [60]. The CZ/NZ ratio increased in rats whose MSCs were treated with EGF and showed improved cardiac function and decreased left ventricular remodeling compared to rats without EGF treatment of MSCs [60].

Another 2009 study involving a rat model of repetitive myocardial ischemia showed that granulocyte-colony stimulating factor (G-CSF), a glycoprotein responsible for hematopoietic cell proliferation and differentiation of neutrophil granulocytes, also stimulates coronary collateral growth [61]. G-CSF mounts a series of defenses against infectious agents, one of which is promotion of neutrophils to release reactive oxygen species (ROS) [61]. This generation of ROS was studied both *in vivo* and *in vitro* and was shown to directly act on injured cardiomyocytes. Cardiomyocytes under the influence of G-CSF-induced ROS generate angiogenic factors that lead to vascular growth and tube formation in levels comparative to cardiomyocytes induced by VEGF [61]. To the surprise of researchers, this study also demonstrated that G-CSF can promote coronary collateral growth without the impetus of repetitive ischemia and hence this cytokine can act as a surrogate for ischemia [61].

Majority of the recent clinical trials in humans purport that stem cell-based therapy adequately facilitates angiogenesis in patients suffering from peripheral arterial disease and promotes wound healing [55]. Specifically, bone marrow-derived stem cell transplantation has shown to improve ischemic symptoms, such as claudication, ischemic rest pain, and has augmented wound healing in ulcer-related conditions [55]. Nonetheless, these studies have been limited by a lack of care standardization, absence of a control group, small sample sizes, dissimilar inclusion criteria, and inconsistencies in methods of outcome assessment [55]. In other cases, the absence of follow-up procedures has prevented elucidation of long-term effects of treating peripheral artery disease with stem cells [55]. While the central issues of public safety and treatment efficacy linger over the field, progress, albeit limited, has been made in the arena of coronary collateral growth.

6. Summary

The process of coronary collateral growth is being better understood year by year. The role that the many chemical factors, mechanical factors, and stem cells play in the process is still incompletely understood. The study of these factors in "normal" preclinical models may be an oversimplification, because under conditions with risk factors for coronary disease, there may be shifts in the normal control mechanisms. We advocate that future studies incorporate models of cardiovascular disease and aging to better understand the mechanisms by which this adaptive process is abrogated in the majority of patients with ischemic heart disease.

Author details

Bhamini Patel, Peter Hopmann, Mansee Desai, Kanithra Sekaran, Kathleen Graham, Liya Yin and William Chilian*

*Address all correspondence to: wchilian@neomed.edu

Department of Integrative Medical Science, Northeast Ohio Medical University, Rootstown, Ohio, USA

References

[1] Cai W, Schaper W. Mechanisms of arteriogenesis. Acta Biochim Biophys Sin (Shanghai). 2008;40(8):681–692.

[2] Heil M, Schaper W. Influence of mechanical, cellular, and molecular factors on collateral artery growth (arteriogenesis). Circ Res. 2004;95(5):449–458.

[3] Pipp F, Boehm S, Cai WJ, Adili F, Ziegler B, Karanovic G, et al. Elevated fluid shear stress enhances postocclusive collateral artery growth and gene expression in the pig hind limb. Arterioscler Thromb Vasc Biol. 2004;24(9):1664–1668.

[4] Buschmann I, Schaper W. Arteriogenesis versus angiogenesis: two mechanisms of vessel growth. News Physiol Sci. 1999;14:121–125.

[5] Schaper W, De Brabander M, Lewi P. DNA synthesis and mitoses in coronary collateral vessels of the dog. Circ Res. 1971;28(6):671–679.

[6] Chilian WM, Mass HJ, Williams SE, Layne SM, Smith EE, Scheel KW. Microvascular occlusions promote coronary collateral growth. Am J Physiol. 1990;258(4 Pt 2):H1103–H1111.

[7] Chalothorn D, Clayton JA, Zhang H, Pomp D, Faber JE. Collateral density, remodeling and VEGF-A expression differ widely between mouse strains. Physiol Genom. 2007.

[8] Clayton JA, Chalothorn D, Faber JE. Vascular endothelial growth factor-A specifies formation of native collaterals and regulates collateral growth in ischemia. Circ Res. 2008;103(9):1027–1036.

[9] Gulec S, Karabulut H, Ozdemir AO, Ozdol C, Turhan S, Altin T, et al. Glu298Asp polymorphism of the eNOS gene is associated with coronary collateral development. Atherosclerosis. 2008;198(2):354–359.

[10] Schaper W, Gorge G, Winkler B, Schaper J. The collateral circulation of the heart. Prog Cardiovasc Dis. 1988;31(1):57–77.

[11] Faber JE, Chilian WM, Deindl E, van Royen N, Simons M. A brief etymology of the collateral circulation. Arterioscler Thromb Vasc Biol. 2014;34(9):1854–1859.

[12] Hara M, Sakata Y, Nakatani D, Suna S, Nishino M, Sato H, et al. Impact of coronary collaterals on in-hospital and 5-year mortality after ST-elevation myocardial infarction in the contemporary percutaneous coronary intervention era: a prospective observational study. BMJ Open. 2016;6(7):e011105.

[13] Fujita M, Sasayama S. Alleviation of myocardial ischemia by the development of coronary collateral circulation. Jpn Circ J. 1989;53(9):1164–1169.

[14] Fujita M, Sasayama S. Reappraisal of functional importance of coronary collateral circulation. Cardiology. 2010;117(4):246–252.

[15] Fujita M, Sasayama S. Coronary collateral growth and its therapeutic application to coronary artery disease. Circ J. 2010;74(7):1283–1289.

[16] Baklanov D, Simons M. Arteriogenesis: lessons learned from clinical trials. Endothelium. 2003;10(4–5):217–223.

[17] Bokeriia LA, Golukhova EZ, Eremeeva MV, Kiselev SL, Aslanidi IP, Vakhromeeva MN, et al. [New approaches to the treatment of ischemic heart disease: therapeutic angiogenesis in combination with surgical revascularization of the myocardium]. Ter Arkh. 2004;76(6):25–30.

[18] Emanueli C, Madeddu P. Angiogenesis gene therapy to rescue ischaemic tissues: achievements and future directions. Br J Pharmacol. 2001;133(7):951–958.

[19] Fujita M, Sasayama S, Asanoi H, Nakajima H, Sakai O, Ohno A. Improvement of treadmill capacity and collateral circulation as a result of exercise with heparin pretreatment in patients with effort angina. Circulation. 1988;77(5):1022–1029.

[20] Mobius-Winkler S, Uhlemann M, Adams V, Sandri M, Erbs S, Lenk K, et al. Coronary collateral growth induced by physical exercise: results of the impact of intensive exercise training on coronary collateral circulation in patients with stable coronary artery disease (EXCITE) trial. Circulation. 2016;133(15):1438–1448; discussion 48.

[21] Meier P, Gloekler S, Zbinden R, Beckh S, de Marchi SF, Zbinden S, et al. Beneficial effect of recruitable collaterals: a 10-year follow-up study in patients with stable coronary artery disease undergoing quantitative collateral measurements. Circulation. 2007;116(9):975–983.

[22] Meier P, Schirmer SH, Lansky AJ, Timmis A, Pitt B, Seiler C. The collateral circulation of the heart. BMC Med. 2013;11:143.

[23] Helfant RH, Vokonas PS, Gorlin R. Functional importance of the human coronary collateral circulation. N Engl J Med. 1971;284(23):1277–1281.

[24] Seiler C, Stoller M, Pitt B, Meier P. The human coronary collateral circulation: development and clinical importance. Eur Heart J. 2013;34(34):2674–2682.

[25] Meier P, Gloekler S, de Marchi SF, Zbinden R, Delacretaz E, Seiler C. An indicator of sudden cardiac death during brief coronary occlusion: electrocardiogram QT time and the role of collaterals. Eur Heart J. 2010;31(10):1197–1204.

[26] Chugh SS, Reinier K, Singh T, Uy-Evanado A, Socoteanu C, Peters D, et al. Determinants of prolonged QT interval and their contribution to sudden death risk in coronary artery disease: the Oregon Sudden Unexpected Death Study. Circulation. 2009;119(5):663–670.

[27] Erdogan T, Kocaman SA, Cetin M, Canga A, Durakoglugil ME, Cicek Y, et al. Relationship of fragmented QRS complexes with inadequate coronary collaterals in patients with chronic total occlusion. J Cardiovasc Med (Hagerstown). 2012;13(8):499–504.

[28] Desch S, de Waha S, Eitel I, Koch A, Gutberlet M, Schuler G, et al. Effect of coronary collaterals on long-term prognosis in patients undergoing primary angioplasty for acute ST-elevation myocardial infarction. Am J Cardiol. 2010;106(5):605–611.

[29] Seiler C, Meier P. Historical aspects and relevance of the human coronary collateral circulation. Curr Cardiol Rev. 2014;10(1):2–16.

[30] van der Hoeven NW, Teunissen PF, Werner GS, Delewi R, Schirmer SH, Traupe T, et al. Clinical parameters associated with collateral development in patients with chronic total coronary occlusion. Heart. 2013;99(15):1100–1105.

[31] Meier P, Hemingway H, Lansky AJ, Knapp G, Pitt B, Seiler C. The impact of the coronary collateral circulation on mortality: a meta-analysis. Eur Heart J. 2012;33(5):614–621.

[32] Fujita M, Tambara K. Recent insights into human coronary collateral development. Heart. 2004;90(3):246–250.

[33] Van Royen N, Piek JJ, Buschmann I, Hoefer I, Voskuil M, Schaper W. Stimulation of arteriogenesis; a new concept for the treatment of arterial occlusive disease. Cardiovasc Res. 2001;49(3):543–553.

[34] Schaper W, Scholz D. Factors regulating arteriogenesis. Arterioscler Thromb Vasc Biol. 2003;23(7):1143–1151.

[35] Kofler NM, Simons M. Angiogenesis versus arteriogenesis: neuropilin 1 modulation of VEGF signaling. F1000Prime Rep. 2015;7:26.

[36] Hollander MR, Horrevoets AJ, van Royen N. Cellular and pharmacological targets to induce coronary arteriogenesis. Curr Cardiol Rev. 2014;10(1):29–37.

[37] Simons M, Schwartz MA. Profilin phosphorylation as a VEGFR effector in angiogenesis. Nat Cell Biol. 2012;14(10):985–987.

[38] Gerber HP, McMurtrey A, Kowalski J, Yan M, Keyt BA, Dixit V, et al. Vascular endothelial growth factor regulates endothelial cell survival through the phosphatidylinositol 3′-kinase/Akt signal transduction pathway. Requirement for Flk-1/KDR activation. J Biol Chem. 1998;273(46):30336–30343.

[39] Mavria G, Vercoulen Y, Yeo M, Paterson H, Karasarides M, Marais R, et al. ERK-MAPK signaling opposes Rho-kinase to promote endothelial cell survival and sprouting during angiogenesis. Cancer Cell. 2006;9(1):33–44.

[40] Toyota E, Warltier DC, Brock T, Ritman E, Kolz C, O'Malley P, et al. Vascular endothelial growth factor is required for coronary collateral growth in the rat. Circulation. 2005;112(14):2108–2113.

[41] Van Royen N, Piek JJ, Schaper W, Bode C, Buschmann I. Arteriogenesis: mechanisms and modulation of collateral artery development. J Nucl Cardiol. 2001;8(6):687–693.

[42] Wu S, Wu X, Zhu W, Cai WJ, Schaper J, Schaper W. Immunohistochemical study of the growth factors, aFGF, bFGF, PDGF-AB, VEGF-A and its receptor (Flk-1) during arteriogenesis. Mol Cell Biochem. 2010;343(1–2):223–229.

[43] Mason IJ. The ins and outs of fibroblast growth factors. Cell. 1994;78(4):547–552.

[44] Tsioumpekou M, Papadopoulos N, Burovic F, Heldin CH, Lennartsson J. Platelet-derived growth factor (PDGF)-induced activation of Erk5 MAP-kinase is dependent on Mekk2, Mek1/2, PKC and PI3-kinase, and affects BMP signaling. Cell Signal. 2016;28(9):1422–1431.

[45] Limbourg A, von Felden J, Jagavelu K, Krishnasamy K, Napp LC, Kapopara PR, et al. MAP-kinase activated protein kinase 2 links endothelial activation and monocyte/macrophage recruitment in arteriogenesis. PLoS One. 2015;10(10):e0138542.

[46] Yang B, Cai B, Deng P, Wu X, Guan Y, Zhang B, et al. Nitric oxide increases arterial endothelial permeability through mediating VE-cadherin expression during arteriogenesis. PLoS One. 2015;10(7):e0127931.

[47] Dai X, Faber JE. Endothelial nitric oxide synthase deficiency causes collateral vessel rarefaction and impairs activation of a cell cycle gene network during arteriogenesis. Circ Res. 2010;106(12):1870–1881.

[48] Matsunaga TDCW, Moniz M, Tessmmer J, Weihrauch D, Chilian WM. Role of nitric oxide and vascular endothelial growth factor in coronary collateral growth. Circulation. 2000;102:3098–3103.

[49] Xu W, Yu H, Li W, Gao W, Guo L, Wang G. Plasma catestatin: a useful biomarker for coronary collateral development with chronic myocardial ischemia. PLoS One. 2016;11(6):e0149062.

[50] Theurl M, Schgoer W, Albrecht K, Jeschke J, Egger M, Beer AG, et al. The neuropeptide catestatin acts as a novel angiogenic cytokine via a basic fibroblast growth factor-dependent mechanism. Circ Res. 2010;107(11):1326–1335.

[51] Hedhli N, Dobrucki LW, Kalinowski A, Zhuang ZW, Wu X, Russell RR, 3rd, et al. Endothelial-derived neuregulin is an important mediator of ischaemia-induced angiogenesis and arteriogenesis. Cardiovasc Res. 2012;93(3):516–524.

[52] Pagel JI, Ziegelhoeffer T, Heil M, Fischer S, Fernandez B, Schaper W, et al. Role of early growth response 1 in arteriogenesis: impact on vascular cell proliferation and leukocyte recruitment in vivo. Thromb Haemost. 2012;107(3):562–574.

[53] Sarateanu CS, Retuerto MA, Beckmann JT, McGregor L, Carbray J, Patejunas G, et al. An Egr-1 master switch for arteriogenesis: studies in Egr-1 homozygous negative and wild-type animals. J Thorac Cardiovasc Surg. 2006;131(1):138–145.

[54] Schwachtgen JL, Houston P, Campbell C, Sukhatme V, Braddock M. Fluid shear stress activation of egr-1 transcription in cultured human endothelial and epithelial cells is mediated via the extracellular signal-related kinase 1/2 mitogen-activated protein kinase pathway. J Clin Invest. 1998;101(11):2540–2549.

[55] Lee KB, Kim DI. Clinical application of stem cells for therapeutic angiogenesis in patients with peripheral arterial disease. Int J Stem Cells. 2009;2(1):11–17.

[56] Deindl E, Schaper W. The art of arteriogenesis. Cell Biochem Biophys. 2005;43(1):1–15.

[57] Yin L, Ohanyan V, Pung YF, Delucia A, Bailey E, Enrick M, et al. Induction of vascular progenitor cells from endothelial cells stimulates coronary collateral growth. Circ Res. 2012;110(2):241–252.

[58] Ziegelhoeffer T, Fernandez B, Kostin S, Heil M, Voswinckel R, Helisch A, et al. Bone marrow-derived cells do not incorporate into the adult growing vasculature. Circ Res. 2004;94(2):230–238.

[59] Heil M, Ziegelhoeffer T, Mees B, Schaper W. A different outlook on the role of bone marrow stem cells in vascular growth: bone marrow delivers software not hardware. Circ Res. 2004;94(5):573–574.

[60] Belmadani S, Matrougui K, Kolz C, Pung YF, Palen D, Prockop DJ, et al. Amplification of coronary arteriogenic capacity of multipotent stromal cells by epidermal growth factor. Arterioscler Thromb Vasc Biol. 2009;29(6):802–808.

[61] Carrao AC, Chilian WM, Yun J, Kolz C, Rocic P, Lehmann K, et al. Stimulation of coronary collateral growth by granulocyte stimulating factor: role of reactive oxygen species. Arterioscler Thromb Vasc Biol. 2009;29(11):1817–1822.

Chapter 9

Angiogenesis and Cardiovascular Diseases: The Emerging Role of HDACs

Ana Moraga, Ka Hou Lao and Lingfang Zeng

Additional information is available at the end of the chapter

http://dx.doi.org/10.5772/66409

Abstract

Cardiovascular diseases (CVD) continue to be the leading cause of death in the world despite recent therapeutic advances. Although many CVDs remain incurable, enormous efforts have been placed in harnessing angiogenesis as therapeutics for these diseases. Epigenetics, the modification of gene expression post-transcriptionally and post-translationally, are important in regulating many biological processes. One of the main post-translational epigenetic modifications, modification of chromatin structure by the acetylation of histone tails within the chromatin by either histone deacetylases (HDACs) or histone acetyltransferases (HATs), is important in modulating gene transcription and has emerged as an important regulatory player from pathogenesis to therapeutics in CVDs. Particularly, HDACs, which are largely involved in promoting chromatin compaction and hence inhibitions of gene transcription, have been implicated in the pathogenic signalling underlying many aspects of CVDs. Recently, histone modifications have been demonstrated to play important roles in the angiogenesis process. Pharmacological inhibitions of HDACs have displayed promising therapeutic potentials in several pre-clinical models of CVDs where angiogenesis is of paramount importance. There are many evidences proving that pro- and anti-angiogenic therapies—and the impact of epigenetics in these processes—can help to artificially reconstruct the vasculature in patients with cardiovascular diseases. Conversely, utilising knowledge of HDACs in angiogenesis might help to develop anti-angiogenic therapies in tackling diseases that are characterised with excessive pathological angiogenesis, including cancer and age-related macular degeneration. Understanding the molecular mechanisms underlying HDACs in modulating angiogenesis will undoubtedly benefit future therapeutics development. This chapter focuses on the emerging role of HDACs in angiogenesis and discuss their potentials and challenges in utilising HDAC inhibitors as therapeutics in several major cardiovascular diseases.

Keywords: angiogenesis, cardiovascular disease, atherosclerosis, histone deacetylase, epigenetics

1. Introduction

Cardiovascular diseases (CVDs) are a worldwide epidemic that have serious implication in public health and constitute a huge amount of healthcare expenditure. Although there are a number of preventable controllable risk factors, such as hypertension, hypercholesterolemia, smoking, obesity, lack of physical activity and diabetes, and others such as age, gender and family history are unmodifiable [1]. Progress in genetic sequencing has allowed the identification of numerous genetic variants associated with specific CVDs [2], but their mechanisms remain unclear. The last few years of research have been a key in understanding how epigenetic mechanisms such as histone modifications are involved in the occurrence and progression of CVDs including atherosclerosis, heart failure, myocardial infarction and cardiac hypertrophy.

Epigenetics represent a phenomenon of altered heritable gene expression without changes to the underlying DNA sequences. The epigenetic alterations can be affected by exogenous stimuli such as diabetes milieu, diets and smoking, while at other times these alterations can subsequently trigger disease initiation [3]. Thus, the impact of epigenetics in CVD is now emerging as an important regulatory key player at different levels from pathophysiology to therapeutics. For instance, histone alterations have been implicated in ECs response to hypoxia and shear stress, in angiogenesis and in endogenous recovery following myocardial infarction (MI) [4]. On the other hand, HDAC inhibitors (HDACi) have been investigated for potential protective effects in heart muscles during acute MI [4, 5].

Tissue repair is one of the main therapeutic challenges facing the scientific community. There are various approaches in improving tissue recovery depending on the pathological conditions, but most of these conditions are initiated by local ischaemia and require a rich network of blood supply for tissue regeneration. Hence, angiogenesis plays a vital part in tissue regeneration in the treatment of CVDs. At present, the promising potentials of angiogenesis therapies are in full swing.

2. Vascular system

2.1. Cardiovascular system

The cardiovascular system consists of three main components: heart, blood vessels (arteries, veins and capillaries) and blood. There are three types of anatomically and functionally distinct blood vessels: arteries, veins and capillaries. The arteries are primarily involved in the delivery of oxygenated blood and nutrients from the heart to target organs and tissues. They have thicker and more elastic vessel walls to complement the higher blood pressure for blood delivery from the heart. The veins carry deoxygenated blood, together with waste products and other factors secreted by the tissues back to the heart. They tend to have larger luminal areas and thinner vessel walls compared to the arteries, and have valves to complement the pressure changes. Connecting these two vessel systems are the capillaries that allow the direct exchanges of oxygen and nutrients with carbon dioxide and waste products between the target tissues and the blood. The walls of all vessels are generally composed of three layers: the tunica intima, tunica media and tunica adventitia. The innermost layer is formed by the tunica intima, which is made up of a single layer of ECs and connective tissues, both of which overlie the internal elastic lamina. The tunica intima has an important function as a selective permeable barrier between the extravascular space, the vascular wall and the blood. The tunica media forms the muscular element of blood vessels that resides between the tunica intima and the tunica adventitia, and comprises circumferentially arranged smooth muscle cells (SMCs) enclosed by a layer of external elastic lamina. They provide supports to the vessels and regulate blood flow and pressure via controlling the luminal diameter. The outermost layer, the tunica adventitia, is made up of connective tissues and matrix-secreting fibroblasts. It is critical to maintaining vascular structure and helps to anchor vessels in place to fit into the surrounding tissues. Capillaries constitute non-muscular vessels and are only made up of an internal elastic lamina covered by a monolayer of ECs, and provide a huge surface area for exchanges of vital blood components and factors between vessels and tissues.

2.2. Endothelial cells and their impairments in CVDs

Vascular endothelial cells (ECs) have a crucial and diverse role, arraying the innermost layer of the entire circulatory system. They act as the semi-selective and non-adherent barrier between the lumen of the vessels and the underlying tissues, regulating tissue perfusion and movement of inflammatory cells between them [6]. They are involved in regulating vascular permeability, blood flow, vascular tone and blood coagulation and are essentially involved in vascular remodelling in responses to diverse physiological and pathological stimuli. Physiologically, ECs exert anti-coagulant and anti-thrombotic effects through the secretion of anti-coagulant factors such as prostacyclin, nitric oxide (NO) and prostaglandin-E_2, and inhibit inflammatory cell adhesion in order to maintain vascular homeostasis [7]. Under pathological states, ECs are activated by vascular insults or pro-inflammatory cytokines, leading to increased permeability, encouraging extravasations of immune cells, which are followed by a series of pathological events leading to eventual vascular remodelling [7]. Decreased EC secretion of the potent vasodilator NO as a result of repressed activity of endothelial NO synthase (eNOS) also contributes to the circus of vascular pathogenesis [8]. These endothelial dysfunctions, whether environmental, genetic or a combination of both, critically contribute to the pathophysiology of many CVDs such as hypertension and atherosclerosis, and represent the discernible therapeutic targets for drug development [9].

3. Angiogenesis

There are three main processes that contribute to the formation of new blood vessels that are termed globally as neovascularisation:

– Vasculogenesis is defined as the de novo formation of vascular structures by the migration of stem cells to the site of vascularisation and differentiation into ECs. Although it was originally thought to be exclusive to embryonic development, it is now widely accepted that the process can also take place in adults, which opens up a new avenue for clinical applications [10].

- Angiogenesis is the formation of new blood vessels by sprouting from pre-existing small vessels in embryonic and adult tissue or by intravascular subdivision process [11]. This process is believed to be induced by angiogenic factors including fibroblast growth factor (FGF) and vascular endothelial growth factor (VEGF).

- Arteriogenesis results from the hypertrophy and luminal distention of pre-existing collateral vessels, which involves specific remodelling of existing nascent EC tubules for greater size, elasticity and stability through the recruitment of and enclosure by SMCs and pericytes that secrete specific extracellular matrices. Therefore, these vessels have fully developed tunica media and tunica adventitia [11].

Angiogenesis is a very complex process that can be simplified into three categories: mechanical, chemical and molecular factors (see Ref. [12] for a more extensive review).

- **Cellular factors**: There are many molecules that can modulate angiogenesis. The most essential angiogenic growth factors are as follows: FGF, VEGF, placenta growth factor, angiopoietin-1 and angiopoietin-2. Several pathological conditions can also initiate angiogenesis. For example, hypoglycaemia increases the expression of critical angiogenic inductor VEGF [13]. It has also been extensively demonstrated that the presence of inflammatory cells, like macrophages and neutrophils, is sufficient to induce angiogenesis [14].

- **Environmental factors**: Angiogenesis can be induced by hypoxia and through increased EC production of NO. Hypoxia stimulates the release of several angiogenic factors including platelet-derived growth factor and FGF-1 and FGF-2 by macrophages. Hypoxia also upregulates VEGF production, which is known to induce the production and secretion of NO from ECs, while eNOS production is amplified during VEGF-induced angiogenesis [15].

- **Mechanical factors**: There are two main factors: haemodynamic and shear stress. Haemodynamic changes trigger an augmentation of blood flow and might therefore stimulate vascular sprouting, maintain patency of the newly formed collateral vessels and provide blood flow to the ischemic area [16]. Shear stress has an important influence on the development of collateral vessel networks in the ischaemic tissues.

4. Epigenetics

The nucleosome is the fundamental subunit of chromatin in eukaryotes. Each nucleosome consists of a 146-bp DNA segment wrapped around an octamer of core histone proteins that includes two molecules of histones H2A, H2B, H3 and H4 associated with a single copy of histone H1. Epigenetics is defined as the study of stable alterations of gene expression without alterations of DNA itself. These alterations include the post-translational addition or removal of methyl groups to DNA as well as methyl, acetyl, sumoyl and phospho groups to histones and other kind of proteins. These changes participate in remodelling chromatin and modifying its accessibility to transcription factors and cofactors [17]. Epigenetic control is one of the main regulatory systems contributing to phenotypic differences between cell types in multicellular organisms. Epigenetic changes may explain why subjects with similar genetic backgrounds and risk factors for particular diseases can differ greatly in clinical manifestation and therapeutic response [18]. It has been reported that epigenetic mechanisms play a critical role in regulating endothelial gene expression [19]. Among these epigenetic changes are the methylation of DNA, RNA-based mechanisms and the posttranslational modification of histone proteins.

DNA methylation

The methylation of DNA involves the covalent modification of the 5-position of cytosine to define the 'fifth base of DNA', 5-methyl-cytosine [20]. In mammals, DNA methylation is almost exclusively restricted to CpG dinucleotides. DNA methylation is catalysed by DNA methyltransferases and regulates biological processes underlying CVD, such as atherosclerosis, inflammation, hypertension, and diabetes [21].

RNA-based mechanisms

1. miRNA therapeutics

   MicroRNAs (miRNA or miR) are short (20–22 nucleotides) non-coding RNAs modulating gene expression further by down-regulating the translation of target mRNAs through the inhibition of post-transcriptional events, through transcript degradation or through direct translational repression.

2. Long non-coding RNAs (lncRNAs)

   Long non-coding RNAs (lncRNAs) are gaining more prominence as regulators of gene expression. The central role that lncRNAs play in heart development is only slowly being recognised [18]. Besides, understanding the function of these molecules in CVD is even further away.

Histone modification

It is well established that histone residues can undergo a wide array of modifications. At least eight different types of modification have been characterised with a range of enzymes identified for each: acetylation, methylation, phosphorylation, ubiquitination, sumoylation, ADP-ribosylation, deimination, and proline isomerisation (**Table 1**).

Histone methylation is modulated by two enzymes: histone methyltransferases and histone demethylases. The acetylation status of histone is fine-tuned by histone acetyltransferases (HATs) and HDACs. HDACs are enzymes that remove acetyl groups from histone lysine residues thereby increasing their negative charges, which lead to chromatin condensation and gene repression [17].

4.1. The HDAC family

Deacetylation of histones in nucleosomes induces chromatin compaction, which represses transcription by preventing the binding of transcription factors and other components of the

Modification type	Amino acid modification	Examples of modifying enzymes	Role
Acetylation	Lysine	Histone acetyl transferases (HATs)	Transcription Repair
		Histone deacetylases (HDACs)	Replication Condensation
Methylation	Lysine	Lysine methyltransferases	Transcription
		Lysine demethylases	Repair
	Arginine	Arginine methyltransferases	Transcription
		Arginine demethylases	
Phosphorylation	Serine	Serine/threonine kinases	Transcription
	Threonine	Dephosphorylated by phosphatases	Repair Condensation
Ubiquitination	Lysine	Ubiquinases (ubiquitin ligases)	Transcription
		Deubiquinating enzymes	Repair
SUMOylation	Lysine	Small ubiquitin-like modifier (SUMO)	Transcription
		De-SUMOylating enzymes: sentrin-specific proteases	
ADP ribosylation	Glutamate	ADP-ribosyltransferases	Transcription
Deimination	Arginine (to Citrulline)	Peptidylarginine deiminases	Transcription
Proline isomerisation	Proline	Proline isomerases	Transcription

Table 1. Types of histone modifications and the enzymes responsible (modified from Ref. [22]).

transcriptional machinery onto the gene promoter and enhancer regions. HDACs are enzymes that remove acetyl groups from hyperacetylated histones, and modification by HDACs leads to a closed chromatin structure and suppression of genes. HDACs are recruited to gene promoters by DNA-binding proteins that recognise certain DNA sequences and in this way provide specific modulation on gene expression.

There are 18 characterised members of the HDAC family in mammals, which can be grouped into four classes depending on their functional similarities and their homology with yeast HDACs. The class I and class II HDACs are considered as the 'classical' HDACs [23].

Class I HDACs comprise nuclear, ubiquitously expressed HDACs 1, 2, 3, and 8. HDAC1, 2, and 8 reside nearly exclusively in the nucleus. HDAC3 is found to shuttle between nucleus and cytoplasm. Because these are ubiquitously expressed and involved in cell proliferation and survival, aberrations in their gene expression have been implicated in a wide range of cancers [24, 25].

Class II HDACs shuttle between the cytoplasm and the nucleus depending on specific cellular signals; they share a tissue-specific expression pattern and are divided into two subgroups:

http://dx.doi.org/10.5772/66409

class IIa (HDACs 4, 5, 7, and 9) and class IIb (HDACs 6 and 10). Class IIa HDACs distinguish themselves with their extended N-terminal regulatory domain, whereas class IIb HDACs contain two catalytic domains. Class IIa HDACs appear to have tissue-specific roles and can shuttle between the cytosol and the nucleus. In fact, the phosphorylation status is a critical event to determine their localisation in the nucleus or cytoplasm and the ability to act as transcriptional co-repressors in the nuclear region. Conversely, class IIb is mostly found in the cytosol [26].

Class III HDACs regroup the ubiquitously expressed silent information regulator 2 (Sir2) family of nicotinamide adenine dinucleotide (NAD+)-dependent HDACs (SIRT1–7), which share structural and functional similarities with the yeast Sir2 protein. Interestingly, these have a critical role in a wide range of cellular processes such as ageing, transcription, cell survival, DNA repair, apoptosis, and inflammation. Sirtuins appear to have contradictory roles in disease. On the one hand, they control many vital functions involved in cellular protection, while on the other hand, they are also involved in several disease pathologies such as metabolic diseases, neurodegenerative disorders, and cancer [27].

Finally, class IV HDAC is the newly discovered HDAC11. HDAC11 is most closely related to class I HDACs. However, since the overall sequence similarities are low, it cannot be grouped into any of the three existing classes. HDAC11 is primarily expressed in heart, smooth muscle, kidney, and brain tissues.

Recent reports suggest that HDACs can deacetylate non-histone proteins as additional functions of HDACs (**Figure 1**). The roles of HDACs in cancer and neurological diseases have

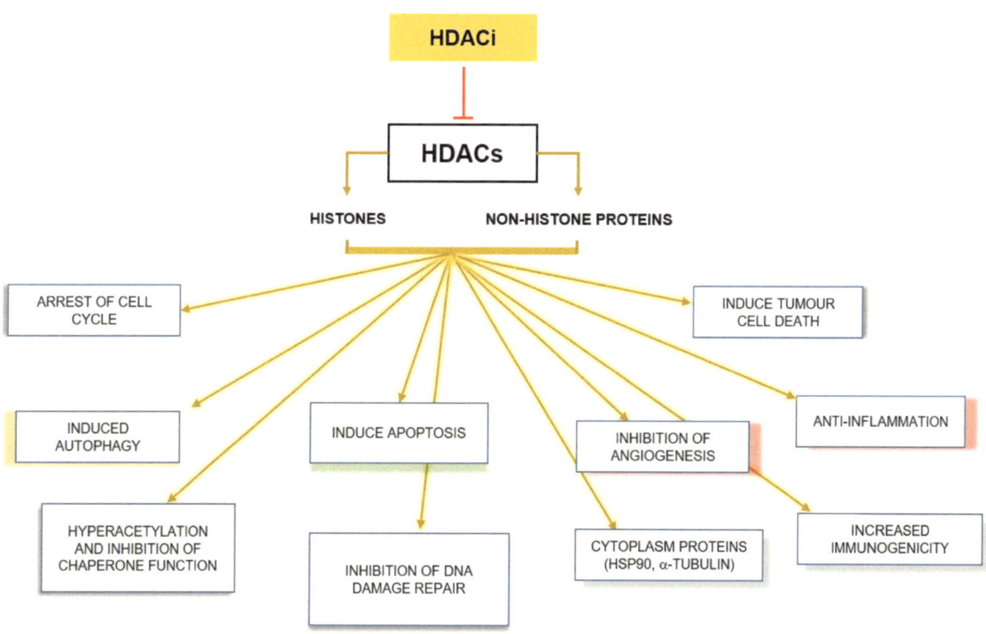

Figure 1. Schematic illustration of HDACi downstream effects. Inhibition of HDACs by HDACi induces acetylation of histone proteins as well as non-histone proteins, which leads to the alteration in various physiological and pathological processes (modified from Refs. [28–30]).

been extensively examined. However, the functions of HDACs in cardiovascular diseases and arteriosclerosis are less explored [23].

4.2. HDAC inhibitors

There has been a breakthrough in the development of HDACi. These HDACi induce acetylation of histone proteins, as well as non-histone proteins, which leads to the alteration and regulation of biological events including angiogenesis, apoptosis/autophagy, cell cycle, fibrogenesis, immune response, inflammation, and metabolism (**Figure 1**). As a result, HDAC inhibitor-based therapies have gained substantial attention as treatments for cardiovascular diseases and cancer.

In the following sections, we will describe the different exerted functions of HDACi in different physiological and pathological conditions.

5. The role of HDACs in angiogenesis: HDAC-regulated ECs functions in vitro

During development of the embryo and the physiological repairs of any tissue damages, the formation of new blood vessels plays a major role. The process can either involve vasculogenesis where ECs may be derived from the differentiation of different kinds of stem cells such as embryonic stem (ES) cells, while angiogenesis requires the proliferation, migration, and sprouting of ECs. Some of these new blood vessel formations are normal and beneficial as seen in wound healing after trauma and ischemic tissue restoration. However, pathological neovascularisation leads to many diseases such as diabetic retinopathy, tumour, and inflammation. Over the past decade, investigations into the role of HDACs in the regulations of these processes have gained some tractions. We have previously shown that the stabilisation of the class I HDAC3 plays an essential role in VEGF receptor 2 (VEGFR2)-mediated endothelial differentiation of mouse ES cells (mESC)-derived Sca-1^+ progenitors [31], while these events can also signal through VEGR2-HDAC3 stabilisation in a ligand-independent manner through exposure to laminar shear flow [32]. These derived EC-like cells display increased angiogenic potential by significantly enhancing re-endothelialisation with the host vessels upon their transplantation into a mouse wire injury model and substantially attenuated the injury-induced neointimal hyperplasia [32]. In addition, HDAC3 is also essential for the survival of ECs under atherogenic disturbed flow, and knock-down of HDAC3 increases neointima formation in the atheroprone ApoE$^{-/-}$ mice [33]. Overall, these show HDAC3 plays a role in the angiogenic processes.

Angiogenic activation of ECs to migrate and to form sprouts is associated with characteristic changes in gene expression profiles [34], which can be modulated by the inhibition of HDAC. HDAC inhibitions by pan-HDAC inhibitors such as suberoylanilide hydroxamic acid (SAHA) and trichostatin A (TSA) can suppress VEGF-induced capillary-like structures formation in human umbilical vein endothelial cells (HUVEC) by suppressing angiogenic factors such as hypoxia-inducible factor 1 alpha (HIF-1α), VEGF, and eNOS while both HDACi also prevent

http://dx.doi.org/10.5772/66409

the sprouting of capillaries from rat aorta [35]. Discrepant reports exist however, as another study has shown that treatment with SAHA or a more class I selective inhibitor valporic acid (VPA) in combination with VEGF indeed resulted in enhanced EC sprouting [36]. These discrepancies could be due to the contrasting roles that other HDACs within the same class and/or from the other classes might play in regulating angiogenesis.

In fact, it is common that completely opposite role has been reported for other HDACs in the regulation of angiogenesis. HDAC4, a class IIa HDAC, was reported to negatively regulate angiogenesis by reducing VEGF expression [37], while others have reported HDAC4 induces angiogenesis through an increase in stability of HIF-1γ [38]. In addition, Zhang et al. showed that HDAC4 inhibition facilitated c-kit+ cardiac stem cells (CSCs) into the differentiation of cardiac lineage commitments with EC potential in vitro [4].

Diverse role has also been reported in another class IIa HDAC HDAC5. On the one hand, HDAC5 has been shown to repress KLF2 an important regulator of EC homeostasis that is normally expressed in the laminar flow-exposed (therefore atheroprotective) segments of the vessels, which results in repressed eNOS expression in ECs [39]. This anti-angiogenic role of HDAC5 was validated by siRNA-mediated knock-down of HDAC5 that promoted migration and sprouting of ECs [40]. Conversely, phosphorylation-dependent nuclear exports of HDAC5 [40] and HDAC7 [41], thereby the de-repression of target genes, are crucial for the expression of VEGF or metalloproteinase-10 in ECs that lead to increased angiogenesis. Moreover, blockade of HDAC7 phosphorylation with a signal-resistant HDAC7 mutant represses EC proliferation and migration in response to VEGF, confirming the important role of both class IIa HDACs plays in VEGF-mediated angiogenesis [42]. In addition, HDAC7 has also been identified as a key modulator of EC migration at least in part by regulating PDGF-B/PDGF-beta gene expression [43].

Evidence from our laboratory demonstrated that mouse HDAC7 undergoes alternative translation during mouse ESCs differentiation, resulting in the production of a 7-amino acid peptide (*Data not publish yet*). This peptide was shown to enhance mouse vascular progenitor cell migration and VEGF-induced differentiation towards the EC lineage in vitro. Overall, HDAC7 appears to be pro-angiogenic, while the mediating role of HDAC5 in angiogenesis could be largely dependent on its translocation within the nucleus.

There is a limited research into the role of class IIb HDAC in angiogenesis, but nevertheless HDAC6 can be classified as a pro-angiogenic factor as it induces cell migration by the deacetylation of cytoskeletal proteins [44, 45]. Class III HDAC SIRT1 is also highly expressed in the vasculature during blood vessel growth where it controls the angiogenic activity of ECs. Loss of SIRT1 function leads to blockage of sprouting angiogenesis [46]. Furthermore, SIRT1 associates with and deacetylates transcription factor Foxo1 and hence restricts its anti-angiogenic activity [46].

6. The role of HDAC in therapeutic angiogenesis

Different strategies for therapeutic angiogenesis, including the direct delivery of angiogenic growth factors and the delivery of cells to ischemic tissues, have been developed. Moreover, there is a recent progress on therapeutic angiogenesis by utilising polymeric biomaterials, combined with stem cell and gene therapy as well as stimulation of endogenous stem cell homing (see Ref. [47] for a more comprehensive review).

Owing to the disadvantage of invasiveness, limited drug diffusion, and lack of selectivity towards targeted tissues, treatments with traditional drugs and surgery are becoming less commonly used [48]. An emerging technique, ultrasound-targeted microbubble destruction (UTMD), has been proposed as a non-invasive and specific targeting approach in angiogenic therapy of CVDs. UTMD might create a series of biological effects, including improving recovery of local tissue damages, improving transient membrane permeability, and extravasation to facilitate the entering of targeted genes or drugs into the tissues or cells of interest.

There are several approaches indicating that inhibition of HDAC protects the heart against injury in different cardiovascular-related diseases, including myocardial infarction, myocardial hypertrophy, and diabetic cardiomyopathy. In addition, HDACi also seem to play a therapeutic role in other CVDs with vascular remodelling as one of their main manifestations. Here, we review the role of HDACs in these diseases one by one in order to better understand the context-dependent effects of HDACs in angiogenesis regulation in these diseases.

6.1. Atherosclerosis

Atherosclerosis of the arteries is a main causative pathogenesis of various CVDs including coronary artery disease (CAD), peripheral vascular disease (PVD), and stroke. It is a chronic pathological condition of the arteries that is characterised by the accumulation of lipids, chronic inflammation, generation of a fibrous cap, proliferation of SMCs, calcification in vascular smooth muscle layer, with the resultant loss of elasticity of arteries. In addition, disturbed shear stress (the tangential force of the flowing blood on the endothelial surface of the blood vessel) contributes to several elements of atherosclerotic disease. As a result of the growth of atheroma, the lumen of the artery is gradually narrowed, which changes the local environment. Activated ECs within the injury lesions produce adhesion molecules [intercellular adhesion molecule (ICAM) and vascular cell adhesion molecule-1 (VCAM-1)], chemotactic proteins [monocyte chemotactic protein-1 (MCP-1)], E- and P-selectin, and growth factors [macrophage colony-stimulating factor (M-CSF)] that create a pro-inflammatory environment. The inflammatory molecules then recruit monocytes to the vessel wall and promote their transmigration across the endothelial monolayer into the intima, where they proliferate, differentiate into macrophages, and foam cells by taking up the lipoproteins, leading to neointimal formation. With time, the foam cells and macrophages die and release lipid-filled contents and tissue factors, contributing to the formation of the lipid-rich necrotic core, which is a key component of unstable plaques. Meanwhile, SMCs migrate from the medial layer and accumulate within the intima, where they synthesise and secrete interstitial collagen and elastin and form the fibrous cap over the lesion. Ultimately, the thin fibrous caps rupture, then expose, and release procoagulant materials into the blood, triggering the thrombosis that impedes blood flow and results in acute stenosis of the arteries, leading to clinical manifestations [49–51].

Because many patients are not candidates for the standard treatments such as angioplasty or bypass surgery, a great enthusiasm has emerged for the utilisation of angiogenesis as a

http://dx.doi.org/10.5772/66409

therapeutic modality for atherosclerotic arterial disease. It must be taken into account that angiogenesis plays a vital part in the pathogenesis and treatment of CVDs and has become one of the hotspots that are being discussed in the past decades. Therapeutic angiogenesis provides a valuable tool for treating cardiovascular diseases by stimulating the growth of new blood vessels from pre-existing vessels.

This avenue needs to be explored with caution however, as the role of angiogenesis in atherosclerosis remains a very contentious topic, and currently, there is no consensus as to whether angiogenesis is a way to treat coronary heart disease or in fact is a key causative factor in the pathogenesis of atherosclerotic plaque formation. The controversy surrounding the role of angiogenesis in ischemic heart disease reflects, in part, the complexity of the underlying disease process. There are lot of studies supporting the therapeutic role of angiogenesis in atherosclerosis since a key therapeutic objective has been to use the angiogenic cytokines such as VEGF or FGF to stimulate collateral blood vessel formation in the ischemic heart and limb [52]. But, on the other hand, the pathogenic role of angiogenesis has been suggested as VEGF, and other angiogenic growth factors can promote atherosclerosis in certain animal models and potentially destabilise coronary plaques by promoting intralesion angiogenesis [53].

Apolipoprotein E-deficient ($ApoE^{-/-}$) mice, created by homologous recombination in ES cells, was first described in 1992 [54, 55]. Since then, this model becomes the most commonly used mouse model of atherosclerosis that is able to develop severe hypercholesterolemia and lesions of atherosclerosis highly similar to those observed in humans. Endogenous SIRT1 has been shown to decrease macrophage foam cell formation and atherogenesis in $ApoE^{-/-}$mice [56], while endothelial-specific overexpression of human SIRT1 reduces atherogenesis in $ApoE^{-/-}$ mice and improves vascular function [57]. So, in the vasculature, *SIRT1* gain-of-function using *SIRT1* overexpression has been shown to improve endothelial function in mice. Subsequently, it was described that SIRT1 does not directly influence endothelium-dependent vascular function in ApoE−/− mice, but it improves vascular function by preventing superoxide production in ECs and reduces the expression of inflammatory adhesion molecules by suppressing NF-κB signalling [58].

HDACi TSA has been shown to exert contradictory role in the formation of atherosclerotic lesion. TSA successfully prevents neointima formation after injury [59, 60]. In contrast, however, several reports have elucidated the proatherogenic effects of TSA [61]. Another example of the discrepancies in TSA roles is the reduction of angiogenesis through the decrease of NO level (a key second messenger in angiogenesis signalling) through downregulation of eNOS [62]. These contrasting findings reinforce the theory of the contesting role angiogenesis plays in atherosclerosis. In addition, it was reported that TSA can reduce the cholesterol biosynthesis by repressing the genes involved in the cholesterol, fatty acids, and glycolysis pathways [63]. These evidences suggest that TSA could be used as a potential therapeutic agent for the control of cholesterol levels as high cholesterol level is one of the main triggers of atherosclerosis.

6.2. Myocardial infarction

Myocardial infarction (MI) occurs when blood flow stops to part of the heart causing damage to the cardiomyocytes. In physiological conditions, oxygen and nutrients are supplied to the ventricular myocytes by the coronary arteries. Under pathological condition, the coronary artery is often occluded by various pathological condition such as the growth of atheroma in the coronary artery, rupture of vulnerable plaque, thrombi from proximal lesions, emboli secondary to atrial fibrillation, or vegetation after endocarditis.

Several gene or protein therapies to deliver angiogenic factors such as VEGF, FGF2, or FGF4, as well as cell therapy using endothelial progenitor cells (EPCs), mesenchymal stem cells (MSCs), or induced pluripotent stem cells (iPSCs), have been developed as potential pro-angiogenic therapeutics for ischemic heart disease and peripheral vascular disease [64, 65]. HDAC4 inhibition has been demonstrated to promote cardiac stem cells mediated cardiac regeneration and improve the restoration of cardiac function in mice [4]. Granger et al. observed that ischemia induces HDAC activity in the heart resulting in increased deacetylation of histones H3/4 in vitro and in vivo that leads to injured cardiomyocytes [66]. Furthermore, HDACi exert direct antifibrotic activities that alter the response to ischemic cardiac injury and reduce infarct size, which are accompanied by improvement in cardiac functions in the mouse infarcted heart. However, it is unclear whether these therapeutic effects have any links with angiogenesis in these earlier studies.

TSA have exerted an increased angiogenic response in vivo in the mouse infarcted hearts. This indicates that TSA preserves cardiac performance and mitigates myocardial remodelling through stimulating cardiac endogenous regeneration that could be dependent on enhanced angiogenesis within the infarcted heart tissues [67]. The repression of ischemia-induced gene expression such as HIF-1α and VEGF has been suggested as possible mechanisms mediated by HDACi to stabilise vascular permeability [66]. Recruitment of stem cells has also been suggested as another main mechanism that TSA mediates through. After 8 weeks of TSA treatment in MI mice with or without c-kit deficiency, significantly improved neovascularisation and cardiac repair accompanied by cardiac functions and reduced cardiac remodelling can be observed in the wildtype infarcted heart compared to the c-kit-deficient mice [68]. It is also important to distinguish between the timing of the HDACi effects. Many reports show that long-term (8 weeks) administration of HDACi induces neovascularisation [67], while acute treatments (12 h) with HDACi inhibit angiogenesis [66].

6.3. Cardiac hypertrophy

Cardiac hypertrophy is a form of remodelling and is an adaptive response to the request for high workload from peripheral tissue or from intrinsic underlying disease conditions such as valvular dysfunction, hypertension, and MI. The heart responds to stresses by undergoing a remodelling process that is associated with myocyte hypertrophy, myocyte death, inflammation, and fibrosis, which often result in impaired cardiac function and heart failure. These are accompanied by activation of the myocyte enhancer factor-2 (MEF2) transcription factor and reprogramming of cardiac gene expression. Recent studies have revealed key roles for HDACs as both positive and negative regulators of pathological cardiac remodelling (**Figure 2**).

Members of MEF2 transcription factors family are some of the key regulators of myocardial hypertrophy. The first connection between HDACs and the regulation of pathological cardiac remodelling was provided by the discovery that class IIa HDACs interact with members of

http://dx.doi.org/10.5772/66409

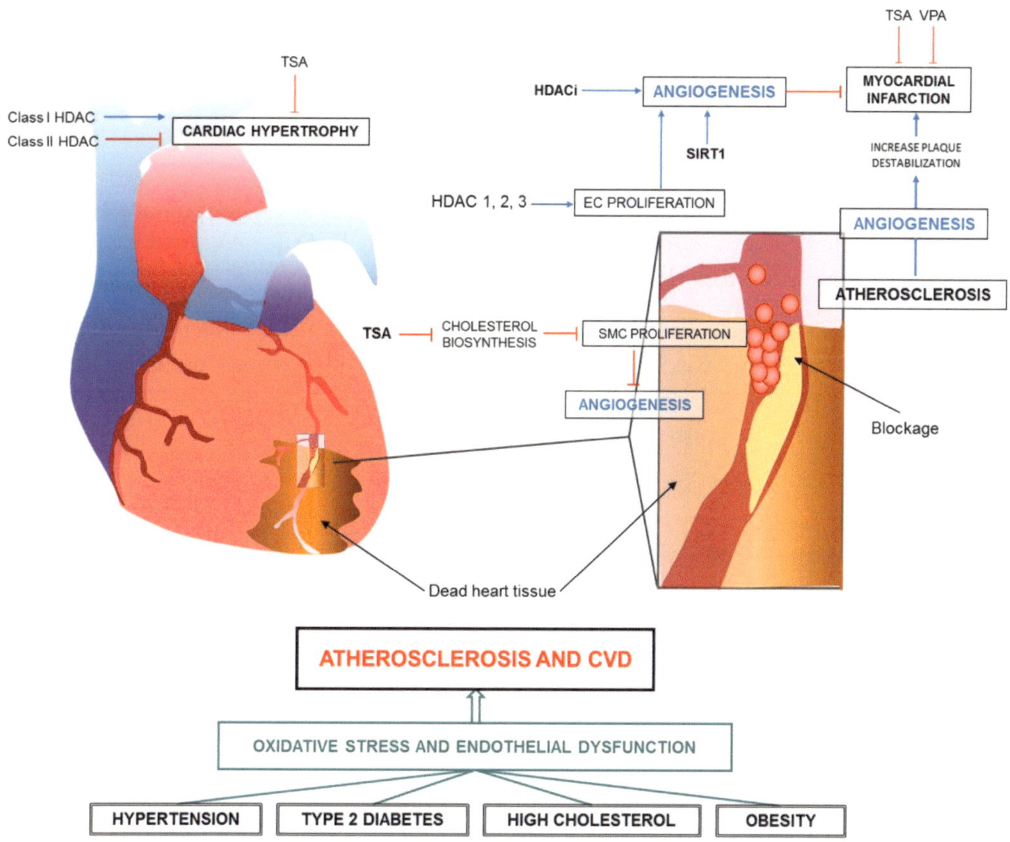

Figure 2. HDACs in cardiovascular disease. Different risk factors lead to the appearance of atheromatous plaques in the coronary arteries, and from these, other cardiovascular diseases such as myocardial infarction occur. The discovery that different HDAC enzymes are involved in processes such as angiogenesis has led to the development of inhibitors to modulate its effect as a therapeutic treatment (→ means induction; ⊣ means inhibition).

MEF2 transcription factor family [69]. The transcriptional activity of MEF2 factors is upregulated in response to pathological stress in the heart, and ectopic overexpression of constitutively active forms of MEF2 in mouse heart causes dilated cardiomyopathy. It was reported that class II HDACs are substrates for a stress-responsive kinase specific for conserved serines that regulate MEF2-HDAC interactions. Those kinases phosphorylate the signal-responsive sites in class II HDACs, and mutant proteins lacking these phosphorylation sites can act as signal-resistant repressors of cardiomyocyte hypertrophy and fetal cardiac gene expression in vitro [70]. These studies support a role for class IIa HDACs as endogenous repressors of cardiac hypertrophy. Conversely, the function of class IIb HDACs in the heart remains largely unknown in heart hypertrophy.

Nevertheless, administration of HDACi TSA 2 weeks after the induction of pressure overload can reverse cardiac hypertrophy in mice [71]. The class I selective HDACi MPT0E014 also improves cardiac contractibility and attenuates structural remodelling in isoproterenol-induced dilated cardiomyopathy [72]. As there is an intrinsic relationship between decreased capillary density and the transition of cardiac hypertrophy to cardiac failure [73], it remains to be investigated whether the cardioprotective effects exerted by HDACi are related to increased angiogenesis within the hypertrophic heart.

6.4. Peripheral artery disease

Peripheral artery disease (PAD) can be defined as the narrowing of the peripheral arteries that are not directly linked to the supply to the heart or the brain. PAD development is a multifactorial process with many different forms [74].

Different action mechanisms have been proposed for different HDACi in terms of regulating angiogenesis in the case of vascular diseases. It was reported in a mouse model of hindlimb ischaemia that the inhibition of class IIa HDACs is pro-angiogenic while class I HDAC inhibition is anti-angiogenic in mouse models of hindlimb ischemia [75].

6.5. Stroke

Stroke is a devastating illness and the second cause of death and disability worldwide after cardiac ischemia. A stroke occurs when a blood vessel that carries oxygen and nutrients to the brain is either blocked by a clot or bursts. As a consequence, part of the brain can die. Post-mortem studies have revealed that angiogenesis can be observed several days after cerebral ischemic stroke; it is noteworthy that higher microvessel density correlates with longer patient survival [76]. Enhanced angiogenesis facilities neurovascular remodelling processes and promotes brain functional recovery after stroke.

There are several studies testing the effects of HDACi in neurovascular remodelling processes and in brain functional recovery after stroke. Sun et al. showed that VPA treatment enhanced post-ischemic angiogenesis by increasing microvessel density, facilitating EC proliferation, and up-regulating rate of cerebral blood flow in the ipsilateral cortex. These events may be associated with up-regulation of HIF-1α and its downstream proangiogenic target VEGF as well as extracellular MMP2/9 [77]. Similar results were obtained by treating rats with VPA during permanent middle cerebral artery occlusion (pMCAO). They exhibit reduced infarct volume, promote functional recovery, enhance angiogenesis by upregulating VEGF [78], and reduce monocytes infiltration [79]. SIRT1 is proangiogenic and increases EC tube formation, especially in post-natal angiogenesis [46]. So loss of SIRT1 reduces angiogenesis and increases brain infarction, while SIRT1 was also demonstrated to play an important role in neuroprotection against brain ischemia by deacetylation and subsequent inhibition of p53-induced and nuclear factor κB-induced inflammatory and apoptotic pathways [80].

After pMCAO, sodium butyrate and TSA induce neurogenesis via HDACi in multiple ischemic brain regions in rats. Sodium butyrate also strongly upregulated VEGF, increasing angiogenesis and functional recovery after stroke. It was also described that sodium butyrate exhibits neuroprotective/neurogenic effects in rat model of neonatal hypoxia-ischemia [81]. All these results highlight that the inhibition of HDAC in brain after stroke enhances angiogenesis, and this may contribute to the long-term functional recovery after stroke.

http://dx.doi.org/10.5772/66409

6.6. HDACs role in angiogenesis in diabetes

Diabetes mellitus is a chronic disease where the lack of insulin leads to anomalies in the substrate metabolism, causing a range of acute and long-term complications. One of the main complication is the loss of small blood vessels. Another related secondary disease is diabetic glomerulomegaly or kidney disease. One of the predominant feature of diabetic glomerulomegaly is an increase in glomerular capillary volume [82], which can be controlled by anti-angiogenic therapies. As there is evidence of genetic association between diabetes and HDACs, treatment with HDACi exerts a reduction in glomerular endothelial markers expression, which demonstrates the anti-angiogenic benefit [83]. This effect seems to be opposite when it applies to the diabetic heart failure model, as another HDACi sodium butyrate exerts improved cardiac functions and increased microvessel density within the diabetic myocardium [84]. Moreover, HDACi also modulates cardiac peroxisome proliferator-activated receptors (PPARs) and fatty acid metabolism in diabetic cardiomyopathy [85].

7. Pathogenic role of angiogenesis

7.1. Cancer

There are more than 200 different kinds of cancers, and each type behaves and responds to treatments in different ways. Epigenetic enzymes are dysregulated in tumours through mutation or altered expression. More importantly, tumourigenesis is largely due to overexpression of oncogenes or the loss of function of tumour suppressor genes. The identification of these proteins has driven the rapid development of small-molecule inhibitors.

As we mention above, the function of HDACs is not solely on modifying histones, but they can also target many different cellular substrates and proteins, including those that are involved in tumour progression. Currently, many HDACi are in clinical trials for cancer therapeutics as HDACi result in hyperacetylation (and therefore repression) of genes related to tumour cell apoptosis, growth arrest, senescence, differentiation, cell invasion, and metastasis [86].

An exemplary role of HDACi play in modulating the tumour cells directly is its action on vasculogenic mimicry (VM). VM refers to the process by which highly aggressive tumour cells mimic ECs to form vessel-like structures that aid in supplying enough nutrients to rapidly growing tumours [87]. HDAC3 has demonstrated an important facilitative role on VM in gliomas, as HDAC3 expression is directly correlated with the number of VM in tumours with worsen tumour grade [88]. HDACi such as SAHA exert significant anti-VM effect in the progressive pancreatic cancer cells through its inhibition of AKT and ERK signalling pathways [89].

The role of HDACs play in tumour angiogenesis has also been studied. It is widely known that hypoxia induces tumour angiogenesis and cell survival through the up-regulation of VEGF expression in tumour cells [90]. Different studies have reported that inhibition of HDAC activity by TSA blocks hypoxia-induced tumour angiogenesis [91]. Other HDACi also exert similar effects, as exemplified by MPT0G157, a potent inhibitor of HDAC1, 2, 3, and 6, which was found to promote HIF-1α degradation followed by the downregulation of VEGF expression [92]. There are also reports of the anti-tumoural effects of other HDACi (TSA, sodium butyrate, and VPA) that are also partly mediated by the reduction of VEGFR-2 expression that might be related to repressing tumour angiogenesis [93].

SIRT1, a class III HDAC, also plays an important role in tumour initiation, progression, and development of drug resistance by hindering senescence, stress-induced apoptosis [94, 95], and activating cell growth and angiogenesis. MiR-34a, whose expression level was found to be reduced in various tumour cell lines [96, 97], was reported to exert its tumour suppression effect via direct binding onto SIRT1 mRNA and regulate cell apoptosis via SIRT1-p53 pathway [98]. miR-34a also exerts its anti-tumoural effect through inhibiting SIRT1 to induce the senescence of EPCs to suppress EPC-mediated tumour angiogenesis [99].

There are emerging HDACi for cancer therapy. HDACi-targeting class I, II, and IV HDACs to be used as anticancer agents are currently under development. One of them, vorinostat, has been approved by FDA for treating cutaneous T-cell lymphoma for patients with persistent or recurrent disease or following two systemic therapies. Other inhibitors, for example, FK228, PXD101, PCI-24781, ITF2357, MGCD0103, MS-275, valproic acid, and LBH589 have also demonstrated therapeutic potential as monotherapy or combination with other anti-tumour drugs [86, 100].

7.2. Age-related macular degeneration

Age-related macular degeneration (AMD) is the leading cause of blindness worldwide. AMD is characterised by the deposition of drusen aggregates under the retinal epithelium. Clusterin is one of the major proteins in drusens [101], and during aging, the expression of clusterin increases [102]. The impact of epigenetic modifications on the pathogenesis of AMD has been reported. It is known that aging affects histone acetylation status, so it is reasonable to presume that the epigenetic regulation might have a role in clusterin expression. It was reported that the treatment with HDACi induces prominent increases in the expression levels of clusterin mRNA and the secretion of clusterin protein. This result indicates that epigenetic factors regulate clusterin expression which could be affecting the pathogenesis of AMD via the inhibition of angiogenesis and inflammation [103].

7.3. Pulmonary arterial hypertension

Pulmonary arterial hypertension (PAH) is a condition characterised by increased pulmonary vascular resistance and pulmonary artery pressure leading to right heart failure and premature death [104]. During the process, there is a vascular remodelling caused by dysregulated cell proliferation, migration, and survival. The cause of PAH is complex, but the excessive proliferation of SMCs and ECs within the pulmonary artery is thought to play an essential role in its pathogenesis.

Elevated levels of HDAC1 and HDAC5 have been observed in the PAH lungs, and treatments with HDACi such as SAHA and VPA reduce disease worsening in rat models of pulmonary hypertension [105]. In addition, MEF2 might have a protective role in PAH progression as the expression of MEF2 and its transcriptional targets are significantly decreased in pulmo-

http://dx.doi.org/10.5772/66409

nary artery ECs from patients with PAH. The impaired MEF2 activity in ECs from PAH was associated with increased nuclear accumulation of HDAC4 and HDAC5. So, increasing MEF2 activity by the selective inhibition of class IIa HDACs by MC1568 seems to suppress excessive EC migration and proliferation by PAH-ECs and can rescue experimental PAH model [106]. Although the increased migration and proliferation of pulmonary artery ECs in PAH are also hallmarks of angiogenesis, it is still contentious to link excessive angiogenesis with the pathogenesis of PAH [107], and any potential anti-angiogenic therapy for PAH should be proceeded with caution.

8. Concluding remarks and future perspectives

The past 15 years of research have significantly advanced our understanding of the functions and modes of regulation of HDACs in CVD. With all the studies discussed above, we can get an idea about how complex it is to translate HDACi as clinical therapeutics as they exert contradictory functions in many occasions. Extensive evidence for HDAC involvement in multiprotein complexes and cell-specific signalling indicates that a deeper understanding of these pathways will be crucial to effective pharmacological targeting in future.

Although angiogenesis seems to be a very promising therapeutic possibility for the majority of CVDs where patients are not responding to conventional treatments, there are also times that angiogenesis participates in the pathological processes. So in some diseases such as MI and diabetic cardiomyopathy, enhancement of angiogenesis is beneficial by improving recovery of injured myocardium. In the other circumstances where aberrant neoangiogensis is one of the main disease manifestations (such as cancer and AMD), potentiation of anti-angiogenic signalling could be beneficial. Thus, the crucial role that angiogenesis can play as a therapy can only be achieved by thoroughly understanding the underlying mechanisms.

In addition, the diverse and contrasting effects that the current available HDACi exert might be due to their low specificity to a particular HDAC. Class IIa HDACs are expressed in limited organs such as the muscles, brain, or bone, whereas class I HDACs exist ubiquitously. Thus, one may question the specificity and adverse effects of unspecific HDACi for therapeutic uses. Therefore in the future, creation of more specific HDACi, armed with better understanding of the underlying mechanisms of specific HDAC in angiogenesis within each pathological condition, could help the development of more targetted treatments to improve vascularisation and tissue repairs with higher efficiency and efficacy.

Alternative methods where HDAC modulation can be utilised in therapeutic angiogenesis are to modulate endothelial differentiation of stem or progenitor cells, which can be applied as cell therapy to enhance angiogenesis within the ischemic tissues. Next-generation gene-editing tool, such as CRISPR-Cas9, can also be extremely useful in accurately targetting specific gene responsible for suppressing or exacerbating angiogenesis depending on the diseases. Moreover, with diseases such as PAH that are characterised by both lack of angiogenesis (within the right ventricles) and excessive angiogenesis (within the pulmonary vasculature), the development of nanoparticles to deliver drugs to specific target tissues can be highly beneficial. This approach will also be extremely useful for patients that manifest both CVD and cancer.

We are currently in an exciting era for translational research with a lot of new inspiring technologies that can truly transform therapeutic approaches. With diligent efforts to devise the role of HDACs underlying angiogenesis robustly in various CVDs, in conjunction with the creation of more selective HDAC inhibitors, advanced engineering solutions, and gene-editing tools to correct genes responsible for repressing angiogenesis, and a commitment in rigorous placebo-controlled clinical trials, superior therapies for CVDs are on the horizon.

Author details

Ana Moraga, Ka Hou Lao and Lingfang Zeng*

*Address all correspondence to: lingfang.zeng@kcl.ac.uk

Cardiovascular Division, Faculty of Life Sciences and Medicine, King's College London, London, UK

References

[1] Goff DC, Lloyd-Jones DM, Bennett G, Coady S, D'Agostino RB, Gibbons R, et al. 2013 ACC/AHA guideline on the assessment of cardiovascular risk: a report of the American College of Cardiology/American Heart Association Task Force on Practice Guidelines. Circulation. 2014;129(25 Suppl 2):S49–73.

[2] O'Donnell CJ, Nabel EG. Genomics of cardiovascular disease. N Engl J Med. 2011;365(22):2098–109.

[3] Jones PA, Baylin SB. The fundamental role of epigenetic events in cancer. Nat Rev Genet. 2002;3(6):415–28.

[4] Zhang LX, DeNicola M, Qin X, Du J, Ma J, Tina Zhao Y, et al. Specific inhibition of HDAC4 in cardiac progenitor cells enhances myocardial repairs. Am J Physiol Cell Physiol. 2014;307(4):C358–72.

[5] Lehmann LH, Worst BC, Stanmore DA, Backs J. Histone deacetylase signaling in cardioprotection. Cell Mol Life Sci. 2014;71(9):1673–90.

[6] Aird WC. Phenotypic heterogeneity of the endothelium: I. Structure, function, and mechanisms. Circ Res. 2007;100(2):158–73.

[7] van Hinsbergh VW. Endothelium—role in regulation of coagulation and inflammation. Semin Immunopathol. 2012;34(1):93–106.

[8] Alderton WK, Cooper CE, Knowles RG. Nitric oxide synthases: structure, function and inhibition. Biochem J. 2001;357(Pt 3):593–615.

http://dx.doi.org/10.5772/66409

[9] Versari D, Daghini E, Virdis A, Ghiadoni L, Taddei S. Endothelial dysfunction as a target for prevention of cardiovascular disease. Diabetes Care. 2009;32 Suppl 2:S314–21.

[10] Risau W, Flamme I. Vasculogenesis. Annu Rev Cell Dev Biol. 1995;11:73–91.

[11] Carmeliet P. Mechanisms of angiogenesis and arteriogenesis. Nat Med. 2000;6(4):389–95.

[12] Al Sabti H. Therapeutic angiogenesis in cardiovascular disease. J Cardiothorac Surg. 2007;2:49.

[13] Sone H, Kawakami Y, Okuda Y, Kondo S, Hanatani M, Suzuki H, et al. Vascular endothelial growth factor is induced by long-term high glucose concentration and up-regulated by acute glucose deprivation in cultured bovine retinal pigmented epithelial cells. Biochem Biophys Res Commun. 1996;221(1):193–8.

[14] Sunderkötter C, Goebeler M, Schulze-Osthoff K, Bhardwaj R, Sorg C. Macrophage-derived angiogenesis factors. Pharmacol Ther. 1991;51(2):195–216.

[15] Tuder RM, Flook BE, Voelkel NF. Increased gene expression for VEGF and the VEGF receptors KDR/Flk and Flt in lungs exposed to acute or to chronic hypoxia. Modulation of gene expression by nitric oxide. J Clin Invest. 1995;95(4):1798–807.

[16] Carmeliet P, Jain RK. Molecular mechanisms and clinical applications of angiogenesis. Nature. 2011;473(7347):298–307.

[17] Fraineau S, Palii CG, Allan DS, Brand M. Epigenetic regulation of endothelial-cell-mediated vascular repair. FEBS J. 2015;282(9):1605–29.

[18] Schiano C, Vietri MT, Grimaldi V, Picascia A, Pascale MR, Napoli C. Epigenetic-related therapeutic challenges in cardiovascular disease. Trends Pharmacol Sci. 2015;36(4):226–35.

[19] Fish JE, Yan MS, Matouk CC, St Bernard R, Ho JJ, Gavryushova A, et al. Hypoxic repression of endothelial nitric-oxide synthase transcription is coupled with eviction of promoter histones. J Biol Chem. 2010;285(2):810–26.

[20] Miranda TB, Jones PA. DNA methylation: the nuts and bolts of repression. J Cell Physiol. 2007;213(2):384–90.

[21] Baccarelli A, Rienstra M, Benjamin EJ. Cardiovascular epigenetics: basic concepts and results from animal and human studies. Circ Cardiovasc Genet. 2010;3(6):567–73.

[22] Bassett SA, Barnett MP. The role of dietary histone deacetylases (HDACs) inhibitors in health and disease. Nutrients. 2014;6(10):4273–301.

[23] Zhou B, Margariti A, Zeng L, Xu Q. Role of histone deacetylases in vascular cell homeostasis and arteriosclerosis. Cardiovasc Res. 2011;90(3):413–20.

[24] Jin KL, Pak JH, Park JY, Choi WH, Lee JY, Kim JH, et al. Expression profile of histone deacetylases 1, 2 and 3 in ovarian cancer tissues. J Gynecol Oncol. 2008;19(3):185–90.

[25] Song Y, Shiota M, Tamiya S, Kuroiwa K, Naito S, Tsuneyoshi M. The significance of strong histone deacetylase 1 expression in the progression of prostate cancer. Histopathology. 2011;58(5):773–80.

[26] de Ruijter AJ, van Gennip AH, Caron HN, Kemp S, van Kuilenburg AB. Histone deacetylases (HDACs): characterization of the classical HDAC family. Biochem J. 2003;370(Pt 3):737–49.

[27] Bosch-Presegué L, Vaquero A. The dual role of sirtuins in cancer. Genes Cancer. 2011;2(6):648–62.

[28] Tang J, Yan H, Zhuang S. Histone deacetylases as targets for treatment of multiple diseases. Clin Sci (Lond). 2013;124(11):651–62.

[29] Yang XJ, Seto E. HATs and HDACs: from structure, function and regulation to novel strategies for therapy and prevention. Oncogene. 2007;26(37):5310–8.

[30] Falkenberg KJ, Johnstone RW. Histone deacetylases and their inhibitors in cancer, neurological diseases and immune disorders. Nat Rev Drug Discov. 2014;13(9):673–91.

[31] Xiao Q, Zeng L, Zhang Z, Margariti A, Ali ZA, Channon KM, et al. Sca-1+ progenitors derived from embryonic stem cells differentiate into endothelial cells capable of vascular repair after arterial injury. Arterioscler Thromb Vasc Biol. 2006;26(10):2244–51.

[32] Zeng L, Xiao Q, Margariti A, Zhang Z, Zampetaki A, Patel S, et al. HDAC3 is crucial in shear- and VEGF-induced stem cell differentiation toward endothelial cells. J Cell Biol. 2006;174(7):1059–69.

[33] Zampetaki A, Zeng L, Margariti A, Xiao Q, Li H, Zhang Z, et al. Histone deacetylase 3 is critical in endothelial survival and atherosclerosis development in response to disturbed flow. Circulation. 2010;121(1):132–42.

[34] Glesne DA, Zhang W, Mandava S, Ursos L, Buell ME, Makowski L, et al. Subtractive transcriptomics: establishing polarity drives in vitro human endothelial morphogenesis. Cancer Res. 2006;66(8):4030–40.

[35] Deroanne CF, Bonjean K, Servotte S, Devy L, Colige A, Clausse N, et al. Histone deacetylases inhibitors as anti-angiogenic agents altering vascular endothelial growth factor signaling. Oncogene. 2002;21(3):427–36.

[36] Jin G, Bausch D, Knightly T, Liu Z, Li Y, Liu B, et al. Histone deacetylase inhibitors enhance endothelial cell sprouting angiogenesis in vitro. Surgery. 2011;150(3):429–35.

[37] Sun X, Wei L, Chen Q, Terek RM. HDAC4 represses vascular endothelial growth factor expression in chondrosarcoma by modulating RUNX2 activity. J Biol Chem. 2009;284(33):21881–90.

[38] Geng H, Harvey CT, Pittsenbarger J, Liu Q, Beer TM, Xue C, et al. HDAC4 protein regulates HIF1α protein lysine acetylation and cancer cell response to hypoxia. J Biol Chem. 2011;286(44):38095–102.

[39] Dekker RJ, van Soest S, Fontijn RD, Salamanca S, de Groot PG, VanBavel E, et al. Prolonged fluid shear stress induces a distinct set of endothelial cell genes, most specifically lung Krüppel-like factor (KLF2). Blood. 2002;100(5):1689–98.

[40] Urbich C, Rössig L, Kaluza D, Potente M, Boeckel JN, Knau A, et al. HDAC5 is a repressor of angiogenesis and determines the angiogenic gene expression pattern of endothelial cells. Blood. 2009;113(22):5669–79.

[41] Margariti A, Zampetaki A, Xiao Q, Zhou B, Karamariti E, Martin D, et al. Histone deacetylase 7 controls endothelial cell growth through modulation of beta-catenin. Circ Res. 2010;106(7):1202–11.

[42] Wang S, Li X, Parra M, Verdin E, Bassel-Duby R, Olson EN. Control of endothelial cell proliferation and migration by VEGF signaling to histone deacetylase 7. Proc Natl Acad Sci USA. 2008;105(22):7738–43.

[43] Mottet D, Bellahcène A, Pirotte S, Waltregny D, Deroanne C, Lamour V, et al. Histone deacetylase 7 silencing alters endothelial cell migration, a key step in angiogenesis. Circ Res. 2007;101(12):1237–46.

[44] Kaluza D, Kroll J, Gesierich S, Yao TP, Boon RA, Hergenreider E, et al. Class IIb HDAC6 regulates endothelial cell migration and angiogenesis by deacetylation of cortactin. EMBO J. 2011;30(20):4142–56.

[45] Li D, Xie S, Ren Y, Huo L, Gao J, Cui D, et al. Microtubule-associated deacetylase HDAC6 promotes angiogenesis by regulating cell migration in an EB1-dependent manner. Protein Cell. 2011;2(2):150–60.

[46] Potente M, Ghaeni L, Baldessari D, Mostoslavsky R, Rossig L, Dequiedt F, et al. SIRT1 controls endothelial angiogenic functions during vascular growth. Genes Dev. 2007;21(20):2644–58.

[47] Deveza L, Choi J, Yang F. Therapeutic angiogenesis for treating cardiovascular diseases. Theranostics. 2012;2(8):801–14.

[48] Liao YY, Chen ZY, Wang YX, Lin Y, Yang F, Zhou QL. New progress in angiogenesis therapy of cardiovascular disease by ultrasound targeted microbubble destruction. Biomed Res Int. 2014;2014:872984.

[49] Libby P, Ridker PM, Hansson GK. Progress and challenges in translating the biology of atherosclerosis. Nature. 2011;473(7347):317–25.

[50] Lusis AJ. Atherosclerosis. Nature. 2000;407(6801):233–41.

[51] Glass CK, Witztum JL. Atherosclerosis. the road ahead. Cell. 2001;104(4):503–16.

[52] Simons M, Ware JA. Therapeutic angiogenesis in cardiovascular disease. Nat Rev Drug Discov. 2003;2(11):863–71.

[53] Celletti FL, Waugh JM, Amabile PG, Brendolan A, Hilfiker PR, Dake MD. Vascular endothelial growth factor enhances atherosclerotic plaque progression. Nat Med. 2001;7(4):425–9.

[54] Plump AS, Smith JD, Hayek T, Aalto-Setälä K, Walsh A, Verstuyft JG, et al. Severe hypercholesterolemia and atherosclerosis in apolipoprotein E-deficient mice created by homologous recombination in ES cells. Cell. 1992;71(2):343–53.

[55] Zhang SH, Reddick RL, Piedrahita JA, Maeda N. Spontaneous hypercholesterolemia and arterial lesions in mice lacking apolipoprotein E. Science. 1992;258(5081):468–71.

[56] Stein S, Lohmann C, Schäfer N, Hofmann J, Rohrer L, Besler C, et al. SIRT1 decreases Lox-1-mediated foam cell formation in atherogenesis. Eur Heart J. 2010;31(18):2301–9.

[57] Zhang QJ, Wang Z, Chen HZ, Zhou S, Zheng W, Liu G, et al. Endothelium-specific overexpression of class III deacetylase SIRT1 decreases atherosclerosis in apolipoprotein E-deficient mice. Cardiovasc Res. 2008;80(2):191–9.

[58] Stein S, Schäfer N, Breitenstein A, Besler C, Winnik S, Lohmann C, et al. SIRT1 reduces endothelial activation without affecting vascular function in ApoE−/− mice. Aging (Albany, NY). 2010;2(6):353–60.

[59] Okamoto H, Fujioka Y, Takahashi A, Takahashi T, Taniguchi T, Ishikawa Y, et al. Trichostatin A, an inhibitor of histone deacetylase, inhibits smooth muscle cell proliferation via induction of p21(WAF1). J Atheroscler Thromb. 2006;13(4):183–91.

[60] Findeisen HM, Gizard F, Zhao Y, Qing H, Heywood EB, Jones KL, et al. Epigenetic regulation of vascular smooth muscle cell proliferation and neointima formation by histone deacetylase inhibition. Arterioscler Thromb Vasc Biol. 2011;31(4):851–60.

[61] Song S, Kang SW, Choi C. Trichostatin A enhances proliferation and migration of vascular smooth muscle cells by downregulating thioredoxin 1. Cardiovasc Res. 2010;85(1):241–9.

[62] Rössig L, Li H, Fisslthaler B, Urbich C, Fleming I, Förstermann U, et al. Inhibitors of histone deacetylation downregulate the expression of endothelial nitric oxide synthase and compromise endothelial cell function in vasorelaxation and angiogenesis. Circ Res. 2002;91(9):837–44.

[63] Chittur SV, Sangster-Guity N, McCormick PJ. Histone deacetylase inhibitors: a new mode for inhibition of cholesterol metabolism. BMC Genomics. 2008;9:507.

[64] Aranguren XL, McCue JD, Hendrickx B, Zhu XH, Du F, Chen E, et al. Multipotent adult progenitor cells sustain function of ischemic limbs in mice. J Clin Invest. 2008;118(2):505–14.

[65] Suzuki H, Shibata R, Kito T, Yamamoto T, Ishii M, Nishio N, et al. Comparative angiogenic activities of induced pluripotent stem cells derived from young and old mice. PLoS One. 2012;7(6):e39562.

[66] Granger A, Abdullah I, Huebner F, Stout A, Wang T, Huebner T, et al. Histone deacetylase inhibition reduces myocardial ischemia-reperfusion injury in mice. FASEB J. 2008;22(10):3549–60.

[67] Zhang L, Qin X, Zhao Y, Fast L, Zhuang S, Liu P, et al. Inhibition of histone deacetylases preserves myocardial performance and prevents cardiac remodeling through stimulation of endogenous angiomyogenesis. J Pharmacol Exp Ther. 2012;341(1):285–93.

http://dx.doi.org/10.5772/66409

[68] Zhang L, Chen B, Zhao Y, Dubielecka PM, Wei L, Qin GJ, et al. Inhibition of histone deacetylase-induced myocardial repair is mediated by c-kit in infarcted hearts. J Biol Chem. 2012;287(47):39338–48.

[69] McKinsey TA, Zhang CL, Olson EN. MEF2: a calcium-dependent regulator of cell division, differentiation and death. Trends Biochem Sci. 2002;27(1):40–7.

[70] Zhang CL, McKinsey TA, Chang S, Antos CL, Hill JA, Olson EN. Class II histone deacetylases act as signal-responsive repressors of cardiac hypertrophy. Cell. 2002;110(4):479–88.

[71] Kee HJ, Sohn IS, Nam KI, Park JE, Qian YR, Yin Z, et al. Inhibition of histone deacetylation blocks cardiac hypertrophy induced by angiotensin II infusion and aortic banding. Circulation. 2006;113(1):51–9.

[72] Kao YH, Liou JP, Chung CC, Lien GS, Kuo CC, Chen SA, et al. Histone deacetylase inhibition improved cardiac functions with direct antifibrotic activity in heart failure. Int J Cardiol. 2013;168(4):4178–83.

[73] Oka T, Akazawa H, Naito AT, Komuro I. Angiogenesis and cardiac hypertrophy: maintenance of cardiac function and causative roles in heart failure. Circ Res. 2014;114(3):565–71.

[74] Lin JB, Phillips EH, Riggins TE, Sangha GS, Chakraborty S, Lee JY, et al. Imaging of small animal peripheral artery disease models: recent advancements and translational potential. Int J Mol Sci. 2015;16(5):11131–77.

[75] Spallotta F, Tardivo S, Nanni S, Rosati JD, Straino S, Mai A, et al. Detrimental effect of class-selective histone deacetylase inhibitors during tissue regeneration following hindlimb ischemia. J Biol Chem. 2013;288(32):22915–29.

[76] Krupinski J, Kaluza J, Kumar P, Kumar S, Wang JM. Role of angiogenesis in patients with cerebral ischemic stroke. Stroke. 1994;25(9):1794–8.

[77] Sun Y, Jin K, Xie L, Childs J, Mao XO, Logvinova A, et al. VEGF-induced neuroprotection, neurogenesis, and angiogenesis after focal cerebral ischemia. J Clin Invest. 2003;111(12):1843–51.

[78] Wang Z, Tsai LK, Munasinghe J, Leng Y, Fessler EB, Chibane F, et al. Chronic valproate treatment enhances postischemic angiogenesis and promotes functional recovery in a rat model of ischemic stroke. Stroke. 2012;43(9):2430–6.

[79] Kim HJ, Rowe M, Ren M, Hong JS, Chen PS, Chuang DM. Histone deacetylase inhibitors exhibit anti-inflammatory and neuroprotective effects in a rat permanent ischemic model of stroke: multiple mechanisms of action. J Pharmacol Exp Ther. 2007;321(3):892–901.

[80] Hernández-Jiménez M, Hurtado O, Cuartero MI, Ballesteros I, Moraga A, Pradillo JM, et al. Silent information regulator 1 protects the brain against cerebral ischemic damage. Stroke. 2013;44(8):2333–7.

[81] Ziemka-Nalecz M, Jaworska J, Sypecka J, Polowy R, Filipkowski RK, Zalewska T. Sodium butyrate, a histone deacetylase inhibitor, exhibits neuroprotective/neurogenic effects in a rat model of neonatal hypoxia-ischemia. Mol Neurobiol. 2016.

[82] Nyengaard JR, Rasch R. The impact of experimental diabetes mellitus in rats on glomerular capillary number and sizes. Diabetologia. 1993;36(3):189–94.

[83] Gilbert RE, Huang Q, Thai K, Advani SL, Lee K, Yuen DA, et al. Histone deacetylase inhibition attenuates diabetes-associated kidney growth: potential role for epigenetic modification of the epidermal growth factor receptor. Kidney Int. 2011;79(12):1312–21.

[84] Chen Y, Du J, Zhao YT, Zhang L, Lv G, Zhuang S, et al. Histone deacetylase (HDAC) inhibition improves myocardial function and prevents cardiac remodeling in diabetic mice. Cardiovasc Diabetol. 2015;14:99.

[85] Lee TI, Kao YH, Tsai WC, Chung CC, Chen YC, Chen YJ. HDAC inhibition modulates cardiac PPARs and fatty acid metabolism in diabetic cardiomyopathy. PPAR Res. 2016;2016:5938740.

[86] West AC, Johnstone RW. New and emerging HDAC inhibitors for cancer treatment. J Clin Invest. 2014;124(1):30–9.

[87] Maniotis AJ, Folberg R, Hess A, Seftor EA, Gardner LM, Pe'er J, et al. Vascular channel formation by human melanoma cells in vivo and in vitro: vasculogenic mimicry. Am J Pathol. 1999;155(3):739–52.

[88] Liu X, Wang JH, Li S, Li LL, Huang M, Zhang YH, et al. Histone deacetylase 3 expression correlates with vasculogenic mimicry through the phosphoinositide3-kinase/ERK-MMP-laminin5γ2 signaling pathway. Cancer Sci. 2015;106(7):857–66.

[89] Xu XD, Yang L, Zheng LY, Pan YY, Cao ZF, Zhang ZQ, et al. Suberoylanilide hydroxamic acid, an inhibitor of histone deacetylase, suppresses vasculogenic mimicry and proliferation of highly aggressive pancreatic cancer PaTu8988 cells. BMC Cancer. 2014;14:373.

[90] Harris AL. Hypoxia—a key regulatory factor in tumour growth. Nat Rev Cancer. 2002;2(1):38–47.

[91] Sawa H, Murakami H, Ohshima Y, Murakami M, Yamazaki I, Tamura Y, et al. Histone deacetylase inhibitors such as sodium butyrate and trichostatin A inhibit vascular endothelial growth factor (VEGF) secretion from human glioblastoma cells. Brain Tumor Pathol. 2002;19(2):77–81.

[92] Huang YC, Huang FI, Mehndiratta S, Lai SC, Liou JP, Yang CR. Anticancer activity of MPT0G157, a derivative of indolylbenzenesulfonamide, inhibits tumor growth and angiogenesis. Oncotarget. 2015;6(21):18590–601.

[93] Hrgovic I, Doll M, Pinter A, Kaufmann R, Kippenberger S, Meissner M. Histone deacetylase inhibitors interfere with angiogenesis by decreasing endothelial VEGFR-2 protein half-life in part via a VE-cadherin dependent mechanism. Exp Dermatol. 2016.

[94] Luo J, Nikolaev AY, Imai S, Chen D, Su F, Shiloh A, et al. Negative control of p53 by Sir2alpha promotes cell survival under stress. Cell. 2001;107(2):137–48.

[95] Huffman DM, Grizzle WE, Bamman MM, Kim JS, Eltoum IA, Elgavish A, et al. SIRT1 is significantly elevated in mouse and human prostate cancer. Cancer Res. 2007;67(14):6612–8.

[96] Li N, Fu H, Tie Y, Hu Z, Kong W, Wu Y, et al. miR-34a inhibits migration and invasion by down-regulation of c-Met expression in human hepatocellular carcinoma cells. Cancer Lett. 2009;275(1):44–53.

[97] Tazawa H, Tsuchiya N, Izumiya M, Nakagama H. Tumor-suppressive miR-34a induces senescence-like growth arrest through modulation of the E2F pathway in human colon cancer cells. Proc Natl Acad Sci USA. 2007;104(39):15472–7.

[98] Yamakuchi M, Lowenstein CJ. MiR-34, SIRT1 and p53: the feedback loop. Cell Cycle. 2009;8(5):712–5.

[99] Zhao T, Li J, Chen AF. MicroRNA-34a induces endothelial progenitor cell senescence and impedes its angiogenesis via suppressing silent information regulator 1. Am J Physiol Endocrinol Metab. 2010;299(1):E110–6.

[100] Tan J, Cang S, Ma Y, Petrillo RL, Liu D. Novel histone deacetylase inhibitors in clinical trials as anti-cancer agents. J Hematol Oncol. 2010;3:5.

[101] Crabb JW, Miyagi M, Gu X, Shadrach K, West KA, Sakaguchi H, et al. Drusen proteome analysis: an approach to the etiology of age-related macular degeneration. Proc Natl Acad Sci USA. 2002;99(23):14682–7.

[102] Trougakos IP, Gonos ES. Regulation of clusterin/apolipoprotein J, a functional homologue to the small heat shock proteins, by oxidative stress in ageing and age-related diseases. Free Radic Res. 2006;40(12):1324–34.

[103] Suuronen T, Nuutinen T, Ryhänen T, Kaarniranta K, Salminen A. Epigenetic regulation of clusterin/apolipoprotein J expression in retinal pigment epithelial cells. Biochem Biophys Res Commun. 2007;357(2):397–401.

[104] Voelkel NF, Gomez-Arroyo J, Abbate A, Bogaard HJ, Nicolls MR. Pathobiology of pulmonary arterial hypertension and right ventricular failure. Eur Respir J. 2012;40(6):1555–65.

[105] Zhao L, Chen CN, Hajji N, Oliver E, Cotroneo E, Wharton J, et al. Histone deacetylation inhibition in pulmonary hypertension: therapeutic potential of valproic acid and suberoylanilide hydroxamic acid. Circulation. 2012;126(4):455–67.

[106] Kim J, Hwangbo +C, Hu X, Kang Y, Papangeli I, Mehrotra D, et al. Restoration of impaired endothelial myocyte enhancer factor 2 function rescues pulmonary arterial hypertension. Circulation. 2015;131(2):190–9.

[107] Voelkel NF, Gomez-Arroyo J. The role of vascular endothelial growth factor in pulmonary arterial hypertension. The angiogenesis paradox. Am J Respir Cell Mol Biol. 2014;51(4):474–84.

Chapter 10

Unique Phenotypes of Endothelial Cells in Developing Arteries: A Lesson from the Ductus Arteriosus

Norika Mengchia Liu and Susumu Minamisawa

Additional information is available at the end of the chapter

http://dx.doi.org/10.5772/66501

Abstract

Endothelial cells (ECs) play a critical role in regulating vascular pathophysiology. Various growth factors and relaxation factors such as vascular endothelial growth factor (VEGF) and nitric oxide (NO), which are derived from ECs, are known to maintain homeostasis and regulate vessel remodeling. Although the inner lumens of all types of vessels are covered by an EC monolayer, the characteristics of ECs differ in each tissue and developing stage of a vessel. Previously, we identified the heterogeneity of ECs of the ductus arteriosus (DA) by analyzing its gene profiles. The DA is a fetal artery that closes immediately after birth due to the changes in concentrations of oxygen and vasoactive factors such as NO and prostaglandin E. Studying the unique gene profile of ECs in the DA can therefore uncover the novel key genes involved in developing vascular function and morphology such as O_2 sensitivity and physiological vascular remodeling. A comprehensive gene analysis identified a number of genes related to morphogenesis and development in the DA. In this chapter, we discuss the heterogeneity of vascular ECs in the developing vessel in the DA.

Keywords: vascular endothelial cells, ductus arteriosus, vascular remodeling, comprehensive gene analysis, oxygen, vitamin A

1. Introduction

The endothelial cells (ECs) in vessels control the vascular tone, permeability, attraction of blood cells, which exhibit both innate and adaptive immunity, and migration/proliferation of underlying cells such as pericytes and smooth muscle cells (SMCs). To accomplish these roles, vascular ECs exhibit phenotypic heterogeneity during development in a time- and tissue-specific manner. The most significant diversity of ECs involves the differences between arteries and veins as well as between large and small vessels. ECs undergo constant changes in phenotype depending on different situations, both physiological and pathological. Physiological angiogenesis occurs during development and repair processes. Many events in vascular development during gestation are reciprocated in the adult neovascularization that takes place in wound healing and ischemic disease treatment. In these cases, ECs must express pro-angiogenic factors. Pathological angiogenesis is often implicated as the abnormal proliferation of ECs such as that seen in tumorigenesis. Accordingly, many cancer studies have focused on vascular endothelial growth factor (VEGF), a pro-angiogenic factor produced from ECs. Endothelial damage and dysfunction causes cardiovascular diseases. For example, endothelial dysfunction reduces nitric oxide (NO) production, which decreases vasodilatory effects on SMCs. In addition, a decrease in NO production is also involved in the attraction of leucocytes and the production of various growth factors that leads to unregulated intimal thickening (**Figure 1**). Therefore, ECs play a central role in modifying the phenotypes of vessels. ECs have different roles depending on where they are located. For instance, in a developing vessel, ECs become tip cells or other stalk cells to regulate different molecular signaling to guide vessel sprouting [1]. Endothelial tip cells coordinate to have less proliferative activity by repressing Notch activity, thus upregulating VEGFR-2 (Flk-1) and other downstream

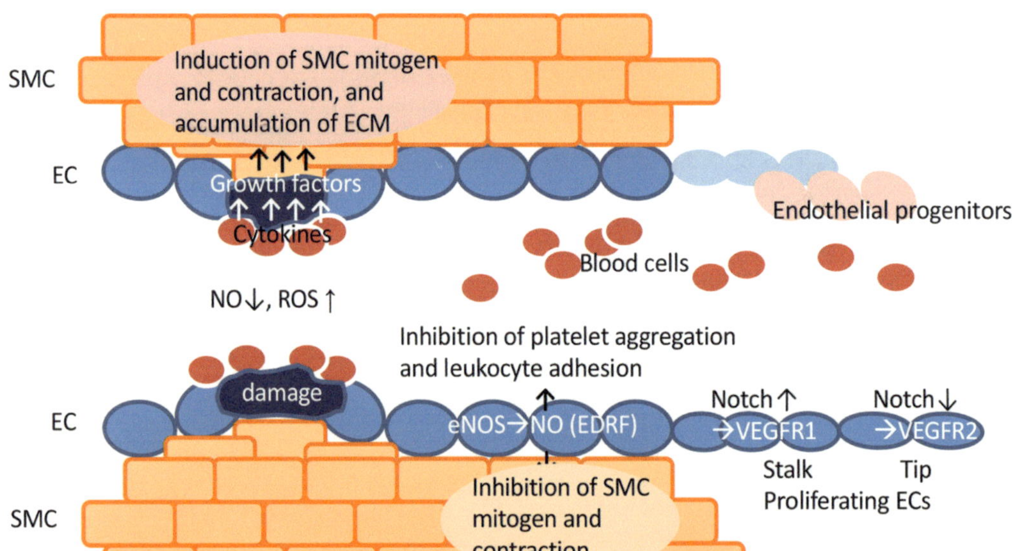

Figure 1. Summarized pathological and physiological vessel response. Damaged ECs are shown in dark blue. Due to the damage, there is a reduction of NO and an increase of ROS, which leads to platelet aggregation or leukocyte adhesion to the intima. Cytokines produced from platelets or leukocytes induce growth factor production and cause SMC hyperplasia and contraction. By contrast, healthy ECs constantly produce EDRF such as NO, so that SMC mitogen and contraction are absent. In developing vessels, ECs are proliferating or deriving from progenitor cells. Proliferating ECs can be distinguished into stalk cells and tip cells, which have different downstream VEGF pathways depending on Notch activity.

http://dx.doi.org/10.5772/66501

Notch transcription factors such as HASER1 [2]. By contrast, Notch signaling is more active and VEGFR-1 (Flt-1) expression is upregulated in stalk ECs. Although Notch and VEGF signals are greatly conserved in vessel sprouting among various tissues and species, how widespread it is in terms of tissue specificity remains to be elucidated (**Figure 1**). Increasing evidence shows that different signaling rules influence tissue-specific vessel sprouting—one study demonstrated that bone morphogenetic protein (BMP) signaling provides the cue for vein-specific angiogenesis during early development, and is independent from canonical VEGF-A signaling [3]. Casanello et al. reported that endothelial diversity is also present in the umbilico-placental vasculature, and emphasized that the heterogeneity of ECs is complicated and cannot be explained simply by comparing the differences between micro- and macro-vasculature, or artery versus vein [4]. Thus, EC shows great heterogeneity in health and disease, and studying the mechanisms of EC heterogeneity would contribute to the understanding of both vascular physiology and pathology.

We previously revealed the unique gene profile of ductus arteriosus (DA)-specific ECs. The DA, a fetal artery that connects the pulmonary artery (PA) and the aorta, is essential for fetuses to bypass the oxygenated blood delivered from the placenta directly to the descending aorta and not through the lung. The DA experiences a dramatic morphological change along with environmental factors after birth, though other connecting arteries remain unchanged. Therefore, even under similar physiological stresses underlying the DA and its connecting arteries, heterogeneity of ECs must exist. In this chapter, we focus on reviewing the unique identified gene profile of DA ECs, which should provide novel insights into heterogeneity in vascular ECs.

Moreover, investigating DA remodeling would potentially help the understanding of diseased vessels, just like other animal models in cardiovascular diseases. For instance, a wire injury model is used for studying pathology of endothelial injury/dysfunction [5]; low-density lipoprotein receptor-deficient mice [6] and apolipoprotein E-deficient mice [7] are commonly used as atherosclerosis models; calcium chloride [8], elastase [9], angiotensin II [10], or microRNA-21 [11] are infused to create an abdominal aortic aneurysms model. Developing a disease model occupies a great deal of scientific findings on pathophysiology, and so the existing models should always open to be refined. The DA can be an alternate model of an occluding vessel, an extracellular matrix (ECM)-enriched vessel, or an oxygen-sensitive vessel. Thus, studying DA ECs would be valuable for understanding an irregular angiogenic pathophysiology.

1.1. Embryonic vasculogenesis

Vasculogenesis and angiogenesis are nomenclaturally similar as they both refer to the genesis of blood vessels [12]. Vasculogenesis is the de novo formation of blood vessels differentiated from mesodermal cells. Angiogenesis is the sprouting of blood vessels that occurs as a result of the proliferation of existing vascular ECs. Despite the difference in these two processes, vasculogenesis and angiogenesis are often compared to further understand their underlying molecular mechanisms. Indeed, a significant amount of knowledge on tumor angiogenesis was achieved by studying embryonic vasculogenesis [13]. Therefore, it is important to study developmental vascular biology and to understand vessel-specific heterogeneity. Moreover, determining the heterogenic diversity of ECs would help open up more options in clinical therapy, ultimately enabling individually designed therapeutic treatments.

The vascular network is the first functional system established in the embryo. A primitive vascular network is formed shortly after gastrulation by deriving endothelial progenitor cells from the mesoderm. This first process is called the formation of angioblasts. Angioblasts then differentiate into ECs by expressing various transcription factors and pan endothelial markers for tubular formation, which is called the primitive vascular plexus [13]. Some of the homeobox (Hox) transcription factors are known to be involved in this process. For instance, Hox A9 regulates the expressions of endothelial NO synthase (eNOS), VEGF-receptor 2 (VEGFR2), and vascular endothelial-cadherin (VE-cadherin), and is responsible for the tubulogenesis of mature ECs [14]. Hox B3 also plays a role in tubulogenesis [15]. Hox D3 induces the differentiation of ECs from angioblasts [16]. The primitive vascular plexus then undergoes complex remodeling accompanied by specification among arteries, veins, and capillaries to become the functional vascular system [13]. Sry-related HMG box (Soxs)-F subgroups Sox7, Sox17, and Sox18, along with vascular endothelial zinc finger-1 (Vezf-1), were found to be essential to the remodeling process [17, 18]. Thus, vasculogenesis in general consists of three steps: formation of angioblasts, formation of the primitive vascular plexus, and vascular remodeling. During these steps, the heterogeneity of vascular ECs is established.

1.2. Physiology of the DA

After the vascular system appears during embryonic development, the heart starts to function, and fetal circulation is established. Fetal circulation is different from adult circulation since the blood is oxygenated in the placenta instead of the lung. Prenatal lungs do not yet need to function so the DA bypasses the pulmonary artery and the descending aorta to send most blood to the body instead of the lungs. Patency of the DA is maintained due to the low oxygen level and high concentration of prostaglandin E_2 (PGE_2) in the blood circulated from the placenta, as well as the production of NO from ECs of the DA. Once the infant has been delivered and lung ventilation has begun, the DA must close properly to enable the transformation to adult circulation. Normal closure happens in two steps: functional closure and anatomical occlusion [19]. The first closure is triggered by an increase in pO_2 and a drop in PGE_2, as well as a drop in blood pressure within the DA caused by the reduction in pulmonary vascular resistance. This functional closure causes the loss of blood flow which therefore induces hypoxia and extensive intimal thickening, followed by fibrosis. The hypoxia on the vessel wall further inhibits endogenous prostaglandin and NO production, which leads to an irreversible closure. Two to three weeks later, the sealed DA eventually becomes a fibrous band called the ligamentum arteriosum (**Figure 2**) [19]. Failed DA closure after birth is a condition called patent DA (PDA), and occurs frequently in premature infants. Medical or surgical treatment of PDA is required when the left-to-right blood shunt is significant.

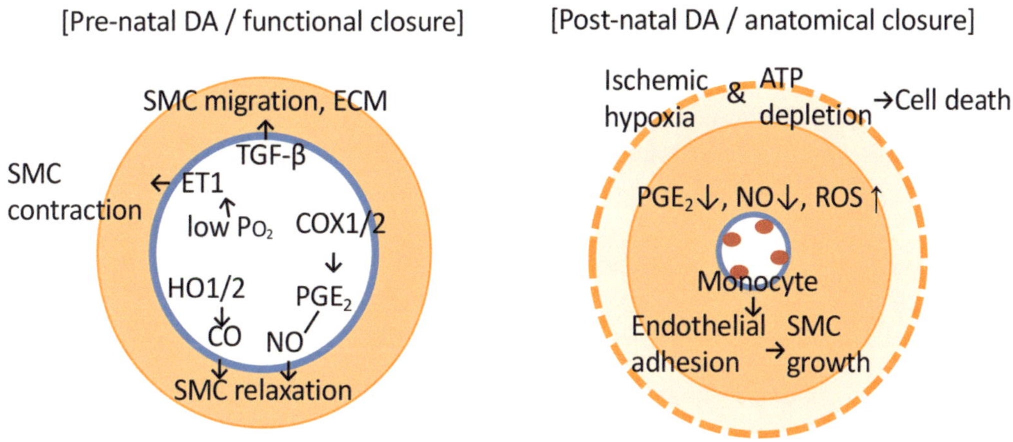

Figure 2. Representative pathways during DA remodeling. In early gestation, the DA remained open due to the high concentration of PGE_2 from placental circulation, and by producing EDHF (NO and CO in the figure). Low oxygen concentration induced ET-1 signaling and TGF-β expression in ECs, leading to functional closure. Postnatal DA is exposed to oxygenated blood that has reduced concentrations of PGE_2 and NO. Due to reduced NO production, ROS are produced and monocytes are attracted to the intima. Monocyte-endothelial interaction induces cytokine and growth factor upregulation, thus promoting SMC growth. Extensive neointimal formation at a later stage causes ischemic hypoxia and ATP depletion, and eventual cell death.

2. Endothelial heterogeneity in terms of the DA

2.1. Current methodologies to study the heterogeneity of DA-specific ECs

The DA is a small shunt vessel in fetuses or neonates. The size of the tissue has always been a study limitation in small mammals such as rodent models. Therefore, although many previous studies used larger mammals such as lamb or pig fetuses, they are inefficient for conducting primary-level research due to the difficulty in handling, low number of offspring, and long gestational period. Rodents overcome these disadvantages, and experimental tools of molecular biology are more available for rodents. Thanks to advancements in technology, there are now more options than ever to overcome the limitation of tissue size in rodents.

2.1.1. Isolation of ECs of the rat DA

DA researchers have used different species, including baboon, pig, sheep, rabbit, chicken, rat, and mouse [20]. These studies focused on a specific population of the cells in the DA and always faced limitations in using rodent animals due to the small size of the fetal tissue. To date, there are only three studies in which pure ECs were successfully isolated from rat DA, including ours. Weber et al. applied a magnetic-activated cell sorting (MACS) method to purify the ECs from collagenase-digested DA tissue [20]. They used von Willebrand factor (vWF) polyclonal antibody in MACS for the isolation. With their experimental method, they succeeded in passaging a pure population of ECs up to three times, which overcame the small number of primary-cultured ECs for further experiments. Following the isolation, they confirmed the purification by flow cytometry and immunohistochemistry analyses. In our previous study, we used a florescence-activated cell sorter (FACS) to purify ECs from collagenase-digested DA tissues [21]. In this experiment, we incubated pooled fresh cells with fluorescein isothiocyanate (FITC)-conjugated anti-CD31 and APC/Cy7-conjugated anti-CD45 antibodies to separate EC and hematopoietic derivation cells, respectively. We confirmed the purity by performing quantitative reverse transcription polymerase chain reaction (RT-PCR) for Tie2 and gamma2-actin expressions, which are markers of ECs and SMCs, respectively. After the FACS sorting, we proceeded directly to RNA isolation from the collected ECs for application to a DNA microarray experiment, which minimized differentiation of the isolated ECs after purification. More recently, a study focused on the heterogeneity of tissue-specific cells that separated ECs and SMCs from the DA using laser-capture microdissection [22].

2.1.2. Comprehensive gene expression analysis of DA tissues

During the past decade, several groups, including ours, have studied comprehensive gene expression in the DA using DNA microarray analysis. One study used human DA specimens, with a broad range of ages [23]. Because of the difficulty involved with human samples of the DA, they could not group the samples with biologic replicates. They found a tendency of expressing more genes that relate to ECM synthesis, which implied the presence of active neointimal proliferation in PDA. Other microarray studies used only rat vessels. Costa et al. compared rat DA samples from embryonic day 19 (E19) and 3 h after birth, examining the effects of oxygen [24]. Our group examined the expression profiles of rat DA and aorta at E19 and E21, and reported that the growth hormone (GH)-receptor signal is predominant in the SMCs of the DA [25]. We also investigated the effect of vitamin A maternal administration on the gene expression pattern of the DA at E19, E21 (full term), and 3–6 h after birth [26]. Moreover, our group utilized the unique phenotype of the Brown-Norway (BN) rat—this strain has been characterized as a novel animal model for PDA possibly due to systemic elastin-related impairments—to compare with vessels of its control strain Fisher 344 [27]. Although all of these studies reported somewhat overlapping results, none could determine the EC-specific gene profiles. As discussed above, the EC layer is maintained to form a single layer; the majority of genes that appear on microarray analysis using whole tissue are therefore from SMC origin.

Because the analysis of the expression profiles of the vascular ECs of the DA is challenging, only two studies have been published to date, including ours [21, 22]. It is difficult to compare these two studies because we used pooled DA ECs purified by FACS, whereas Bokenkamp et al. used laser-capture microdissection to isolate DA ECs from a frozen sample. Accordingly, some of the study results are inconsistent. For example, Bokenkamp et al. demonstrated that the expression of Rgs5 mRNA was higher in the DA compared to the aorta [22], whereas we did not find a difference in Rgs5 expression between DA ECs and aortic ECs. In our study, we divided samples into four groups: the DA and aorta of E21 fetals (F group) and neonates 30 min after birth (N group) rats. We further categorized the microarray data with GeneGo MetaCore software to clarify the meaning of enriched gene expressions. Interestingly, the majority of the identified DA-dominant genes had not previously been reported in previous DA-related studies. We review the unique gene profiles of DA-specific ECs in the following sections.

http://dx.doi.org/10.5772/66501

2.2. Characteristics of DA-specific ECs in DA remodeling

As mentioned in the earlier section, the DA has special remodeling processes that differ from other vessels. Most research on DA remodeling has been conducted using the whole tissue or its SMCs. The importance of signals generated from blood or ECs has, however, begun to be realized.

2.2.1. *Extracellular matrix remodeling of the DA*

In the late 1980s, Rabinovitch's group discovered that the intimal cushion formation of the DA is attributed to a special character in its cells [28, 29]. Using *in vitro* cells from lamb tissues, they demonstrated that there are 10-fold and five-fold increased incorporations of hyaluronan and heparansulfate in the ECM of DA ECs, respectively, compared to cells of the adjacent aorta or pulmonary artery (PA). They further found that this remodeling, which involves the increased hyaluronan accumulation in DA ECs, contributes to the migration of DA SMCs [30], and is transforming growth factor-beta (TGF-β)-dependent [31]. About a decade later, the same group reported that TGF-β1 expression in DA ECs was upregulated in the early gestation of fetal lambs compared to aortic ECs, but was downregulated to the same level as aortic ECs by late gestation [32]. This dynamic modification in the DA EC was explained to relate to stability in the translation and transcription of its mRNA. This second study provided some of the first evidence showing that there are tissue-specific and developmental patterns of expression in DA ECs.

The comprehensive gene analysis study identified significantly high expressions of N-deacetylase/N-sulfotransferase (Ndst3), Glipican 3(Gpc3), and heparan-sulfate 6-O-sulfotransferase 2 (Hs6st2), all of which are involved in heparasulfate synthesis, in DA ECs in both full-term fetal and neonatal periods [21]. Ndst3 is the most important heparin-sulfate synthase among the three members of the NDST family [33]. Other genes that are known to relate to ECM, especially collagen synthesis, were also found to show higher expression levels in DA ECs than aortic ECs: the glycosyltransferase25 domain containing 2 (Glt25d2), which is known to strengthen collagen activity [34]; growth differentiation factor (Gdf6), and microfibrillar-associated protein 5 (Mfap5), which promotes collagen production [35, 36]; Mfap4, which stabilizes collagen activity [37]; anthrax toxin receptor 1 (Antxr1), which provides a link between collagen I and actin cytoskeleton [38]; and prolyl 4-hydroxylase-alpha polypeptide (P4ha1), which is related to the procollagen process [39]. ADAM metallopeptidase with thrombospondin type 1 motif-17 preproprotein (Adamts17), plasminogen activator tissue (Plat), and fibrillin 1 (Fbn1), which are also categorized as related to ECM formation, were upregulated in DA ECs [21]. Interestingly, connective tissue growth factor (CTGF) was found to show higher expression in DA ECs than in aortic ECs in the postnatal period, whereas there was no difference in the fetal period [21]. CTGF is a well-known downstream mediator of TGF-β1 in various cells and it exhibits diverse functions, such as cell proliferation, apoptosis, cell adhesion, ECM or collagen production, and angiogenesis [40, 41]. Moreover, a recent study demonstrated that, via stimulation of TGF-β1, CTGF binds to VEGF, and that the complex inhibited VEGF-mediated angiogenesis in cardiac cells [42]. Although further studies are needed, these results imply that there are intricate regulations among TGF-β1, CTGF, and VEGF in the DA remodeling after birth.

2.2.2. PGE_2, *endothelial-derived relaxation, and hyperpolarizing factors in the DA*

PGE_2 is a potent vasodilator for the DA. It is generated by the enzyme cyclooxygenase (COX). There are two isoforms, COX-1 and COX-2. Although COX-2 is an inducible isoform that requires cytokine, both COX-1 and COX-2 are known to be involved in fetal development [43]. The expression levels of these two vary among species as well as the term of gestation. For instance, COX-2 is barely detected in the DA of fetal pig, but more dominantly regulates DA tone in fetal lamb by expressing it in ECs [43]. Another study found that there is a cooperative interaction between PGE_2 and NO, an endothelial-derived relaxation factor (EDRF) [44]. Several studies showed that NO is more potent than PGE_2 in the preterm DA, whereas the opposite relationship is seen at term [45–47]. Another EDRF that is found to be related to controlling DA tone is carbon monoxide (CO). CO is naturally formed in the body from the enzymatic activity of heme oxygenase (HO-1/2). Coceani et al. demonstrated that CO formed by HO (ECs of DA only express HO-1 in rat and pig fetuses) interfered with the reaction with the cytochrome P450-based monooxygenase and inhibited the synthesis of endothelin-1 (ET-1), which is a potent vasoconstrictor that is also critical in DA tone [48–50]. CO generated from HO-1, but not HO-2, is known to have a protective effect on ECs of various vessels [51], and induces angiogenesis [52]. Importantly, compensatory mechanisms among PGE_2, NO, and CO were elucidated by using eNOS, COX, or HO-2-mutant mice [53]. The study showed that there is no narrowing of the DA in each mutant, and that endothelial-derived hyperpolarizing factor (EDHF) additionally exhibits a large reciprocal effect [53]. In addition to bradykinin, which has been shown to have the same relaxation effect as EDHF, there could be more agents potentially qualified as EDHF. A more recent study reported that hydrogen sulfide (H_2S) also acts as EDHF by expressing its synthetic enzymes cystathionine-γ-lyase (CSE) and cystathionine-β-synthase (CBS) in the intima, likely ECs of the DA [54].

2.2.3. *Inflammatory response in DA ECs during anatomic remodeling*

Anatomic remodeling of the full-term DA shares similar features of inflammatory vascular disorders such as atherosclerosis. As a consequence of the functional closure of the DA, ischemic hypoxia of the muscle media is induced due to the loss of luminal and vasa vasorum blood flow. Therefore, ATP depletion causes cell death [55, 56] and VEGF induction increases the penetration of vasa vasorum into the DA muscle media [57]. Clyman's group examined the inflammatory processes involved in the postnatal constriction of the DA [58]. They found that VLA4 integrin expressing mononuclear cells ($CD14^+/CD163^+$ cells [59]), in which the ligand is vascular cell adhesion molecule-1 (VCAM-1) in ECs, increased to adhere to the lumen of the DA after birth. Along with the increased monocytes recruitment, VCAM-1 and E-selectin expressions were also elevated in DA ECs after birth [58]. Unlike the pathophysiology of atherosclerosis, the upregulation of P-selectin and intracellular adhesion molecule-1 (ICAM-1) induced by monocytes adhesion was not seen in the DA. Interestingly, $VLA4^+$ mononuclear cell adhesion was found to predominantly regulate the extent of neointimal remodeling of the DA after birth, with T-lymphocyte adhesion to a lesser extent, but no neutrophil or platelet adhesion [58]. VCAM-1 and E-selectin were also induced by VEGF and several cytokines, such as TNF-α, IFN-γ, and CD154, likely due to the profound hypoxia in the DA wall after birth. These responses are also seen in atherosclerotic remodeling, but the pattern of gene

http://dx.doi.org/10.5772/66501

expression modification seemed less in DA closure since IL-1 and MCP-1 were not expressed in the closing DA [58]. Some researchers argue, however, that the inflammatory response during DA closure may cause a failure in constriction after birth [58], because TNF-α and IL-6 are known to have potent vasodilatory effects [60–63].

The monocyte-endothelial cell interaction has been implicated to play a critical role in vascular pathogenesis by inducing platelet-derived growth factor (PDGF) secretion that promotes the migration of SMCs into neointima [64]. Indeed, PDGF-B chain expression upregulation was confirmed in DA tissues after birth, and was inhibited by blocking monocyte adhesion using anti-VLA-4 monoclonal antibody treatment [59]. Moreover, the regulator of G-protein signaling 5 (Rgs5) that was found to be enriched in both ECs and SMCs of DA at full-term gestation compared to adjacent aortic cells [22] was suggested to be negatively regulated by PDGF [65]. PDGF-dependent repression of Rgs5 leads to SMC migration and G protein-coupled receptor-mediated-signaling pathways, such as mitogen-activated protein kinase activation, thus contributing to vessel contraction and remodeling [65]. The Rgs5 expression level in DA tissue after birth has not been studied, but it is reasonable to hypothesize that it would be decreased, likely due to increased PDGF secretion after birth. Further studies are required to elucidate the intricate effects of DA remodeling.

2.2.4. *Epithelial/endothelial-to-mesenchymal transition-related gene expressions in the DA*

Recent studies have suggested that epithelial/endothelial-to-mesenchymal transition (EMT/EndMT)-related genes play an important role in DA closure [21, 66]. Our microarray study on FACS isolated ECs from rat DA revealed that Tgfb2, actin alpha 2 smooth muscle aorta (ACTA2), N-cadherin (cadherin 2 or Cdh2), and met proto-oncogene (hepatocyte growth factor receptor or Met), which are known to be related to the EMT process, are significantly expressed compared to the aortic ECs [21]. In accordance with this finding, ACTA2 mutation is well characterized in PDA [67]. Another study that showed the importance of BMP9 and BMP10 as circulating growth factors in DA postnatal closure also found that they induced expressions of EMT/EndMT-initiating transcription factors SNAI1, SNAI2, ZEB2, TWIST1, and FOXC2 in ECs [66]. The study found that treatment with a neutralizing anti-BMP10 antibody on BMP9 knockout mice led to reopening of the DA. BMP9 and BMP10 are members of the TGF-β family, and are known to be elevated in mice around birth [68]. They have high affinity to bind to activin receptor-like kinase 1(ALK1), which is an EC-specific receptor [69], and additionally upregulate the expressions of BMPR2, ActR2A, and the co-receptor endoglin as well in the DA [66]. Moreover, BMP9 is reported to upregulate COX-2 and hyaluronic acid synthase 2 (HAS2) expressions, but not COX-1 [66, 70, 71]. Therefore, EMT or EndMT induced by BMP9 and BMP10 is thought to be a necessary process for anatomical closure of the DA.

Although it remains to be proved whether ECs at the lumen of closing DA would differentiate into mesenchymal cells, Levet et al. observed that there is a loss of EC-specific marker (PECAM or CD31)-positive cells at the lumen [66]. Since those cells at the lumen had an autophagic appearance, the authors speculated that the loss of ECs is at least partially due to cell death. However, it is also reasonable to assume that the EC loss is attributed to EndMT which resulted in loss of the EC characteristics.

2.3. Genetic responses to external stimuli on the DA and other vessels

The DA encounters great environmental changes during the perinatal period. Interestingly, the DA dramatically changes its morphology despite other neighboring arteries remaining unchanged. Therefore, it is reasonable to assume that the DA is sensitive to external or internal stimuli, which are primarily received by cells at the lumen, more than other neighboring arteries.

2.3.1. Response to oxygen

In fetal life when the lungs are not yet ventilated, the resistance of pulmonary vessels is high. Therefore, most of the blood that is oxygenated from the placenta passes to the descending aorta through the DA. At birth, in accordance with lung expansion, the blood passing via the DA is reduced, since the resistance of the pulmonary arteries is lower than that of the systemic arteries. In addition, an increase in oxygen concentration of the blood and a decrease in PGE_2 levels trigger the contraction of the DA. Our previous study demonstrated that α1G, a T-type voltage-dependent Ca^{2+} channel, mediates oxygenation-induced closure of the DA after birth [72].

Furthermore, as the neonatal period progresses, the DA constricts more and the vascular cells undergo hypoxic changes. As a result of hypoxia, reactive oxygen species (ROS) are generated by converting O_2 to $O_2^{\bullet -}$ by NADPH oxidase in ECs. Further activated redox-signaling pathways increase the tyrosine and serine/threonine phosphorylation of proteins, and result in various physiological and pathophysiological responses that are reviewed elsewhere [73]. VEGF is one of the best known genes that are elevated in response to hypoxia in the DA, which contributes to the ingrowth of vasa vasorum and neointimal proliferation [57].

Our microarray analysis identified a significant number of genes that more closely relate to oxygen in DA ECs than in aortic ECs. Aldehyde dehydrogenase 1 family-member A1 (Aldh1a1), aldolase C-fructose-bisphosphate (Aldoc), and CD38 are oxygen-related enzymes, and Vegfa, Tgfb2, and Ctgf are oxygen-related receptor ligands [21]. CD38 has been recently implicated to regulate Ca^{2+} signaling in response to ROS generation in pulmonary arterial SMCs [74]. Therefore, it would be interesting to examine the importance of CD38 in the DA.

2.3.2. Response to retinoic acid

Retinoic acid (RA), a metabolite of vitamin A, plays a critical role in organogenesis, such as the formation of the face, heart, eyes, limbs, and nervous systems [75]. Vitamin A maternal administration has been proven to increase the activities of vessel-contractile proteins and to accelerate the development of the O_2-sensing mechanism in the DA [76]. Yokoyama et al. compared gene expression profiles by microarray in the DA in the presence or absence of maternal vitamin A administration at different developmental stages, and found that 91 genes in total responded to the treatment [26]. In addition to the genes that were previously demonstrated to be induced by RA, such as fibronectin-1 and HAS2, the study also found that vitamin A treatment promoted the maturation of functions and structure of the DA. They also identified that VEGFA was increased by vitamin A administration.

Our microarray study on ECs from the DA versus the aorta also revealed the response to vitamin A to be one of the most dominant biological processes that worked in DA ECs [21]. TGF-beta 2, CD38, Ald1a1, Sp100, paired-like homeodomain 2-transcript variant 2 (Pitx2), fatty acid desaturase 1 (Fads1), and dickkopf homolog 1 (Dkk1) were listed in the category. Although the MetaCore system did not mention it, lecithin-retinol acyltransferase (Lrat) was also increased in DA ECs. Indeed, Lrat was identified as one of the most significant expressions in DA ECs, as it had a more than five-fold increase compared to aortic ECs. Given the fact that Lrat is the predominant enzyme in retinoid absorption [77], it is reasonable to think that this gene could play a great role in the DA having higher sensitivity to RA.

2.4. Other genes uniquely expressed in DA ECs

Our previous study identified more than 80 genes that were expressed more than two-fold or greater in ECs of the DA compared to those of the aorta, in both terms (F and N) [21]. In this section, DA EC-unique genes that were not mentioned in the earlier section will be summarized.

2.4.1. Neural crest cell-related genes during development

The DA derives from neural crest cells that are located in the sixth pharyngeal arch artery [78, 79], which is one of the progenitors of the second heart field [78, 79]. We identified that Tbx1, a major transcriptional factor in the second heart field, was expressed approximately four-fold more in DA ECs compared to aortic ECs. Pitx2 and Fgf10, which are known to co-express with Tbx1 [80, 81], also showed more than two-fold expressions in DA ECs than in aortic ECs. Indeed, Momma suggested that the deletion of human chromosome 22q11.2, where Tbx1 is, increased DA anomalies [82]. Moreover, cadherin 2 (Cdh2), which is known to work downstream of Pitx2 [83], and Ephrin B1 (Efnb1), Hs6st2, and Isl1, which are known to be in the Fgf10 signaling pathway [84–86], were also expressed dominantly in DA ECs [21].

2.4.2. Solute carrier family 38, member 1 (Slc38a1)

Slc38a1 is a highly homologous protein subtype of placental system A, a Na^{+}-dependent amino acid transporter that contributes to nutrient fetal growth, by expressing in the placenta [87]. Placental system A activity increases along with the progression of pregnancy and therefore coincides with demands of fetal nutrient [88]. Slc38a1 was found to be one of the most dominant genes in DA ECs compared to aortic ECs [21]. Slc38a1 itself has not been fully characterized yet and has not been implicated in studies in the DA. Recently, using siRNA technology on cytotrophoblast cells, Slc38a1 was revealed to be a key contributor to total system A activity in term placenta [87]. Hence, the fact that Slc38a1 expressed approximately seven-fold more in DA ECs than in aortic ECs at full-term gestation implies its involvement in the vascular remodeling of the DA. Further study is needed to identify the role of Slc38a1 in the DA during development.

2.4.3. Calpain-6

The calpain family is a calcium-dependent cysteine protease that is ubiquitously expressed in human tissues. Calpain-6 was identified about two decades ago; it has special features that make it stand out from other family members [89]. Calpain-6 is the only family member that lacks a calmodulin-like domain; it therefore has no protease active site [89]. Calpain-6 was exclusively but highly expressed during embryogenesis [90] and in placenta in 50 adult tissues [89] (no DA examination). Our microarray study identified that calpain-6 was also one of the most strongly expressed genes in DA ECs compared to aortic ECs, especially in fetal tissue [21]. Calpain-6 was recently implicated in tumor angiogenesis. Specifically, calpain-6 is suggested to play an important role in bone tumorigenesis and metastasis [91]. In the study, calpain-6 was found to be upregulated by ET-1, and to provide a protective effect against cell apoptosis and promote cell proliferation [91]. As mentioned earlier, ET-1 is increased in the DA to regulate its vasoconstriction [48–50]. Therefore, calpain-6 might be a newly identified gene in ET-1 signaling generated in DA ECs.

3. Conclusion

Studying EC heterogeneity aids our understanding of the physiology and pathophysiology of angiogenesis. It also has great potential to identify novel ways to regulate angiogenesis for treatment purposes. Comprehensive gene analysis using a microarray made it possible to reveal many genes that were previously functionally unidentified in tissue or disease. Molecular analyses using whole tissues hinder the data on specific cell types. ECs are the key cells responsible for primarily generating signaling pathways to modulate the functions or structure of a vessel. Vessels mainly consist of a medial layer (the majority of which is composed of SMCs), and a single layer of ECs. The separation of ECs would therefore be the first hurdle to overcome in order to acquire data on ECs.

This chapter focused on reviewing the current knowledge of DA ECs, since we believe that the DA could be utilized as a vessel model for studying the mechanisms of both neointimal formation and apoptosis in addition to embryonic vasculogenesis. DA-specific ECs are highly unique compared to aortic ECs in terms of their heterogeneity. DA ECs have a great number of specific genes related to ECM formation, inflammatory response, EMT or EndMT, and oxygen and retinoic acid response. DA ECs also have more genes that are conserved from embryogenesis compared to adjacent aortic ECs. In our previous study, Slac38a1, Capn6, and Lrat were found to be the most significantly expressed genes in DA ECs. Although much more research is required to validate the importance of these newly identified dominant genes in DA ECs, we expect that these findings will promote further studies on PDA, therapeutic angiogenesis, and cancer treatment.

Acknowledgements

We would like to thank Dr. Hua Cai for supporting N.M. Liu's continuing research at the University of California, Los Angeles, as well as the fellowship support from the American Heart Association, Western States Affiliate Winter 2014 Predoctoral Fellowship (Award#14PRE20380184), and the American Association of Japanese University Women 2016. This work was also supported by grants from the Ministry of Education, Culture, Sports, Science and Technology of Japan (S.M.), the Vehicle Racing Commemorative Foundation (S.M.), The Jikei University Graduate Research Fund (SM) and the Miyata Cardiology Research Promotion Foundation (S.M.).

Author details

Norika Mengchia Liu[1] and Susumu Minamisawa[2]*

*Address all correspondence to: sminamis@jikei.ac.jp

1 University of California, Los Angeles, CA, USA

2 The Jikei Medical University, Tokyo, Japan

References

[1] Chappell JC, Wiley DM, Bautch VL. (2011) Regulation of blood vessel sprouting. *Seminars in Cell & Developmental Biology* **22:** 1005–1011.

[2] Holderfield MT, Henderson Anderson AM, Kokubo H, Chin MT, Johnson RL, Hughes CC. (2006) HESR1/CHF2 suppresses VEGFR2 transcription independent of binding to E-boxes. *Biochemical and Biophysical Research Communications* **346:** 637–648.

[3] Wiley DM, Kim JD, Hao J, Hong CC, Bautch VL, Jin SW. (2011) Distinct signalling pathways regulate sprouting angiogenesis from the dorsal aorta and the axial vein. *Nature Cell Biology* **13:** 686–692.

[4] Casanello P, Schneider D, Herrera EA, Uauy R, Krause BJ. (2014) Endothelial heterogeneity in the umbilico-placental unit: DNA methylation as an innuendo of epigenetic diversity. *Frontiers in Pharmacology* **5:** 49.

[5] Sata M, Maejima Y, Adachi F, et al. (2000) A mouse model of vascular injury that induces rapid onset of medial cell apoptosis followed by reproducible neointimal hyperplasia. *Journal of Molecular and Cellular Cardiology* **32:** 2097–2104.

[6] Bentzon JF, Falk E. (2010) Atherosclerotic lesions in mouse and man: is it the same disease? *Current Opinion in Lipidology* **21:** 434–440.

[7] Zhang SH, Reddick RL, Piedrahita JA, Maeda N. (1992) Spontaneous hypercholesterolemia and arterial lesions in mice lacking apolipoprotein E. *Science* **258:** 468–471.

[8] Freest-one T, Turner RJ, Higman DJ, Lever MJ, Powell JT. (1997) Influence of hypercholesterolemia and adventitial inflammation on the development of aortic aneurysm in rabbits. *Arteriosclerosis, Thrombosis, and Vascular Biology* **17:** 10–17.

[9] Pyo R, Lee JK, Shipley JM, et al. (2000) Targeted gene disruption of matrix metalloproteinase-9 (gelatinase B) suppresses development of experimental abdominal aortic aneurysms. *The Journal of Clinical Investigation* **105:** 1641–1649.

[10] Daugherty A, Cassis LA. (2004) Mouse models of abdominal aortic aneurysms. *Arteriosclerosis, Thrombosis, and Vascular Biology* **24:** 429–434.

[11] Maegdefessel L, Azuma J, Toh R, et al. (2012) MicroRNA-21 blocks abdominal aortic aneurysm development and nicotine-augmented expansion. *Science Translational Medicine* **4:** 122ra122.

[12] Drake CJ. (2003) Embryonic and adult vasculogenesis. *Birth Defects Research. Part C, Embryo Today: Reviews* **69:** 73–82.

[13] Dejana E, Taddei A, Randi AM. (2007) Foxs and Ets in the transcriptional regulation of endothelial cell differentiation and angiogenesis. *Biochimica et Biophysica Acta* **1775:** 298–312.

[14] Rossig L, Urbich C, Bruhl T, et al. (2005) Histone deacetylase activity is essential for the expression of HoxA9 and for endothelial commitment of progenitor cells. *Journal of Experimental Medicine* **201:** 1825–1835.

[15] Myers C, Charboneau A, Boudreau N. (2000) Homeobox B3 promotes capillary morphogenesis and angiogenesis. *The Journal of Cell Biology* **148:** 343–351.

[16] Gorski DH, Walsh K. (2000) The role of homeobox genes in vascular remodeling and angiogenesis. *Circulation Research* **87:** 865–872.

[17] Downes M, Koopman P. (2001) SOX18 and the transcriptional regulation of blood vessel development. *Trends in Cardiovascular Medicine* **11:** 318–324.

[18] Kuhnert F, Campagnolo L, Xiong JW, et al. (2005) Dosage-dependent requirement for mouse Vezf1 in vascular system development. *Developmental Biology* **283:** 140–156.

[19] Gournay V. (2011) The ductus arteriosus: physiology, regulation, and functional and congenital anomalies. *Archives of Cardiovascular Diseases* **104:** 578–585.

[20] Weber SC, Gratopp A, Akanbi S, et al. (2011) Isolation and culture of fibroblasts, vascular smooth muscle, and endothelial cells from the fetal rat ductus arteriosus. *Pediatric Research* **70:** 236–241.

[21] Liu NM, Yokota T, Maekawa S, et al. (2013) Transcription profiles of endothelial cells in the rat ductus arteriosus during a perinatal period. *PloS One* **8:** e73685.

[22] Bokenkamp R, van Brempt R, van Munsteren JC, et al. (2014) Dlx1 and Rgs5 in the ductus arteriosus: vessel-specific genes identified by transcriptional profiling of laser-capture microdissected endothelial and smooth muscle cells. *PLoS One* **9:** e86892.

[23] Mueller PP, Drynda A, Goltz D, Hoehn R, Hauser H, Peuster M. (2009) Common signatures for gene expression in postnatal patients with patent arterial ducts and stented arteries. *Cardiology in the Young* **19:** 352–359.

[24] Costa M, Barogi S, Socci ND, et al. (2006) Gene expression in ductus arteriosus and aorta: comparison of birth and oxygen effects. *Physiological Genomics* **25:** 250–262.

[25] Jin MH, Yokoyama U, Sato Y, et al. (2011) DNA microarray profiling identified a new role of growth hormone in vascular remodeling of rat ductus arteriosus. *The Journal of Physiological Sciences: JPS* **61:** 167–179.

[26] Yokoyama U, Sato Y, Akaike T, et al. (2007) Maternal vitamin A alters gene profiles and structural maturation of the rat ductus arteriosus. *Physiological Genomics* **31:** 139–157.

[27] Hsieh YT, Liu NM, Ohmori E, et al. (2014) Transcription profiles of the ductus arteriosus in Brown-Norway rats with irregular elastic fiber formation. *Circulation Journal: Official Journal of the Japanese Circulation Society* **78:** 1224–1233.

[28] Rabinovitch M, Beharry S, Bothwell T, Jackowski G. (1988) Qualitative and quantitative differences in protein synthesis comparing fetal lamb ductus arteriosus endothelium and smooth muscle with cells from adjacent vascular sites. *Developmental Biology* **130:** 250–258.

[29] Rabinovitch M, Boudreau N, Vella G, Coceani F, Olley PM. (1989) Oxygen-related prostaglandin synthesis in ductus arteriosus and other vascular cells. *Pediatric Research* **26:** 330–335.

[30] Boudreau N, Turley E, Rabinovitch M. (1991) Fibronectin, hyaluronan, and a hyaluronan binding protein contribute to increased ductus arteriosus smooth muscle cell migration. *Developmental Biology* **143:** 235–247.

[31] Boudreau N, Clausell N, Boyle J, Rabinovitch M. (1992) Transforming growth factor-beta regulates increased ductus arteriosus endothelial glycosaminoglycan synthesis and a post-transcriptional mechanism controls increased smooth muscle fibronectin, features associated with intimal proliferation. *Laboratory Investigation; A Journal of Technical Methods and Pathology* **67:** 350–359.

[32] Zhou B, Coulber C, Rabinovitch M. (1998) Tissue-specific and developmental regulation of transforming growth factor-beta1 expression in fetal lamb ductus arteriosus endothelial cells. *Pediatric Research* **44:** 865–872.

[33] Pallerla SR, Lawrence R, Lewejohann L, et al. (2008) Altered heparan sulfate structure in mice with deleted NDST3 gene function. *The Journal of Biological Chemistry* **283:** 16885–16894.

[34] Schegg B, Hulsmeier AJ, Rutschmann C, Maag C, Hennet T. (2009) Core glycosylation of collagen is initiated by two beta(1-O)galactosyltransferases. *Molecular and Cellular Biology* **29:** 943–952.

[35] Albig AR, Becenti DJ, Roy TG, Schiemann WP. (2008) Microfibril-associate glycoprotein-2 (MAGP-2) promotes angiogenic cell sprouting by blocking notch signaling in endothelial cells. *Microvascular Research* **76:** 7–14.

[36] Mikic B, Rossmeier K, Bierwert L. (2009) Identification of a tendon phenotype in GDF6 deficient mice. *Anatomical Record* **292:** 396–400.

[37] Lausen M, Lynch N, Schlosser A, et al. (1999) Microfibril-associated protein 4 is present in lung washings and binds to the collagen region of lung surfactant protein D. *The Journal of Biological Chemistry* **274:** 32234–32240.

[38] Garlick KM, Batty S, Mogridge J. (2012) Binding of filamentous actin to anthrax toxin receptor 1 decreases its association with protective antigen. *Biochemistry* **51:** 1249–1256.

[39] Li L, Zhang K, Cai XJ, Feng M, Zhang Y, Zhang M. (2011) Adiponectin upregulates prolyl-4-hydroxylase alpha1 expression in interleukin 6-stimulated human aortic smooth muscle cells by regulating ERK 1/2 and Sp1. *PLoS One* **6:** e22819.

[40] Chen MM, Lam A, Abraham JA, Schreiner GF, Joly AH. (2000) CTGF expression is induced by TGF- beta in cardiac fibroblasts and cardiac myocytes: a potential role in heart fibrosis. *Journal of Molecular and Cellular Cardiology* **32:** 1805–1819.

[41] Szeto CC, Lai KB, Chow KM, Szeto CY, Wong TY, Li PK. (2005) Differential effects of transforming growth factor-beta on the synthesis of connective tissue growth factor and vascular endothelial growth factor by peritoneal mesothelial cell. *Nephron. Experimental Nephrology* **99:** e95–e104.

[42] Lai KB, Sanderson JE, Yu CM. (2013) The regulatory effect of norepinephrine on connective tissue growth factor (CTGF) and vascular endothelial growth factor (VEGF) expression in cultured cardiac fibroblasts. *International Journal of Cardiology* **163:** 183–189.

[43] Clyman RI, Hardy P, Waleh N, et al. (1999) Cyclooxygenase-2 plays a significant role in regulating the tone of the fetal lamb ductus arteriosus. *The American Journal of Physiology* **276:** R913–921.

[44] Baragatti B, Brizzi F, Ackerley C, Barogi S, Ballou LR, Coceani F. (2003) Cyclooxygenase-1 and cyclooxygenase-2 in the mouse ductus arteriosus: individual activity and functional coupling with nitric oxide synthase. *British Journal of Pharmacology* **139:** 1505–1515.

[45] Momma K, Toyono M. (1999) The role of nitric oxide in dilating the fetal ductus arteriosus in rats. *Pediatric Research* **46:** 311–315.

[46] Richard C, Gao J, LaFleur B, et al. (2004) Patency of the preterm fetal ductus arteriosus is regulated by endothelial nitric oxide synthase and is independent of vasa vasorum in the mouse. *American Journal of Physiology. Regulatory, Integrative and Comparative Physiology* **287:** R652–660.

[47] Takizawa T, Kihara T, Kamata A. (2001) Increased constriction of the ductus arteriosus with combined administration of indomethacin and L-NAME in fetal rats. *Biology of the Neonate* **80:** 64–67.

[48] Coceani F, Kelsey L, Seidlitz E. (1996) Carbon monoxide-induced relaxation of the ductus arteriosus in the lamb: evidence against the prime role of guanylyl cyclase. *British Journal of Pharmacology* **118:** 1689–1696.

[49] Coceani F, Kelsey L, Seidlitz E, Korzekwa K. (1996) Inhibition of the contraction of the ductus arteriosus to oxygen by 1-aminobenzotriazole, a mechanism-based inactivator of cytochrome P450. *British Journal of Pharmacology* **117:** 1586–1592.

[50] Coceani F, Kelsey L, Seidlitz E, et al. (1997) Carbon monoxide formation in the ductus arteriosus in the lamb: implications for the regulation of muscle tone. *British Journal of Pharmacology* **120:** 599–608.

http://dx.doi.org/10.5772/66501

[51] Brouard S, Otterbein LE, Anrather J, et al. (2000) Carbon monoxide generated by heme oxygenase 1 suppresses endothelial cell apoptosis. The *Journal of Experimental Medicine* **192:** 1015–1025.

[52] Li Volti G, Sacerdoti D, Sangras B, et al. (2005) Carbon monoxide signaling in promoting angiogenesis in human microvessel endothelial cells. *Antioxidants & Redox Signaling* **7:** 704–710.

[53] Baragatti B, Brizzi F, Barogi S, et al. (2007) Interactions between NO, CO and an endothelium-derived hyperpolarizing factor (EDHF) in maintaining patency of the ductus arteriosus in the mouse. *British Journal of Pharmacology* **151:** 54–62.

[54] Baragatti B, Ciofini E, Sodini D, Luin S, Scebba F, Coceani F. (2013) Hydrogen sulfide in the mouse ductus arteriosus: a naturally occurring relaxant with potential EDHF function. *American Journal of Physiology. Heart and Circulatory Physiology* **304:** H927–934.

[55] Goldbarg S, Quinn T, Waleh N, et al. (2003) Effects of hypoxia, hypoglycemia, and muscle shortening on cell death in the sheep ductus arteriosus. *Pediatric Research* **54:** 204–211.

[56] Levin M, Goldbarg S, Lindqvist A, et al. (2005) ATP depletion and cell death in the neonatal lamb ductus arteriosus. *Pediatric Research* **57:** 801–805.

[57] Clyman RI, Seidner SR, Kajino H, et al. (2002) VEGF regulates remodeling during permanent anatomic closure of the ductus arteriosus. *American Journal of Physiology. Regulatory, Integrative and Comparative Physiology* **282:** R199–206.

[58] Waleh N, Seidner S, McCurnin D, et al. (2005) The role of monocyte-derived cells and inflammation in baboon ductus arteriosus remodeling. *Pediatric Research* **57:** 254–262.

[59] Waleh N, Seidner S, McCurnin D, et al. (2011) Anatomic closure of the premature patent ductus arteriosus: the role of CD14+/CD163+ mononuclear cells and VEGF in neointimal mound formation. *Pediatric Research* **70:** 332–338.

[60] Hollenberg SM, Cunnion RE, Parrillo JE. (1991) The effect of tumor necrosis factor on vascular smooth muscle. In vitro studies using rat aortic rings. *Chest* **100:** 1133–1137.

[61] Johns DG, Webb RC. (1998) TNF-alpha-induced endothelium-independent vasodilation: a role for phospholipase A2-dependent ceramide signaling. *The American Journal of Physiology* **275:** H1592–1598.

[62] Minghini A, Britt LD, Hill MA. (1998) Interleukin-1 and interleukin-6 mediated skeletal muscle arteriolar vasodilation: in vitro versus in vivo studies. *Shock* **9:** 210–215.

[63] Patel JN, Jager A, Schalkwijk C, et al. (2002) Effects of tumour necrosis factor-alpha in the human forearm: blood flow and endothelin-1 release. *Clinical Science* **103:** 409–415.

[64] Funayama H, Ikeda U, Takahashi M, et al. (1998) Human monocyte-endothelial cell interaction induces platelet-derived growth factor expression. *Cardiovascular Research* **37:** 216–224.

[65] Gunaje JJ, Bahrami AJ, Schwartz SM, Daum G, Mahoney WM, Jr. (2011) PDGF-dependent regulation of regulator of G protein signaling-5 expression and vascular smooth muscle cell functionality. *American Journal of Physiology. Cell Physiology* **301:** C478–489.

[66] Levet S, Ouarne M, Ciais D, et al. (2015) BMP9 and BMP10 are necessary for proper closure of the ductus arteriosus. *Proceedings of the National Academy of Sciences of the United States of America* **112:** E3207–3215.

[67] Hajj H, Dagle JM. (2012) Genetics of patent ductus arteriosus susceptibility and treatment. *Seminars in Perinatology* **36:** 98–104.

[68] Ricard N, Ciais D, Levet S, et al. (2012) BMP9 and BMP10 are critical for postnatal retinal vascular remodeling. *Blood* **119:** 6162–6171.

[69] David L, Mallet C, Mazerbourg S, Feige JJ, Bailly S. (2007) Identification of BMP9 and BMP10 as functional activators of the orphan activin receptor-like kinase 1 (ALK1) in endothelial cells. *Blood* **109:** 1953–1961.

[70] Loftin CD, Trivedi DB, Tiano HF, et al. (2001) Failure of ductus arteriosus closure and remodeling in neonatal mice deficient in cyclooxygenase-1 and cyclooxygenase-2. *Proceedings of the National Academy of Sciences of the United States of America* **98:** 1059–1064.

[71] Yokoyama U, Minamisawa S, Quan H, et al. (2006) Chronic activation of the prostaglandin receptor EP4 promotes hyaluronan-mediated neointimal formation in the ductus arteriosus. *The Journal of Clinical Investigation* **116:** 3026–3034.

[72] Akaike T, Jin MH, Yokoyama U, et al. (2009) T-type Ca2+ channels promote oxygenation-induced closure of the rat ductus arteriosus not only by vasoconstriction but also by neointima formation. *The Journal of Biological Chemistry* **284:** 24025–24034.

[73] Frey RS, Ushio-Fukai M, Malik AB. (2009) NADPH oxidase-dependent signaling in endothelial cells: role in physiology and pathophysiology. *Antioxidants & Redox Signaling* **11:** 791–810.

[74] Lee S, Paudel O, Jiang Y, Yang XR, Sham JS. (2015) CD38 mediates angiotensin II-induced intracellular Ca^{2+} release in rat pulmonary arterial smooth muscle cells. *American Journal of Respiratory Cell and Molecular Biology* **52:** 332–341.

[75] Smith SM, Dickman ED, Power SC, Lancman J. (1998) Retinoids and their receptors in vertebrate embryogenesis. *The Journal of Nutrition* **128:** 467S–470S.

[76] Wu GR, Jing S, Momma K, Nakanishi T. (2001) The effect of vitamin A on contraction of the ductus arteriosus in fetal rat. *Pediatric Research* **49:** 747–754.

[77] O'Byrne SM, Wongsiriroj N, Libien J, et al. (2005) Retinoid absorption and storage is impaired in mice lacking lecithin:retinol acyltransferase (LRAT). *The Journal of Biological Chemistry* **280:** 35647–35657.

[78] Bergwerff M, DeRuiter MC, Gittenberger-de Groot AC. (1999) Comparative anatomy and ontogeny of the ductus arteriosus, a vascular outsider. *Anatomy and Embryology* **200:** 559–571.

[79] Ivey KN, Sutcliffe D, Richardson J, Clyman RI, Garcia JA, Srivastava D. (2008) Transcriptional regulation during development of the ductus arteriosus. *Circulation Research* **103:** 388–395.

[80] Hu T, Yamagishi H, Maeda J, McAnally J, Yamagishi C, Srivastava D. (2004) Tbx1 regulates fibroblast growth factors in the anterior heart field through a reinforcing autoregulatory loop involving forkhead transcription factors. *Development* **131:** 5491–5502.

[81] Nowotschin S, Liao J, Gage PJ, Epstein JA, Campione M, Morrow BE. (2006) Tbx1 affects asymmetric cardiac morphogenesis by regulating Pitx2 in the secondary heart field. *Development* **133:** 1565–1573.

[82] Momma K. (2010) Cardiovascular anomalies associated with chromosome 22q11.2 deletion syndrome. *The American Journal of Cardiology* **105:** 1617–1624.

[83] Plageman TF, Jr., Zacharias AL, Gage PJ, Lang RA. (2011) Shroom3 and a Pitx2-N-cadherin pathway function cooperatively to generate asymmetric cell shape changes during gut morphogenesis. *Developmental Biology* **357:** 227–234.

[84] Golzio C, Havis E, Daubas P, et al. (2012) ISL1 directly regulates FGF10 transcription during human cardiac outflow formation. *PLoS One* **7:** e30677.

[85] Morriss-Kay GM, Wilkie AO. (2005) Growth of the normal skull vault and its alteration in craniosynostosis: insights from human genetics and experimental studies. *Journal of Anatomy* **207:** 637–653.

[86] Qu X, Carbe C, Tao C, et al. (2011) Lacrimal gland development and Fgf10-Fgfr2b signaling are controlled by 2-O- and 6-O-sulfated heparan sulfate. *The Journal of Biological Chemistry* **286:** 14435–14444.

[87] Desforges M, Greenwood SL, Glazier JD, Westwood M, Sibley CP. (2010) The contribution of SNAT1 to system A amino acid transporter activity in human placental trophoblast. *Biochemical and Biophysical Research Communications* **398:** 130–134.

[88] Mahendran D, Byrne S, Donnai P, et al. (1994) Na+ transport, H+ concentration gradient dissipation, and system A amino acid transporter activity in purified microvillous plasma membrane isolated from first-trimester human placenta: comparison with the term microvillous membrane. *American Journal of Obstetrics and Gynecology* **171:** 1534–1540.

[89] Dear N, Matena K, Vingron M, Boehm T. (1997) A new subfamily of vertebrate calpains lacking a calmodulin-like domain: implications for calpain regulation and evolution. *Genomics* **45:** 175–184.

[90] Dear TN, Boehm T. (1999) Diverse mRNA expression patterns of the mouse calpain genes Capn5, Capn6 and Capn11 during development. *Mechanisms of Development* **89:** 201–209.

[91] Marion A, Dieudonne FX, Patino-Garcia A, Lecanda F, Marie PJ, Modrowski D. (2012) Calpain-6 is an endothelin-1 signaling dependent protective factor in chemoresistant osteosarcoma. *International Journal of Cancer* **130:** 2514–2525.

Chapter 11

Vascular Repair and Remodeling: A Review

Nicolás F. Renna, Rodrigo Garcia, Jesica Ramirez and
Roberto M. Miatello

Additional information is available at the end of the chapter

http://dx.doi.org/10.5772/67485

Abstract

Vascular remodeling is alterations in the structure of resistance vessels contributing to elevated systemic vascular resistance in hypertension. In this review, physiopathology of vascular remodeling is discussed, and the impact of antihypertensive drug treatment on remodeling is described, emphasizing on human data, fundamentally as an independent predictor of cardiovascular risk in hypertensive patients. Then we discussed a vascular repair by endothelial progenitor cells (EPCs) that play important roles in the regeneration of the vascular endothelial cells (ECs). The normal arterial vessel wall is mostly composed of ECs, vascular smooth muscle cells (VSMCs), and macrophages. Endothelial impairment is a major contributor to atherosclerosis and restenosis after percutaneous coronary intervention (PCI). Reendothelialization can effectively inhibit VSMC migration and proliferation and decrease neointimal thickening.

Keywords: endothelial progenitor cells, fructose-fed hypertensive rats, metabolic syndrome, hypertension, oxidative stress, vascular remodeling

1. Role of endothelial progenitor cells in vascular repair

Vascular diseases, including atherosclerosis, media calcification, and microangiopathy, are prevalent in patients with diabetes mellitus and are considered to be primary causes of death and disability in these individuals [1]. Atherosclerosis occurs earlier in patients with diabetes, frequently with greater severity and a more diffuse distribution. Patients with diabetes have increased prevalence of vascular disease and, as a result, increased morbimortality from acute myocardial infarction. Diabetes and metabolic syndrome (MS) are associated with vascular function abnormalities and ensuing morphological changes associated with vascular remodeling and atherosclerosis [2, 3].

The arterial vessel wall is mostly composed of endothelial cells (ECs), vascular smooth muscle cells (VSMCs), adventitial connective tissue and macrophages. Endothelial impairment is believed to be a major contributor to atherosclerosis or restenosis after percutaneous coronary intervention (PCI). Reendothelialization with ECs can effectively inhibit VSMC migration and proliferation and decrease neointimal thickening. It is for this reason that we studied a mechanism to achieve a rapid reendothelialization, through, for example, autologous translators of endothelial progenitor cells (EPC), mature or immature, as a fundamental hypothesis in the prevention of these two pathologies: atherosclerosis and restenosis, which derive in the same clinical entity: acute coronary syndrome.

EPCs are divided into different evolutionary stages from mother cells to mature ECs. Both early and late EPCs can repair blood vessels, but late EPCs that have a strong proliferation capacity are more involved in the formation of new vessels or angiogenesis. By measuring EPC in patients by flow cytometry in patients by flow cytometry, we found that in patients with atherosclerosis are decreased compared to control subjects without atherosclerosis [4–6]. Several studies show that EPCs can be recruited to sites of endothelial injury then mature in site, changing cluster of differentiation (CD), and playing a major role in reendothelialization [7–9].

Atherosclerosis is an inflammatory disease with leukocyte infiltration, accumulation of smooth muscle cells, and formation of neointima. Damage of the endothelial monolayer triggers the development of thrombosis with consequent occlusion versus arterial subocclusion. Recent studies demonstrated the recruitment and incorporation of EPC into atherosclerotic lesions and therefore provided evidence supporting the role of vascular cells in the pathophysiology of atherosclerosis. Moreover, there is evidence that EPC are capable of regenerating cells, vascular grafts, and native vessels [10, 11].

The EPCs can mediate vascular repair and attenuate atherosclerosis progression even in the continued presence of vascular injury. Although the mechanisms involved are still not clear, EPCs seem to contribute to the restoration of the endothelial monolayer [12]. In addition to bone marrow, spleen-derived EPCs also have the capacity to repair damaged endothelium [13]. EPCs derived from spleen homogenates also enhanced reendothelialization and reduce neointima formation after induction of endothelial cell damage using the carotid artery model [14].

Other models have also been used, such as the balloon injury model, mobilization of circulating EPCs, and accelerated repair of the nude endothelium [15]. In addition, autologous EPCs that overexpress endothelial nitric oxide synthase (eNOS) ameliorates endothelial integrity when transplanted into mice after carotid artery balloon injury. Increased NO bioavailability significantly strengthens the vasoprotective properties of the reconstituted endothelium, leading to inhibition of neointimal hyperplasia [16].

Transfer of progenitor cells is not always beneficial. ApoE KO mice receiving mononuclear bone marrow cells, following induced hind limb ischemia, showed increased neovascularization, accelerated atherosclerotic plaque formation, and lesion size compared to control groups [17]. In an alternate study, because of proinflammatory properties of these cells, as reduction in IL-10 levels in the atherosclerotic aortas was observed accelerated atherosclerosis along with reduced plaque stability [18]. Similarly, even though implantation of an arteriovenous anti-CD34-ePTFE graft in pigs, it also stimulated intimal hyperplasia [19, 20]. Besides obvious differences in various experimental models, it is difficult to reconcile these findings and it seems that excessive mobilization of progenitor cells may lead to restenosis, but its absence may impair reendothelialization [21]. It is important to mention term EPC is loosely used to describe a vastly heterogenic cell population that is consisted of different progenitors. Recent studies have highlighted the impact of cell isolation protocols on the functional capacity, that is, different phenotypes.

2. Flow cytometric characteristics of EPC

EPCs are identified by expression of CD34, CD133, or VEGFR2. Their accurate characterization is very difficult, because as these cells may originate from multiple precursors: the hemangioblast, nonhematopoietic mesenchymal precursors, such as the bone marrow, monocytic cells, and also tissue resident stem cells. Two methods for isolation of EPCs from the peripheral blood have been described [22]:

1. From isolated monocytic cells onto fibronectin-coated plates and cultured in the presence of growth factors, form colonies after 5–7 days, denominated endothelial cell colony-forming units (CFU-EC) [23].
2. From monocytic cells from peripheral blood plated onto collagen-I-coated plates in endothelial growth media (EGM-2) can give rise to CFU-EC after 14–21 days [24]. The expression of VEGFR2 on peripheral blood monocytes is essential for their endothelial-like function [25].

How was it exposed beforehand, there are two distinct phenotypes: early EPCs and late outgrowth EPCs [26, 27] which differ fundamentally from each other their proliferation potential. The first, that are derived from monocytic cells, have low proliferative capacity but express of eNOS and they fail to form perfused vessels in vivo. The late outgrowth EPCs have a high proliferation rate and can be maintained in culture extensively. These cells play a key role in angiogenesis [22]. Some studies further identified these cells as $CD34^{+}CD45^{-}$ precursors [28] and clarified their origin from the peripheral blood monocytes. $CD14^{+}$ cells seem to give rise to early EPCs, whereas late EPCs develop exclusively from the $CD14^{-}$ subpopulation [29].

In experimental studies, where EPCs are infused into ischemic lower limbs, only a small number of these can be seen in capillaries of the patient, although the perfusion improves considerably [30–33]. This suggests the potential release paracrine of angiogenic factors. This supportive function of EPCs may be crucial in ensuring the survival of tissue-residing cells and enhancing blood vessel formation and tissue repair. Early outgrowth EPCs produce higher levels of growth factors [34, 35]. To summary, it can say that EPC phenotype vary depending on their origin and their clutters of differentiation, with different functions:

1. immature EPCs that have proliferative ability
2. mature EPCs that can physically engraft into neoendothelial layer
3. supportive EPCs that produce growth factors to promote endothelial repair.

3. Angiogenesis in the vessel wall

An interesting question could be: How do the vessel wall progenitor cells migrate to the endothelial and intima layer of the vessel? The answer is the vasa vasorum. These play a significant role in transporting cells to the intimal region and have positively correlated with the development of atherosclerosis [35, 36]. In atherosclerotic lesions abundant microvessels can be observed. The vasa vasorum are considered to significantly contribute to:

1. atherosclerosis progression
2. plaque instability
3. also authors, support that contribute to plaque regression.

The real thing is that decreased blood supply through the adventitial vasa vasorum can trigger atherogenic intima thickening [37, 38]. Using the Lac-Z mice, Xu et al. [10] provided unique insights into the formation of these microvessels. It was clearly demonstrated that endothelial cells of microvessels within allografted vessels were derived from bone marrow progenitor cells (**Figure 1**). These results suggest a potentially dual role of EPCs in transplant atherosclerosis, protective through the repair of the denuded endothelium and promoting plaque

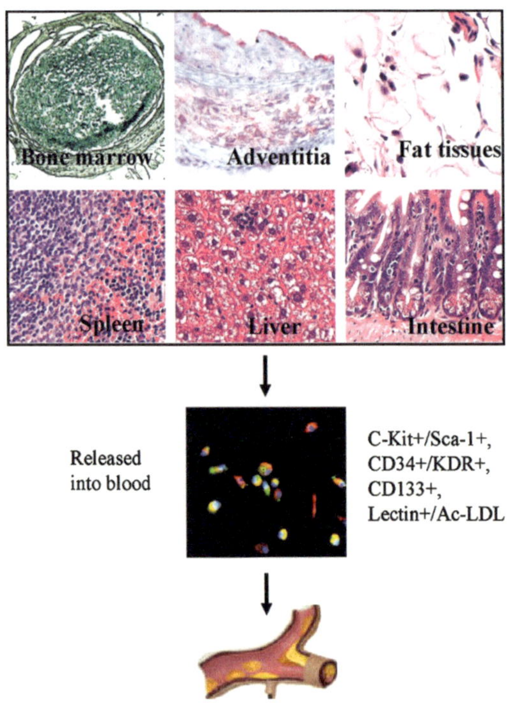

Figure 1. EPC origins. EPCs could be released from bone marrow, fat tissues, vessel wall, especially adventitia and spleen, liver, and intestine, where they form a circulating EPC pool. They can then contribute to the repair of damaged vessels in pathological conditions.

angiogenesis. Some studies have shown the potential detrimental EPC transplantation as lung cancer or multiple myeloma [38]. Additional experiments are required to fully delineate the functional significance of stem cell incorporation into the microvasculature and define the role of progenitors in tipping the balance between atheroprotection and atherogenesis.

4. Definition of vascular remodeling

The vascular wall is formed by endothelium cells, smooth muscle cells, and fibroblasts interacting to form an autocrine-paracrine complex. During vascularization, the vascular wall cells detects changes in the environment, releasing communication signals as growth factors, inflammation mediators, and paracrine mediators that influences on vascular structure and function. The results are vascular remodeling. This is an active process of structural change that involves changes in at least four cellular processes: cell growth, cell apoptosis, cell migration, and the synthesis or degradation of extracellular matrix.

Vascular remodeling is dependent on dynamic interactions between: (1) local growth factors, (2) vasoactive substances, and (3) hemodynamic stimuli, and is an active process that occurs in response to long-standing changes in afterload conditions; that it may subsequently contribute to the pathophysiology of vascular diseases and circulatory disorders [39].

Increased peripheral vascular resistance in hypertension was uniformly ascribed to a higher volume of wall material per unit length of vessel or "hypertrophy." It was always thought that the process of vascular hypertrophy was only due to increased muscle cells, as in the left ventricle, the term remodeling was first applied to the resistance vessels by Baumbach and Heistad to indicate a structural rearrangement of existing wall material around a smaller lumen [39–41].

Mulvany proposed that vascular remodeling should encompass any change in diameter noted in a fully relaxed vessel, not explained by a change in transmural pressure or compliance, and therefore due to structural factors [42–44]. With the objective of to be operational, the classification necessitates appropriate methods for the measurement of resistance vessels dimensions, supplying factors either removed or controlled for: (i) vascular tone, (ii) transmural pressure, and (iii) vessel compliance [38, 45].

5. Classification of vascular remodeling

Consideration of morphological changes has changed over time. Gibbons proposed a classification based on the response to increased blood pressure. These changes are displayed predominantly in media-to-lumen ratio (M/L), changing the vessel wall width for increased muscle mass (**Figure 2A**) or in the reorganization of cellular and noncellular elements (**Figure 2B**). These changes increase vascular reactivity, thus enhancing peripheral resistance. Another mechanism are mainly involves changes in the dimensions of the lumen (**Figure 2C** and **D**). In this case, the restructuring of the active components and cell signals does not

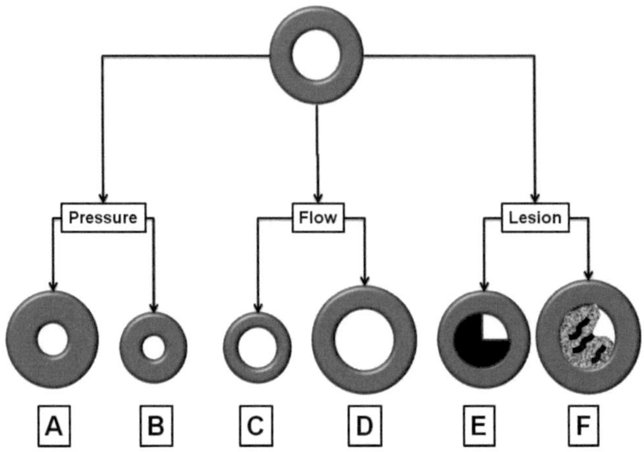

Figure 2. Changes are predominantly in media-to-lumen ratio (M/L), changing the vessel wall width for increased muscle mass (A) or in the reorganization of cellular and noncellular elements (B). Another mechanism of remodeling are mainly involves changes in the dimensions of the lumen (C) and (D). In this case, the restructuring of the active components and cell signals does not result in significant changes in the dimensions of the vascular lumen. Another form of vascular remodeling is microcirculation rarefaction (E) and (F).

result in significant changes in the dimensions of the vascular lumen; the changes in vessel wall thickness are relatively small. Clinical examples of this type of restructuring include the dilation of vascular remodeling associated with a constantly high blood flow (**Figure 2D**) (e.g. arteriovenous fistula) or the loss of cellularity and extracellular matrix proteolysis, resulting in the formation of an aneurysm. Equally, a reduction in the diameter of the vascular mass results from a long-term reduction in blood flow (**Figure 2C**). In fact, microcirculation rarefaction is another form of vascular remodeling that promotes hypertension and ischemic tissue. The vascular wall is also markedly changed in response to vascular injury (**Figure 2E** and **F**). In neointima, forms of reparative response to injury, as thrombosis, migration and vascular smooth muscle cells (VSMCs) proliferation, increased matrix production, and infiltration of inflammatory cells also exist.

Hypertension is associated with structural changes in the resistance vessels such as reduction in lumen diameter and increase in M/L ratio. This mode of structural change has been called "remodeling" [46].

Structural changes in resistance vessels are described as a rearrangement process to understand the pathogenesis of the disease and its therapeutic approach. However, it has been discussed that the term "remodeling" is not ideal because it is frequently used to describe any change in the structure of the vessel or myocardium. To avoid this difficulty, some authors make four proposals [47].

First, the term "remodeling" is limited to situations where there is a change in the lumen of a relaxed vessel, as measured under standard intravascular pressure. The changes in the characteristics of the wall material do not take into account the change in the vascular lumen.

Second, the process of changing the vessel wall without changes in the amount or characteristics of the materials are termed eutrophic remodeling. This process can be characteristic from

http://dx.doi.org/10.5772/67485

situations involving an increase in the amount of material (hypertrophic remodeling) and those involving a reduction in the amount of material (hypotrophic remodeling).

Third, changes associated with decreased or an increased in lumen diameter should be classified as internal remodeling and external remodeling, respectively.

Finally, the remodeling process should be quantified. The term "remodeling index" refers to the variations of lumen referred to as eutrophic remodeling, depending on the changes in the wall section area.

The four proposals above allow for accurate terminology. Thus, the increase in the M/L ratio and decrease in the lumen diameter in resistance vessels of patients with essential hypertension without any change in the amount of wall material is called inner eutrophic remodeling. The decrease in the lumen diameter of the renal afferent arteriole with a decrease in the amount of wall material is called inner hypotrophic remodeling.

Chronic changes in hemodynamic forces structurally alter the vascular wall. In addition, hemodynamic changes are not the only production mechanisms of vascular remodeling. The inflammatory response and changes in the components of the matrix have been suggested as important mediators in the vascular adaptation process [48].

Figure 3 highlights schematically the adaptation of these changes in different pathologies, including structural changes to the intima layer that contribute to remodeling of the vascular wall. Thus, outward remodeling compensates for atherosclerotic plaque growth and delays the progression of blood flow limitation during stenosis, whereas during restenosis, intimal hyperplasia causes a narrowing of the lumen.

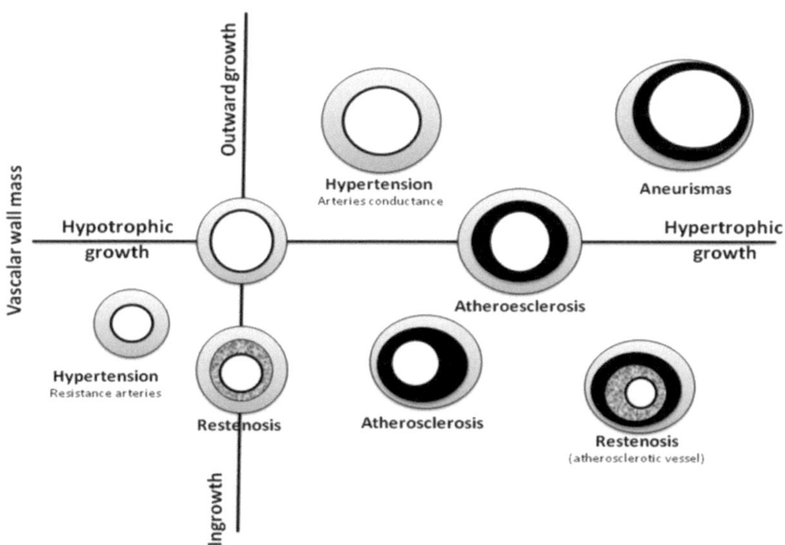

Figure 3. Schematic adaptation of changes in different pathologies, including structural changes to the intima layer that contribute to remodeling of the vascular wall. Thus, outward remodeling compensates for atherosclerotic plaque growth and delays the progression of blood flow limitation during stenosis, whereas during restenosis, intimal hyperplasia causes a narrowing of the lumen.

In summary, vascular wall remodeling is the result of changes in cellular and noncellular components, depending on the disease process causing the changes. Changes in the growth and migration of VSMC, endothelial dysfunction, inflammatory processes, and the synthesis or degradation of extracellular matrix components may be present during the disease process.

6. Pathophysiology of vascular remodeling in hypertension

6.1. Hypothesis of inflammatory and endothelial dysfunction

The traditional view of atherosclerosis as a lipid storage disease is crumbling with growing evidence that inflammation is involved during all stages, from the initial injury to the final stage of thrombotic complications. The narrowing of the arterial lumen is not necessarily a sign of myocardial infarction, and treating narrowed blood vessels does not prolong life. Although invasive procedures are needed in some cases, we understand that medical treatment and lifestyle modification (diet and physical activity) produce benefits that may result from reductions in inflammatory processes [49].

Usually, endothelial cells (EC) prevent leukocyte adhesion. However, the triggers of atherosclerosis can initiate the expression of adhesion molecules on EC, mediating leukocyte adhesion to the arterial wall. A key part of this interaction is VCAM-1. It is likely that oxidized lipids can induce gene expression via the pathway initiated by the nuclear transcription factor-kB (NF-kB), such as IL-1β and TNF-α [50].

This concept of vascular inflammatory disease allows a new approach for risk stratification and treatment. Increased levels of CAM are predictive of cardiac events and are an independent risk factor in men with coronary disease [51]. In our previous study, we demonstrated the presence of the endothelium as well as the products of NF-kB signaling and VCAM-1 in an experimental model of metabolic syndrome in hypertensive rats receiving a fructose-rich diet fructose-fed hypertensive rats (FFHR) [52].

Chemokines are low molecular weight cytokines responsible for mediating the maturation, differentiation, and migration of cells involved in the inflammatory response. In addition to this role, chemokines could promote reactive oxygen species (ROS) production and other cytokines during leukocyte infiltration of the vessel wall. Monocyte chemotactic protein-1 (MCP-1) is a chemokine that regulates the migration and infiltration of monocytes and macrophages into the site of inflammation. It is overexpressed in the presence of cardiovascular risk factors, especially in atherosclerotic lesions. Differential activation induces nuclear transcription factors such as NF-kB and AP-1, which leads to the release of IL-6 and the proliferation of VSMC [53].

Cytokines are soluble proteins that form a complex signaling network critical in the regulation of innate and adaptive inflammatory response. Cytokines modulate the inflammatory response through their influence on the growth, development and activation of leukocytes, and other inflammatory cells. TNF-α is a key mediator in systemic inflammation with a significant role in the Th1 inflammatory pathway. The activity of TNF-α is varied and includes the production of interleukin CAM expression, cell migration and activation, and activation of metalloproteinases (MMP) and COX activity, promoting the procoagulant state. TNF-α is detected in endothelial cells and smooth muscle cells at all stages of the formation of atheromatous plaques [54].

There are over 30 members of the interleukin family. They are subdivided by the similar structure or homology of the receptor. The transformation from a vascular homeostasis inflammatory state is influenced by an imbalance between the pro-inflammatory and anti-inflammatory activities of interleukins. The role of IL-1 includes the stimulation of CAM, chemokines, growth factors, tissue factor, and other cytokines. The expression levels of the receptor antagonist IL-1Ra significantly increase in unstable angina compared with stable angina. Decreased levels of IL-1Ra after coronary stent placement may be linked to a low association with recurrent ischemia [55]. IL-6 is a multifunctional cytokine with a central role in inflammation. Elevated levels of IL-6 increase the risk of myocardial infarction and mortality in patients with coronary heart disease [56].

IL-10 has pleiotropic properties and influences different cell populations. Its most important role is in inflammatory vascular disease as part of the Th2 response. The expression of IL-10 decreases the expression of inflammatory cytokines, decreasing the Th1 phenotype. IL-10 also decreases NF-kB signaling reducing synthesis of pro-inflammatory cytokines, CAM, chemoattractants, and growth factors [57, 58].

Endothelial dysfunction in FFHR causes an increase in the expression of NF-kB and AP-1 and the posttranscriptional product VCAM-1. The expression of NF-kB (p65) and AP-1 (c-fos) predominates throughout the vessel wall. Increased VCAM-1, as discussed in the literature, is a marker of vascular inflammation, vascular permeability, and endothelial dysfunction.

This experimental model produced an increased expression of several cytokines. This finding demonstrates that the vascular bed FFHR model presents a pro-inflammatory and proatherogenic microenvironment that favors vascular remodeling. C-reactive protein (CRP) was used to evaluate whether this local inflammatory process is also systemic and revealed significantly increased IL-6 expression in the liver.

The potential importance of vascular wall inflammation as a therapeutic target remains an area not yet fully explored, where understanding the involvement of inflammatory mediators in vascular remodeling is relevant. The data suggest that oxidative stress and the subsequent activation of genes involved in the inflammatory process are actively involved in organ damage at the vascular level.

6.2. Vascular remodeling and extracellular matrix metalloproteinases

MMPs are tools for maintaining the homeostasis of extracellular structures. Their synthesis is induced by cytokines as well as cell-cell and cell-matrix interactions. Acute coronary syndromes are an example of an increase in clinical conditions, specifically in the vulnerable region of the plaque [59]. Exposure to oxidized low-density lipoproteins or TNF-α induces the expression of MT3-MMP, a protease that degrades atherosclerotic plaques and is expressed in macrophages [60, 61].

MMPs with accessory signaling molecules can modulate cell-cell interactions through the activation of signal transmission and release of cytokines and chemokines. By these effects, accessory signaling molecules can propagate the inflammatory response.

6.3. Vascular remodeling and acute phase reactants

The production of acute phase reactants is a normal physiological response to cytokine release in acute and chronic inflammatory conditions. Ultrasensitive quantification of CRP, when it is below the detection limits of the common assay, has a very important role in the detection of vascular inflammation and cardiovascular risk prediction. There is evidence that CRP is involved in atherosclerosis, especially during the early stages. It stimulates the production of pro-inflammatory cytokines in monocytes and macrophages [62] and mediates the expression of CAM, allowing for increased leukocyte adhesion and migration. Their increased expression suppresses endothelial nitric oxide synthase [34] and promotes a procoagulant state.

Multiple studies have determined that increases in CRP are an independent risk factor for developing atherosclerosis. Data from clinical studies indicate that this association is less important when viewed in healthy subjects and controls inflammatory markers such as IL-6 and fibrinogen [63, 64], whereas another study identified CRP as a predictor of diabetes mellitus independent of established risk factors. CRP also indicated a correlation with the risk of cardiovascular events in women with metabolic syndrome [65].

6.4. Vascular remodeling and the renin-angiotensin-aldosterone system

Another important pillar in the vascular remodeling process is the renin-angiotensin-aldosterone system (RAAS) [66, 67]. To evaluate its participation, we studied the expression of AT1R and AT2R at the vascular level. In the experimental model of FFHR, we observed increased expression of AT1R and decreased expression of AT2R, promoting growth, vascular hypertrophy, and endothelial dysfunction. The release of ROS and initiation of vascular inflammation through different intracellular signaling cascades foster interconnections with other routes such as NAD(P)H oxidase and the growth factor receptor associated with insulin (IGFR).

Figure 4 allows us to appreciate the AT1R-associated intracellular cascades. In this experimental model, the route associated with the satellite receptor and the IGFR subunit associated with NAD(P)H oxidase are the most important pathophysiological mechanisms. The FAK pathways PI3K and JAK2 generate stimuli and trigger contraction, migration and cell adhesion via intranuclear promoters that synthesize ICAM-1 and VCAM-1. Endothelial Growth Factor Receptor (EGFR) and Insulin Growth Factor Receptor (IGFR) amplified pathways are associated with cellular growth and hypertrophy as a result of insulinogenic stimuli and permit activation of collagenase, which modifies the extracellular matrix. Finally, the oxidative stress pathway stimulated by angiotensin activates redox-sensitive inflammatory molecules such as AP-1 and NF-kB, which amplify the inflammatory response by cytokines, chemokines, and lymphokines to ultimately induce more vascular inflammation.

Angiotensin II is the main effector of the RAAS in the homeostatic regulation of the cardiovascular system and in the pathogenesis of cardiovascular disease. Aldosterone interacts with mineralocorticoid receptors (MR), causing endothelial dysfunction, facilitating thrombosis,

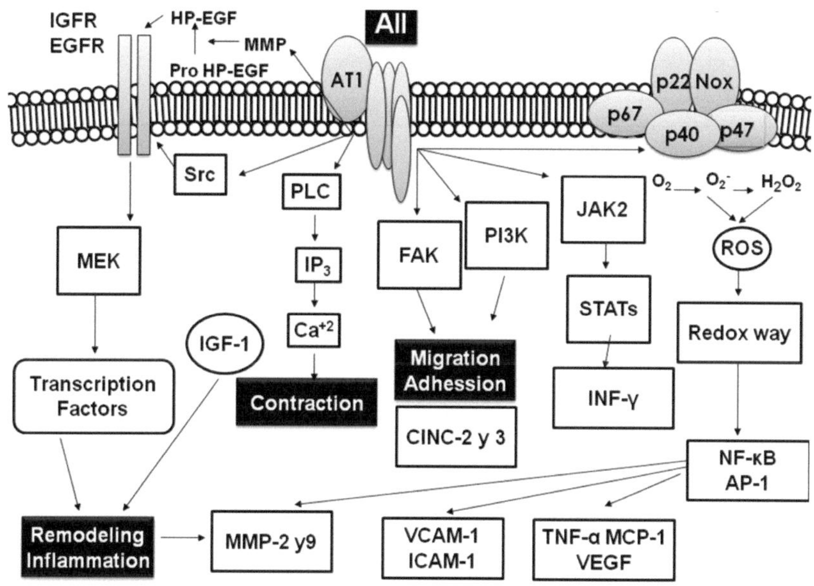

Figure 4. Associated intracellular cascades to physiopathology of vascular remodeling. In FFHR experimental model, the route associated with the satellite receptor and the IGFR subunit associated with NAD(P)H oxidase are the most important pathophysiological mechanisms. Also, the oxidative stress pathway stimulated by angiotensin activates redox-sensitive inflammatory molecules such as AP-1 and NF-kB, which amplify vascular inflammatory response.

reducing complacence, causing vascular hypertrophy and cardiac fibrosis, and generating pathological remodeling. Aldosterone also induces the growth and proliferation of VSMC. A classical genomic action of aldosterone on MR is the translocation of this Aldo-MR complex into the nucleus, where it interacts with promoters to post-transcriptionally regulate gene and protein expression. For this path, increased Ki-ras2A expression (small and monomeric GTP-binding protein), which is associated with cardiac remodeling, generates fibrosis, and cell proliferation by ERK1/2 possibly [68]. Recently, some authors have demonstrated that aldosterone stimulates EGFR intracellularly in CHO cells. The transactivation of this receptor has also been described as a crucial step in the cascade of MAPK signaling activated by angiotensin II. This pathway allows for "cross-talk" and mutual activation that allows the development of cardiovascular injury and subsequent remodeling. The latter route is via "fast" activation, which is different from genomic stimulation and stimulates MKP-1 and Ki-generated ras2A proliferation and vascular remodeling; this discovery explains the changes previously observed in other studies [69].

Noting the role of aldosterone in vascular remodeling in FFHR, we observed that chronic administration of spironolactone did not change the variables of metabolic syndrome that were partially reversed by oxidative stress. This can be explained by the relationship between aldosterone and the angiotensin II receptor AT1R, which sensitizes the effects and increased the post-receptor response [67].

In summary, abundant evidences indicate the involvement of the RAAS in the pathophysiology of vascular remodeling; our observations in experimental pathology highlight the structural and functional changes.

In this special issue, different authors have tried to demonstrate the involvement of different pathophysiological mechanisms to clarify the vascular changes associated with hypertension and metabolic syndrome.

7. Clinical data

The most feasible possibility for studies of resistance vessels in humans relies on the examination of small muscular arteries from biopsies of subcutaneous gluteal fat. Small arteries can also be obtained from omental fat [70–73]. The dissected vessels are mounted in a wire or pressure myograph, but due to the invasive character of these procedures, most relevant studies are of modest size [74–76]. In other cases, untreated hypertensives in place of patients newly diagnosed. In this studies, a data indicate that small subcutaneous arteries of nondiabetic hypertensives undergo inward eutrophic remodeling. Evidence suggests that diabetes, on top of essential hypertension, is associated with media hypertrophy (eutrophy remodeling). The same hypertrophy was also shown by one of these studies in normotensive diabetics, supporting a pressure-independent effect.

Finally, hypertension secondary as renovascular disease could promote media growth in arteries [77–80].

When evaluating the clinical data, there are two problems.

1. sampling problem.
2. subcutaneous vasculature is not necessarily representative of other vascular beds. In opposition to this idea, a positive correlation has been found in hypertensive patients between coronary flow reserve and the M/L ratio of subcutaneous arteries, indeed supporting that hypertensive changes of microvascular structure were not limited to the subcutis tissue.

Author details

Nicolás F. Renna[1,2*], Rodrigo Garcia[2], Jesica Ramirez[3] and Roberto M. Miatello[1,2]

*Address all correspondence to: nicolasfede@gmail.com

1 Department of Pathology, School of Medicine, National University of Cuyo, Mendoza, Argentina

2 Institute of Experimental Medicine and Biology of Cuyo (IMBECU), CONICET, Mendoza, Argentina

3 Genetics Institute, School of Medicine, National University of Cuyo, Mendoza, Argentina

References

[1] Werner N, Nickenig G. Endothelial progenitor cells in health and atherosclerotic disease. Ann Med 2007;39:82–90.

[2] Tepper OM, Galiano RD, Capla JM, Kalka C, Gagne PJ, Jacobowitz GR, et al. Human endothelial progenitor cells from type II diabetics exhibit impaired proliferation, adhesion, and incorporation into vascular structures. Circulation 2002;106:2781–2786.

[3] Ghani U, Shuaib A, Salam A, Nasir A, Shuaib U, Jeerakathil T, et al. Endothelial progenitor cells during cerebrovascular disease. Stroke 2005;36:151–153.

[4] Cubbon RM, Rajwani A, Wheatcroft SB. The impact of insulin resistance on endothelial function, progenitor cells and repair. Diab Vasc Dis Res 2007;4:103–111.

[5] Xiao Q, Kiechl S, Patel S, Oberhollenzer F, Weger S, Mayr A, et al. Endothelial progenitor cells, cardiovascular risk factors, cytokine levels and atherosclerosis—results from a large population-based study. PLoS ONE 2007;2:e975.

[6] Fadini GP, Agostini C, Sartore S, Avogaro A. Endothelial progenitor cells in the natural history of atherosclerosis. Atherosclerosis 2007;194:46–54.

[7] Heiss C, Keymel S, Niesler U, Ziemann J, Kelm M, Kalka C. Impaired progenitor cell activity in age-related endothelial dysfunction. J Am Coll Cardiol 2005;45:1441–1448.

[8] Vasa M, Fichtlscherer S, Aicher A, Adler K, Urbich C, Martin H, et al. Number and migratory activity of circulating endothelial progenitor cells inversely correlate with risk factors for coronary artery disease. Circ Res 2001;89:E1–E7.

[9] Kissel CK, Lehmann R, Assmus B, Aicher A, Honold J, Fischer-Rasokat U, et al. Selective functional exhaustion of hematopoietic progenitor cells in the bone marrow of patients with postinfarction heart failure. J Am Coll Cardiol 2007;49:2341–2349.

[10] Xu Q Mouse models of arteriosclerosis: from arterial injuries to vascular grafts. Am J Pathol 2004;165:1–10.

[11] Hu Y, Davison F, Zhang ZG, Xu Q. Endothelial replacement and angiogenesis in arteriosclerotic lesions of allografts are contributed by circulating progenitor cells. Circulation 2003;108:3122–3127.

[12] Xu Q, Zhang Z, Davison F, Hu Y. Circulating progenitor cells regenerate endothelium of vein graft atherosclerosis, which is diminished in apoE-deficient mice. Circ Res 2003;93:e76–e86.

[13] Rauscher FM, Goldschmidt-Clermont PJ, Davis BH, Wang T, Gregg D, Ramaswami P, et al. Aging, progenitor cell exhaustion, and atherosclerosis. Circulation 2003;108:457–463.

[14] Wassmann S, Werner N, Czech T, Nickenig G. Improvement of endothelial function by systemic transfusion of vascular progenitor cells. Circ Res 2006;99:e74–e83.

[15] Werner N, Junk S, Laufs U, Link A, Walenta K, Bohm M, et al. Intravenous transfusion of endothelial progenitor cells reduces neointima formation after vascular injury. Circ Res 2003;93:e17–e24.

[16] Kong D, Melo LG, Gnecchi M, Zhang L, Mostoslavsky G, Liew CC, et al. Cytokine-induced mobilization of circulating endothelial progenitor cells enhances repair of injured arteries. Circulation 2004;110:2039–2046.

[17] Griese DP, Ehsan A, Melo LG, Kong D, Zhang L, Mann MJ, et al. Isolation and transplantation of autologous circulating endothelial cells into denuded vessels and prosthetic grafts: implications for cell-based vascular therapy. Circulation 2003;108:2710–2715.

[18] Silvestre JS, Gojova A, Brun V, Potteaux S, Esposito B, Duriez M, et al. Transplantation of bone marrow-derived mononuclear cells in ischemic apolipoprotein E-knockout mice accelerates atherosclerosis without altering plaque composition. Circulation 2003;108:2839–2842.

[19] George J, Afek A, Abashidze A, Shmilovich H, Deutsch V, Kopolovich J, et al. Transfer of endothelial progenitor and bone marrow cells influences atherosclerotic plaque size and composition in apolipoprotein E knockout mice. Arterioscler Thromb Vasc Biol 2005;25:2636–2641.

[20] Rotmans JI, Heyligers JM, Verhagen HJ, Velema E, Nagtegaal MM, de Kleijn DP, et al. In vivo cell seeding with anti-CD34 antibodies successfully accelerates endothelialization but stimulates intimal hyperplasia in porcine arteriovenous expanded polytetrafluoroethylene grafts. Circulation 2005;112:12–18.

[21] Yeh ET, Zhang S, Wu HD, Korbling M, Willerson JT, Estrov Z. Transdifferentiation of human peripheral blood CD34+-enriched cell population into cardiomyocytes, endothelial cells, and smooth muscle cells in vivo. Circulation 2003;108:2070–2073.

[22] Seeger FH, Tonn T, Krzossok N, Zeiher AM, Dimmeler S. Cell isolation procedures matter: a comparison of different isolation protocols of bone marrow mononuclear cells used for cell therapy in patients with acute myocardial infarction. Eur Heart J 2007;28:766–772.

[23] Yoder MC, Mead LE, Prater D, Krier TR, Mroueh KN, Li F, et al. Redefining endothelial progenitor cells via clonal analysis and hematopoietic stem/progenitor cell principals. Blood 2007;109:1801–1809.

[24] Hur J, Yang HM, Yoon CH, Lee CS, Park KW, Kim JH, et al. Identification of a novel role of T cells in postnatal vasculogenesis: characterization of endothelial progenitor cell colonies. Circulation 2007;116:1671–1682.

[25] Urbich C, Heeschen C, Aicher A, Dernbach E, Zeiher AM, Dimmeler S. Relevance of monocytic features for neovascularization capacity of circulating endothelial progenitor cells. Circulation 2003;108:2511–2516.

[26] Elsheikh E, Uzunel M, He Z, Holgersson J, Nowak G, Sumitran-Holgersson S. Only a specific subset of human peripheral-blood monocytes has endothelial-like functional capacity. Blood 2005;106:2347–2355.

[27] Gehling UM, Ergun S, Schumacher U, Wagener C, Pantel K, Otte M, et al. In vitro differentiation of endothelial cells from AC133-positive progenitor cells. Blood 2000;95:3106–3112.

[28] Lin Y, Weisdorf DJ, Solovey A, Hebbel RP. Origins of circulating endothelial cells and endothelial outgrowth from blood. J Clin Invest 2000;105:71–77.

[29] Timmermans F, Van Hauwermeiren F, De Smedt M, Raedt R, Plasschaert F, De Buyzere ML, et al. Endothelial outgrowth cells are not derived from CD133+ cells or CD45+ hematopoietic precursors. Arterioscler Thromb Vasc Biol 2007;27:1572–1579.

[30] Gulati R, Jevremovic D, Peterson TE, Chatterjee S, Shah V, Vile RG, et al. Diverse origin and function of cells with endothelial phenotype obtained from adult human blood. Circ Res 2003;93:1023–1025.

[31] Crosby JR, Kaminski WE, Schatteman G, Martin PJ, Raines EW, Seifert RA, et al. Endothelial cells of hematopoietic origin make a significant contribution to adult blood vessel formation. Circ Res 2000;87:728–730.

[32] Gothert JR, Gustin SE, van Eekelen JA, Schmidt U, Hall MA, Jane SM, et al. Genetically tagging endothelial cells in vivo: bone marrow-derived cells do not contribute to tumor endothelium. Blood 2004;104:1769–1777.

[33] Peters BA, Diaz LA, Polyak K, Meszler L, Romans K, Guinan EC, et al. Contribution of bone marrow-derived endothelial cells to human tumor vasculature. Nat Med 2005;11:261–262.

[34] Zentilin L, Tafuro S, Zacchigna S, Arsic N, Pattarini L, Sinigaglia M, et al. Bone marrow mononuclear cells are recruited to the sites of VEGF-induced neovascularization but are not incorporated into the newly formed vessels. Blood 2006;107:3546–3554.

[35] Calvi LM, Adams GB, Weibrecht KW, Weber JM, Olson DP, Knight MC, et al. Osteoblastic cells regulate the haematopoietic stem cell niche. Nature 2003;425:841–846.

[36] Asahara T, Takahashi T, Masuda H, Kalka C, Chen D, Iwaguro H, et al. VEGF contributes to postnatal neovascularization by mobilizing bone marrow-derived endothelial progenitor cells. Embo J 1999;18:3964–3972.

[37] Hanahan D, Folkman J. Patterns and emerging mechanisms of the angiogenic switch during tumorigenesis. Cell 1996;86:353–364.

[38] Baumbach GL, Heistad DD. Remodeling of cerebral arterioles in chronic hypertension. Hypertension 1989;13:968–972.

[39] Mulvany MJ. Vascular remodelling of resistance vessels: can we define this? Cardiovasc Res 1999;41:9–13.

[40] Bund SJ, Lee RM. Arterial structural changes in hypertension: a consideration of methodology, terminology and functional consequence. J Vasc Res 2003;40:547–557.

[41] Mulvany MJ. Structural abnormalities of the resistance vasculature in hypertension. J Vasc Res 2003;40:558–560.

[42] Dunn WR, Gardiner SM. Differential alteration in vascular structure of resistance arteries isolated from the cerebral and mesenteric vascular beds of transgenic [(mRen-2)27], hypertensive rats. Hypertension 1997;29:1140–1147.

[43] Hashimoto H, Prewitt RL, Efaw CW. Alterations in the microvasculature of one-kidney, one-clip hypertensive rats. Am J Physiol 1987;253: H933–H940.

[44] Korsgaard N, Mulvany MJ. Cellular hypertrophy in mesenteric resistance vessels from renal hypertensive rats. Hypertension 1988;12:162–167.

[45] Intengan HD, Deng LY, Li JS, Schiffrin EL. Mechanics and composition of human subcutaneous resistance arteries in essential hypertension. Hypertension 1999;33:569–574.

[46] Heagerty AM, Aalkjaer C, Bund SJ, Korsgaard N, Mulvany MJ, Small artery structure in hypertension: dual processes of remodeling and growth. Hypertension 1993;21: 391–397.

[47] Pasterkamp, G, Galis ZS, de Kleijn DPV. Expansive arterial remodeling: location, location, location. Arterioscler Thromb Vasc Biol 2004;24(4):650–657.

[48] Libby, P. Inflammation and cardiovascular disease mechanisms. Am J Clin Nutr 2006;83(2):456S–460.

[49] Nakane, H, et al. Gene transfer of endothelial nitric oxide synthase reduces angiotensin II-induced endothelial dysfunction. Hypertension 2000;35(2):595–601.

[50] Lopez Garcia CM, Perez Gonzalez PA. Handbook on metabolic syndrome: classification, risk factors and health impact. 1 ed. Vascular Repair by Endothelial Progenitor Cells in an Experimental Model of Metabolic Syndrome, ed. Endocrinology Research and Clinical Developments, 2012. NY: Nova Science Publishers, Inc. 450.

[51] Viedt, C, et al. Monocyte chemoattractant protein-1 induces proliferation and interleukin-6 production in human smooth muscle cells by differential activation of nuclear factor-{kappa}b and activator protein-1. Arterioscler Thromb Vasc Biol 2002;22(6):914–920.

[52] Sack, M. Tumor necrosis factor-alpha in cardiovascular biology and the potential for anti-tumor necrosis factor-alpha therapy in heart disease. Pharmacol Ther 2002;94:123–135.

[53] Giuseppe, P, et al. Prognostic value of interleukin-1 receptor antagonist in patients undergoing percutaneous coronary intervention. Am J Cardiol 2002;89(4):372–376.

[54] Hernandez-Rodriguez, J, et al. Elevated production of interleukin-6 is associated with a lower incidence of disease-related ischemic events in patients with giant-cell arteritis: angiogenic activity of interleukin-6 as a potential protective mechanism. Circulation 2003;107(19):2428–2434.

[55] de Waal Malefyt, R, et al. Interleukin 10(IL-10) inhibits cytokine synthesis by human monocytes: an autoregulatory role of IL-10 produced by monocytes. J Exp Med 1991;174(5):1209–1220.

[56] Galis, ZS, et al. Increased expression of matrix metalloproteinases and matrix degrading activity in vulnerable regions of human atherosclerotic plaques. J Clin Investig 1994;94(6): 2493–2503.

[57] Uzui, H, et al. Increased expression of membrane type 3-matrix metalloproteinase in human atherosclerotic plaque: role of activated macrophages and inflammatory cytokines. Circulation 2002;106(24):3024–3030.

[58] Pasceri, V, Willerson JT, Yeh ETH. Direct proinflammatory effect of C-reactive protein on human endothelial cells. Circulation 2000;102(18):2165–2168.

[59] Venugopal, SK, et al. Demonstration that C-reactive protein decreases eNOS expression and bioactivity in human aortic endothelial cells. Circulation 2002;106(12):1439–1441.

[60] Luc, G, et al. C-reactive protein, interleukin-6, and fibrinogen as predictors of coronary heart disease: the PRIME study. Arterioscler Thromb Vasc Biol 2003;23(7):1255–1261.

[61] van der Meer, IM, et al. The value of C-reactive protein in cardiovascular risk prediction: the Rotterdam study. Arch Intern Med 2003;163(11):1323–1328.

[62] Freeman, DJ, et al. C-reactive protein is an independent predictor of risk for the development of diabetes in the West of Scotland Coronary Prevention Study. Diabetes 2002;51(5):1596–1600.

[63] Touyz, RM, et al. Differential activation of extracellular signal-regulated protein kinase 1/2 and p38 mitogen activated-protein kinase by AT1 receptors in vascular smooth muscle cells from Wistar-Kyoto rats and spontaneously hypertensive rats. J Hypertens 2001;19(3):553–559.

[64] Min, L-J, et al. Cross-talk between aldosterone and angiotensin II in vascular smooth muscle cell senescence. Cardio Res 2007;76(3):506–516.

[65] Min, L-J, et al. Aldosterone and angiotensin II synergistically induce mitogenic response in vascular smooth muscle cells. Circ Res 2005;97(5):434–442.

[66] Brown, NJ, Aldosterone and vascular inflammation. Hypertension 2008;51(2):161–167.

[67] Rizzoni D, Porteri E, Boari GE, De Ciuceis C, Sleiman I, Muiesan ML et al. Prognostic significance of small-artery structure in hypertension. Circulation 2003;108:2230–2235.

[68] Mathiassen ON, Buus NH, Sihm I, Thybo NK, Morn B, Schroeder AP et al. Small artery structure is an independent predictor of cardiovascular events in essential hypertension. J Hypertens 2007;25:1021–1026.

[69] Aalkjaer C, Heagerty AM, Bailey I, Mulvany MJ, Swales JD. Studies of isolated resistance vessels from offspring of essential hypertensive patients. Hypertension 1987;9:III155–III158.

[70] Korsgaard N, Aalkjaer C, Heagerty AM, Izzard AS, Mulvany MJ. Histology of subcutaneous small arteries from patients with essential hypertension. Hypertension 1993;22:523–526.

[71] Izzard AS, Cragoe EJ Jr, Heagerty AM. Intracellular pH in human resistance arteries in essential hypertension. Hypertension 1991;17:780–786.

[72] Thurmann PA, Stephens N, Heagerty AM, Kenedi P, Weidinger G,Rietbrock N. Influence of isradipine and spirapril on left ventricular hypertrophy and resistance arteries. Hypertension 1996;28:450–456.

[73] Schofield I, Malik R, Izzard A, Austin C, Heagerty A. Vascular structural and functional changes in type 2 diabetes mellitus: evidence for the roles of abnormal myogenic responsiveness and dyslipidemia. Circulation 2002;106:3037–3043.

[74] Kvist S, Mulvany MJ. Reduced medication and normalization of vascular structure, but continued hypertension in renovascular patients after revascularization. Cardiovasc Res 2001;52:136–142.

[75] Schiffrin EL, Deng LY. Structure and function of resistance arteries of hypertensive patients treated with a beta-blocker or a calcium channel antagonist. J Hypertens 1996;14:1247–1255.

[76] Schiffrin EL, Park JB, Intengan HD, Touyz RM. Correction of arterial structure and endothelial dysfunction in human essential hypertension by the angiotensin receptor antagonist losartan. Circulation 2000;101:1653–1659.

[77] Park JB, Schiffrin EL. Small artery remodeling is the most prevalent (earliest?) form of target organ damage in mild essential hypertension. J Hypertens 2001;19:921–930.

[78] Harazny JM, Ritt M, Baleanu D, Ott C, Heckmann J, Schlaich MP et al. Increased wall: lumen ratio of retinal arteriole s in male patients with a history of a cerebrovascular event. Hypertension 2007;50:623–629.

[79] Lee RM. Vascular changes at the prehypertensive phase in the mesenteric arteries from spontaneously hypertensive rats. Blood Vessels 1985;22:105–126.

[80] Takeshita A, Imaizumi T, Ashihara T, Yamamoto K, Hoka S, Nakamura M. Limited maximal vasodilator capacity of forearm resistance vessels in normotensive young men with a familial predisposition to hypertension. Circ Res 1982;50:671–677.

Section 3

Mechanisms of Tumor Angiogenesis

Chapter 12

Tumor Angiogenesis: A Focus on the Role of Cancer Stem Cells

Keiko Fujita and Masumi Akita

Additional information is available at the end of the chapter

http://dx.doi.org/10.5772/66402

Abstract

Angiogenesis is the process of growth of new blood vessels. Tumor angiogenesis plays pivotal roles in tumor development, progression, and metastasis. The conventional notion of tumor vasculature is that new tumor blood vessels sprout from preexisting vasculature near the tumor; hence, tumor endothelial cells are derived from normal endothelial cells. However, recent evidence suggests that CD133-positive cancer stem cells (CSCs) in glioblastomas generate tumor endothelial progenitor cells, which further differentiate into tumor endothelial cells. This chapter offers an overview of current knowledge on the role of CSCs in tumor angiogenesis. Furthermore, we discuss our recent discoveries related to human hepatoblastoma stem cells. Future efforts to elucidate the characteristics of tumor angiogenesis should enable the development of effective new anti-angiogenic therapies.

Keywords: tumor angiogenesis, cancer stem cells, hepatoblastoma, cell culture

1. Introduction

Angiogenesis is an essential process by which new blood vessels are formed. In malignancies, tumor growth and metastasis are angiogenesis dependent. It is widely accepted that new tumor blood vessels sprout from preexisting vasculature. Therefore, tumor endothelial cells are considered to be derived from normal endothelial cells. However, over the last few years, different processes by which tumor vascularization occurs have been documented. It has been shown that endothelial cells in the tumor vasculature arise from a small population of tumor cells known as cancer stem cells (CSCs) or tumor-initiating cells. Since John Dick and others identified leukemia cells in 1994 [1], the presence of CSCs with similar properties to normal stem cells has been discovered. CSCs have the ability to undergo self-renewal and differentiation into diverse cancer cells and are capable of becoming malignant. CD133 (or

Prominin1), a cell surface glycoprotein used widely as a marker for normal stem cells, is additionally recognized as a marker for CSCs. Recent reports suggest that CD133-positive CSCs in glioblastomas generate tumor endothelial progenitor cells, which further differentiate into tumor endothelial cells [2–4].

What is the origin of endothelial cells and pericytes lining tumor blood vessels? Can CSCs give rise to tumor endothelial cells? The origin of tumor endothelial cells is the main focus of this chapter. We will provide an overview of current studies and discuss the role of CSCs in tumor angiogenesis. We have investigated the relationship between tumor endothelial cells and CSCs in human hepatoblastoma, which is the most frequent type of malignant tumor to occur in the pediatric liver. Our findings are reported in this chapter.

2. Characteristics of tumor blood vessels

The field of angiogenesis research arose following a publication by Folkman in 1971. The future of anticancer therapy was emphasized in that the potential utility of angiogenesis inhibitors against cancer was identified. The term "anti-angiogenesis" was proposed by Folkman's research group to refer to the inhibition of new vessel sprouts from penetrating into an early tumor implant [5].

Tumor endothelial cells lining the inner layer of blood vessels are the main targets of anti-angiogenic therapy. It is believed that new tumor vessels generally sprout from preexisting vasculature; accordingly, new tumor vessels are considered structurally and functionally normal. However, recent studies have reported that tumor blood vessels differ morphologically and phenotypically from normal blood vessels [6]. A common feature in the architecture of the normal vasculature is a hierarchical and regular branching pattern. In contrast, tumor blood vessels are structurally distinct from normal blood vessels. Tumor endothelial cells, which are not comprised of regular monolayers, do not function as a normal barrier [7]. The pericytes form abnormally loose associations with these cells and extend cytoplasmic processes deep into the tumor tissue [8]. An inner layer of tumor blood vessels is composed of a specific phenotype of tumor-associated blood endothelial cells. Furthermore, the tumor endothelial cells are heterogeneous according to the malignancy status of tumor [9].

3. Tumor-specific angiogenesis

3.1. Cancer stem cells (CSCs) or tumor-initiating cells

The American Association for Cancer Research (AACR) defined CSCs as subpopulations of cells within a tumor that possess the capacity for self-renewal and generation of heterogeneous lineages of cancer cells that constitute the tumor [10].

The cancer stem cell theory provides an attractive explanation for tumor proliferation and progression. According to this theory, tumors retain subsets of cells with functional heterogeneity. However, the putative relationship between CSCs and tumor angiogenesis remains poorly understood [11].

http://dx.doi.org/10.5772/66402

3.2. The origin of the endothelial cells in the tumor vasculature

The origin of endothelial cells in the tumor vasculature is not yet known [12]. Some studies suggest that CSCs play an important role in tumor vascularization. The tumor stem cells defined as CSCs or tumor-initiating cells are considered the source of tumor cells. Moreover, novel findings, which suggest that CSCs also give rise to endothelial cells in the tumor vasculature, have been described in recent reports [2–4]. A proportion of endothelial cells that contribute to blood vessels in glioblastomas originate from the tumor itself, having differentiated from CSCs. A subset of endothelial cells that constitute tumor vessels carries genetic aberrations found in the tumor cells themselves. It has been shown that a glioblastoma cell population that could differentiate into endothelial cells and form blood vessels was enriched in cells expressing the tumor stem cell marker CD133.

3.3. The origin of pericytes in the tumor vasculature

Pericytes are mural cells that wrap around the endothelial cells of capillaries and venules. Vascular pericytes play important roles in supporting vascular structure and function. As communication between pericytes and endothelial cells has been demonstrated to occur, it is considered that pericytes may prove a novel target for tumor therapy [13]. A recent study has reported that glioblastoma stem cells give rise to vascular pericytes that support vessel function and tumor growth. These results suggest that CSCs from glioblastomas generate the majority of vascular pericytes [14].

4. Tumor angiogenesis via endothelial differentiation of human hepatoblastoma stem cells

We have investigated the relationship between tumor endothelial cells and CSCs in human hepatoblastoma, which is the most frequent type of malignant tumor that occurs in the pediatric liver.

4.1. Characteristics of human hepatoblastoma cells

4.1.1. CD133

CSCs exhibit specific cell membrane markers; CD133 is considered a stem-like cell marker in various cancers [15–17]. In human hepatocellular carcinoma (HCC) and HCC cell lines, CD133 is expressed by only a minority of the tumor cell population. CD133+ cells exhibit the ability to self-renew, produce differentiated progenies, and form new tumors [18, 19].

4.1.2. Cell culture

Human hepatoblastoma cell line (HuH-6 clone 5, well-differentiated type, JCRB0401) was procured from the Health Science Research Resources Bank (Osaka, Japan) and cultured in Dulbecco's modified Eagle's medium (DMEM) containing 10% fetal bovine serum (FBS) and 50 μg/mL gentamicin, according to a previously described protocol [20].

4.1.3. SEM and TEM

For SEM observation, the samples were fixed in 0.1 M phosphate buffer (pH 7.2) containing 2.5% glutaraldehyde for 1 h and subsequently fixed in 0.1 M phosphate buffer (pH 7.2) containing 1% OsO_4 for 1 h, dehydrated in graded ethanol, and critical-point air-dried after treatment with isoamyl acetate. The samples were sputter-coated with OsO_4 and observed under a SEM (Hitachi, S-4800; Tokyo, Japan) [21].

For TEM, the cells were fixed in 0.1 M phosphate buffer (pH 7.2) containing 2.5% glutaraldehyde for 1 h, followed by fixation in 0.1 M phosphate buffer (pH 7.2) containing 1% OsO_4 for another hour. The specimens were dehydrated in graded ethanol, embedded in epoxy resin, cut into ultrathin sections, and stained with uranyl acetate and lead citrate. The stained ultrathin sections were observed under a TEM (JEM-1010; Tokyo, Japan) [21].

4.1.4. Distribution of CD133 in human hepatoblastoma cells

We investigated CD133 distribution in human hepatoblastoma cells. CD133 was mainly localized in membrane ruffles in the peripheral regions of the cell. Examination of the CD133-positive sites using SEM revealed that they coincided with filopodia and lamellipodia. TEM revealed that CD133 was preferentially concentrated in a complex structure formed by filopodia and lamellipodia [21] (**Figure 1**).

4.2. Isolation and identification of human hepatoblastoma stem cells

A key challenge in the study of CSCs is the development of reproducible and reliable methods for CSC isolation and identification. The side population (SP) assay identifies the fraction of cells that efflux Hoechst dye through ATP-binding cassette (ABC) transporters. We identified hepatoblastoma stem cells based on their ability to efflux Hoechst 33342 dye using flow cytometry, as described in Hayashi et al. [22]. A fraction of SP cells was analyzed by flow cytometry (FACS Vantage SE, BD, Tokyo, Japan) (**Figure 2**). SP cells were injected subcutaneously into immunodeficient NOD/SCID mice (male, 4-week-old: Charles River Japan Inc.), and tumor growth was evaluated. All animal experiments were approved by the Institutional Animal Care and Use Committee of Saitama Medical University.

4.3. Sphere formation assay and three-dimensional collagen gel culture system

Digested xenograft tumor fragments were cultured, and tumor sphere assay was carried out. The spheres were cultivated using three-dimensional collagen gel culture methods, referring to the previous reports [23–25]. The spheres were fixed with 4% paraformaldehyde/phosphate buffer saline (PBS) and then embedded in Technovit 8100 (T8100, Heraeus Kulzer, Wehrheim, Germany) according to the manufacturer's instructions.

4.4. Immunohistochemical detection of CD133

The location of CD133 expression was examined in Technovit-embedded sections (**Figure 3**). Some spheres were observed to form capillary-like structures (**Figure 4**).

http://dx.doi.org/10.5772/66402

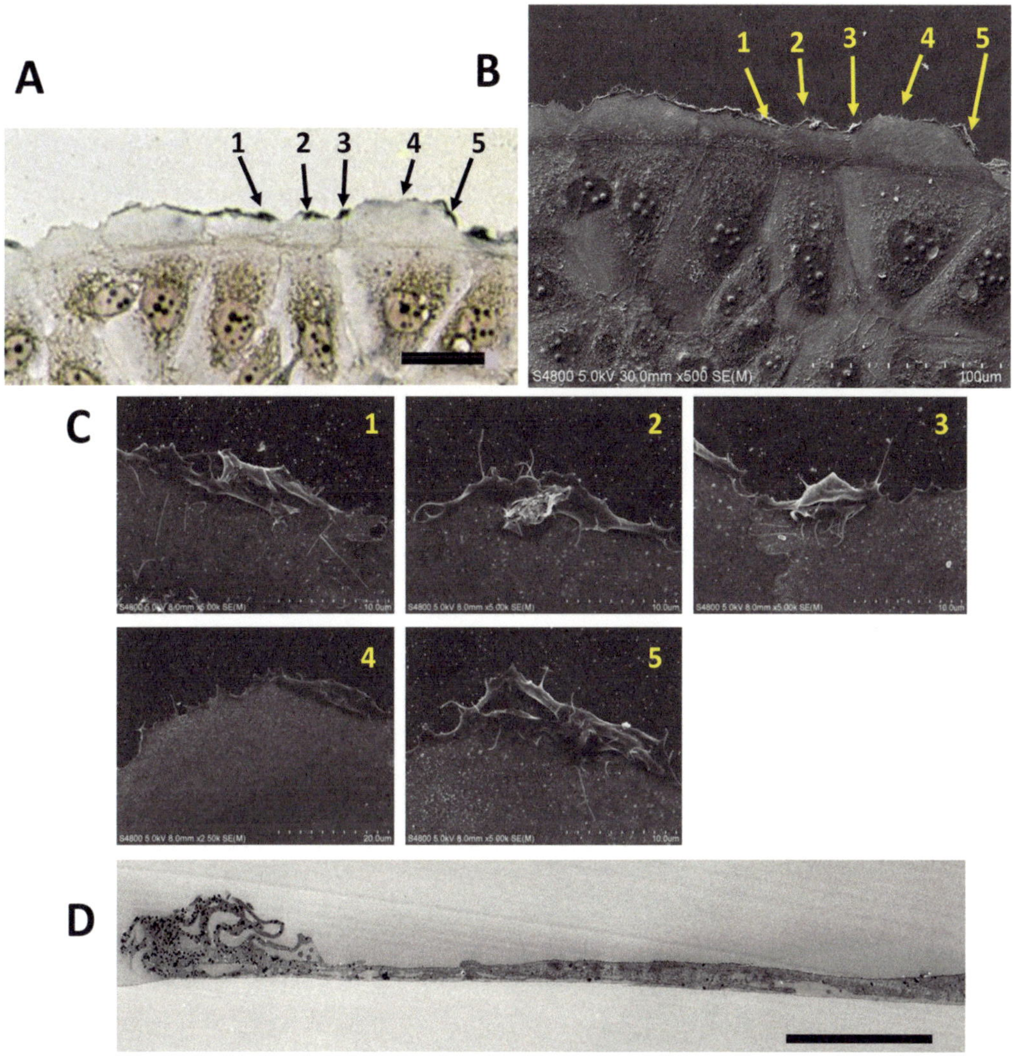

Figure 1. Immunohistochemical analyses of CD133 in hepatoblastoma cells by light microscopy, scanning electron microscopy (SEM), and transmission electron microscopy (TEM). (**A**) Intense immunolabeling of CD133 was observed at the peripheral regions of cells (arrow numbers 1, 2, 3, and 5) by light microscopy. Nanogold labeling was followed by gold enhancement for 20 min. Arrow number 4 indicated a negative site; scale bar: 50 μm. (**B**) SEM image of the sample shown in **A**; the peripheral region of cells (arrow numbers 1, 2, 3, and 5) coincided with the positive sites observed in **A**. (**C**) Higher magnification of SEM images of the positive sites shown in **B**; the positive sites were composed of a complex structure of filopodia and lamellipodia. (**D**) TEM analysis: CD133 was preferentially concentrated in the complex filopodial structure and at the leading edge of lamellipodia. The clustered particles form black spots; scale bar: 5 μm. (Modified from Akita et al. [21]).

Immunostaining for correlative observation by light microscopy and electron microscopy was performed, according to previously described methods [21], to detect the expression of CD133 in these capillary-like structures. The spheres were incubated with primary anti-CD133 antibody (Santa Cruz Biotechnology, CA). Alexa Fluor 488- and 1.4-nm nanogold-conjugated goat

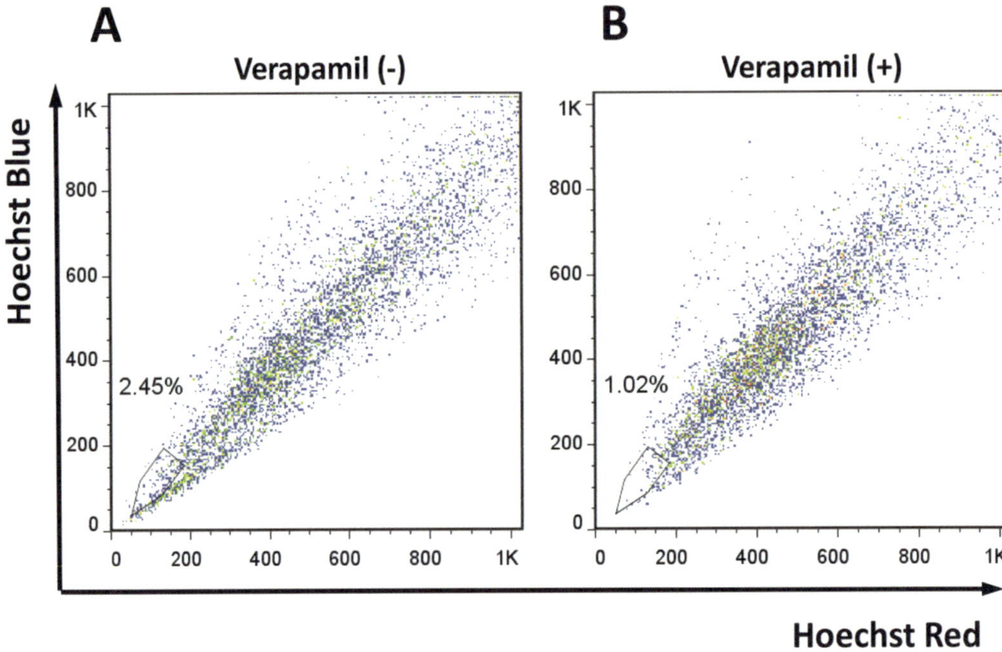

Figure 2. Identification and characterization of side population (SP) cells from a hepatoblastoma cell line. The SP cells in hepatoblastoma cells were identified by flow cytometry using a Hoechst33342-based staining procedure. (**A**) The SP cells displayed in plots show a tail-like subpopulation close to the G0/G1 phase (on the left). Representative images of dot plot analysis by FACS demonstrating the presence of 2.45% SP cells. (**B**) The ABC transporter inhibitor verapamil effectively blocks the export of the Hoechst dye, thus leading to the disappearance of the SP subpopulation. SP cells were reduced to 1.02% upon treatment with verapamil.

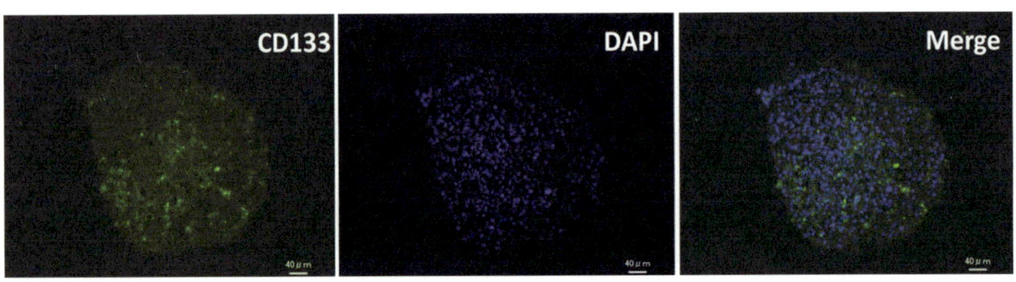

Figure 3. Immunofluorescence of hepatoblastoma tumor sphere. Immunofluorescence of tumor sphere labeled with anti-CD133 antibody (green); nuclei stained with DAPI (blue). The overlaid image is shown in the right panel (merge); scale bar: 40 μm.

anti-rabbit IgG (Nanoprobes, Yaphank, NY, USA) were used as secondary antibodies. The nanogold signal was enhanced using GoldEnhance EM (Nanoprobes) for 20 min. The spheres were analyzed by light microscopy (**Figure 5**, inset). The spheres of interest were subjected to the gold-enlargement procedure using GoldEnhance EM (Nanoprobes, Yaphank, NY, USA) to an appropriate size for TEM analysis, according to the manufacturer's instructions. Some spheres formed CD133-positive capillary-like structures. TEM imaging of these structures confirmed the presence of identifiable lumens (**Figure 5**, bottom).

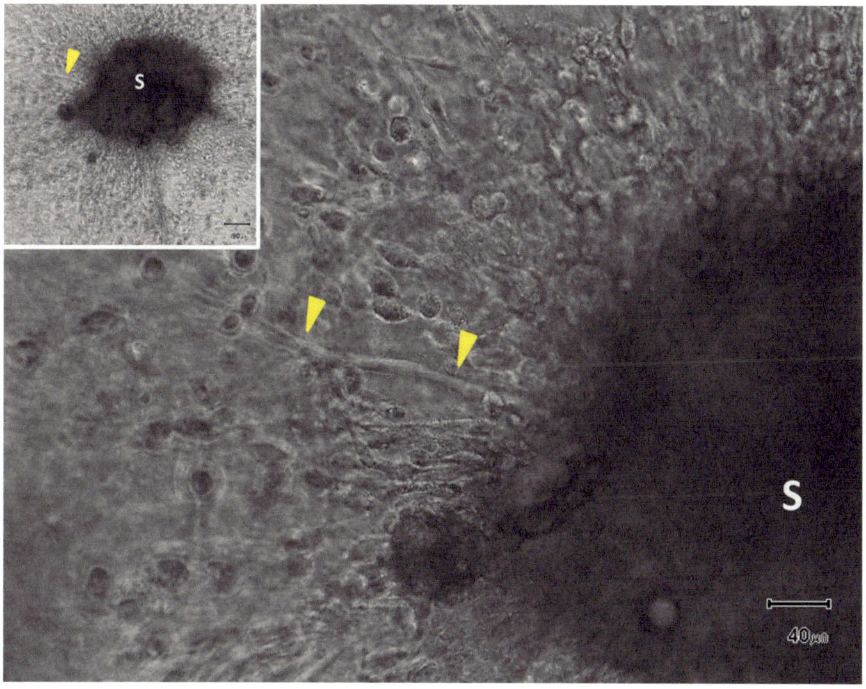

Figure 4. Tube formation assay of hepatoblastoma tumor sphere. Phase-contrast microscopy shows a tubular structure sprouting (arrowheads) from hepatoblastoma tumor sphere (S) in a three-dimensional collagen gel. Higher magnification of the inset indicated bottom; scale bar: 90 μm (inset), 40 μm (bottom).

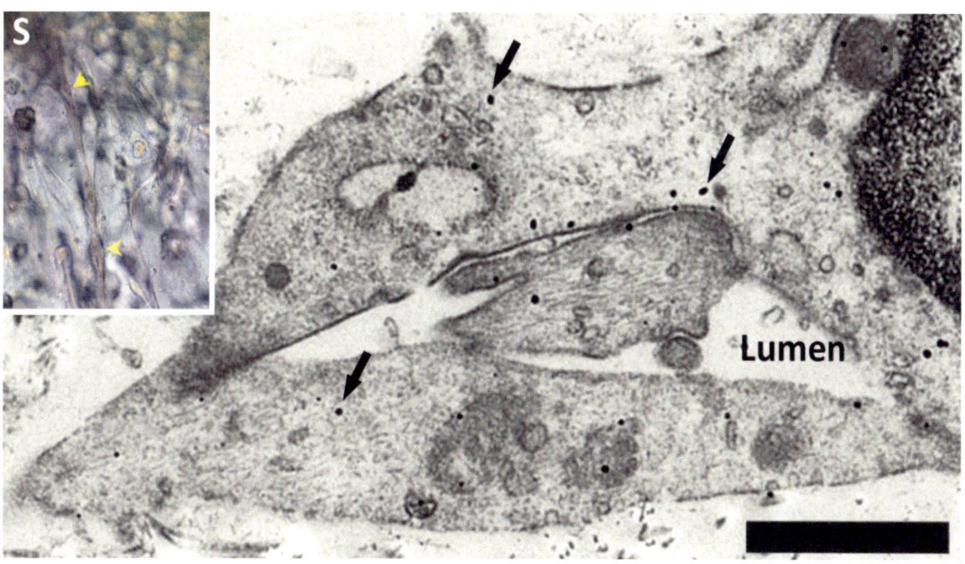

Figure 5. Immunohistochemical detection of CD133 in capillary tubes. (**Inset**) Light microscopy showed that the capillary tube formed from the hepatoblastoma tumor sphere (S) in the collagen gel was positive for CD133 (arrowheads). Nanogold labeling was followed by gold enhancement for 20 min. (**Bottom**) Transmission electron microscopy (TEM) image of the sample shown in the inset; the cross section of this tube is shown. CD133 was detected in the capillary tube. The clustered particles form black spots (arrows); scale bar: 1 μm.

5. Conclusions and perspectives

Tumor angiogenesis has been widely mentioned as a process that new blood vessels are developed from preexisting host blood vessels surrounding the tumors. However, we propose a paradigm change. Our results suggest that CD133-positive CSCs differentiate into tumor vascular endothelial cells and might be able to form tumor vessels.

Since Folkman hypothesized the notion of targeting tumor endothelial cells with anti-angiogenic therapy, numerous anti-angiogenic drugs have been discovered. Previously, we reported that CD133-positive capillary tubes were formed in vitro. Statins, which are widely used as cholesterol-lowering agents, strongly inhibited the capillary tube formation [26]. Statin diminished intraplaque angiogenesis [27] and reduced the growth and spread of many cancers [28, 29]. Khaidakov et al. suggested that statin had anti-angiogenic effects [30]. We propose that the anti-angiogenic effects of statins can be considered for the cancer therapy.

Acknowledgements

This work was supported in part by JSPS KAKENHI Grant Numbers JP25462779 and JP16K11353.

Author details

Keiko Fujita[1]* and Masumi Akita[2]

*Address all correspondence to: kfujita@saitama-med.ac.jp

1 Department of Anatomy, Faculty of Medicine, Saitama Medical University, Saitama, Japan

2 Division of Morphological Science, Faculty of Medicine, Biomedical Research Center, Saitama Medical University, Saitama, Japan

References

[1] Lapidot T, Sirard C, Vormoor J, Murdoch B, Hoang T, Caceres-Cortes J, Minden M, Paterson B, Caligiuri MA, Dick JE. A cell initiating human acute myeloid leukemia after transplantation into SCID mice. Nature. 1994;367:645–648. doi:10.1038/367645a0

[2] Bautch VL. Cancer: Tumour stem cells switch sides. Nature. 2010;468:770–771. doi:10.1038/468770a

[3] Ricci-Vitiani L, Pallini R, Biffoni M, Todaro M, Invernici G, Cenci T, Maira G, Parati EA, Stassi G, Larocca LM, De Maria R. Tumour vascularization via endothelial differentiation of glioblastoma stem-like cells. Nature. 2010;468:824–828. doi:10.1038/nature09557

[4] Wang R, Chadalavada K, Wilshire J, Kowalik U, Hovinga KE, Geber A, Fligelman B, Leversha M, Brennan C, Tabar V. Glioblastoma stem-like cells give rise to tumour endothelium. Nature. 2010;468:829–833. doi:10.1038/nature09624

[5] Folkman J. Tumor angiogenesis: therapeutic implications. N Engl J Med. 1971;285:1182–1186. doi:10.1056/NEJM197111182852108

[6] Hida K, Maishi N, Torii C, Hida Y. Tumor angiogenesis—characteristics of tumor endothelial cells. Int J Clin Oncol. 2016;21:206–212. doi:10.1007/s10147-016-0957-1

[7] Hashizume H, Baluk P, Morikawa S, McLean JW, Thurston G, Roberge S, Jain RK, McDonald DM. Openings between defective endothelial cells explain tumor vessel leakiness. Am J Pathol. 2000;156:1363–1380. doi:10.1016/S0002-9440(10)65006-7

[8] Baluk P, Hashizume H, McDonald DM. Cellular abnormalities of blood vessels as targets in cancer. Curr Opin Genet Dev. 2005;15:102–111. doi:10.1016/j.gde.2004.12.005

[9] Hida K, Maishi N, Sakurai Y, Hida Y, Harashima H. Heterogeneity of tumor endothelial cells and drug delivery. Adv Drug Deliv Rev. 2016;99:140–147. doi:10.1016/j.addr.2015.11.008

[10] Clarke MF, Dick JE, Dirks PB, Eaves CJ, Jamieson CH, Jones DL, Visvader J, Weissman IL, Wahl GM. Cancer stem cells—perspectives on current status and future directions: AACR Workshop on cancer stem cells. Cancer Res. 2006;66:9339–9344. doi:10.1158/0008-5472.CAN-06-3126

[11] Li S, Li Q. Cancer stem cells and tumor metastasis. Int J Oncol. 2014;44:1806–1812. doi:10.3892/ijo.2014.2362

[12] Krishna Priya S, Nagare RP, Sneha VS, Sidhanth C, Bindhya S, Manasa P, Ganesan TS. Tumour angiogenesis-Origin of blood vessels. Int J Cancer. 2016;139:729–735. doi:10.1002/ijc.30067

[13] Kang E, Shin JW. Pericyte-targeting drug delivery and tissue engineering. Int J Nanomedicine. 2016;11:2397–2406. doi:10.2147/IJN.S105274

[14] Cheng L, Huang Z, Zhou W, Wu Q, Donnola S, Liu JK, Fang X, Sloan AE, Mao Y, Lathia JD, Min W, McLendon RE, Rich JN, Bao S. Glioblastoma stem cells generate vascular pericytes to support vessel function and tumor growth. Cell. 2013;153:139–152. doi:10.1016/j.cell.2013.02.021

[15] Ricci-Vitiani L, Lombardi DG, Pilozzi E, Biffoni M, Todaro M, Peschle C, De Maria R. Identification and expansion of human colon-cancer-initiating cells. Nature. 2007;445:111–115. doi:10.1038/nature05384

[16] Brungs D, Aghmesheh M, Vine KL, Becker TM, Carolan MG, Ranson M. Gastric cancer stem cells: evidence, potential markers, and clinical implications. J Gastroenterol. 2016;51:313–326. doi:10.1007/s00535-015-1125-5

[17] Konishi H, Asano N, Imatani A, Kimura O, Kondo Y, Jin X, Kanno T, Hatta W, Ara N, Asanuma K, Koike T, Shimosegawa T. Notch1 directly induced CD133 expression

in human diffuse type gastric cancers. Oncotarget. 2016;7:56598-56607. doi:10.18632/oncotarget.10967

[18] Suetsugu A, Nagaki M, Aoki H, Motohashi T, Kunisada T, Moriwaki H. Characterization of CD133+ hepatocellular carcinoma cells as cancer stem/progenitor cells. Biochem Biophys Res Commun. 2006;351:820–824. doi:10.1016/j.bbrc.2006.10.128

[19] Ma S, Chan KW, Hu L, Lee TK, Wo JY, Ng IO, Zheng BJ, Guan XY. Identification and characterization of tumorigenic liver cancer stem/progenitor cells. Gastroenterology. 2007;132:2542–2556. doi:10.1053/j.gastro.2007.04.025

[20] Morimura T, Fujita K, Akita M, Nagashima M, Satomi A. The proton pump inhibitor inhibits cell growth and induces apoptosis in human hepatoblastoma. Pediatr Surg Int. 2008;24:1087–1094. doi:10.1007/s00383-008-2229-2

[21] Akita M, Tanaka K, Murai N, Matsumoto S, Fujita K, Takaki T, Nishiyama H. Detection of CD133 (prominin-1) in a human hepatoblastoma cell line (HuH-6 clone 5). Microsc Res Tech. 2013;76:844–852. doi:10.1002/jemt.22237

[22] Hayashi S, Fujita K, Matsumoto S, Akita M, Satomi A. Isolation and identification of cancer stem cells from a side population of a human hepatoblastoma cell line, HuH-6 clone-5. Pediatr Surg Int. 2011;27:9–16. doi:10.1007/s00383-010-2719-x

[23] Akita M, Murata E, Merker H-J, Kaneko K. Morphology of capillary-like structures in a three-dimensional aorta/collagen gel culture. Ann Anat. 1997;179:127–136. doi:10.1016/S0940-9602(97)80087-8

[24] Akita M, Murata E, Merker H-J, Kaneko K. Formation of new capillary-like tubes in a three-dimensional in vitro model (Aorta/Collagen Gel). Ann Anat. 1997;179:137–147. doi:10.1016/S0940-9602(97)80088-X

[25] Fujita K, Asami Y, Tanaka K, Akita M, Merker H-J. Anti-angiogenic effects of thalidomide: expression of apoptosis-inducible active-caspase-3 in a three-dimensional collagen gel culture of aorta. Histochem Cell Biol. 2004;122:27–33. doi:10.1007/s00418-004-0669-x

[26] Akita M, Tanaka K, Matsumoto S, Komatsu K, Fujita K. Detection of the hematopoietic stem and progenitor cell marker CD133 during angiogenesis in three-dimensional collagen gel culture. Stem Cells Int. 2013;2013:Article ID 927403,10 pages http://dx.doi.org/10.1155/2013/927403

[27] Karthikeyan VJ, Lip GY. Statins and intra-plaque angiogenesis in carotid artery disease. Atherosclerosis. 2007;192:455–456. doi:10.1016/j.atherosclerosis.2007.01.018

[28] Poynter JN, Gruber SB, Higgins PD, Almog R, Bonner JD, Rennert HS, Low M, Greenson JK, Rennert G. Statins and the risk of colorectal cancer. N Engl J Med. 2005;352:2184–2192. doi:10.1056/NEJMoa043792

[29] Friis S, Poulsen AH, Johnsen SP, McLaughlin JK, Fryzek JP, Dalton SO, Sørensen HT, Olsen JH. Cancer risk among statin users: a population-based cohort study. Int J Cancer. 2005;114:643–647. doi:10.1002/ijc.20758

[30] Khaidakov M, Wang W, Khan JA, Kang BY, Hermonat PL, Mehta JL. Statins and angiogenesis: is it about connections? Biochem Biophys Res Commun. 2009;387:543–547. doi:10.1016/j.bbrc.2009.07.057

Chapter 13

VEGF-Mediated Signal Transduction in Tumor Angiogenesis

Lucia Napione, Maria Alvaro and Federico Bussolino

Additional information is available at the end of the chapter

http://dx.doi.org/10.5772/66764

Abstract

The vascular endothelial growth factor-A (VEGF) plays a crucial role in tumor angiogenesis. Through its primary receptor VEGFR-2, VEGF exerts the activity of a multitasking cytokine, which is able to stimulate endothelial cell survival, invasion and migration into surrounding tissues, proliferation, as well as vascular permeability and inflammation. The core components of VEGF signaling delineate well-defined intracellular routes. However, the whole scenario is complicated by the fact that cascades of signals converge and branch at many points in VEGF signaling, thus depicting a complex signal transduction network that is also finely regulated by different mechanisms. In this chapter, we present a careful collection of the best-characterized VEGF-induced signal transduction pathways, attempting to offer an overview of the complexity of VEGF signaling in the context of tumor angiogenesis.

Keywords: VEGF, signaling, angiogenesis, endothelial cells

1. Introduction

It has been over four decades that Judah Folkman hypothesized, demonstrated and emphasized the critical importance of angiogenesis in tumor growth [1]. His experimental studies showed that in the absence of vascularization a tumor would grow only to a finite size of few thousand cells, restricted by the inability of oxygen and nutrients to penetrate the tissue beyond the diffusion limits of approximately 1–2 mm. To overcome this passive diffusion-limited size, the tumor must perturb the physiological state of its environment inducing the so-called angiogenic switch that implicates the transition from quiescent to active endothelium leading to the vascularization of the growing cell mass. The angiogenic switch was initially hypothesized to be triggered by the production and release of a growth factor called TAF (tumor angiogenesis factor) by tumor cells [2]. Indeed, the explosive growth in tumor angiogenesis research identified and characterized a number of angiogenic inducers. Among them, vascular endothelial growth factor (VEGF) is recognized as the major tumor angiogenesis factor [3].

VEGF family consists of five secreted proteins (VEGF-A, VEGF-B, VEGF-C, VEGF-D and placental growth factor). In terms of endothelial biology and tumor angiogenesis, VEGF-A (hereafter referred as VEGF)—in particular VEGF-A_{165}—is considered to be the most physiologically relevant form. VEGF angiogenic potential is strictly dependent on its multifunctional activity. Indeed, the coordinated arrangement of endothelial cells to form and maintain new vascular tubes requires the induction of vascular permeability, endothelial cell migration, proliferation and survival. These biological responses take place in the endothelium via a complex network of intracellular signal transduction pathways, mainly mediated by VEGF-induced VEGF receptor 2 (VEGFR-2) activation [4].

In this chapter, after a short historical synopsis of Judah Folkman's hypotheses and main discoveries in the field of tumor angiogenesis, we will present a careful collection of the best characterized VEGF-induced signal transduction mechanisms, attempting to offer an overview of the complexity of VEGF signaling. The most intriguing aspect is that cascades of kinases, activity of other enzymes and recruitment of adapter proteins converge and branch at many points in VEGF signaling, emphasizing how linear pathways can integrate to form a complex signal transduction network. If multitasking and integrated signaling go some way toward an understanding of the functional versatility of VEGF, it becomes quite complicated to elucidate how specific information is processed through these pathways and how signaling events are regulated in order to trigger a specific cellular behavior.

2. Historical synopsis of Judah Folkman's hypotheses and main discoveries in the field of tumor angiogenesis

Judah Folkman's scientific achievements in angiogenesis research revolutionized biomedical research and clinical drug development. Until the early 1970s and for some years thereafter, the conventional wisdom was that tumor vasculature was an inflammatory reaction to dying tumor cells. In 1971, Folkman articulated several "visionary" hypotheses on tumor angiogenesis which are now widely accepted. His ideas were based not only on his own work, but also on some studies of a small number of investigators [5–7]. As well summarized in a Cancer Research Commentary recently written by Augustin [8], Folkman published his hypothesis article in 1971, (i) predicting that tumors would be restricted to microscopic size in the absence of angiogenesis, (ii) suggesting that tumors secrete diffusible angiogenic molecules, (iii) describing a model of tumor dormancy due to the blocked angiogenesis, (iv) proposing the term anti-angiogenesis for the prevention of new capillary sprouts from being recruited

http://dx.doi.org/10.5772/66764

into a growing tumor, (v) envisaging the future discovery of angiogenesis inhibitors and (vi) proposing the idea that an antibody to a tumor angiogenic factor could be an anticancer drug.

Folkman and collaborators obtained the first evidence of the existence of the avascular and vascular phases of solid tumor growth in 1963, on the basis of experiments in isolated perfused organs [9]. A rabbit's thyroid gland was seeded with cancer cells from mice and perfused with a blood substitute. Tiny tumors formed, but they grew to the same size, then stopped and never became vascularized. When tumors were transplanted into live mice, they rapidly vascularized and grew vigorously. This lab work and some clinical observations (in particular those regarding retinoblastoma in children) help Folkman develop and sustain the hypothesis that tumor growth is angiogenesis dependent.

In the decade following the 1971 report, research in the tumor angiogenesis field attracted little scientific interest, but Folkman and his team preserved in their investigations, providing convincing evidences for dependence of tumor growth on neovascularization [10–14]. This was achieved in particular thanks to the development and use of bioassays devoted to angiogenesis research, such as the model of eye transplant and chick embryo chorioallantoic membrane. Of note, one of the major steps in allowing scientific appreciation of the role of tumor angiogenesis and demonstrating angiogenesis in vitro was developing methods for passage of endothelial cells. In 1979, Folkman's laboratory reported long-term passage of endothelial cells [15], and the following year, they demonstrated angiogenesis in vitro using endothelial cell cultures exposed to tumor conditioned media [16].

After the developments of the late 1970s, many other scientists entered the field of angiogenesis and Folkman's skeptics became his competitors [17]. In particular, the 1980s were an intense period of hunting for the hypothesized TAF [8]. In 1983, Dvorak and collaborators reported the isolation of a tumor-derived factor that they called "vascular permeability factor" (VPF) on the basis of its capability to induce blood vessel leakage [18]. However, at that time, VPF was not completely purified and therefore not fully identified. In 1989, Ferrara purified a novel angiogenic protein that he termed "vascular endothelial growth factor" (VEGF) on the basis of its observed growth-promoting activity toward only vascular endothelial cells [19]. Around the same time, Folkman's laboratory isolated an angiogenic protein that resulted to be identical to that purified by Ferrara [20]. By 1990, it was realized that VEGF and VPF were in fact the same protein. There is no doubt that it was the discovery of VEGF to set in motion a revolution in the field of angiogenic research.

From 1980 to 2005, Folkman's laboratory reported the discovery of eleven angiogenesis inhibitors, eight of them are endogenous angiogenesis inhibitors [21]. Effort persisted in this area and new anti-angiogenic molecules are continuously being developed. They essentially fall into two distinct types: (i) antibody directed toward angiogenic factors such as VEGF, for example, Avastin (Bevacizumab, Genentech) and (ii) small molecules inhibiting cellular signaling by targeting multiple receptor tyrosine kinases among them VEGFR-2, for example, Sutent (Sunitinib, Pfizer) and Nexavar (Sorafenib, Bayer and Onyx Pharmaceuticals) [17].

Targeting VEGF and VEGFR-2 offers benefit to patients with at least some types of cancer and provides proof of principle that attacking the vasculature is a valid approach to cancer therapy [22]. At present, however, despite important results, the overall clinical benefits of anti-VEGF/VEGFR-2 therapy are still relatively modest: not all cancer patients respond to anti-VEGF treatments, and when they do increased survival may only be measured in weeks or months [17]. This is realistically due to a number of different and not yet fully clarified reasons, which open discussion going beyond the topic of this chapter. Here, we will only mention, as reported by Van Epps in 2005, that one of Folkman's hopes for the future was that anti-angiogenesis therapy could be initiated—based on diagnostic biomarkers—even before the tumor reveals its location in the body, thus stopping cancer before it really gets started [23, 24].

3. VEGF-mediated signal transduction

In vivo angiogenic response to VEGF is mainly mediated via activation of VEGFR-2, expressed primarily in endothelial cells. VEGFR-2 activation initiates several intricate signaling paths, which eventually lead to different endothelial responses: cell survival, proliferation, migration, invasion into the surrounding tissue, vascular permeability and vascular inflammation [25]. These responses involve (i) a number of pivotal effectors such as phosphoinositide 3 kinase (PI3K), phospholipase Cγ (PLCγ), SRC, focal adhesion kinase (FAK) and Rho family of GTPases; (ii) several multifunctional docking proteins and adaptors; and (iii) VEGFR-2 partners such as Neuropilin 1 (NRP1), integrins and vascular endothelial (VE)-cadherin. It is apparent that these proteins orchestrate a complex signaling network leading to the integration of the different VEGF-induced endothelial responses that allows tumor angiogenesis to take place. **Figure 1** illustrates, in a simplified manner, VEGF-mediated signal transduction, showing signal core components along with the main well-defined intracellular routes leading to different endothelial responses.

3.1. VEGFR-2 activation

VEGFR-2 is a tyrosine kinase receptor (RTK). Binding of VEGF to VEGFR-2 promotes receptor dimerization, allowing trans/autophosphorylation of intracellular tyrosine residues. Among the 19 tyrosine residues present in the intracellular domain of VEGFR-2, there are five major phosphorylation sites: Y951, Y1054, Y1059, Y1175 and Y1214. The Y1054 and Y1059 are located in the kinase domain activation loop, and their phosphorylation is critical for receptor catalytic activity [26]. Y951 is located in the kinase insert domain, and its phosphorylation serves as a binding site for T cell-specific adaptor (TSAD) also known as VEGFR-2-associated protein (VRAP) [27, 28]. The Y1175 and Y1214 are located in the carboxy-terminal domain. Phosphorylation of Y1175 creates a binding site for PLCγ [29], p85 subunit of PI3K [30], the adaptor proteins SHB [31] and SCK [32]. This residue is well-recognized as a critical mediator of VEGFR-2 signaling. Phosphorylated Y1214 has been described to bind the adaptor protein NCK [33].

VEGFR-2 activation and downstream signaling are modulated by different mechanisms. The main of them involve (i) receptor interaction with NRP1, specific integrins and VE-cadherin

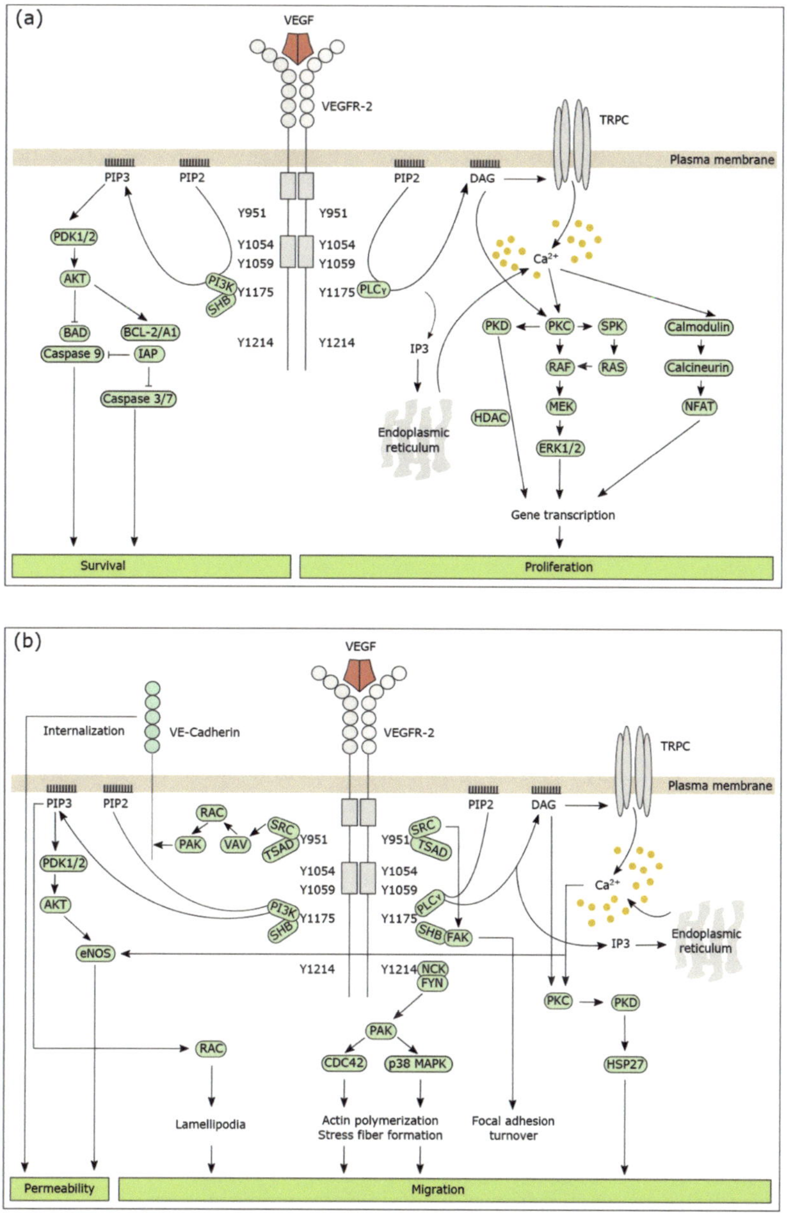

Figure 1. Signal transduction mediated by VEGF/VEGFR-2. Core signaling pathways involved in VEGF-induced (a) cell survival and proliferation and (b) vascular permeability and cell migration. See text for details.

(see Section 3.7) and (ii) the activity of the protein tyrosine phosphatases (PTPs) such as vascular endothelial PTP (VEPTP), SRC homology 2 domain PTP (SHP2) and PTP1B [34]. VEGFR-2 activation may also be influenced by the presence of heparin sulfate glycoproteins that modulate VEGF-VEGFR-2 binding and signaling amplitude [35, 36]. Indeed, a change in ligand-receptor affinity may highly influence RTK signaling. We recently reported that

VEGF-VEGFR2 affinity may vary from low to high based on the endothelial cell density state that we also reported to influence the number of total and surface VEGFR-2 [37]. In particular, by combining wet-lab experiments, theoretical insights and mathematical modeling, we found that ligand-receptor affinity is reduced in long-confluent compare to sparse endothelial cells, which recapitulate in vitro the condition of quiescent and angiogenic endothelium in vivo.

3.2. PLCγ signaling

Activated VEGFR-2 directly recruits PLCγ, which is in turn phosphorylated [38, 39]. Phosphorylated PLCγ hydrolyzes the membrane phospholipid phosphatidylinositol-4,5-bi-phosphate (PIP2), generating diacylglycerol (DAG) and inositol 1,4,5-trisphosphate (IP3). This latter mobilizes Ca^{2+} from the endoplasmic reticulum, thus leading to an increase in intracellular Ca^{2+}. IP3-mediated Ca^{2+} increase supports DAG-induced activation of PKC, from which it is triggered the RAF1-MEK-ERK1/2 mitogen-activated protein (MAP) kinase cascade, that is, the best characterized pathway propagated downstream to VEGF/VEGFR-2/PLCγ axis resulting, in particular, in endothelial cell proliferation trough the ERK1/2-dependent regulation of gene transcription.

Most RTKs are known to utilize the classical GRB2-SOS-RAS activation of the RAF1-MEK-ERK1/2 cascade. Conflicting results exist in the literature with respect to the interaction of VEGFR-2 with SHC or GRB2, which recruit the RAS activating nucleotide-exchange factor SOS to the receptor, and the significance of the classical RAS-mediated MAP kinase cascade downstream to VEGFR-2 is unclear [32, 40]. Indeed, it is well-accepted that, after VEGF stimulation, most of the MAP kinase activation is mediated via the PLCγ-activated PKC as first reported by Takahashi and coworkers [39, 41]. These authors described the pathway as RAS-independent; however, considering the same pathway, Shu and colleagues reported the involvement of sphingosine kinase (SPK), found to link PKC to RAS activation in a manner independent of RAS nucleotide-exchange factor [42].

VEGF-induced activation of PKC also results in activation of protein kinase D (PKD), found to influence ERK1/2 activation and cell proliferation [43]. In response to VEGF, gene repressive action of histone deacetylases (HDAC) 5 and 7 in endothelial cells is overcome by the PLCγ-PKC-PKD pathway-dependent HDAC 5 and 7 phosphorylation and nuclear export, resulting in the regulation of gene transcription, cell proliferation and migration [44, 45]. Moreover, VEGF-induced PKC-dependent activation of PKD has also been reported to induce HSP27 phosphorylation and mediate cell migration without involving the p38 MAP kinase (p38 MAPK)/MAP kinase-activated protein kinase 2 signaling cascade [46].

As mentioned above, PLCγ activation induced an increase in intracellular Ca^{2+}. Ca^{2+} signaling is crucial in VEGF/VEGFR-2 signal transduction, not only for PLCγ/PKC-mediated pathways but also for activation of other molecular players such as, in particular, the endothelial nitric oxide synthase (eNOS) and the nuclear factor of activated T-cell (NFAT) family of transcription factors. eNOS plays a crucial role in the control of vascular homeostasis and permeability; its activity is regulated by a complex combination of protein–protein interactions and signal transduction cascades involving Ca^{2+} mobilization and phosphorylation events

[47]. VEGF stimulates both Ca^{2+} and phosphorylation-dependent regulation of eNOS activity. VEGF stimulation in endothelial cells first leads to the Ca^{2+}-calmodulin disruption of the caveolin-eNOS complex and promotes the association between eNOS and the chaperon protein HSP90; eNOS-bound HSP90 can then recruit VEGF-activated AKT to the complex, which in turn can phosphorylate eNOS, resulting in potentiation of its activity [48]. NFAT proteins—extensively studied in the immune system—are functional in several cell types, including cancer cells, endothelial cells and infiltrating immune cells [49]. The multiple functions attributed to NFAT include cell growth, survival, invasion and angiogenesis. These transcription factors are activated through a Ca^{2+}- and calmodulin-activated calcineurin-dependent mechanism. In endothelial cells, VEGF stimulates receptor-mediated activation of PLCγ leading to an increase in intracellular Ca^{2+}, calcineurin activation and NFAT nuclear translocation that in turn leads to the transactivation of genes that are essential for angiogenesis [49, 50], such as COX-2 resulting in synthesis of PGE2, a mediator of endothelial cell migration and tube formation [51]. Moreover, in endothelial cells, VEGF-mediated NFAT activation induces a gene repertoire that includes an inherent inflammatory component, similar to that of interleukin 1 [52]. In addition, it has been recently reported that endothelial cells decode VEGF-mediated Ca^{2+} signaling patterns to produce distinct functional responses: cell proliferation and cell migration involving NFAT and myosin light chain kinase, respectively [53].

VEGFR-2/PLCγ signaling also involves TRPC channels, which are Ca^{2+}-permeable nonselective cation channels. Indeed, VEGF induces Ca^{2+} elevation through both Ca^{2+} release from intracellular stores and extracellular Ca^{2+} entry. In particular, VEGFR-2/PLCγ axis activates TRPC3 and TRPC6 in a DAG-dependent manner [54]. TRPC6 has been reported to be required for VEGF-mediated Ca^{2+} increase and the subsequent signaling that lead to processes associated with angiogenesis, such as cell migration, proliferation and tube formation [55, 56].

Overall, PLCγ appears as a regulator of a number of pathways, leading to cell proliferation and migration and contributing to vascular permeability. Thus, a better understanding of its downregulation may be of interest in further elucidating the regulation of VEGF-induced signaling, as well as in the development of new anti-angiogenic therapies. Indeed, very little is known about the regulation of PLCγ activity. Singh and colleagues have been reported that VEGF-induced PLCγ ubiquitination inhibits its tyrosine phosphorylation, thus providing a negative feedback to prevent sustained PLCγ stimulation [57]. In addition, we have previously reported the essential role of PTPs on VEGF-induced PLCγ activation, suggesting the existence of at least one—not yet characterized—PTP directly targeting PLCγ and counteracting receptor-mediated signal [37].

3.3. PI3K signaling

VEGF/VEGFR-2 axis activates PI3K in different ways, including direct or indirect (i.e., through adaptor and scaffold proteins) binding of PI3K to the receptor, and the involvement of SRC (see Sections 3.4 and 3.6). The activated PI3K converts the plasma membrane lipid PIP2 to phosphatidylinositol-3,4,5-trisphosphate (PIP3), and signaling proteins with pleckstrin homology (PH) domains accumulate at site of PI3K activation by directly binding to PIP3 [58]. Among these signaling proteins of particular interest are the serine-threonine kinases

AKT and phosphoinositide-dependent kinase 1 (PDK1). Phosphorylation of AKT by PDK1 and PDK2 allows the full activation of AKT, resulting in the phosphorylation of a number of proteins [59]. Other PH domain-containing proteins that are activated by PIP3 include GDP-GTP exchange factors for the small GTPase RAC [58, 60].

PI3K/AKT pathway is considered the main mechanism by which VEGF induces endothelial cell survival. AKT mediates both short- and long-term cell survival effects by inhibiting (through direct phosphorylation) pro-apoptotic proteins such as BAD, caspase 9 and forkhead transcription factors, and by upregulating anti-apoptotic proteins such as BCL-2 [61, 62]. In 1998, Gerber and coworkers were the first to report that VEGF regulates endothelial cell survival through the PI3K/AKT signal transduction pathway and that VEGF also induces expression of the anti-apoptotic proteins BCL-2 and A1 in endothelial cells [63, 64]. In the following year, Tran and colleagues reported a marked induction of the IAP family anti-apoptotic proteins survivin and XIAP—which inhibit caspase 3, 7 and 9—by VEGF in endothelial cells [65].

Although crucial for its function in cell survival, AKT is not simply a regulator of cell survival but a multifunctional protein playing a pivotal role in both cancer cells and endothelial cells. In addition to cell survival, AKT activation has been linked to tumor angiogenesis via several other biological processes, including vascular permeability, cell proliferation, synthesis and release of matrix metalloproteinases and induction of VEGF production by cancer cells [59]. Beyond the pro-survival effect and considering the VEGF/VEGFR-2 signal transduction in the endothelium, the main contribution exerted by AKT resides in the direct phosphorylation of eNOS, thus contributing to the control of endothelial permeability [48, 66].

3.4. SRC and FAK

The SRC family of protein tyrosine kinases (SFKs) plays key roles in regulating signal transduction by a diverse set of cell surface receptors in the context of a variety of cellular environments [67]. Endothelial SFKs includes SRC, YES and FYN. Many of the VEGF-mediated pathways involve SRC activity. Moreover, SRC is intimately involved in the modulation of the activity of FAK through direct phosphorylation (see below). VEGFR-2 activates SRC according to different mechanisms: (i) by direct binding to Y951 in the receptor [27], (ii) through the adaptor protein TSAD [68] or (iii) involving the scaffold protein GAB1 and GAB2 [69].

VEGF-induced SRC activity is involved in the activation of different signaling proteins, such as PI3K, FAK and eNOS. Holmqvist and colleagues reported that activated VEGFR-2 recruits SHB and SRC and that this latter phosphorylates SHB, which allows the subsequent activation of PI3K and phosphorylation of FAK at Y576 [31]. Duval and coworkers reported that VEGF induces phosphorylation of VEGFR-2-associated HSP90, which is dependent on receptor internalization and on SRC kinase activation; furthermore, they demonstrated that SRC directly phosphorylates HSP90 and that this event is essential for VEGF-stimulated eNOS association to HSP90 and thus NO release from endothelial cells [70]. In response to VEGF, Src may also activate members of the MAP kinase cascade such as RAF1 [71] and b-RAF [72]; this latter is activated in a manner dependent of SRC-mediated phosphorylation of the scaffold protein IQ motif-containing GTPase-activating protein 1 (IQGAP1).

In parallel with the effect exerted on intracellular signaling proteins, SRC plays a pivotal role in the disorganization of cadherin-dependent cell-cell contacts and in integrin-VEGFR-2 cross-activation. In response to VEGF, SRC phosphorylates VE-cadherin in adherens junctions, allowing endothelial cell migration and inducing vascular permeability [73–76]. Mahabeleshwar and coworkers reported that there is an intimate and coordinated relationship between VEGFR-2 and $\alpha v\beta 3$ integrin involving SRC activity [77]. In particular, they demonstrated that (i) adhesion- and growth factor-induced $\beta 3$ integrin tyrosine phosphorylation is directly mediated by SRC, (ii) SRC-dependent $\beta 3$ integrin tyrosine phosphorylation is critical for interaction between VEGFR-2 and $\beta 3$ integrin, and (iii) SRC mediates growth factor-induced $\beta 3$ integrin activation, ligand binding and $\alpha v\beta 3$ integrin-dependent cellular adhesion, directional migration of endothelial cells and initiation of angiogenic programming in endothelial cells.

As mentioned above, SRC is involved in the modulation of FAK activity through direct phosphorylation. The non-receptor tyrosine kinase FAK—well recognized as an important regulator of cell migration—is localized in focal adhesions, established as a consequence of integrin ligation to the extracellular matrix. Upon integrin-dependent cell adhesion, phosphorylation of FAK and its catalytic activity are stimulated. FAK possesses six tyrosyl residues (i. e., Y397, Y407, Y576, Y577, Y861 and Y925) that are differentially phosphorylated by diverse agonists and that are implicated in transmitting different signals and effects. Y397 is an autophosphorylation site that recruits SH2 domain-containing proteins, including members of SKFs, PLCγ and the p85 subunit of PI3K [78]. It appears that SRC is first recruited to Y397 and then involved in transphosphorylation of other tyrosyl residues within FAK, such as Y576 and Y577; this confers maximal activation of FAK and signaling in response to adhesion [79, 80]. In particular, upon VEGF stimulation, Y576 and Y861 are both phosphorylated in a SRC-dependent manner [31, 81], while Y407 is phosphorylated in a SRC-independent manner that involves the recruitment of HSP90 to the receptor, followed by the activation of RHOA and that of RHO activated kinase (ROCK) [81]. This results in phosphorylation of FAK on S732 that allows FAK-related kinase PYK2-mediated phosphorylation of FAK on Y407, promoting cell migration [82].

3.5. Rho family GTPases

The RHO family GTPases—shuttling between inactive GDP-bound and active GTP-bound forms—include RHO, RAC and CDC42, which are known to regulate primarily the reorganization of actin cytoskeletal systems such as actin stress fibers and focal adhesions, lamellipodia and filopodia, respectively [83]. A growing body of evidence indicates a crucial role for VEGF-induced RHO GTPases activity in endothelial cell during the processes involved in angiogenesis such as, in particular, cell migration and vascular permeability [84]. VEGF/VEGFR-2 axis stimulates the activities of RHO [81, 85], RAC [86, 87] and CDC42 [88]. As reported in Section 3.4, VEGF-induced RHO activity stimulates FAK activation promoting cell migration [81]. VEGF-induced RAC activation has been linked to both endothelial permeability and cell migration. Gavard and Gutkind reported that RAC takes part in a signaling pathway by which VEGF stimulation promotes the rapid endocytosis of VE-cadherin, thereby disrupting the endothelial barrier function [86]. In particular, they demonstrated that VEGFR-2 activates RAC through the SRC-dependent phosphorylation of the nucleotide-exchange factor VAV2 and that RAC activation, in turn, promotes the p21-activated kinase (PAK)-mediated phosphorylation of VE-cadherin resulting in the recruitment of beta-arrestin 2 to phosphorylated VE-cadherin, thereby promoting its internalization into clathrin-coated vesicles and the consequent disassembly of intercellular junctions. To complement this study, Garrett and coworkers reported that VEGF-induced SRC-dependent VAV2 phosphorylation and downstream activation of RAC1 are also responsible for endothelial cell migration and wound closure [87]. The involvement of CDC42 in VEGF signaling has been reported in particular by Lamalice and colleagues [33, 88]. They proposed a model according to which, upon VEGFR-2 activation phosphorylated Y1214 within the receptor recruits the adaptor protein NCK that becomes phosphorylated providing a recruitment site for FYN that is also phosphorylated and required for the phosphorylation of NCK and that of the p21-activated protein kinase PAK-2, an effector of CDC42; then, this early molecular complex containing VEGFR-2·NCK·FYN·PAK-2 triggers the sequential activation of CDC42 and p38 MAPK leading to actin polymerization, stress fiber formation and endothelial cell migration.

3.6. Key docking, adaptor and scaffold proteins

As it emerges from what above described, it is evident that, beyond a number of kinases and other enzymes, VEGFR-2 signaling involves several key docking, adaptor and scaffold proteins including SHB, TSAD, NCK, IQGAP1 and GAB1. In the following, we briefly summarize their main involvement downstream to VEGF/VEGFR-2 axis.

The adapter protein SHB contains at least four different domains responsible for protein-protein interactions (i.e., the proline-rich motifs in its N-terminus, the phospho-tyrosine binding (PTB) domain, potential tyrosine phosphorylation sites and the C-terminal SH2 domain) and has been shown to operate downstream of several RTKs exerting versatile effects on a number of signaling pathways [89]. SHB binds to phosphorylate Y1175 in VEGFR-2 and is phosphorylated by SRC; this allows the subsequent activation of PI3K and phosphorylation of FAK at Y576 in the kinase domain, regulating the migratory response in endothelial cells [31]. Along this pathway, it is possible that SHB is required for VEGF-mediated activation of FAK by allowing SRC to phosphorylate Y576. Indeed, it has been demonstrated that the PTB domain of SHB can bind directly to FAK and regulate its activity in response to FGFR-1 activation in endothelial cells [90].

TSAD is an adaptor protein containing a SH2 domain, tyrosines in protein binding motifs and a proline-rich domain allowing SH3-dependent interactions. TSAD interacts with and modulates the activity of some SFKs such as LCK and SRC [68, 91], and has been found to control actin polymerization events in both T cells and endothelial cells [27, 92]. TSAD binds to phosphorylate Y951 in VEGFR-2 via its SH2 domain and to SRC via its proline-rich domain. TSAD has been reported as an important docking mechanism for SRC to VEGFR-2, involved in the regulation of cell migration, endothelial cell junctions and vascular permeability, but not cell proliferation [27, 68].

NCK is an adapter protein consisting of one SH2 domain and three SH3 domains. A main function of NCK is to link receptor and receptor-associated tyrosine kinases with proteins that directly or indirectly regulate remodeling and reorganization of the actin cytoskeleton [93]. According to the model proposed by Lamalice and colleagues, upon phosphorylation on Y1214 in VEGFR-2, NCK is recruited to the receptor thus allowing the formation of a molecular complex containing VEGFR-2·NCK·FYN·PAK-2 that convey the sequential activation of CDC42 and p38 MAPK leading to actin polymerization, stress fiber formation and endothelial cell migration [33]. Moreover, it has been reported that NCK participates with PAK in the signaling pathway by which VEGF stimulates the assembly of focal adhesions [94].

The multidomain scaffold protein IQGAP1 binds to several structural and signaling proteins. For example, interactions of the IQGAP1 calponin homology domain (CHD) with F-actin and the GAP-related domain (GRD) with small GTPases regulate the cytoskeleton to promote actin binding or polymerization that regulates cell migration, stability of cell-cell contacts and cytokinesis; moreover, IQGAPs also scaffold molecules form signaling complexes, such as components of the MAP kinase cascade, thus promoting their activity [95]. Along VEGF signal transduction, IQGAP1 becomes phosphorylated by SRC and activates b-RAF, contributing to cell proliferation [72]. Moreover, IQGAP1 has been implicated in regulation of cell migration and cell-cell contacts [96, 97]. In particular, Yamaoka-Tojo and colleagues suggested that IQGAP1 may function as a scaffold to link VEGFR-2 to the adherens junctions through binding to VEGFR-2 and VE-cadherin/β-catenin complex, thereby dissociating α-catenin from the adherens junctional complex and contributing to VEGF-stimulated loss of cell-cell contacts in endothelial cell [97].

GAB1 is the prototype of a subfamily of large multiadapter proteins sharing an N-terminal PH domain, two proline-rich regions involved in constitutive binding to GRB2 and multiple tyrosine phosphorylation sites [98]. Downstream to VEGF/VEGFR-2 axis, GAB1—recruited through an amplification loop involving PIP3 and its PH domain—has been proposed to be a primary actor in coupling VEGFR-2 to PI3K/AKT [98]. In response to VEGF, it has been reported that GAB1 is phosphorylated and associates not only with PI3K, but also with GRB2, SHP2, SHC and PLCγ influencing the signaling downstream to VEGFR-2 and, in particular, cell migration and capillary formation [99].

3.7. Neuropilin 1, integrins and Vascular Endothelial Cadherin

VEGF signaling is complicated by the fact that VEGFR-2 interact with additional cellular proteins such as, in particular, NRP1, specific integrins and VE-cadherin [100]. This modulates the signal strength induced by VEGFR-2 on the basis of the extracellular cues arising from the soluble ligand, cell-substratum and cell-cell interactions.

NRP1 is a transmembrane receptor for VEGF and the neuronal guidance cue SEMA3A, with essential roles in both vascular and neuronal development, as well as in pathological angiogenesis [101, 102]. The precise mechanism of VEGF-VEGFR-2-NRP1 interaction and the functional consequences of this molecular complex are still being explored. The most widely accepted model of NRP1 function in angiogenesis postulates that it forms a VEGF-dependent complex with VEGFR-2 to enhance the activation of a wide variety of intracellular signal transduction pathways, including those that involve ERK1/2, AKT, SRC and p38 MAPK [103]. Moreover, it has been reported that NRP1 promotes VEGFR-2 trafficking through RAB11 vesicles thereby specifying signal output [104].

Integrins link intracellular signaling pathways induced by soluble factor to output elicited by cellular interactions with extracellular matrix. Specific integrins, particularly integrin β1 and β3, act as important partners for VEGFR-2. An intimate and coordinated relationship between VEGFR-2 and αvβ3 has been reported by Mahabeleshwar and coworkers (see Section 3.4) [77]. In particular, the relationship between VEGFR-2 and β3 integrin appears to be synergistic, because VEGFR-2 activation induces β3 integrin tyrosine phosphorylation, which, in turn, is crucial for maximum phosphorylation of VEGFR-2 [77]. Exposure of endothelial cells to matrix-bound VEGF promotes VEGFR-2-integrin β1 complex formation, redistribution to focal adhesion, prolonged activation of VEGFR-2 with differential phosphorylation of Y1214 and extended activation kinetics of p38 MAPK [105].

VE-cadherin is involved in the formation of adherens junctions in endothelial cells and plays a crucial role in VEGF signaling. In resting endothelial cells, VE-cadherin complexes with VEGFR-2 at cell-cell contacts and attenuates VEGFR-2 phosphorylation through the phosphatase DEP1 [106]. Upon VEGF stimulation, VEC is phosphorylated and in turn internalized, thereby disrupting the endothelial barrier function (see Sections 3.4 and 3.5).

3.8. VEGFR-2 internalization

It is well known that VEGFR-2 undergoes internalization and trafficking upon VEGF stimulation. Emerging evidences suggest that VEGFR-2 internalization and trafficking are tightly controlled processes that influence the sensitivity of endothelial cells to VEGF and the signaling propagated downstream to the receptor. Although the mechanisms regulating VEGFR-2 internalization and trafficking and their exerted effects on signaling are still not fully understood, it is apparent that a pivotal role is played by VEGFR-2 interaction with specific protein partners such as, in particular but not only, VE-cadherin and NRP1.

In endothelial cells, VEGFR-2 is located in different subcellular pools, including receptors diffusely distributed in the plasma membrane, engaged in cell-cell junctions through the interaction with VE-cadherin and associated with various intracellular compartments. Resting endothelial cells have two surface pools of VEGFR-2: a stable pool that is complexed with VE-cadherin, and a flux pool that is constantly cycling between the surface and the endocytic compartment in a VEGF independent manner [107, 108]. VE-cadherin prevents internalization of VEGFR-2 by physical interaction and recruitment of the DEP-1 phosphatase [106]. VEGF stimulation results in clathrin-dependent internalization of VEGFR-2. The clathrin-coated vesicles fuse with early endosomes and then proceed through a series of steps that can either direct their recycling back to the plasma membrane via the fast (RAB4) or slow (RAB11) recycling pathways or target them for degradation into lysosome via the RAB7 pathway [109]. Ballmer-Hofer and colleagues reported that when complexed with NRP1, internalized VEGFR-2 is recycled through RAB4 and RAB11 positive vesicles; while in the absence of NRP1, internalized VEGFR-2 bypassed RAB11 vesicles and rapidly accumulated in RAB7

http://dx.doi.org/10.5772/66764

vesicles indicative of receptor degradation [104]. They also showed that VEGFR-2 is dephosphorylated before entry into the RAB11 compartment and then targeted to the plasma membrane where it presumably initiates a new round of ligand binding and receptor activation thereby prolonging VEGF signaling to downstream targets [104]. Furthermore, there are also evidences that when activated VEGFR-2—not yet dephosphorylated—is trapped inside endosomes, it is still capable of stimulating some downstream signaling proteins such as those belonging to the MAP kinase cascade [110].

4. Synopsis of VEGF-induced endothelial responses and their role in tumor angiogenesis

VEGF/VEGFR-2 signal transduction leads to six major endothelial responses: cell survival, invasion and migration into the surrounding tissue, proliferation, vascular permeability and vascular inflammation. These endothelial responses are tightly integrated to allow tumor angiogenesis to progress successfully.

Vascular permeability—crucial for normal tissue homeostasis—is a prerequisite for VEGF-induced angiogenesis. Endothelial permeability is mediated by the so-called transcellular and paracellular pathways, that is, solutes and cells can pass through (transcellular) or between (paracellular) endothelial cells. Transcellular passage requires cell fenestration and/or a complex system of transport vesicles that includes organelles called vesiculo-vacuolar organelles, while the paracellular pathway depends on the coordinated opening and closure of endothelial cell-to-cell junctions, combined with cell retraction. VEGF is involved in both transcellular and paracellular permeability. VEGF/VEGFR-2 axis induces increased endothelial permeability mainly through SRC-mediated signaling of VE-cadherin internalization (see Sections 3.4 and 3.5) that disrupts the endothelial barrier function, and by activation of PLCγ that mediates an increase in intracellular Ca^{2+} resulting in Ca^{2+}-calmodulin-dependent regulation of eNOS (see Section 3.2). Activation of eNOS—also achieved by AKT-mediated phosphorylation—promotes an increase in vascular permeability by NO production that is followed by vasodilatation. VEGF-induced vascular permeability contributes to the dissemination of extracellular proteases and the deposition of a fibrin gel provisional stroma that changes the extracellular matrix of normal tissues from anti- to pro-angiogenic and stromagenic, favoring and supporting inward migration of endothelial cells and the growth of new endothelial sprouts [111]. In addition, the reduced vessel integrity may promote leukocyte extravasation and facilitate exit of metastasis from the primary tumors.

VEGF-induced vascular permeability goes in parallel with vascular inflammation. Although VEGF is not an inflammatory cytokine, VEGF-induced gene transcription—in particular through NFAT activation—includes a conspicuous inflammatory component (see Section 3.2). This could conceivably promote attraction of inflammatory cells that may contribute to the angiogenic response. Indeed, it is well established that tumor angiogenesis is linked to inflammation. On the one hand, tumor cells can be killed by the immune system; on the other hand, tumor can use leukocytes to supports its expansion.

Endothelial cell invasion into the surrounding tissue is made possible by means of the release of MMPs, which degrade the basal membrane and the extracellular matrix and allow the migration of endothelial cells to form capillary sprouts. Endothelial cells express different MMPs, and it has been reported that their expression is induced by VEGF and regulated by Ets transcription factors [112, 113]. Signaling pathways, such as MAP kinase cascade, PI3K/AKT axis, and Ca^{2+}-specific signals, converge on the Ets transcription factors, controlling their activity.

VEGF-induced endothelial cell migration and proliferation are tightly regulated and coordinated spatio-temporal behaviors, which—in parallel with sustained cell survival—enable angiogenic sprouting and capillary lumen formation, necessary to create the new vessels devoted to support tumor growth and metastasis spread. VEGF-induced endothelial survival and proliferation are stimulated primarily via PI3K/AKT and PLCγ/ERK pathways, respectively, involving—as above described—several signaling intermediates. VEGF-induced endothelial cell migration appears to be regulated by a larger number of pathways, including the involvement of PLCγ, PI3K, RHO GTPases, SRC and FAK activities.

5. Conclusions

In this chapter, we attempted in particular to describe the best characterized signal transduction events downstream to VEGF/VEGFR-2 axis involved in tumor angiogenesis. Multiple VEGF-induced signaling pathways take part in the promotion of different biological responses in endothelial cells. Although it is possible to recognize distinct patterns along VEGF-induced signaling, they are intricate, characterized by the involvement of a number of enzymes and adaptor/scaffold proteins—whose activity converges and branches at many point—and by the presence of VEGFR-2 molecular partners influencing endothelial cell sensitivity to VEGF and receptor signal output. This depicts a complex signal network induced by VEGF, where the apparent redundancy in operating signaling pathways is likely to reflect a need for a fine-tuning and a differential control of the biological effects in response to VEGF [25]. Although past decade has seen an important advancement in our understanding of VEGF signaling, there is still a lack of insight in many aspects of VEGF/VEGFR-2 signal transduction, in particular for what concerns its fine regulation. A further elucidation of the multifaced VEGF signaling network in the context of endothelial biology is crucial for developing new potential anti-angiogenic therapies. In parallel with current therapies that directly target VEGF and VEGFR-2, agents able to influence key molecular player—proximal, median or distal to VEGFR-2—could be of clinical interest.

Acknowledgement

Publication costs have been supported by "Associazione Italiana per la Ricerca sul Cancro" (AIRC), project code 12182.

Author details

Lucia Napione[1,2,*], Maria Alvaro[1,2] and Federico Bussolino[1,2]

*Address all correspondence to: lucia.napione@ircc.it

1 Laboratory of Vascular Oncology, Candiolo Cancer Institute – IRCCS, Candiolo, Italy

2 Department of Oncology, University of Torino, Candiolo, Italy

References

[1] Folkman J. Tumor angiogenesis: therapeutic implications. N Engl J Med. 1971; 285(21):1182–6.

[2] Folkman J. Proceedings: tumor angiogenesis factor. Cancer Res. 1974;34(8):2109–13.

[3] Ferrara N, Gerber HP, LeCouter J. The biology of VEGF and its receptors. Nat Med. 2003;9(6):669–76.

[4] Koch S, Claesson-Welsh L. Signal transduction by vascular endothelial growth factor receptors. Cold Spring Harb Perspect Med. 2012;2(7):a006502.

[5] Algire G, Chalkley H. Vascular reactions of normal and malignant tissues in vivo. I. Vascular reactions of mice to wounds and to normal and neoplastic implants. J Natl Cancer Inst. 1945. p. 73–85.

[6] Greenblatt M, Shubi P. Tumor angiogenesis: transfilter diffusion studies in the hamster by the transparent chamber technique. J Natl Cancer Inst. 1968;41(1):111–24.

[7] Warren BA, Shubik P. The growth of the blood supply to melanoma transplants in the hamster cheek pouch. Lab Invest. 1966;15(2):464–78.

[8] Augustin HG. Commentary on Folkman: "How is blood vessel growth regulated in normal and neoplastic tissue?". Cancer Res. 2016;76(10):2854–6.

[9] Ribatti D. Judah Folkman, a pioneer in the study of angiogenesis. Angiogenesis. 2008; 11(1):3–10.

[10] Gimbrone MA, Leapman SB, Cotran RS, Folkman J. Tumor dormancy in vivo by prevention of neovascularization. J Exp Med. 1972;136(2):261–76.

[11] Gimbrone MA, Leapman SB, Cotran RS, Folkman J. Tumor angiogenesis: iris neovascularization at a distance from experimental intraocular tumors. J Natl Cancer Inst. 1973;50(1):219–28.

[12] Gimbrone MA, Cotran RS, Leapman SB, Folkman J. Tumor growth and neovascularization: an experimental model using the rabbit cornea. J Natl Cancer Inst. 1974;52(2):413–27.

[13] Knighton D, Ausprunk D, Tapper D, Folkman J. Avascular and vascular phases of tumour growth in the chick embryo. Br J Cancer. 1977;35(3):347–56.

[14] Brem S, Brem H, Folkman J, Finkelstein D, Patz A. Prolonged tumor dormancy by prevention of neovascularization in the vitreous. Cancer Res. 1976;36(8):2807–12.

[15] Folkman J, Haudenschild CC, Zetter BR. Long-term culture of capillary endothelial cells. Proc Natl Acad Sci U S A. 1979;76(10):5217–21.

[16] Folkman J, Haudenschild C. Angiogenesis in vitro. Nature. 1980;288(5791):551–6.

[17] Stephenson J, Goddard J, Al-Taan O, Dennison A, Morgan B. Tumor Angiogenesis: a growth area—from John Hunter to Judah Folkman and beyond. J Cancer Res: Hindawi Publishing Corporation; 2013. pp. 1–6.

[18] Senger DR, Galli SJ, Dvorak AM, Perruzzi CA, Harvey VS, Dvorak HF. Tumor cells secrete a vascular permeability factor that promotes accumulation of ascites fluid. Science. 1983;219(4587):983–5.

[19] Leung DW, Cachianes G, Kuang WJ, Goeddel DV, Ferrara N. Vascular endothelial growth factor is a secreted angiogenic mitogen. Science. 1989;246(4935):1306–9.

[20] Rosenthal RA, Megyesi JF, Henzel WJ, Ferrara N, Folkman J. Conditioned medium from mouse sarcoma 180 cells contains vascular endothelial growth factor. Growth Factors. 1990;4(1):53–9.

[21] Folkman J. Endogenous angiogenesis inhibitors. APMIS. 2004;112(7–8):496–507.

[22] Sitohy B, Nagy JA, Dvorak HF. Anti-VEGF/VEGFR therapy for cancer: reassessing the target. Cancer Res. 2012;72(8):1909–14.

[23] Van Epps H. What tumors need: a brief history of angiogenesis. J Exp Med. 2005. p. 1024.

[24] Folkman J. Angiogenesis: an organizing principle for drug discovery? Nat Rev Drug Discov. 2007;6(4):273–86.

[25] Claesson-Welsh L, Welsh M. VEGFA and tumour angiogenesis. J Intern Med. 2013;273(2): 114–27.

[26] Kendall RL, Rutledge RZ, Mao X, Tebben AJ, Hungate RW, Thomas KA. Vascular endothelial growth factor receptor KDR tyrosine kinase activity is increased by autophosphorylation of two activation loop tyrosine residues. J Biol Chem. 1999;274(10):6453–60.

[27] Matsumoto T, Bohman S, Dixelius J, Berge T, Dimberg A, Magnusson P, et al. VEGF receptor-2 Y951 signaling and a role for the adapter molecule TSAd in tumor angiogenesis. EMBO J. 2005;24(13):2342–53.

[28] Wu LW, Mayo LD, Dunbar JD, Kessler KM, Ozes ON, Warren RS, et al. VRAP is an adaptor protein that binds KDR, a receptor for vascular endothelial cell growth factor. J Biol Chem. 2000;275(9):6059–62.

[29] Takahashi T, Yamaguchi S, Chida K, Shibuya M. A single autophosphorylation site on KDR/Flk-1 is essential for VEGF-A-dependent activation of PLC-gamma and DNA synthesis in vascular endothelial cells. EMBO J. 2001;20(11):2768–78.

[30] Dayanir V, Meyer RD, Lashkari K, Rahimi N. Identification of tyrosine residues in vascular endothelial growth factor receptor-2/FLK-1 involved in activation of phosphatidylinositol 3-kinase and cell proliferation. J Biol Chem. 2001;276(21):17686–92.

[31] Holmqvist K, Cross MJ, Rolny C, Hägerkvist R, Rahimi N, Matsumoto T, et al. The adaptor protein shb binds to tyrosine 1175 in vascular endothelial growth factor (VEGF) receptor-2 and regulates VEGF-dependent cellular migration. J Biol Chem. 2004;279(21):22267–75.

[32] Warner AJ, Lopez-Dee J, Knight EL, Feramisco JR, Prigent SA. The Shc-related adaptor protein, Sck, forms a complex with the vascular-endothelial-growth-factor receptor KDR in transfected cells. Biochem J. 2000;347(Pt 2):501–9.

[33] Lamalice L, Houle F, Huot J. Phosphorylation of Tyr1214 within VEGFR-2 triggers the recruitment of Nck and activation of Fyn leading to SAPK2/p38 activation and endothelial cell migration in response to VEGF. J Biol Chem. 2006;281(45):34009–20.

[34] Kappert K, Peters KG, Böhmer FD, Ostman A. Tyrosine phosphatases in vessel wall signaling. Cardiovasc Res. 2005;65(3):587–98.

[35] Gitay-Goren H, Soker S, Vlodavsky I, Neufeld G. The binding of vascular endothelial growth factor to its receptors is dependent on cell surface-associated heparin-like molecules. J Biol Chem. 1992;267(9):6093–8.

[36] Jakobsson L, Kreuger J, Holmborn K, Lundin L, Eriksson I, Kjellén L, et al. Heparan sulfate in trans potentiates VEGFR-mediated angiogenesis. Dev Cell. 2006;10(5):625–34.

[37] Napione L, Pavan S, Veglio A, Picco A, Boffetta G, Celani A, et al. Unraveling the influence of endothelial cell density on VEGF-A signaling. Blood. 2012;119(23):5599–607.

[38] Olsson AK, Dimberg A, Kreuger J, Claesson-Welsh L. VEGF receptor signalling—in control of vascular function. Nat Rev Mol Cell Biol. 2006;7(5):359–71.

[39] Takahashi T, Shibuya M. The 230 kDa mature form of KDR/Flk-1 (VEGF receptor-2) activates the PLC-gamma pathway and partially induces mitotic signals in NIH3T3 fibroblasts. Oncogene. 1997;14(17):2079–89.

[40] Kroll J, Waltenberger J. The vascular endothelial growth factor receptor KDR activates multiple signal transduction pathways in porcine aortic endothelial cells. J Biol Chem. 1997;272(51):32521–7.

[41] Takahashi T, Ueno H, Shibuya M. VEGF activates protein kinase C-dependent, but Ras-independent Raf-MEK-MAP kinase pathway for DNA synthesis in primary endothelial cells. Oncogene. 1999;18(13):2221–30.

[42] Shu X, Wu W, Mosteller RD, Broek D. Sphingosine kinase mediates vascular endothelial growth factor-induced activation of ras and mitogen-activated protein kinases. Mol Cell Biol. 2002;22(22):7758–68.

[43] Wong C, Jin ZG. Protein kinase C-dependent protein kinase D activation modulates ERK signal pathway and endothelial cell proliferation by vascular endothelial growth factor. J Biol Chem. 2005;280(39):33262–9.

[44] Ha CH, Wang W, Jhun BS, Wong C, Hausser A, Pfizenmaier K, et al. Protein kinase D-dependent phosphorylation and nuclear export of histone deacetylase 5 mediates vascular endothelial growth factor-induced gene expression and angiogenesis. J Biol Chem. 2008;283(21):14590–9.

[45] Wang S, Li X, Parra M, Verdin E, Bassel-Duby R, Olson EN. Control of endothelial cell proliferation and migration by VEGF signaling to histone deacetylase 7. Proc Natl Acad Sci U S A. 2008;105(22):7738–43.

[46] Evans IM, Britton G, Zachary IC. Vascular endothelial growth factor induces heat shock protein (HSP) 27 serine 82 phosphorylation and endothelial tubulogenesis via protein kinase D and independent of p38 kinase. Cell Signal. 2008;20(7):1375–84.

[47] Shaul PW. Regulation of endothelial nitric oxide synthase: location, location, location. Annu Rev Physiol. 2002;64:749–74.

[48] Brouet A, Sonveaux P, Dessy C, Balligand JL, Feron O. Hsp90 ensures the transition from the early Ca^{2+}-dependent to the late phosphorylation-dependent activation of the endothelial nitric-oxide synthase in vascular endothelial growth factor-exposed endothelial cells. J Biol Chem. 2001;276(35):32663–9.

[49] Mancini M, Toker A. NFAT proteins: emerging roles in cancer progression. Nat Rev Cancer. 2009;9(11):810–20.

[50] Suehiro J, Kanki Y, Makihara C, Schadler K, Miura M, Manabe Y, et al. Genome-wide approaches reveal functional vascular endothelial growth factor (VEGF)-inducible nuclear factor of activated T cells (NFAT) c1 binding to angiogenesis-related genes in the endothelium. J Biol Chem. 2014;289(42):29044–59.

[51] Hernández GL, Volpert OV, Iñiguez MA, Lorenzo E, Martínez-Martínez S, Grau R, et al. Selective inhibition of vascular endothelial growth factor-mediated angiogenesis by cyclosporin A: roles of the nuclear factor of activated T cells and cyclooxygenase 2. J Exp Med. 2001;193(5):607–20.

[52] Schweighofer B, Testori J, Sturtzel C, Sattler S, Mayer H, Wagner O, et al. The VEGF-induced transcriptional response comprises gene clusters at the crossroad of angiogenesis and inflammation. Thromb Haemost. 2009;102(3):544–54.

[53] Noren DP, Chou WH, Lee SH, Qutub AA, Warmflash A, Wagner DS, et al. Endothelial cells decode VEGF-mediated Ca^{2+} signaling patterns to produce distinct functional responses. Sci Signal. 2016;9(416):ra20.

[54] Cheng HW, James AF, Foster RR, Hancox JC, Bates DO. VEGF activates receptor-operated cation channels in human microvascular endothelial cells. Arterioscler Thromb Vasc Biol. 2006;26(8):1768–76.

[55] Ge R, Tai Y, Sun Y, Zhou K, Yang S, Cheng T, et al. Critical role of TRPC6 channels in VEGF-mediated angiogenesis. Cancer Lett. 2009;283(1):43–51.

[56] Hamdollah Zadeh MA, Glass CA, Magnussen A, Hancox JC, Bates DO. VEGF-mediated elevated intracellular calcium and angiogenesis in human microvascular endothelial cells in vitro are inhibited by dominant negative TRPC6. Microcirculation. 2008;15(7):605–14.

[57] Singh AJ, Meyer RD, Navruzbekov G, Shelke R, Duan L, Band H, et al. A critical role for the E3-ligase activity of c-Cbl in VEGFR-2-mediated PLCgamma1 activation and angiogenesis. Proc Natl Acad Sci U S A. 2007;104(13):5413–8.

[58] Cantley LC. The phosphoinositide 3-kinase pathway. Science. 2002;296(5573):1655–7.

[59] Jiang BH, Liu LZ. PI3K/PTEN signaling in angiogenesis and tumorigenesis. Adv Cancer Res. 2009;102:19–65.

[60] Missy K, Van Poucke V, Raynal P, Viala C, Mauco G, Plantavid M, et al. Lipid products of phosphoinositide 3-kinase interact with Rac1 GTPase and stimulate GDP dissociation. J Biol Chem. 1998;273(46):30279–86.

[61] Vivanco I, Sawyers CL. The phosphatidylinositol 3-kinase AKT pathway in human cancer. Nat Rev Cancer. 2002;2(7):489–501.

[62] Pugazhenthi S, Nesterova A, Sable C, Heidenreich KA, Boxer LM, Heasley LE, et al. Akt/protein kinase B up-regulates Bcl-2 expression through cAMP-response element-binding protein. J Biol Chem. 2000;275(15):10761–6.

[63] Gerber HP, McMurtrey A, Kowalski J, Yan M, Keyt BA, Dixit V, et al. Vascular endothelial growth factor regulates endothelial cell survival through the phosphatidylinositol 3′-kinase/Akt signal transduction pathway. Requirement for Flk-1/KDR activation. J Biol Chem. 1998;273(46):30336–43.

[64] Gerber HP, Dixit V, Ferrara N. Vascular endothelial growth factor induces expression of the antiapoptotic proteins Bcl-2 and A1 in vascular endothelial cells. J Biol Chem. 1998;273(21):13313–6.

[65] Tran J, Rak J, Sheehan C, Saibil SD, LaCasse E, Korneluk RG, et al. Marked induction of the IAP family antiapoptotic proteins survivin and XIAP by VEGF in vascular endothelial cells. Biochem Biophys Res Commun. 1999;264(3):781–8.

[66] Dimmeler S, Fleming I, Fisslthaler B, Hermann C, Busse R, Zeiher AM. Activation of nitric oxide synthase in endothelial cells by Akt-dependent phosphorylation. Nature. 1999;399(6736):601–5.

[67] Parsons SJ, Parsons JT. Src family kinases, key regulators of signal transduction. Oncogene. 2004;23(48):7906–9.

[68] Sun Z, Li X, Massena S, Kutschera S, Padhan N, Gualandi L, et al. VEGFR2 induces c-Src signaling and vascular permeability in vivo via the adaptor protein TSAd. J Exp Med. 2012;209(7):1363–77.

[69] Caron C, Spring K, Laramée M, Chabot C, Cloutier M, Gu H, et al. Non-redundant roles of the Gab1 and Gab2 scaffolding adapters in VEGF-mediated signalling, migration, and survival of endothelial cells. Cell Signal. 2009;21(6):943–53.

[70] Duval M, Le Boeuf F, Huot J, Gratton JP. Src-mediated phosphorylation of Hsp90 in response to vascular endothelial growth factor (VEGF) is required for VEGF receptor-2 signaling to endothelial NO synthase. Mol Biol Cell. 2007;18(11):4659–68.

[71] Alavi A, Hood JD, Frausto R, Stupack DG, Cheresh DA. Role of Raf in vascular protection from distinct apoptotic stimuli. Science. 2003;301(5629):94–6.

[72] Meyer RD, Sacks DB, Rahimi N. IQGAP1-dependent signaling pathway regulates endothelial cell proliferation and angiogenesis. PLoS One. 2008;3(12):e3848.

[73] Eliceiri BP, Paul R, Schwartzberg PL, Hood JD, Leng J, Cheresh DA. Selective requirement for Src kinases during VEGF-induced angiogenesis and vascular permeability. Mol Cell. 1999;4(6):915–24.

[74] Weis S, Shintani S, Weber A, Kirchmair R, Wood M, Cravens A, et al. Src blockade stabilizes a Flk/cadherin complex, reducing edema and tissue injury following myocardial infarction. J Clin Invest. 2004;113(6):885–94.

[75] Wallez Y, Cand F, Cruzalegui F, Wernstedt C, Souchelnytskyi S, Vilgrain I, et al. Src kinase phosphorylates vascular endothelial-cadherin in response to vascular endothelial growth factor: identification of tyrosine 685 as the unique target site. Oncogene. 2007;26(7):1067–77.

[76] Dejana E, Tournier-Lasserve E, Weinstein BM. The control of vascular integrity by endothelial cell junctions: molecular basis and pathological implications. Dev Cell. 2009;16(2):209–21.

[77] Mahabeleshwar GH, Feng W, Reddy K, Plow EF, Byzova TV. Mechanisms of integrin-vascular endothelial growth factor receptor cross-activation in angiogenesis. Circ Res. 2007;101(6):570–80.

[78] Mitra SK, Hanson DA, Schlaepfer DD. Focal adhesion kinase: in command and control of cell motility. Nat Rev Mol Cell Biol. 2005;6(1):56–68.

[79] Calalb MB, Polte TR, Hanks SK. Tyrosine phosphorylation of focal adhesion kinase at sites in the catalytic domain regulates kinase activity: a role for Src family kinases. Mol Cell Biol. 1995;15(2):954–63.

[80] Owen JD, Ruest PJ, Fry DW, Hanks SK. Induced focal adhesion kinase (FAK) expression in FAK-null cells enhances cell spreading and migration requiring both auto- and activation loop phosphorylation sites and inhibits adhesion-dependent tyrosine phosphorylation of Pyk2. Mol Cell Biol. 1999;19(7):4806–18.

[81] Le Boeuf F, Houle F, Huot J. Regulation of vascular endothelial growth factor receptor 2-mediated phosphorylation of focal adhesion kinase by heat shock protein 90 and Src kinase activities. J Biol Chem. 2004;279(37):39175–85.

[82] Le Boeuf F, Houle F, Sussman M, Huot J. Phosphorylation of focal adhesion kinase (FAK) on Ser732 is induced by rho-dependent kinase and is essential for proline-rich tyrosine kinase-2-mediated phosphorylation of FAK on Tyr407 in response to vascular endothelial growth factor. Mol Biol Cell. 2006;17(8):3508–20.

[83] Takai Y, Sasaki T, Matozaki T. Small GTP-binding proteins. Physiol Rev. 2001;81(1): 153–208.

[84] van der Meel R, Symons MH, Kudernatsch R, Kok RJ, Schiffelers RM, Storm G, et al. The VEGF/Rho GTPase signalling pathway: a promising target for anti-angiogenic/anti-invasion therapy. Drug Discov Today. 2011;16(5–6):219–28.

[85] Sulpice E, Ding S, Muscatelli-Groux B, Bergé M, Han ZC, Plouet J, et al. Cross-talk between the VEGF-A and HGF signalling pathways in endothelial cells. Biol Cell. 2009;101(9):525–39.

[86] Gavard J, Gutkind JS. VEGF controls endothelial-cell permeability by promoting the beta-arrestin-dependent endocytosis of VE-cadherin. Nat Cell Biol. 2006;8(11): 1223–34.

[87] Garrett TA, Van Buul JD, Burridge K. VEGF-induced Rac1 activation in endothelial cells is regulated by the guanine nucleotide exchange factor Vav2. Exp Cell Res. 2007;313(15):3285–97.

[88] Lamalice L, Houle F, Jourdan G, Huot J. Phosphorylation of tyrosine 1214 on VEGFR2 is required for VEGF-induced activation of Cdc42 upstream of SAPK2/p38. Oncogene. 2004;23(2):434–45.

[89] Annerén C, Lindholm CK, Kriz V, Welsh M. The FRK/RAK-SHB signaling cascade: a versatile signal-transduction pathway that regulates cell survival, differentiation and proliferation. Curr Mol Med. 2003;3(4):313–24.

[90] Holmqvist K, Cross M, Riley D, Welsh M. The Shb adaptor protein causes Src-dependent cell spreading and activation of focal adhesion kinase in murine brain endothelial cells. Cell Signal. 2003;15(2):171–9.

[91] Granum S, Andersen TC, Sørlie M, Jørgensen M, Koll L, Berge T, et al. Modulation of Lck function through multisite docking to T cell-specific adapter protein. J Biol Chem. 2008;283(32):21909–19.

[92] Berge T, Sundvold-Gjerstad V, Granum S, Andersen TC, Holthe GB, Claesson-Welsh L, et al. T cell specific adapter protein (TSAd) interacts with Tec kinase ITK to promote CXCL12 induced migration of human and murine T cells. PLoS One. 2010;5(3):e9761.

[93] Lettau M, Pieper J, Gerneth A, Lengl-Janssen B, Voss M, Linkermann A, et al. The adapter protein Nck: role of individual SH3 and SH2 binding modules for protein interactions in T lymphocytes. Protein Sci. 2010;19(4):658–69.

[94] Stoletov KV, Ratcliffe KE, Spring SC, Terman BI. NCK and PAK participate in the signaling pathway by which vascular endothelial growth factor stimulates the assembly of focal adhesions. J Biol Chem. 2001;276(25):22748–55.

[95] Hedman AC, Smith JM, Sacks DB. The biology of IQGAP proteins: beyond the cytoskeleton. EMBO Rep. 2015;16(4):427–46.

[96] Yamaoka-Tojo M, Ushio-Fukai M, Hilenski L, Dikalov SI, Chen YE, Tojo T, et al. IQGAP1, a novel vascular endothelial growth factor receptor binding protein, is involved in reactive oxygen species-dependent endothelial migration and proliferation. Circ Res. 2004;95(3):276–83.

[97] Yamaoka-Tojo M, Tojo T, Kim HW, Hilenski L, Patrushev NA, Zhang L, et al. IQGAP1 mediates VE-cadherin-based cell-cell contacts and VEGF signaling at adherence junctions linked to angiogenesis. Arterioscler Thromb Vasc Biol. 2006;26(9):1991–7.

[98] Dance M, Montagner A, Yart A, Masri B, Audigier Y, Perret B, et al. The adaptor protein Gab1 couples the stimulation of vascular endothelial growth factor receptor-2 to the activation of phosphoinositide 3-kinase. J Biol Chem. 2006;281(32):23285–95.

[99] Laramée M, Chabot C, Cloutier M, Stenne R, Holgado-Madruga M, Wong AJ, et al. The scaffolding adapter Gab1 mediates vascular endothelial growth factor signaling and is required for endothelial cell migration and capillary formation. J Biol Chem. 2007;282(11):7758–69.

[100] Cébe-Suarez S, Zehnder-Fjällman A, Ballmer-Hofer K. The role of VEGF receptors in angiogenesis; complex partnerships. Cell Mol Life Sci. 2006;63(5):601–15.

[101] Raimondi C, Ruhrberg C. Neuropilin signalling in vessels, neurons and tumours. Semin Cell Dev Biol. 2013;24(3):172–8.

[102] Fantin A, Herzog B, Mahmoud M, Yamaji M, Plein A, Denti L, et al. Neuropilin 1 (NRP1) hypomorphism combined with defective VEGF-A binding reveals novel roles for NRP1 in developmental and pathological angiogenesis. Development. 2014;141(3):556–62.

[103] Plein A, Fantin A, Ruhrberg C. Neuropilin regulation of angiogenesis, arteriogenesis, and vascular permeability. Microcirculation. 2014;21(4):315–23.

[104] Ballmer-Hofer K, Andersson AE, Ratcliffe LE, Berger P. Neuropilin-1 promotes VEGFR-2 trafficking through Rab11 vesicles thereby specifying signal output. Blood. 2011;118(3):816–26.

[105] Chen TT, Luque A, Lee S, Anderson SM, Segura T, Iruela-Arispe ML. Anchorage of VEGF to the extracellular matrix conveys differential signaling responses to endothelial cells. J Cell Biol. 2010;188(4):595–609.

[106] Grazia Lampugnani M, Zanetti A, Corada M, Takahashi T, Balconi G, Breviario F, et al. Contact inhibition of VEGF-induced proliferation requires vascular endothelial cadherin, beta-catenin, and the phosphatase DEP-1/CD148. J Cell Biol. 2003;161(4):793–804.

[107] Gampel A, Moss L, Jones MC, Brunton V, Norman JC, Mellor H. VEGF regulates the mobilization of VEGFR2/KDR from an intracellular endothelial storage compartment. Blood. 2006;108(8):2624–31.

[108] Scott A, Mellor H. VEGF receptor trafficking in angiogenesis. Biochem Soc Trans. 2009;37(Pt 6):1184–8.

[109] Simons M, Gordon E, Claesson-Welsh L. Mechanisms and regulation of endothelial VEGF receptor signalling. Nat Rev Mol Cell Biol. 2016;17(10):611–25.

[110] Lampugnani MG, Orsenigo F, Gagliani MC, Tacchetti C, Dejana E. Vascular endothelial cadherin controls VEGFR-2 internalization and signaling from intracellular compartments. J Cell Biol. 2006;174(4):593–604.

[111] Nagy JA, Dvorak AM, Dvorak HF. Vascular hyperpermeability, angiogenesis, and stroma generation. Cold Spring Harb Perspect Med. 2012;2(2):a006544.

[112] Oda N, Abe M, Sato Y. ETS-1 converts endothelial cells to the angiogenic phenotype by inducing the expression of matrix metalloproteinases and integrin beta3. J Cell Physiol. 1999;178(2):121–32.

[113] Heo SH, Choi YJ, Ryoo HM, Cho JY. Expression profiling of ETS and MMP factors in VEGF-activated endothelial cells: role of MMP-10 in VEGF-induced angiogenesis. J Cell Physiol. 2010;224(3):734–42.

Chapter 14

Noncoding RNAs in Lung Cancer Angiogenesis

Ioana Berindan-Neagoe, Cornelia Braicu,
Diana Gulei, Ciprian Tomuleasa and
George Adrian Calin

Additional information is available at the end of the chapter

http://dx.doi.org/10.5772/66529

Abstract

Lung cancer is the major death-related cancer in both men and women, due to late diagnostic and limited treatment efficacy. The angiogenic process that is responsible for the support of tumor progression and metastasis represents one of the main hallmarks of cancer. The role of VEGF signaling in angiogenesis is well-established, and we summarize the role of semaphorins and their related receptors or hypoxia-related factors role as prone of tumor microenvironment in angiogenic mechanisms. Newly, noncoding RNA transcripts (ncRNA) were identified to have vital functions in miscellaneous biological processes, including lung cancer angiogenesis. Therefore, due to their capacity to regulate almost all molecular pathways related with altered key genes, including those involved in angiogenesis and its microenvironment, ncRNAs can serve as diagnosis and prognosis markers or therapeutic targets. We intend to summarize the latest progress in the field of ncRNAs in lung cancer and their relation with hypoxia-related factors and angiogenic genes, with a particular focus on ncRNAs relation to semaphorins.

Keywords: noncoding RNAs, angiogenesis, lung cancer, semaphorins, therapy

1. Introduction

1.1. Noncoding RNAs (ncRNAs)—definition, biogenesis and classification

The noncoding RNAs evolved in the last few years as important regulators of numerous physiological and pathological processes with increased attention regarding cancer diagnosis, prognosis, and therapeutics [1]. The concept known as "dark matter" defined by the lack of function and lack of genetic information is now long gone, being replaced by the regulatory ncRNAs involved in cancer development and progression [1]. The transcription of the noncoding regions produces RNA sequences that can vary in size, short, mid-size, and long noncoding RNAs, and are able to influence the expression of tumor suppressor or tumor promoting coding genes, activity that further classifies this class of RNAs into oncogenic or tumor suppressor sequences [2].

The noncoding niche is rapidly expanding as new sequences are discovered and characterized. The ncRNAs, as their name underline, are RNAs that do not codify for proteins but new molecular concepts are revealed regarding the interplay between these types of RNA sequences and protein coding genes [3]. ncRNAs are also known as regulatory RNAs.

One of the most studied ncRNAs class is represented by microRNAs (miRNAs) that are small single-stranded nucleotide sequences (18–22 nucleotide length) capable of gene regulation through sequence complementarity [2], being involved in all hallmarks of cancer [4]. The biogenesis mechanism is presented in **Figure 1**. The discovery of miRNAs has enabled new

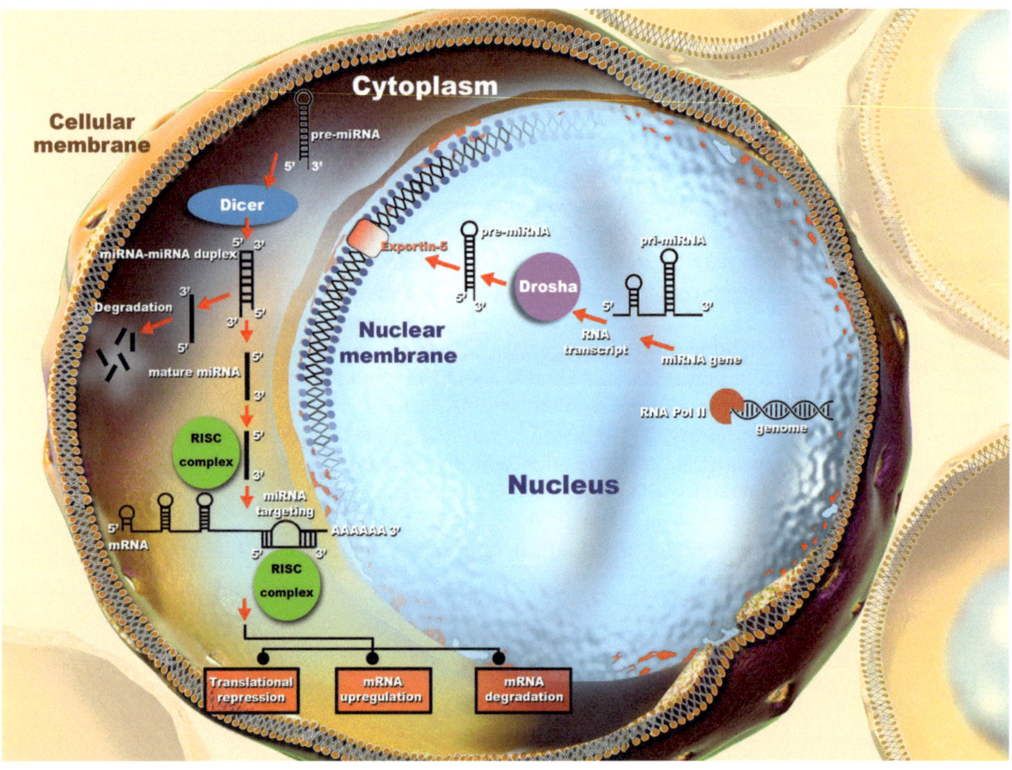

Figure 1. miRNA biogenesis mechanism. microRNAs are situated in the genome of the host as individual transcriptional units but also as clusters of a number of distinct microRNAs. For the first step, RNA polymerase II transcribes the target sequence resulting in a primary transcript named pri-miRNAs. This unprocessed sequence is then subjected to the activity of RNase III-type enzyme Drosha that transforms the pri-miRNA sequence into a transcript of approximatively 70 nt, pre-miRNA. This precursor is then transferred in the cytoplasm via Exportin-5, followed by another miRNA manipulation step governed by the RNase III protein Dicer, resulting in a double stranded RNA called miRNA-miRNA duplex. The less stable strand is further captured by the RISC complex, association that facilitates specific gene regulation through complementary interactions.

http://dx.doi.org/10.5772/66529

noninvasive diagnosis methods and also has conducted towards the development of more targeted therapeutics alternatives in a large number of cancers and other pathological states [4, 5]. Despite numerous discoveries in the ncRNA field, the two main noncoding fronts in cancer are still represented by microRNAs and the more recent characterized long noncoding RNAs (lncRNAs) [6]. As the technology advances, these last sequences are increasingly mentioned in pathological contexts, where differential expression levels are associated with malignant states and other diseases [6]. Despite the associations between lncRNAs expression patterns and different types of cancers, there are still many unknowns regarding the complex mechanism of action.

MiRNAs revolution has stimulated the investigation of other types of small ncRNAs such as small interfering RNAs (siRNAs), and Piwi-interacting RNAs (piRNAs) [3, 7, 8]. These last two types of molecules are similar to miRNAs in length and function, where siRNAs mediate posttranscriptional inhibitory processes and piRNAs act particularly on transposable elements and are capable of forming complexes with Piwi proteins [7, 8]. piRNAs transcribed from kiwi clusters together with Piwi proteins are capable of transposon modulation through interruption of the specific transcript that will be no longer able to exercise their specific activity. Other types of ncRNAs, circularRNA (ciRNA) are formed through base pairing of intronic repeats that ends up with a complete circular fragment that is able to act as a miRNA sponge through complementary interactions [3, 9].

Supplementing the complex regulatory networks of miRNAs, ciRNAs have recently emerged as new cancer modeling tools through miRNA targeting, escaping from the initial characterization as transcriptional "noise" [9, 10]. These types of transcripts are ubiquitous present in eukaryotic cells and competitively bind microRNAs sequences, functioning like an inhibitory sponge; process that could attribute a significant therapeutic potential to these circular fragments [9, 10, 11, 12]. In this sense, specific microRNAs are eliminated from the regulatory networks, influencing the expression scheme of target genes. Competitive endogenous RNA (ceRNA) describes a new mechanism of gene regulation, being involved in physiological and pathological processes [13].

The traditional concept that RNA molecules are just intermediary sequences between DNA and proteins is now replaced with more advanced molecular data, where short- and long-noncoding sequences play a key role in normal development and disease progression [14]. SiRNAs and miRNAs are similar in length, approximatively 22 nucleotides, and are both processed by Dicer through cleavage. SiRNAs are derived from complementary dsRNA duplexes, where miRNAs originate from imperfect RNA hairpins from short introns or long transcripts [15–18]. Both small noncoding types of sequences associate with Argonaute proteins in order to manipulate gene expression (generally through 3'UTRs) [19], although siRNAs are also involved in viral defense and transposon regulation. piRNAs are the longest fragments from the small RNAs group, having approximatively 26–30 in length. This class associates with PIWI-clade Argonaute proteins in order to guide transposon activity and chromatin status [15, 17]. Long noncoding RNA group consist in all RNA sequences that are not responsible for protein generation and their length exceed

200 nucleotides, being further grouped in concordance with their genomic localization: intronic, intergenic, sense, and antisense ncRNAs to host gene locus [6, 20]. Biogenesis of lncRNAs is very similar with the processing activity of mRNAs molecule, being transcribed by RNA Pol II and also being subjected to the same epigenetic modifications and splicing signals. The functional roles of lncRNAs are more extended than in the case of small ncRNAs, a significant part being still incompletely understood. Briefly, this type of sequences is not so well conserved as miRNAs and also can control gene activity at different levels in a more complex scheme [2, 6, 16].

2. Lung cancer—molecular classification and survival rates

Lung cancer occupies the first place regarding the mortality rates from the oncological field, being characterized by an aggressive profile that ends with numerous deadly metastatic sites. One of the main reasons for the high mortality rates consists in the late diagnosis [21]. According to the characteristics of the cancer cells, this malignancy presents itself in two major forms, one being *small-cell lung cancer* (SCLC), and the other being named *non-small-cell lung cancer* (NSCLC) according to the histological classification and another rare subtype, *lung carcinoid tumor* (*LCT*) [22, 23]. NSCLC ranks as the number one diagnosed type of lung cancer in the oncological field, being further divided into three histologic types: *squamous cell carcinoma, large-cell carcinoma, and adenocarcinoma. Adenocarcinomas* represent the most common subtype of NSCLC, with an incidence of 35–40% from all lung cancer cases, being the most lethal type of cancer in male population, and the second in women. This type of pulmonary malignancy frequently presents distant metastases and pleural effusions. Between a quarter and 30% of all lung cancer cases belong to the squamous cell carcinoma category. These particular tumors are mostly located in the central areas of the lungs, and were shown to be connected to tobacco smoking [24]. Lung carcinoid tumors are very rare and represent about 5% of the lung cancers which grows very slowly and are rarely associated with metastasis [25]. Despite the frequency drop, pulmonary tumors remain the major cause of death and morbidity around the world, being very aggressive and refractory to standard oncologic therapy [26], due to the late diagnostic [27].

Environmental and occupational exposure to different agents and an individual's susceptibility for these agents were associated with a risk of lung cancer in approximately 9–15% of cases. The cigarette smoke is the primary risk factor for the development of lung cancer and is estimated to be responsible for approximately 90% of all lung cancers [24], followed by asbestos [28], and radon [27]. More than 300 harmful substances with 40 known potent carcinogens were discovered in tobacco smoke.

The classical therapeutic strategies like surgery and chemotherapy or radiation fail to accomplish their purpose in advanced pathological states. In the case of patients diagnosed early in the disease, the chances of survival are more promising, being observed a partial response to drugs based on platinum. However, even in this case, the final outcome is not necessary a positive one due to acquisition of treatment resistance. According to National Cancer Institute, survival rates for early stages of NSCLC are extremely low compared to other types of cancer, where the rate for the late stages of the same malignancy can reach even 1%: the 5 years survival rate for stage IA is approximately 49%, 45% for stage IB, 30% for stage IIA and 31% for IIB. The next stages, IIIA and IIIB, are associated with even more dramatically numbers, 14% and 5% respectively (**Figure 2**). For the case of metastatic lung cancer, where the tumor has spread within different body sites, the survival rates are extremely low (1%) [29, 30]. Therefore, a critical part of lung cancer management is represented by the discovery of specific molecular carcinogenic pathways in order to precisely target key molecules that are responsible for tumor development and avoid treatment resistance. ncRNAs study represents an important research direction for achieving these goals.

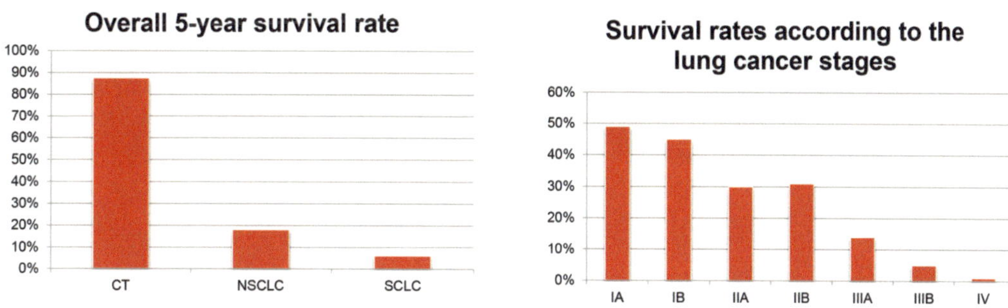

Figure 2. The overall survival rates associated with different lung cancer subtypes (NSCLC, SCLC) and the 5-year survival rate based on lung cancer stages.

3. Angiogenesis—beyond hallmarks of lung cancer

Nowadays, the cancer hallmarks are at the center of carcinogenesis: prolonged proliferation signals, escaping of growth inhibitors, apoptosis inhibition, indefinite replicative potential, vascular network development (angiogenesis) and activation of cell invasion, and thus metastasis (**Figure 3**) [31]. Although all of these hallmarks represent key elements without which tumorigenesis could not more or less advance, angiogenesis surpasses this listing of malignant processes: without the ability to receive oxygen and nutrients and evacuate waste products, the spreading of the tumor is naturally restricted. Moreover, the vessel network is one of the invasion routes used by transformed mesenchymal cell in order to evade from the original carcinogenic site and invade other tissues [31]. All these features stand at the base of the therapeutic concept, where angiogenesis is one of the main signaling pathway targeted in the treatment of cancer patients, including individuals with lung cancer. Inhibition of this malignant progression pathway through exogenous administration of targeted agents in the form of ncRNAs/anti-ncRNAs will enable the proper management of tumor spreading and will serve as a feasible therapeutic strategy for lung cancer [33].

The most promising proangiogenic target in lung cancer is VEGF (vascular endothelial growth factor), more precisely the interaction of VEGF with the transmembrane receptors or receptors downstream the signaling pathways. However, prolonged exposure to VEGF/VEGFR inhibitors may force tumor cells to find alternative pathways for vascular

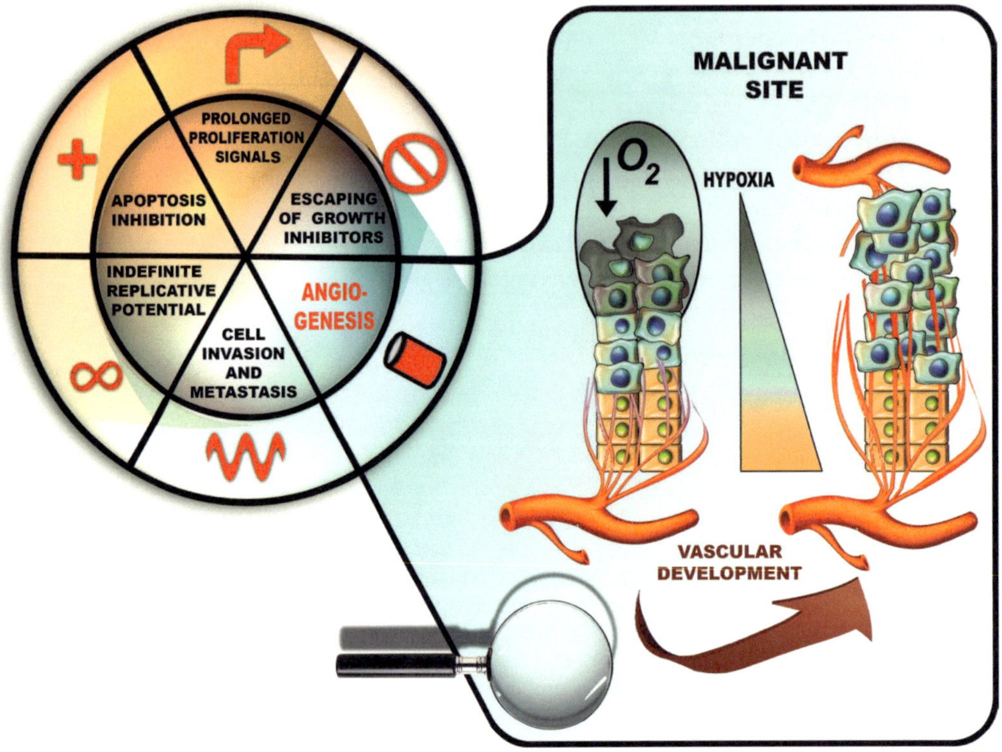

Figure 3. Lung cancer hallmarks with focus on angiogenesis.

development [34]. Additionally, some other angiogenic pathways have been explored with the same purpose, where FGFRs (fibroblast growth factor receptors), angiopoietin, PDGFRs (platelet-derived growth factor receptors), and, in the last few years, semaphorins and the related receptors captured the attention [32, 34]. The metastatic cascade, a multievent process that leads to the spreading of the tumor cells to numerous sites in the organism and causes death, represents the main challenge in cancer treatment and angiogenesis plays a major role in this progression [35].

3.1. Implication of ncRNAs in regulation of lung cancer angiogenesis

As a result of the limited success of the classical antiangiogenic therapies targeting VEGF and its related receptors [35, 36], researchers have deepened their knowledge by analyzing the expression of ncRNAs sequences in this pathology (**Figure 4**) [37, 38]. The mechanism of lung cancer angiogenesis is far from being completely deciphered and implicit the process of therapeutic inhibition via ncRNAs remains to be further investigated. Targeting ncRNAs will enable a more precise treatment and will avoid compensatory mechanisms retrieved in lung cancer [2, 37, 38].

http://dx.doi.org/10.5772/66529

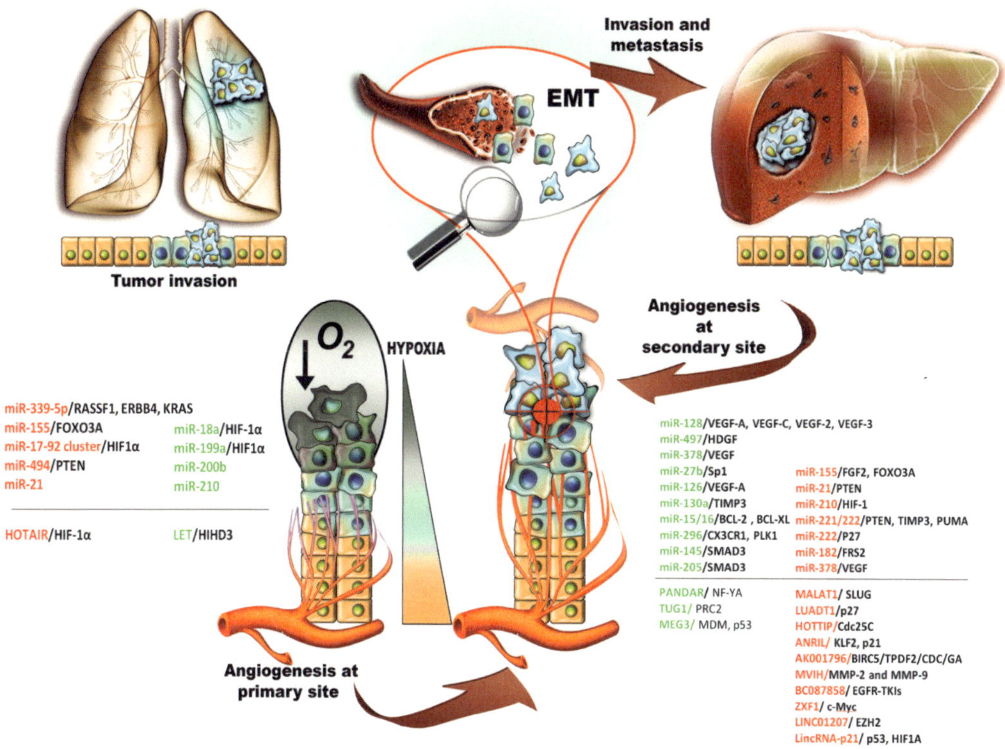

Figure 4. Evolution of vascular network within lung cancer. Malignant cells lacking nutrients and oxygen enter in hypoxic stress, state that promotes the signaling pathways related to angiogenesis in order to sustain cell proliferation. The same process is present at the metastatic sites, where mesenchymal cells that went through epithelial to mesenchymal transition are establishing new malignant formations. The complex malignant scheme is strictly regulated by noncoding RNAs (miRNAs and lncRNAs). Red - overexpressed ncRNAs; Green- downregulated ncRNAs.

3.2. miRNAs related to lung cancer angiogenesis

Among all types of ncRNAs, miRNAs molecules are the most intensive studied in what regards novel cancer therapies. Although the majority of the studies are concentrated on oncogenic miRNA inhibition via exogenous delivery of complementary (antisense) sequences through different vectors, it seems that another therapeutic alternative consists in miRNA replacement. This last type of targeted treatment may be even more effective due to the fact that the predominant pathological model consists more in dowregulated tumor suppressor sequences than overexpressed oncogenic genes [5, 21, 39].

Until this moment, several miRNA patterns involved in different lung cancer processes such as cell proliferation, resistance to therapy, invasion, metastasis, and angiogenesis have been identified. We will focus on some important miRNAs that presented the most aberrant expression related to lung cancer angiogenesis (**Tables 1** and **2**).

No.	Name	Location	Length (nucleotides)	Expression level	Target gene	Activity	Possible role in lung cancer angiogenesis	Clinical potential	References
1	miR-27b	9q22.32	22	▼	Sp1	Possible key miRNA regarding the development of lung cancer; ectopic expression reduced the cell growth and invasion	Sp1, a target gene of miR-27b, was associated with the angiogenic phenotype in gastric cancer, with key roles in the manipulation of this process; patients with high levels of Sp1 presented a more vascularized phenotype	Therapeutic target	[40, 41]
2	miR-126	9q34.3	22	▼	VEGF-A	Low expression of this miRNA is associated with high vascular density in NSCLC; this data were also observed in vitro	Due to direct targeting of miR-126 on VEGF-A, overexpression of this miRNA could be suitable for anti-angiogenic therapies	Therapeutic target and also prognosis tool	[42]
3	miR-130a	11q12.1	21	▼	MET	miR-130a downregulates the expression levels of two oncogenic miRNAs, miR-221 and miR-222; MET suppression	MET represents a key factor for vascular development and miR-221/222 cluster could also play an important role in angiogenesis due to the direct down regulation of TIMP3, an inhibitor of MET; miR-130 is able to reduce the levels of both this systems	Important therapeutic potential	[43, 44]
4	miR-15/16	13q14.3	–	▼	BCL-2 and BCL-XL	MiR-15/16 cluster was found as downregulated in NSCLCs; miR-15 directly targets BCL-2 and BCL-XL	BCL-2 has a suppressive action on VEGF and TP in lung cancer, both strongly implicated in angiogenesis development	Contradictory results; further studies needed	[45–47]
5	miR-378	5q32	21	▼	VEGF	Inhibition of lung cancer angiogenesis through VEGF targeting	Regulator of a central element in lung cancer angiogenesis	*In vivo* demonstrated therapeutic target	[48, 49]
6	miR-296	20q13.32	21	▼	CX3CR1, PLK1	Tumor suppressor role in lung cancer development targeting chemosensitivity and cell viability	MIR-296 has been associated with angiogenesis	Potential therapeutic target	[50–52]

http://dx.doi.org/10.5772/66529

No.	Name	Location	Length (nucleotides)	Expression level	Target gene	Activity	Possible role in lung cancer angiogenesis	Clinical potential	References
7	miR-128	2q21.3	23	▼	VEGF-A, VEGF-C, VEGF-2, VEGF-3	*In vitro* and *in vivo* overexpression of miR-128 led to significant suppression of angiogenesis due to down regulation of the target genes; furthermore miR-128 expression is correlated with the development stages of lung cancer	Current data shows that miR-128 could be used effectively as therapeutic target or prognostic tool	Therapeutic target for enhanced expression and prognosis tool	[53]
8	miR-497	17p13.1	20	▼	HDGF	Ectopic expression of this sequence in an animal model demonstrated positive effects through inhibition of cell proliferation and angiogenesis	Experimental data shows that miR-497 could be used with success as an antiangiogenic agent for lung cancer	Therapeutic target	[54]
9	let-7b	22q13.31	21	▼	RAS	Lung cancer tumors tissue revealed a downregulated pattern and was associated with increased vascular density	The collected data suggest a possible role for miR-7b as antiangiogenic tool in the moment of ectopic expression	Prognosis and therapeutic tool	[55]
10	miR-145	5q32	22	▼	SMAD3	Implicated in EMT and invasion	Enhancement of this miR expression could serve as a therapeutic strategy for lung cancer	Possible therapeutic target	[56]
11	miR-205	1q32.2	20	▼	VEGF	Implicated in EMT and invasion	Enhancement of this miR expression could serve as a therapeutic strategy for lung cancer	Possible therapeutic target	[57]

Table 1. The main tumor suppressor altered miRNAs implicated in lung cancer angiogenesis.

No	Name	Location	Length (nucleotides)	Expression level	Target gene	Activity	Possible role in lung cancer angiogenesis	Clinical potential	References
1	miR-221 miR-222	Xp11.3	23	▲	PTEN, TIMP3	Highly expressed in lung cancer cells; promotes invasion and migration	miR-221/222 cluster could have a role in angiogenesis promotion through down regulation of TIMP3, an inhibitor of MET, an angiogenesis promoter	Therapeutic target and patients stratification toll	[58]
					PUMA	Co-modulation of the two miRNAs on PUMA promotes cell proliferation and inhibits apoptosis			[59]
2	miR-222	Xp11.3	23	▲	P27	Increased miR-221/222 expression promotes H460 cells viability and proliferation	Considering the possible in vivo role of p27, where the overexpression of this gene impaired angiogenesis, miR-222 that inhibits the expression of p27 could become a potent therapeutic target regarding antiangiogenic strategies	Therapeutic target for inhibition	[60, 61]
3	miR-210	11p15.5	22	▲		Significantly up-regulated in lung cancer tissues and associated with angiogenic potential in other types of cancers	Due to the regulation by HIF-1 involved in hypoxia (event that triggers angiogenesis development), miR-210 could also become a therapeutic target	Still limited data	[62, 63]
4	miR-155	21q21.3	22	▲/▼	FGF2	MIR-155 expression is correlated with FGF2 levels, an important molecule for lung cancer angiogenesis. Also, mimR-155 was correlated with VEGF-A in the N+ subgroup of NSCLC	Several studies have investigated the role of this miR in angiogenesis	Prognosis and therapeutic tool	[64, 65]
					FOXO3A, SOCS1, SOCS6, and PTEN	Hypoxia promotes miR-155 increased expression concomitant with the downregulation of FOXO3A target			[65, 66]

http://dx.doi.org/10.5772/66529

No	Name	Location	Length (nucleotides)	Expression level	Target gene	Activity	Possible role in lung cancer angiogenesis	Clinical potential	References
5	miR-21	17q23.1	21	▲	PTEN, SOCS1, and, SOCS6	After antiangiogenic therapy this miR was observed as downregulated	Possible role in lung cancer angiogenesis observed after the post-antiangiogenic down regulation	Possible therapeutic target	[66]
6	miR-182	7q32.2	23	▲	FRS2	miR-182 directly targets FRS2 in lung cancer, gene that represents a key molecule for NSLC progression and antigenesis	N/A	Therapeutic and diagnosis tool	[67]
7	miR-106a	Xq26.2	22	▲	–	Augmented expression of miR-106 in NSCLC was reported in several studies	Previously associated with hypoxia progression in colon and breast cancer that could enable a possible role in lung cancer hypoxia/ angiogenesis	Possible therapeutic target	[67–69]

Table 2. The main oncogenic miRNAs involved in lung cancer angiogenesis.

3.3. LncRNAs related to lung cancer angiogenesis

The number of lncRNAs has significantly increased due to the progresses offered by sequencing methods in genomic research. Long noncoding transcripts act as gene regulators via a wide range of mechanism [70], those related to lung cancer being summarized in **Table 3**. The first long noncoding sequence associated with lung cancer was MALAT1 that through increased expression and gene targeting (caspase-8, caspase-3, BCL-XL, BCL-2, and BAX) promotes the proliferation and invasiveness of cancer cells. Recently it was emphasized to target SLUG gene via a competitively "sponging" miR-204 [71]. Following this initial lncRNA, a significant list of lncRNA was associated with lung cancer progression or inhibition through modulation of key mechanisms involved in the hallmarks of lung pathology. The regulatory process is complex, lncRNAs being able to escort chromatin modifying enzymes to target loci within the genome, to bind the promoter of genes and modify the transcription process, to be processed into miRNAs and further act as short noncoding transcripts, and finally to modify the stability of specific mRNAs through direct binding [70].

Recent evidences suggested the role of PANDAR in lung cancer cell proliferation through p53/PANDAR/NF-YA/Bcl-2 axis [72]. Another lncRNA positively regulated by p53 is TUG1, whose downregulation is associated with increased cell proliferation and poor survival rate in lung cancer patients [73]. Also, considering the antiangiogenetic role of the p53 gene and the positive correlation between the two sequences, there is a possible role for TUG1 in angiogenesis suppression, however further investigations are necessary. HOTTIP is a long noncoding transcript that is associated with tumor growth [74], process that involves the formation of new blood vessel network, fact that could transform HOTTIP into a new target for antiangiogenetic therapies. MVIH is associated with microvascular invasion in HCC, being upregulated in this type of cancer with an increased oncogenic potential. Further studies have investigated the possible role of the same lncRNA in lung cancer and the results were increasingly similar with the previous pathology, MVIH representing a biomarker for poor prognosis and associated tumor cell proliferation [75]. There are also other lncRNAs with tumor suppressor or tumor promoting roles in lung cancer malignancies, like MEG3 (tumor suppressor), ANRIL, and AK001796 (oncogenic role) that are involved in cell proliferation and cell viability, processes that go hand in hand with the angiogenetic transformation [76–78]. lnRNA BC087858 is overexpressed in NSCLC and was demonstrated to be connected with drug resistance via EGFR-TKIs axis [80]. MEG3 was proved to be downregulated in tumoral tissue, and directly related with high tumoral stage. Preclinical studies demonstrated a reduced proliferation rate in the case of MEG3 overexpression, by targeting MDM2 and p53 proteins. MEG3 is presented not only as prognostic marker but also as important therapeutic target [76]. ANRIL is overexpressed in lung cancer tissue, being correlated with tumor-node-metastasis stages and tumor size, but until now there are not presented data with a direct connection with angiogenesis [78].

3.4. Ultraconserved regions (UCRs)

Ultraconserved regions (UCRs) are genome sequences longer than 200 bp and, as the name suggests, are conserved within humans, rats, and mouse, preserving their nucleotide

lncRNA	Target gene	Biological role	Reference
TUG1	PRC2	Tumor suppressor lncRNA regulated by p53, gene that promotes the expression of TUG1	[73]
MEG3	MDM and p53	Tumor suppressor role through cell proliferation reduction and increased survival. P53 expression is frequently correlated with the expression of the MEG3, with possible cumulative role in angiogenesis suppression	[76]
MALAT1	SLUG	Promoter of EMT and metastasis, via miR-204	[71]
PANDAR	NF-YA	Inhibits tumor cell proliferation in the moment of overexpression through p53/PANDAR/NF-YA/Bcl-2 axis	[72]
LUADT1	p27	Oncogenic role through promotion of cell proliferation; knockdown of the target gene significantly contribute to the reduced tumor size by inhibition of cell expansion	[79]
HOTTIP	Cdc25C	Promotes tumor growth and is overexpressed in lung cancers	[74]
ANRIL	KLF2 and p21	Oncogenic role; knockdown of this lncRNA reduced proliferation and increased apoptosis	[78]
MEG3	MDM and p53	Tumor suppressor role exercised through cell proliferation reduction and increased survival. P53 expression is frequently correlated with the expression of the MEG3, with possible cumulative role in angiogenesis suppression	[76]
AK001796	BIRC5/TPDF2/CDC/GA	Oncogenic role; involved in maintaining the tumor cell viability through complex mechanisms	[77]
MVIH	MMP-2 and MMP-9	Overexpressed in lung malignancies, being associated with increased cell proliferation and poor prognosis; previously recognized as angiogenesis promoter in HCCs	[75]
BC087858	EGFR-TKIs	Promotes cells invasion and induces drug resistance to EGFR-TKIs by activating PI3K/AKT and MEK/ERK pathways and EMT via up-regulating ZEB1 and Snail	[80]
ZXF1	c-Myc	LncRNA ZXF1overexpression was connected with a relatively poor prognosis; Knockdown by siRNA has no effect on cell proliferation, but decreased the migration and invasion of lung cancer cells	[81, 82]
LINC01207	EZH2	Cancer initiation and progression	[83]
LincRNA-p21	p53 and HIF1A	Regulation of TP53-dependent apoptosis and Warburg effect and angiogenesis	[84]

Table 3. The main lncRNAs involved in lung cancer angiogenesis and possible therapeutic targets for inhibiting lung cancers.

succession during the evolution [85, 86]. Until this moment there are a number of 481 conserved sequences, a part of them being situated at sensitive sites regarding cancer susceptibility and are further transcribed (T-UCR) into pathological expression patterns. Considering this recent discovery, it has been postulated that the differential expression pattern could serve as stratification tool in the oncology domain, being able to differentiate between human cancers and possible between molecular subtypes of carcinomas [85, 86].

The exact mechanism that leads to aberrant expression of T-UCR is not fully deciphered, although it is thought that the primary regulation models are represented by miRNAs interactions and epigenetic modifications in CpG islands hypermethylation [85].

Calin et. al. were the first to discover the T-UCR spectrum in malignant cells compared with healthy ones and found significant differences between the two states [85]. So far, molecular analysis have revealed different T-UCR signatures in a number of carcinomas, including prostate, hepatocellular, and colorectal cancer, as well as in chronic lymphocytic leukemia and neuroblastoma. Presently was observed upregulation of several T-UCRs and demonstrated by multiple investigations to be related with increased risks for tumour occurrence and a high metastatic rate. Therefore, the main investigation area is focused on integration of synthetic antisense oligonucleotides (ASOs) to inhibit T-UCR functions [85]. In lung cancer, an important number of T-UCRs need to be characterized and then used for developing novel therapies. In spite of the interest on the T-UCR, there are only few investigations on T-UCR therapy.

4. ncRNAs related to hypoxia in lung cancer

Hypoxia is a preangiogenetic process driven by specific gene modifications, alterations that are able to induce the installation of the mesenchymal phenotype through epithelial to mesenchymal transition (EMT), acquisition of drug and radiation resistance, and propagation of lung cancer stem cells [87, 88]. Compared to other cancers, lung malignancy is severely sustained by the installation of hypoxia through complex interactions between specific molecules (HIF1α and miRNAs or other ncRNAs, as displayed in **Tables 4** and **5**) and establishment of noncoding regulatory networks related to connection with the cell cycle regulation, apoptosis or autophagy [88].

In terms of lung cancer hypoxia, miRNAs play a pivotal role through the ability to orchestrate extensive signaling networks involved in this carcinogenic step. MiR-200 family has been extensively characterized in numerous malignant scenarios and miR-200b member seems to have a role that could be exploited in the context of the clinical area regarding hypoxia induced EMT where cells acquire motility characteristic and are able to invade secondary sites within the organism promoting lung cancer metastasis [89]. Reinforced expression of the tumor suppressor miRNAs inhibited EMT through regulation of key genes involved in this pathway [88]. Another possible therapeutic target is represented by miR-21, that is elevated in NSCLC-derived cells grown under hypoxic conditions [90]. Hypoxic conditions also triggered miR-155 overexpression and downregulation of FOXO3A target gene, and protects lung cancer cells to irradiation, elucidating a possible course of treatment through inhibition of miR-155 combined with radiotherapy [65].

Type of miRNA	Expression level	Name	Target gene	miRNA role in lung cancer hypoxia	Possible clinical role of miRNAs in lung cancer	References
Tumor suppressor miRNAs	▼	miR-200b	–	Hypoxia-induced EMT in lung cancer, influencing the activity of key genes involved in mesenchymal transition miR-200 mimic blocks hypoxia-induced EMT	Novel therapeutic strategy via Nobiletin delivery	[89]
	▼	miR-210	–	Regulate cellular response under hypoxic conditions High levels connected with a positive outcome in NSCLC patients	Biomarker for prognosis and patient stratification	[63, 91]
	▼	miR-18a	HIF-1α	Connected with lung metastasis of breast cancer cells ability to decrease the hypoxic stress *in vitro* and reduce cell invasiveness	Possible prognosis factor of lung metastasis in breast cancer	[92]
	▼	miR-199a	HIF1α	Inhibition of cancer cell hypoxia induced proliferation in NSCLC cells	Possible prognosis factor	[93]
Oncogenic miRNAs	▲	miR-21	–	NSCLC derived cell lines grown under hypoxic condition showed an elevated miR-21 expression; modulates radiation resistance via hypoxic mechanism	Possible therapeutic and prognosis role	[87, 90]
	▲	miR-339	RASSF1, ERBB4, KRAS	Activity correlated with the process of response to hypoxia	Possible target for therapeutic strategies	[94]
	▲	miR-155	FOXO3A	Correlates with poor prognosis and protects hypoxic lung cancer cells to irradiation and conversely	Therapeutic potential for radio sensitization of hypoxic lung cancer cells	[65]
	▲	miR-17-92 cluster	HIF1α	Downregulation of HIF1α does not affect the cellular adaptation to hypoxia	Possible prognosis factor	[95]
	▲	miR-494	PTEN	Promotes angiogenesis through direct targeting of PTEN and activation of Akt/eNOS pathway; expression is induced during hypoxia	Possible prognosis and therapeutic tool	[96]

Table 4. Tumor suppressor and oncogenic miRNAs involved in lung cancer hypoxia with possible roles in diagnosis, prognosis, and therapy.

Type of lncRNA	Expression level	Name	Target gene	lncRNA role in lung cancer hypoxia	Possible clinical role of lncRNAs in lung cancer	References
Tumor supressor lncRNAs	▼	lncRNA-LET (Low expression in tumor)	HIHD3; hypoxia-induced histone deacetylase 3	Squamous-cell lung carcinomas downregulated by HIHD3 promotes hypoxia-induced cancer cell invasion	New methods for therapeutic intervention	[97]
	▼	GAS5-AS1	–	Downregulation of GAS5-AS1 contributes to hypoxia tumor metastasis in non-small cell lung cancer	Prognosis and therapeutic marker	[98]
	▼	LincRNA-p21	TP53 and HIF-1α	Target angiogenic mechanisms	Prognosis marker	[84]
Oncogenic lncRNAs	▲	HOTAIR (HOX transcript antisense intergenic RNA)	HIF-1α	HOTAIR is upregulated in hypoxic conditions and is a direct target of HIF-1α; Promotion of cancer cell proliferation and ability to migrate and invade other sites	Novel therapeutic target	[99, 100]
	▲	H19	HIF-1α	Possess oncogenic properties triggered by hypoxic stress Correlates with p53 tumor suppressor status	Prognosis/ Diagnosis marker	[101]

Table 5. LncRNAs involved in lung cancer hypoxia with possible roles in diagnosis, prognosis, and therapy.

Hypoxia management has led to reduced angiogenesis and thus obtuse the malignant cell proliferation and survival due to deprivation of nutrients and oxygen via various molecules including the noncoding transcripts represented by miRNAs and lncRNAs. Multiple targeting through ncRNAs that are able to influence the fate of the hypoxic microenvironment will bring new insights into the pathogenesis of lung cancer, permitting the development of new clinical tools for cancer management, improving the concerning survival rate of this pathology. The list of miRNAs and lncRNAs implicated in the vascular invasion of the pulmonary malignancy is presented in **Tables 4** and **5**.

LncRNAs have recently emerged as important prognosis and therapeutic tolls in different malignancies and even for specific carcinogenic processes as lung cancer hypoxia. One of the main studied lncRNAs is HOTAIR, pathological expressed in numerous malignant scenarios, being associated with tumor promoting roles and a negative outcome in oncological patients. It was demonstrated that this lncRNA is a direct target for HIF-1α that act as an enhancer of expression and contribute together to the securitization of hypoxia followed by cell proliferation, migration, and metastasis. This information could transform HOTAIR in a possible therapeutic target under hypoxic conditions for NSCLC, that is limited in what regards the therapeutic options [99, 100]. Another newly discovered lncRNAs in lung cancer hypoxia that is lncRNA-LET targeted by HIHDR. The interaction between these two molecules ends with reduction of histone acetylation at the promoter region of the noncoding transcripts and thus decreased expression. Moreover, the downregulation process secures the expression of nuclear factor 90 proteins, a key element for cell migration induced by hypoxia. This data suggest that lncRNA-LET can be used as a clinical tool against cancer promotion [97].

LincRNA-p21 impacts prognosis in resected nonsmall-cell lung cancer patients through angiogenesis regulation. LincRNA-p21 was proved to be activated by TP53 and HIF1A [84]. It was proved to target the apoptosis pathway via regulation by p53 and the Warburg effect. LincRNA-p21 is downregulated in tumor tissue, and has effect on the lung cancer patients via angiogenesis regulation [84].

Other important ncRNA structures with a significant role in the development of novel molecular therapies are represented by PIWI-interacting RNAs (piRNAs). piRNAs are recognized to be involved in transposon silencing and gene expression during development and the complete role on the somatic cells remains to be deciphered [8]. In a recent paper were emphases a different piRNASs expression profiles between normal bronchial epithelial cells and lung cancer cells. The most downregulated piRNAs in lung cancer cells was piRNA-like-163 (piR-L-163) having as direct target the phosphorylated ERM (p-ERM) [102]. S100A4-small interfering RNA (S100A4-siRNA) was proved to activate the apoptosis and increase the radiosensitivity of A549 lung cells. S100A4 may promote A549 cell proliferation but also invasion, and metastasis by regulating the expression of E-cadherin and p53 protein [103].

5. ncRNAs targeting semaphorines and its related receptors in lung cancer

Semaphorins are guidance molecules which were characterized initially as directing elements for axon outgrowth; however advances in genomic and translational medicine revealed a more complex role for these proteins, being involved in cell migration, vascular network, and tissue development [32, 104]. Considering their vital role in physiological processes is not surprising that these guidance proteins are also involved in similar pathological processes especially from the oncologic area, where they exercise the same functions, but in a negative manner [32]. Therefore, semaphorins are implicated in carcinogenic establishment, metastasis, and especially angiogenesis in numerous cancers, including lung cancer. Regarding their role in angiogenesis, the family of semaphorins is divided into two main pathological classes: tumor suppressors inhibiting the angiogenic process and oncogenes through promotion of vascular invasion. Therefore, loss of expression in the case of antiangiogenic semaphorins and/or increased expression pattern for the procarcinogenic ones translates into sustaining of the malignant cells [106]. Immediately after the establishment of their newly discovered role, *in vitro* and *in vivo* studies confirmed the ability of semaphorins to serve as therapeutic targets in the form of suppression or enhancement [32]. Despite the fact that their role in pulmonary malignant processes is quite extensively studied, little is known about the ncRNAs regulatory action on the expression pattern of semaphorins. Deciphering the regulatory noncoding sequence panel for these proteins will enable a more advanced and specific molecular management of lung cancer, especially in angiogenesis that has a vital role regarding the maintenance of tumor cells integrity and proliferation.

The process of angiogenesis, can also occur through semaphorin receptors, neuropilins, and plexins (**Figure 5**). In the case of neuropilins, we encounter a multiple ligation system, this membrane proteins being able to bind both class-3 semaphorins, VEGF and growth factors. Also, this type of receptors that are essential to proper vascular development during organism development are generally mutated in lung cancer. On the other hand, *in vivo* suppression of neuropilins led to improper vascular network.

Among the first studies that elucidated the role of neuropilins in vascular development is the research where the authors observed that overexpressing of *Nrp1* was lethal for embryos due to extensive vascular defects like overdevelopment of blood vessel network and deformed hearts [107]. This discovery paved the way for further research in the area of cancer management with focus on targeted therapy. Therefore, it has been proven that a combined form of therapy represented by neuropilins inhibitors (semaphorin, anti-NRP, soluble NRP - B domain, and VEGF mimetics) administrated concomitant with anti-VEGF signaling molecules (kinase inhibitors, anti-VEGF, anti-VEGFR-2, and soluble VEGFR for VEGF) is more efficient than the classical antiangiogenic therapeutic strategy targeted towards VEGF alone [104]. Research studies demonstrated a role for NRP1 and NRP2 in lung cancer progression and angiogenesis where these two molecules were observed as normally expressed in bronchial basal cells, and as it progressed in the severity of the cell lesions, the level of neuropilins increased significantly, concomitant with VEGF expression [104]. NRP1 has been previously associated with cancer angiogenesis: overexpression of NRP1 in AT2.1 cells (*in vitro* model of prostate cancer) resulted in advanced vascular density, cell proliferation, and also inhibited apoptosis [108]; rat estrogen-induced pituitary tumors presented increased levels of NRP1, level that was also correlated in a positive manner with the aggressiveness of angiogenesis development [109].

The competitive binding of class-3 semaphorins and VEGF that in physiological conditions leads to the proper development of the vascular platform is changed during malignant scenarios where proangiogenic VEGF takes the lead due to mutations in the structure of the binding domain that decreases the complementarity with semaphorins or enhances the expression of receptors. Therefore, an alternative therapeutic pathway could be represented by the

http://dx.doi.org/10.5772/66529

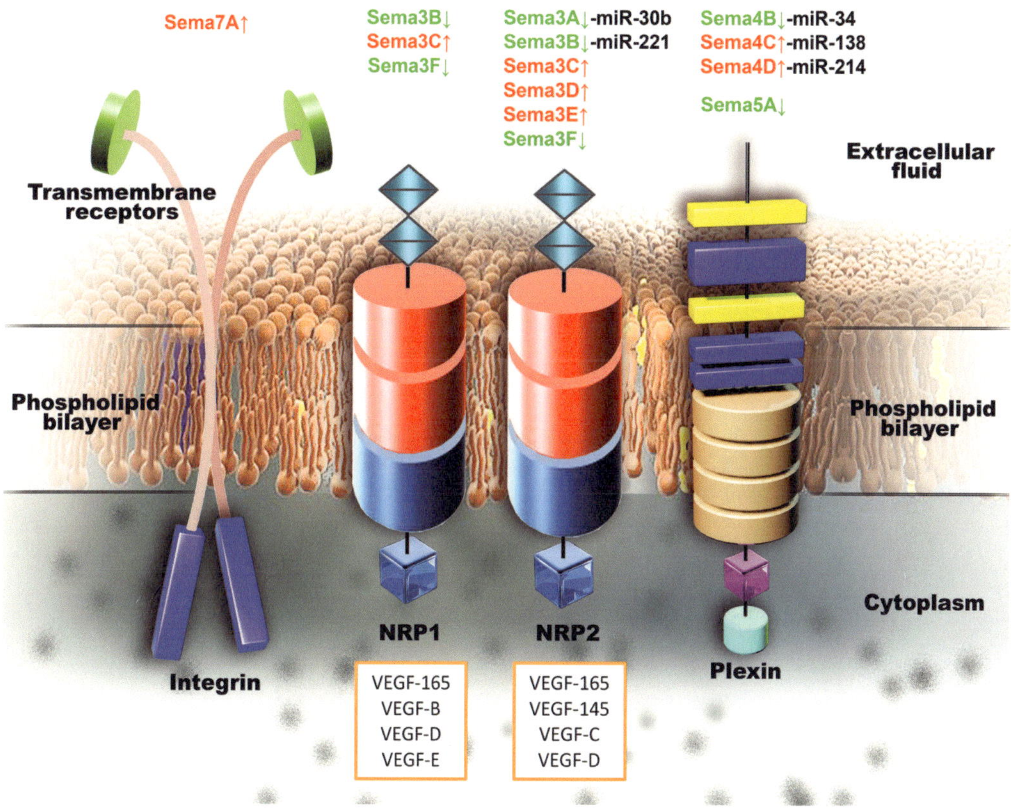

Figure 5. Semaphorin receptors and ncRNAs regulation. Green – downregulated genes; Red – overexpressed genes.

modulation of neuropilins (NRPs) expression. Furthermore, the specific malignant expression is most likely influenced by other molecules such as miRNAs and lncRNAs (**Table 6**).

Lung cancer therapies focused on semaphorins and their receptors are still an insufficiently explored domain that could hold great promises regarding the inhibition of cancer spreading. Considering the competitive binding between class-3 semaphorins and VEGF in vascular development, antiangiogenic strategies as antibodies for VEGF or NRP inhibition, soluble NRP or NRP blocking peptides have been tested with effective results [104, 106]. A more recent treatment compromising both VEGF and SEMA3A inhibitors have been applied *in vitro* and *in vivo* for colon cancer [105]. Another type of action could be represented by the induced internalization of the neuropilins through administration of dextran sulfate and fucoidan that significantly decreased the number of endothelial surface receptors, including VEGFR [131]. Although anti-VEGF molecules are well-known as efficient angiogenesis inhibitors, combining the modulation of VEGF/VEGFR with SEMA/NRP may hold significant clinical usage. Moreover, extension of the molecular insight regarding noncoding RNAs regulation of semaphorins and their receptor could improve even more the inhibition of angiogenesis if we take in consideration the ability of noncoding RNAs to regulate waste singling networks that involve more than one target gene.

Semaphorin	Regulatory miRNAs	Predicted targeting miRNAs	Role in lung cancer	Potential clinical role in lung cancer	Ref.
Semaphorin 3A (SEMA 3A)	miR-30b	miR-95-3p miR-589-5p	NSCLC-anticarcinogenic activity; low expression of SEMA 3A correlates with lymph node metastasis	Biomarker for prognosis	[104, 110]
Semaphorin 3B (SEMA 3B)	miR-221	miR-155-5p miR-107 miR-187-5p miR-18a-3p miR-708 miR-3074-5p miR-106b-3p miR-340-3p miR-3074-5p	Cell proliferation and invasion Small-cell lung cancer-tumor suppressor role via induction of apoptosis and inhibition of angiogenesis	Marker for cancer progression	[111, 112]
Semaphorin 3C (SEMA 3C)	–	miR-4746-5p miR-500a-5p miR-187-5p miR-301a-5p miR-21-3p miR-106a-3p miR-4677-3p miR-3074-5p let-7g-3p miR-183-3p miR-29a-3p miR-519a-5p miR-200c-5p miR-4668-3p miR-16-2-3p miR-193a-3p miR-4326 miR-4417 miR-3664-3p miR-155-5p miR-590-5p miR-616-3p miR-3182 miR-103a-2-5p miR-501-5p miR-362-3p miR-330-5p miR-30e-5p	A549 lung cancer cells -p65-SEMA3C (cleaved SEMA3C) – protumorigenic activities	Novel antitumorigenic drug	[113]
Semaphorin 3D (SEMA 3D)	–	miR-484 miR-15b-3p miR-16-2-3pmiR-32-3p miR-32-5p miR-33a-5p miR-33b-3p miR-340-5p miR-4668-3p miR-345-5p miR-629-5p miR-18a-5p miR-1306-5p	Proangiogenic and metastatic role	Prediction of response and survival	[114, 115]

Semaphorin	Regulatory miRNAs	Predicted targeting miRNAs	Role in lung cancer	Potential clinical role in lung cancer	Ref.
		let-7a-3p miR-183-3p miR-21-3p miR-21-5p miR-4742-5p miR-425-5p miR-200a-5p miR-301a-5p miR-3619-3p miR-589-5p miR-3614-3p miR-141-5p miR-106a-3p miR-93-3p			
Semaphorin 3E (SEMA 3E)	–	miR-340-5p miR-1306-5p miR-15b-3p let-7d-5p miR-1307-3p miR-629-5p miR-629-3p miR-4677-3p let-7g-3p miR-301a-5p miR-15b-5p miR-19a-3p miR-16-2-3p miR-105-3p miR-18a-5p miR-1306-5p miR-19a-3p miR-1307-5p miR-505-5p	*In vivo* promotion of lung metastasis and tumor progression	Possible target for therapeutic strategies	[116]
Semaphoring 3F (SEMA 3F)	–	miR-29c-3p miR-191-3p miR-29b-1-5p miR-18a-5p miR-20a-5p miR-29b-2-5p miR-200c-5p let-7g-3p let-7a-3p let-7d-5p miR-7-5p miR-3619-3p miR-590-5p miR-29b-2-5p miR-30e-5p miR-676-3p miR-135b-3p miR-30c-1-3p miR-140-3p miR-135b-3p miR-140-3p	Role in TGF-beta1-induced EMT Antitumor role; Downregulated in lung cancer Targets HIF-1 and VEGF	Possible prognosis biomarker and therapeutic target	[117, 118]

Semaphorin	Regulatory miRNAs	Predicted targeting miRNAs	Role in lung cancer	Potential clinical role in lung cancer	Ref.
Semaphorin 4B (SEMA 4B)	miR-34	miR-34	NSCLC—inhibition of invasion and growth—prevention of metastasis-direct target of hypoxia-inducible factor 1 (HIF-1) miR-34/p53 axis	Novel therapeutic target for inhibition of metastasis and growth -Novel therapeutic target through inhibition of HIF-1	[119–121]
Semaphorin 4C (SEMA 4C)	miR-138	miR-138	NSCLC-cell proliferation and EMT	New target or prognosis marker for lung cancer treatment	[122]
Semaphorin 4D (SEMA 4D)	miR-214	miR-199b-3p miR-127-3p miR-185-5p miR-421 miR-500a-5p miR-22-3p miR-500a-5p miR-22-3p miR-505-5p let-7g-3p miR-1269a miR-18a-5p miR-3614-3p miR-331-3p miR-18a-5p miR-18a-3p	Highly expressed in lung cancer; promotion of angiogenesis; NSCLC-*in vitro* inhibition of cell proliferation, migration, and invasion	Possible early prognosis tool and therapeutic target	[124–126]
Semaphorin 5A (SEMA 5A)	-	miR-3677-3p miR-3200-3p miR-32-5p miR-29b-1-5p miR-183-3p miR-345-5p miR-454-5p miR-3614-3p miR-18a-3p miR-500a-5p miR-106b-3p miR-27b-5p let-7g-3p miR-660-5p miR-135b-3p miR-1306-5p miR-29a-3p miR-29b-2-5p miR-425-3p miR-365a-5p miR-3136-3p miR-93-3p miR-4787-3p miR-19a-3p	NSCLC-tumor suppressor role; low levels associated with poor survival rate	New biomarker for NSCLC	[127]

Semaphorin	Regulatory miRNAs	Predicted targeting miRNAs	Role in lung cancer	Potential clinical role in lung cancer	Ref.
Semaphorin 6A (SEMA 6A)	miR-27a/b	miR-1307-3p miR-940 miR-3187-3p miR-33a-5p miR-425-3p miR-99b-5p miR-99b-3p miR-183-3p miR-3176 miR-760 miR-345-5p miR-4461	Endothelial cell repulsion	New therapeutic target through manipulation of miR-27a/b expression	[128, 129]
Semaphorin 7A (SEMA 7A)	–	22_40957679_40957783 (novel miRNA)	Promotion of tumor microenvironment and metastasis through regulation of prototypic chitinase-like protein (Chi3l1)	Possible role as therapeutic target	[130]

Table 6. Semaphorin and the targeting miRNAs with implication in lung cancer.

6. ncRNAs therapies targeting lung cancer angiogenesis

Once considered the "trash" of the genome, the noncoding RNA sequences are now emerging as important therapeutic targets (**Table 7**). Due to the complex regulatory network involving ncRNAs and also because of the personalized pathological expression pattern among cancer types, subtypes and malignant stages, ncRNAs are subjected to numerous preclinical studies regarding their silencing or induced expression [2]. A lipid-based delivery vehicle for tumor suppressor miR-34 was developed in order to enhance the expression of the specific molecule in a mouse model of non-small-cell lung cancer [132]. This approach has demonstrated to be efficient in both locally and systemically administration, being observed a reinforced miR expression concomitant with downregulation of the specific targets. Moreover, the intravenous delivery of miR-34 mimic did not produce an immune reaction in mice, but unfortunately this was not the case in humans. Very recently, MRX34, the miR-34 mimic, was stopped to be administrated in a cancer clinical trial due to major immune reactions [133].

Another therapeutic alternative that is currently on the scientific spotlight consist in the manipulation of the ciRNAs that can function as microRNA sponges, modulating their oncogenic or tumor suppressor activity [136]. Despite the fact that there is a number of research studies focused on this type of noncoding RNAs, relatively little is known about the regulatory mechanism of circRNAs in cancer development. Future perspectives imply ciRNAs-based therapy that can stand as "super-sponges" and modulate the activity of extended regulatory miRNA networks, influencing at a superior level the carcinoma progression [136].

miRNAs	Lung cancer subtype	Experimental model	Therapeutic approach	Delivery system	Target gene	Obtained results	References
miR-128	NSCLC	NSCLC cells	Ectopic miR-128 overexpression		VEGF-C	Inhibition of VEGF-C expression concomitant with angiogenesis restriction	[53]
		HUVECs and NSCLC cells			VEGF-A, VEGFR-2 and VEGFR-3	Low expression of the target genes that are critical factors for angiogenesis	
		Nude mice (A549 cells)	*In vivo* replacement therapy			Inhibition of lymphangiogenesis	
miR-497	NSCLC	NSCLC cells	Over expression of the miRNA		VEGF-A	Decreases in the levels of VEGF-A protein with no significant changes for the VEGF-A mRNA; inhibition of cell invasion	[123]
			miRNA inhibition			Increased levels of VEGF-A protein with no significant changes for the VEGF-A mRNA; increased cell invasion	
		NSCLC cells SCID mouse xenograft model	Ectopic expression of the miRNA sequence		HDGF	Restoration of the miR-497 levels reduced tumor development and angiogenesis in both *in vitro* and *in vivo* experimental models	[54]
miR-378	NSCLC	Swiss nude immunodeficient murine model (NCI-H292-Luc cells overexpressing miR-378—subcutaneous xenografts)	Overexpression of miR-378	Lentiviral vectors particles (pEZX-MR03 backbone)	HMOX1	mir-378 over expression models presented tumors with decreased vascularisation compared to the models with HMOX1 induced over expression; increased oxygen partial pressure; increased MUC5AC, Ang-1,MMP12 levels and decreased TNF-α and IL-1β levels - all essential genes for angiogenesis	[48]
miR-126		A549, Y-90 and SPC-A1 cells	Overexpression of miR-126	mir-126 expression vector (LV-miR-126)	VEGF-A	Dowregulation of VEGF-A gene correlated with inhibited cell growth	[42]
		Tumor xenograft model (A549 infected with LV-miR-126)	mir-126 expression vector (LV-miR-126)				

miRNAs	Lung cancer subtype	Experimental model	Therapeutic approach	Delivery system	Target gene	Obtained results	References
miR-222	NSCLC	H460 cells	Inhibition of miR-222 expression	miR-222 inhibitor	p27 (*in vivo* over expression of p27 impaired angiogenesis)	Inhibition of oncogenic miR expression resulted in decreased cell viability and proliferation	[60, 61]
miR-27b	NSCLC	HEK293 cells	Cotransfection of miR-27b mimics and WT Sp1 in order to express both miRNA and target gene	psiCHECK-2 vector	Sp1	Expression of miR-27b resulted in suppression of cell growth and reduced invasion	[128]
miR-130a	NSCLC	A549,CALU-1, H1299 and A459 cells	Transfection with miR-130a in order to increase the endogenous levels of this sequence	pre-miR 130a	MET	Strong reduction of MET (angiogenesis promoter) mRNA and protein levels; down regulation of miR-221 and miR-222, that are able to inhibit TIMP3 expression, molecule that in turn inhibits MET	[44]
miR-210	Adenocarcinoma	A549 cells	Knocked down of miR-210 in hypoxic parameters	antimiR-210	SDHD (positive-regulatory loop between miR-210 and HIF-1α)	Decreased cell survival and alteration of mitochondrial phenotype	[63]
miR-155	Adenocarcinoma	A549 and H460 cells	Inhibition of miR-155 levels in cells preserved in hypoxic conditions	Synthetic antimiR-155	FOXO3A (associated with roles in angiogenesis)	miR-155 inhibition exercise a positive role through radiosensitization of the cells	[65, 134]
miR-21	NSCLC	A549	*In vitro* inhibition of miR-21	miR-21-sponge	PDCD4 (associated with angiogenesis development)	Inhibition of miR-21 ameliorates cell proliferation, migration, and invasion through PDCD4 modulation; knockdown of PDCD4 has been demonstrated to stimulate angiogenesis through positive regulation of Ang-2 (negative prognostic factor in lung cancer)	[66, 135]

Table 7. Some relevant miRNAs tested on cell culture and animal models as potential therapeutic agents in lung cancer.

The discovery of lncRNAs as regulators of cancer development has naturally conducted towards potential therapeutic alternatives using these long fragments as direct targets. The expression pattern of these sequences has been also investigated in lung cancer and the list of oncogenic and tumor suppressor pathological expressed lncRNAs is continuously growing. Administration of siRNA, shRNA, and miRNAs or antisense oligonucleotides in order to inhibit oncogenic lncRNAs is currently under investigation [137]. HOTAIR has been on the spotlight of artificial knockdown via siRNA delivery with great rates of success in lung cancer and also breast and pancreatic malignancies [100].

Moreover, the same approaches have been shown to be effective for the reverse of cisplatin resistance through reduced expression of p21 [138]. Downregulation of MALAT1 through shRNA delivery is also a potent therapeutic approach for lung cancer as it was shown reduced cell viability after this type of treatment [71]. MALAT1 has been also inhibited by exogenous antisense oligonucleotides, approach that induced reduced cancer progression through cell cycle arrest [151]. Considering that in lung cancer there are also downregulated tumor suppressor lncRNAs, the replacement therapy could also stand as an effective therapeutic approach for this type of carcinoma, but nonetheless the scientific information are quite limited regarding this area.

The discovery that miRNA sequences can act as key regulators in cancer pathways through aberrant expression has led to the idea that these fragments could serve as potent therapeutic targets [139]. In this sense, several strategies have been implemented until now: inhibition strategies—inhibitory antisense oligonucleotides and delivery vectors (miRNA sponges) and enhancement strategies—miRNA replacement therapy (**Figure 6**) [139, 140].

For the case of therapeutics that follow an antagonistic pattern, the activity of tumor promoting miRNAs that are hazardous expressed is inhibited via administration of single stranded oligonucleotides complementary with the specific molecule or with the target binding site on the mRNA molecule; in either situation, the interaction between miRNAs and mRNA molecules is blocked and the downstream pathological pathway is strongly affected [140].

Delivery of anti-miRNA oligonucleotides (AMOs) in the context of preclinical studies is still a problematic area considering the necessity of target administration, prolonged stability, and increased pharmacokinetic properties [140]. In this means, there is an urgent need for efficient delivery vectors/vehicles that are able to fulfill the reminded request in order to accomplish the treatment purpose. The majority of the freely administrated oligonucleotides is retrieved in the liver and kidneys and then eliminated through the urine. Also, the necessary dose of synthetic sequences is usually very high and the chance for off-target delivery is also increasing. Establishment of an effective delivery system will break the grounds of miRNAs therapeutics and also other noncoding treatment strategies [139]. The current strategy for *in vivo* administration implies conjugation-based methods, where miRNA sequences are conjugated with different molecules like cholesterol [141] and α-tocopherol [142]. Although these studies have demonstrated promising results, the efficiency of miRNA targeting is still limited. Another type of delivery method consists in liposome-mediated delivery of siRNAs, where the first attempt [143] was to inhibit the replication of hepatitis B virus (HBV) in an animal model through administration of siRNAs integrated in as polyethylene glycol (PEG)–lipid conjugate (SNALP). Since then, different liposome-based vehicles have been tested and the results are encouraging considering that the administration dose is significantly decreased

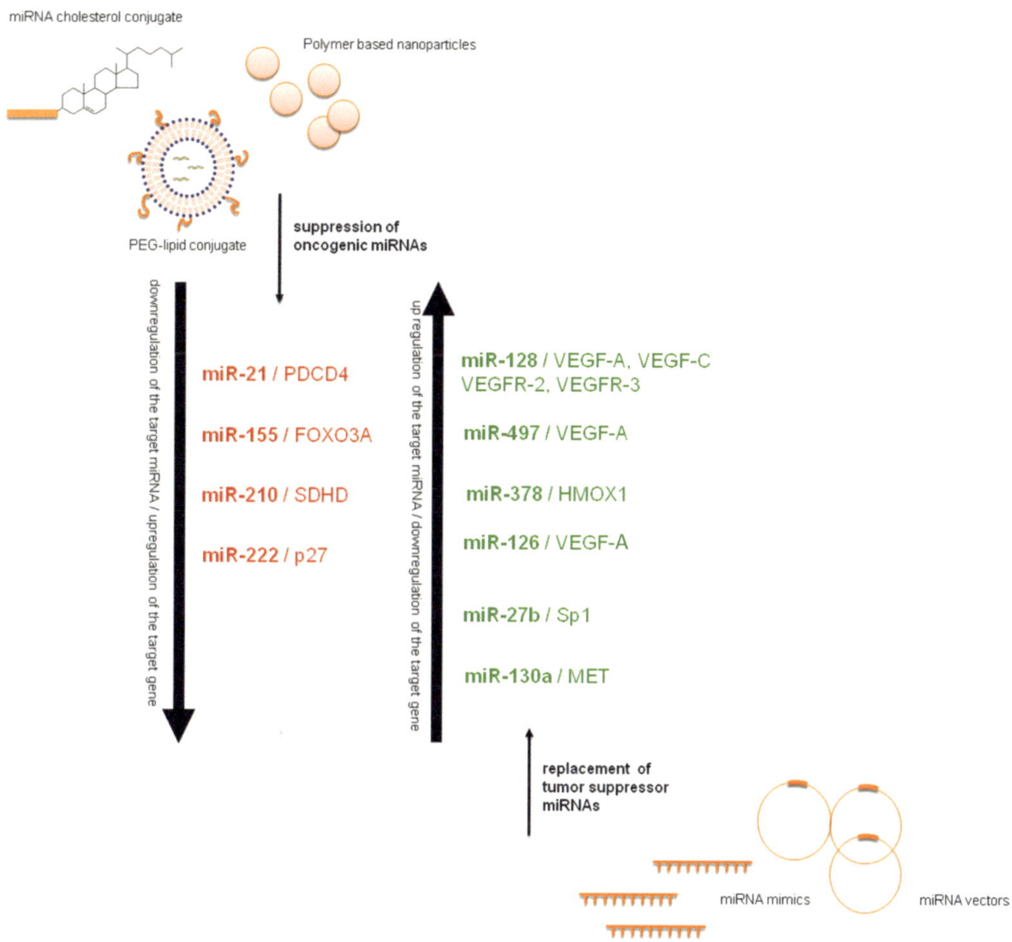

Figure 6. MicroRNAs have emerged as important regulators of lung cancer angiogenesis and also as key therapeutic targets regarding inhibition or enhancement strategies. MiRNAs sequences that are marked with green composed the tumor suppressor group that have been tested in the context of replacement therapies; the genes marked with the same color represent the target genes that have been downregulated after therapeutic modulation of miRNAs. Inversely, miRNAs sequences marked with red are oncogenic ones proposed for inhibition in what regards antiangiogenic programs; the genes marked with the same color also represent the target genes, but in this case their expression has been augmented.

comparing to the naked oligonucleotides [144–147]. Progresses in the area of material science produced a promising *in vivo* delivery system in the form of polymer-based nanoparticles that are more flexible than liposomes and also can be produced in a more homogenous manner regarding their size and form [139]. In respect of siRNAs and anti-miRs delivery, the size of the vehicle is very important in order to permit the passing through cellular compartments, where nanoparticles can fulfill this request having a size between 10 and 100 nm [139]. Moreover, in order to avoid the stimulation of the immune system, cyclodextrin–PEG conjugated nanoparticles have been developed and tested for the inhibition of EWS–FLI1 in an *in vivo* model of Ewing's sarcoma [148]. Attracting strategies for targeted therapies consist in the conjugation of siRNAs or anti-miR sequences with specific antibodies able to conduct the small fragments towards distinctive cells expressing the desired antigen [147, 149, 150].

MiRNA replacement therapy is more limited regarding the current attempts and results, although it seems to emerge as a more efficient form of treatment considering that the majority of pathological expressed miRNAs consist in downregulated or inhibited tumor suppressor sequences [140]. Even if the success of this therapeutic strategy could be greater than miRNA inhibition workflows, the requirements for the structure and composition of the replacement fragment are much more stringent considering the necessity of RISC uptake. Furthermore, the impediments regarding the delivery system for these oligonucleotides are the same as in the case of inhibitory antisense attempts.

7. Conclusions and future perspectives

Lung cancer remains the most deadly disease from the oncological field, being an aggressive form of cancer that is usually diagnosed in late stages with minimal therapeutic alternatives. Even in the case of early discovery, the classical treatments have failed numerous times due to compensatory mechanisms developed within the tumor environment leading to the same negative outcome. Therefore, we face a crisis situation where we need to develop new therapeutic tools for lung cancer management able to target key elements/pathways, but avoid in the same time the possibility of alternative carcinogenic pathways activation. One of the hallmarks of cancer is represented by angiogenesis, process that is in the sight of researchers for some time, but the classical inhibition of central molecules like VEGF has failed to deliver long-lasting results. Therefore, ncRNAs have emerged as potential lifesaving agents due to the capacity of extensive modulation, where the same ncRNA is able to target multiple genes and regulate their function. Also the same microRNA, or more recently discovered, the lncRNA can be encounter in different consecutive processes in pulmonary carcinogenesis, as in the case of hypoxia and angiogenesis. Development of novel therapeutic tools able to transform the pathological expression of ncRNAs, mainly through silencing of upregulated patterns, will enable a more extensive, and in the same time, specific approach that will probably excludes the installation of compensatory mechanism and significantly contribute to a better outcome in lung cancer patients. The concept of noncoding RNAs as therapeutic targets in the clinical context is now more feasible than ever, being supported by numerous preclinical studies. One of the main approaches should involve manipulation of miRNAs that are actively implicated in the regulation of VEGF genes expression, genes that hold a key role in the vascular development process. Even more, a heterogeneous approach that implies the administration of different miRNA sequences able to target multiple genes and naturally multiple pathological pathways within the angiogenic process will represent a more extended form of therapy that could modify extensive regulatory networks. This type of targeting will also minimize the compensatory mechanisms that are usually encountered after the implementation of classical therapeutic strategies due to concomitant regulation of multiple signaling pathways. Additionally, some other approaches may be used for the inhibition of angiogenesis. For example, semaphorins are now emerging as important regulators of vascular density in malignancies, with possible roles as prognostic tools or even therapeutic targets. Inhibition of procarcinogenic semaphorins would represent a novel course of action regarding cancer treatment considering their central role in vascular density. Moreover, the

http://dx.doi.org/10.5772/66529

receptors associated with semaphorins contain binding sites for both semaphorins and VEGF molecules, engaging the competitive binding between these types of molecules. Managing the expression of VEGF via miRNA therapy concomitant with the levels of neuropilins (semaphorins receptors) will enable a more dramatic approach that could have more drastic results for cancer development.

Current therapeutic programs are promoting the effectiveness of specific sequence inhibition or enhancement through administration of antisense oligonucleotides or supplementation of the same sequence through exogenous enhancement. Development of chemically modified oligonucleotides under the form of medication for individuals diagnosed with cancer is now at the close horizon. Administration of synthetic oligonucleotides for noncoding RNAs inhibition or upregulation will enhance the effect of the current therapeutic strategies by modulation of specific gene expression able to influence the carcinogenic process or even reverse the malignant installation. In this sense, it is now clearly understood that the major strategy towards cancer treatment is focused on taking advantage of the key roles of noncoding sequences regarding the modulation of entire aberrant regulatory networks through manipulation of central molecules.

Acknowledgments

This work was supported by the POC-P_37_796 grant, entitled "Clinical and economical impact of personalized targeted anti-microRNA therapies in reconverting lung cancer chemoresistance"-CANTEMIR.

Author details

Ioana Berindan-Neagoe[1,2,3*], Cornelia Braicu[1], Diana Gulei[2], Ciprian Tomuleasa[1,4] and George Adrian Calin[5]

*Address all correspondence to: ioana.neagoe@umfcluj.ro

1 Research Center for Functional Genomics, Biomedicine and Translational Medicine, "Iuliu Hatieganu", University of Medicine and Pharmacy Iuliu-Hatieganu, Cluj-Napoca, Romania

2 Medfuture—Research Center for Advanced Medicine, University of Medicine and Pharmacy Iuliu-Hatieganu, Cluj-Napoca, Romania

3 Department of Functional Genomics and Experimental Pathology, The Oncological Institute "Prof. Dr. Ion Chiricuta", Cluj-Napoca, Romania

4 Department of Hematology, The Oncological Institute "Prof. Dr. Ion Chiricuta", Cluj-Napoca, Romania

5 Department of Experimental Therapeutics, The University of Texas M.D. Anderson Cancer Center, Houston, TX, USA

References

[1] Mattick, J.S. and I.V. Makunin, *Non-coding RNA*. Hum Mol Genet, 2006. **15 Spec No 1**: pp. R17–29.

[2] Braicu, C., et al., *NCRNA combined therapy as future treatment option for cancer*. Curr Pharm Des, 2014. **20**(42): pp. 6565–74.

[3] Choudhuri, S., *Small noncoding RNAs: biogenesis, function, and emerging significance in toxicology*. J Biochem Mol Toxicol, 2010. **24**(3): pp. 195–216.

[4] Berindan-Neagoe, I., et al., *MicroRNAome genome: a treasure for cancer diagnosis and therapy*. CA Cancer J Clin, 2014. **64**(5): pp. 311–36.

[5] Berindan-Neagoe, I. and G.A. Calin, *Molecular pathways: microRNAs, cancer cells, and microenvironment*. Clin Cancer Res, 2014. **20**(24): pp. 6247–53.

[6] Kung, J.T., D. Colognori, and J.T. Lee, *Long noncoding RNAs: past, present, and future*. Genetics, 2013. **193**(3): pp. 651–69.

[7] Liu, Y. *MicroRNAs and PIWI-interacting RNAs in oncology*. Oncol Lett, 2016. **12**(4): pp. 2289–2292.

[8] Ng, K.W., C. Anderson, E.A. Marshall, B.C. Minatel, K.S. Enfield, H.L. Saprunoff, W.L. Lam, and V.D. Martinez, *Piwi-interacting RNAs in cancer: emerging functions and clinical utility*. Mol Cancer, 2016. **15**: p. 5.

[9] Hansen, T.B., J. Kjems, and C.K. Damgaard, *Circular RNA and miR-7 in cancer*. Cancer Res, 2013. **73**(18): pp. 5609–12.

[10] Peng, L., X.Q. Yuan, and G.C. Li, *The emerging landscape of circular RNA ciRS-7 in cancer (Review)*. Oncol Rep, 2015. **33**(6): pp. 2669–74.

[11] Ebbesen, K.K., T.B. Hansen, and J. Kjems, *Insights into circular RNA biology*. RNA Biol, 2016 Dec 16:0. [Epub ahead of print]

[12] Hansen, T.B., et al., *Natural RNA circles function as efficient microRNA sponges*. Nature, 2013. **495**(7441): pp. 384–8.

[13] Shao, T., et al., *Identification of module biomarkers from the dysregulated ceRNA-ceRNA interaction network in lung adenocarcinoma*. Mol Biosyst, 2015. **11**(11): pp. 3048–58.

[14] Taft, R.J., et al., *Non-coding RNAs: regulators of disease*. J Pathol, 2010. **220**(2): pp. 126–39.

[15] Malone, C.D. and G.J. Hannon, *Small RNAs as guardians of the genome*. Cell, 2009. **136**(4): pp. 656–68.

[16] Carthew, R.W. and E.J. Sontheimer, *Origins and mechanisms of miRNAs and siRNAs*. Cell, 2009. **136**(4): pp. 642–55.

[17] Ghildiyal, M. and P.D. Zamore, *Small silencing RNAs: an expanding universe*. Nat Rev Genet, 2009. **10**(2): pp. 94–108.

[18] Sobecka, A., W. Barczak, and W.M. Suchorska. *RNA interference in head and neck oncology*. Oncol Lett., 2016. **12**(5): pp. 3035–3040.

[19] Meister, G. *Argonaute proteins: functional insights and emerging roles*. Nat Rev Genet, 2013. 14(7): pp. 447–59.

[20] Tordonato, C., P.P. Di Fiore, and F. Nicassio, *The role of non-coding RNAs in the regulation of stem cells and progenitors in the normal mammary gland and in breast tumors*. Front Genet, 2015. **6**: p. 72.

[21] Kilgoz, H.O., et al., *KRAS and the reality of personalized medicine in non-small cell lung cancer*. Mol Med, 2016. **22**.

[22] Nicholson, S.A., et al., *Small cell lung carcinoma (SCLC): a clinicopathologic study of 100 cases with surgical specimens*. Am J Surg Pathol, 2002. **26**(9): pp. 1184–97.

[23] Nicholson, A.G., et al., *The international association for the study of lung cancer lung cancer staging project: proposals for the revision of the clinical and pathologic staging of small cell lung cancer in the forthcoming eighth edition of the TNM classification for lung cancer*. J Thorac Oncol, 2016. **11**(3): pp. 300–11.

[24] Cheng, T.D., et al., *The international epidemiology of lung cancer: latest trends, disparities, and tumor characteristics*. J Thorac Oncol, 2016. 11(10):1653–71.

[25] Okereke, I.C., et al., *Outcomes after surgical resection of pulmonary carcinoid tumors*. J Cardiothorac Surg, 2016. **11**: p. 35.

[26] Govindan, R., et al., *Changing epidemiology of small-cell lung cancer in the United States over the last 30 years: analysis of the surveillance, epidemiologic, and end results database*. J Clin Oncol, 2006. **24**(28): pp. 4539–44.

[27] Urman, A. and H.D. Hosgood, *Curbing the burden of lung cancer*. Front Med, 2016. **10**(2): pp. 228–32.

[28] Landrigan, P.J., *Comments on the 2014 Helsinki Consensus Report on Asbestos*. Ann Glob Health, 2016. **82**(1): pp. 217–20.

[29] http://www.cancer.org/cancer/lungcancer-non-smallcell/detailedguide/non-small-cell-lung-cancer-survival-rates, accessed, august 2016

[30] http://globocan.iarc.fr/old/FactSheets/cancers/lung-new.asp, accessed, august 2016

[31] Hanahan, D. and R.A. Weinberg, *Hallmarks of cancer: the next generation*. Cell, 2011. **144**(5): pp. 646–74.

[32] Neufeld, G., N. Shraga-Heled, T. Lange, N. Guttmann-Raviv, Y. Herzog, and O. Kessler, *Semaphorins in cancer*. Front Biosci, 2005. **10**: pp. 751–60.

[33] Piperdi, B., A. Merla, and R. Perez-Soler, *Targeting angiogenesis in squamous non-small cell lung cancer*. Drugs, 2014. **74**(4): pp. 403–13.

[34] Cabebe, E. and H. Wakelee, *Role of anti-angiogenesis agents in treating NSCLC: focus on bevacizumab and VEGFR tyrosine kinase inhibitors*. Curr Treat Options Oncol, 2007. **8**(1): pp. 15–27.

[35] Lee, S.M., et al., *Anti-angiogenic therapy using thalidomide combined with chemotherapy in small cell lung cancer: a randomized, double-blind, placebo-controlled trial*. J Natl Cancer Inst, 2009. **101**(15): pp. 1049–57.

[36] Arnedos, M., et al., *Personalized treatments of cancer patients: a reality in daily practice, a costly dream or a shared vision of the future from the oncology community?* Cancer Treat Rev, 2014. **40**(10): pp. 1192–8.

[37] Li, H. and X. Lv, *Functional annotation of noncoding variants and prioritization of cancer-associated lncRNAs in lung cancer*. Oncol Lett, 2016. **12**(1): pp. 222–230.

[38] Stenvang, J., M. Lindow, and S. Kauppinen, *Targeting of microRNAs for therapeutics*. Biochem Soc Trans, 2008. **36**(Pt 6): pp. 1197–200.

[39] Zhang, B., X. Pan, G.P. Cobb and T.A. Anderson, *microRNAs as oncogenes and tumor suppressors*. Dev Biol, 2007 Feb 1. **302**(1): pp. 1–12.

[40] Wang, L., et al., *Altered expression of transcription factor Sp1 critically impacts the angiogenic phenotype of human gastric cancer*. Clin Exp Metastasis, 2005. **22**(3): pp. 205–13.

[41] Safe S. *MicroRNA-Specificity Protein (Sp) Transcription factor interactions and significance in carcinogenesis*. Curr Pharmacol Rep, 2015. **1**(2): pp. 73–78.

[42] Liu, B., et al., *MiR-126 restoration down-regulate VEGF and inhibit the growth of lung cancer cell lines in vitro and in vivo*. Lung Cancer, 2009. **66**(2): pp. 169–75.

[43] Zhou, Y.M., J. Liu, and W. Sun, *MiR-130a overcomes gefitinib resistance by targeting met in non-small cell lung cancer cell lines*. Asian Pac J Cancer Prev, 2014. **15**(3): pp. 1391–6.

[44] Acunzo, M., et al., *miR-130a targets MET and induces TRAIL-sensitivity in NSCLC by downregulating miR-221 and 222*. Oncogene, 2012. **31**(5): pp. 634–42.

[45] Sun, C.Y., X.M. She, Y. Qin, Z.B. Chu, L. Chen, L.S. Ai, L. Zhang, and Y. Hu. *miR-15a and miR-16 affect the angiogenesis of multiple myeloma by targeting VEGF*. Carcinogenesis, 2013. **34**(2): pp. 426–35.

[46] Tafsiri, E., et al., *Expression of miRNAs in non-small-cell lung carcinomas and their association with clinicopathological features*. Tumour Biol, 2015. **36**(3): pp. 1603–12.

[47] Koukourakis, M.I., et al., *bcl-2 and c-erbB-2 proteins are involved in the regulation of VEGF and of thymidine phosphorylase angiogenic activity in non-small-cell lung cancer*. Clin Exp Metastasis, 1999. **17**(7): pp. 545–54.

[48] Skrzypek, K., et al., *Interplay between heme oxygenase-1 and miR-378 affects non-small cell lung carcinoma growth, vascularization, and metastasis*. Antioxid Redox Signal, 2013. **19**(7): pp. 644–60.

[49] Chen, L.T., et al., *MicroRNA-378 is associated with non-small cell lung cancer brain metastasis by promoting cell migration, invasion and tumor angiogenesis*. Med Oncol, 2012. **29**(3): pp. 1673–80.

[50] Luo, W., et al., *miRNA-296-3p modulates chemosensitivity of lung cancer cells by targeting CX3CR1*. Am J Transl Res, 2016. **8**(4): pp. 1848–56.

[51] Xu, C., et al., *miR-296-5p suppresses cell viability by directly targeting PLK1 in non-small cell lung cancer*. Oncol Rep, 2016. **35**(1): pp. 497–503.

[52] Suarez, Y. and W.C. Sessa, *MicroRNAs as novel regulators of angiogenesis*. Circ Res, 2009. **104**(4): pp. 442–54.

[53] Hu, J., et al., *microRNA-128 plays a critical role in human non-small cell lung cancer tumourigenesis, angiogenesis and lymphangiogenesis by directly targeting vascular endothelial growth factor-C*. Eur J Cancer, 2014. **50**(13): pp. 2336–50.

[54] Zhao, W.Y., et al., *Downregulation of miR-497 promotes tumor growth and angiogenesis by targeting HDGF in non-small cell lung cancer*. Biochem Biophys Res Commun, 2013. **435**(3): pp. 466–71.

[55] Xia, X.M., W.Y. Jin, R.Z. Shi, Y.F. Zhang, and J. Chen. *Clinical significance and the correlation of expression between Let-7 and K-ras in non-small cell lung cancer*. Oncol Lett, 2010. **1**(6): pp. 1045–1047.

[56] Hu, H., et al., *MiR-145 and miR-203 represses TGF-beta-induced epithelial-mesenchymal transition and invasion by inhibiting SMAD3 in non-small cell lung cancer cells*. Lung Cancer, 2016. **97**: pp. 87–94.

[57] Li, J., et al., *The role of miR-205 in the VEGF-mediated promotion of human ovarian cancer cell invasion*. Gynecol Oncol. 2015. **137**: pp. 125–133.

[58] Garofalo, M., et al., *miR-221&222 regulate TRAIL resistance and enhance tumorigenicity through PTEN and TIMP3 downregulation*. Cancer Cell, 2009. **16**(6): pp. 498–509.

[59] Zhang, C., et al., *PUMA is a novel target of miR-221/222 in human epithelial cancers*. Int J Oncol, 2010. **37**(6): pp. 1621–6.

[60] Zhong, C., et al., *MicroRNA-222 promotes human non-small cell lung cancer H460 growth by targeting p27*. Int J Clin Exp Med, 2015. **8**(4): pp. 5534–40.

[61] Goukassian, D., et al., *Overexpression of p27(Kip1) by doxycycline-regulated adenoviral vectors inhibits endothelial cell proliferation and migration and impairs angiogenesis*. FASEB J, 2001. **15**(11): pp. 1877–85.

[62] Devlin, C., et al., *miR-210: More than a silent player in hypoxia*. IUBMB Life, 2011. **63**(2): pp. 94–100.

[63] Puissegur, M.P., et al., *miR-210 is overexpressed in late stages of lung cancer and mediates mitochondrial alterations associated with modulation of HIF-1 activity*. Cell Death Differ, 2011. **18**(3): pp. 465–78.

[64] Donnem, T., et al., *Prognostic impact of MiR-155 in non-small cell lung cancer evaluated by in situ hybridization*. J Transl Med, 2011. **9**: p. 6.

[65] Babar, I.A., et al., *Inhibition of hypoxia-induced miR-155 radiosensitizes hypoxic lung cancer cells*. Cancer Biol Ther, 2011. **12**(10): pp. 908–14.

[66] Xue, X., Y. Liu, Y. Wang, M. Meng, K. Wang, X. Zang, et al. MiR-21 and MiR-155 promote non-small cell lung cancer progression by downregulating SOCS1, SOCS6, and PTEN. Oncotarget, 2016.

[67] Yanaihara, N., et al., *Unique microRNA molecular profiles in lung cancer diagnosis and prognosis*. Cancer Cell, 2006. **9**(3): pp. 189–98.

[68] Donnem, T., et al., *MicroRNA signatures in tumor tissue related to angiogenesis in non-small cell lung cancer*. PLoS One, 2012. **7**(1): pp. e29671.

[69] Patnaik, S.K., et al., *Evaluation of microRNA expression profiles that may predict recurrence of localized stage I non-small cell lung cancer after surgical resection*. Cancer Res, 2010. **70**(1): pp. 36–45.

[70] Sang, H., et al., *Long non-coding RNA functions in lung cancer*. Tumour Biol, 2015. **36**(6): pp. 4027–37.

[71] Li, J., et al., *LncRNA MALAT1 exerts oncogenic functions in lung adenocarcinoma by targeting miR-204*. Am J Cancer Res, 2016. **6**(5): pp. 1099–107.

[72] Han, L., et al., *Low expression of long noncoding RNA PANDAR predicts a poor prognosis of non-small cell lung cancer and affects cell apoptosis by regulating Bcl-2*. Cell Death Dis, 2015. **6**: p. e1665.

[73] Zhang, E.B., et al., *P53-regulated long non-coding RNA TUG1 affects cell proliferation in human non-small cell lung cancer, partly through epigenetically regulating HOXB7 expression*. Cell Death Dis, 2014. **5**: p. e1243

[74] Deng, H.P., et al., *Long non-coding RNA HOTTIP promotes tumor growth and inhibits cell apoptosis in lung cancer*. Cell Mol Biol (Noisy-le-grand), 2015. **61**(4): pp. 34–40.

[75] Nie, F.Q., et al., *Long non-coding RNA MVIH indicates a poor prognosis for non-small cell lung cancer and promotes cell proliferation and invasion*. Tumour Biol, 2014. **35**(8): pp. 7587–94.

[76] Lu, K.H., et al., *Long non-coding RNA MEG3 inhibits NSCLC cells proliferation and induces apoptosis by affecting p53 expression*. BMC Cancer, 2013. **13**: pp. 461.

[77] Yang, Q., et al., *A novel long noncoding RNA AK001796 acts as an oncogene and is involved in cell growth inhibition by resveratrol in lung cancer*. Toxicol Appl Pharmacol, 2015. **285**(2): pp. 79–88.

[78] Nie, F.Q., et al., *Long noncoding RNA ANRIL promotes non-small cell lung cancer cell proliferation and inhibits apoptosis by silencing KLF2 and P21 expression*. Mol Cancer Ther, 2015. **14**(1): pp. 268–77.

[79] Qiu, M., et al., *A novel lncRNA, LUADT1, promotes lung adenocarcinoma proliferation via the epigenetic suppression of p27*. Cell Death Dis, 2015. **6**: pp. e1858.

[80] Pan, H., et al., *Long non-coding RNA BC087858 induces non-T790M mutation acquired resistance to EGFR-TKIs by activating PI3K/AKT and MEK/ERK pathways and EMT in non-small-cell lung cancer*. Oncotarget, 2016. **7**(31): pp. 49948–60.

[81] Zhang, L., et al., *Enhanced expression of long non-coding RNA ZXF1 promoted the invasion and metastasis in lung adenocarcinoma*. Biomed Pharmacother, 2014. **68**(4): pp. 401–7.

[82] Yang, Z.T., et al., *Overexpression of Long Non-Coding RNA ZXF2 Promotes Lung Adenocarcinoma Progression Through c-Myc Pathway*. Cell Physiol Biochem, 2015. **35**(6): pp. 2360–70.

[83] Wang, G., H. Chen, and J. Liu, *The long noncoding RNA LINC01207 promotes proliferation of lung adenocarcinoma*. Am J Cancer Res, 2015. **5**(10): pp. 3162–73.

[84] Castellano, J.J., et al., *LincRNA-p21 impacts prognosis in resected non-small-cell lung cancer patients through angiogenesis regulation*. J Thorac Oncol, 2016. **11**(12):2173–82

[85] Calin, G.A., et al., *Ultraconserved regions encoding ncRNAs are altered in human leukemias and carcinomas*. Cancer Cell. **12**(3): pp. 215–229.

[86] Peng, J.C., J. Shen, and Z.H. Ran, *Transcribed ultraconserved region in human cancers*. RNA Biol, 2013. **10**(12): pp. 1771–7

[87] Jiang, S., et al., *MicroRNA-21 modulates radiation resistance through upregulation of hypoxia-inducible factor-1alpha-promoted glycolysis in non-small cell lung cancer cells*. Mol Med Rep, 2016. **13**(5): pp. 4101–7.

[88] Kenneth, Niall S. and S. Rocha, *Regulation of gene expression by hypoxia*. Biochem J, 2008. **414**(1): pp. 19–29.

[89] Gao, X.J., et al., *Nobiletin inhibited hypoxia-induced epithelial-mesenchymal transition of lung cancer cells by inactivating of Notch-1 signaling and switching on miR-200b*. Pharmazie, 2015. **70**(4): pp. 256–62.

[90] Haigl, B., et al., *Expression of microRNA-21 in non-small cell lung cancer tissue increases with disease progression and is likely caused by growth conditional changes during malignant transformation*. Int J Oncol, 2014. **44**(4): pp. 1325–34.

[91] Eilertsen, M., et al., *Positive prognostic impact of miR-210 in non-small cell lung cancer*. Lung Cancer, 2014. **83**(2): pp. 272–8.

[92] Krutilina, R., et al., *MicroRNA-18a inhibits hypoxia-inducible factor 1alpha activity and lung metastasis in basal breast cancers*. Breast Cancer Res, 2014. **16**(4): p. R78.

[93] Ding, G., et al., *MiR-199a suppresses the hypoxia-induced proliferation of non-small cell lung cancer cells through targeting HIF1alpha*. Mol Cell Biochem, 2013. **384**(1–2): pp. 173–80.

[94] Guo, W.G., et al., *Bioinformatics analyses combined microarray identify the desregulated microRNAs in lung cancer*. Eur Rev Med Pharmacol Sci, 2013. **17**(11): pp. 1509–16.

[95] Taguchi, A., et al., *Identification of hypoxia-inducible factor-1 alpha as a novel target for miR-17-92 microRNA cluster*. Cancer Res, 2008. **68**(14): pp. 5540–5.

[96] Mao, G., et al., *Tumor-derived microRNA-494 promotes angiogenesis in non-small cell lung cancer*. Angiogenesis, 2015. **18**(3): pp. 373–82.

[97] Yang, F., et al., *Repression of the long noncoding RNA-LET by histone deacetylase 3 contributes to hypoxia-mediated metastasis*. Mol Cell, 2013. **49**(6): pp. 1083–96.

[98] Wu, Y., et al., *Downregulation of the long noncoding RNA GAS5-AS1 contributes to tumor metastasis in non-small cell lung cancer*. Sci Rep, 2016, **6**: p. 31093.

[99] Zhou, C., et al., *Long noncoding RNA HOTAIR, a hypoxia-inducible factor-1alpha activated driver of malignancy, enhances hypoxic cancer cell proliferation, migration, and invasion in non-small cell lung cancer*. Tumour Biol, 2015. **36**(12): pp. 9179–88.

[100] Yao, Y., J. Li, and L. Wang, *Large intervening non-coding RNA HOTAIR is an indicator of poor prognosis and a therapeutic target in human cancers*. Int J Mol Sci, 2014. **15**(10): pp. 18985–99.

[101] Matouk, I.J., et al., *The oncofetal H19 RNA connection: hypoxia, p53 and cancer*. Biochim Biophys Acta, 2010. **1803**(4): pp. 443–51.

[102] Mei, Y., et al., *A piRNA-like small RNA interacts with and modulates p-ERM proteins in human somatic cells*. Nat Commun, 2015. **6**: p. 7316.

[103] Qi, R., T. Qiao, and X. Zhuang, *Small interfering RNA targeting S100A4 sensitizes non-small-cell lung cancer cells (A549) to radiation treatment*. Onco Targets Ther, 2016. **9**: pp. 3753–62.

[104] Geretti, E. and M. Klagsbrun, *Neuropilins: novel targets for anti-angiogenesis therapies*. Cell Adh Migr, 2007. **1**(2): pp. 56–61.

[105] Nguyen, Q.D., et al., *Inhibition of vascular endothelial growth factor (VEGF)-165 and semaphorin 3A-mediated cellular invasion and tumor growth by the VEGF signaling inhibitor ZD4190 in human colon cancer cells and xenografts*. Mol Cancer Ther, 2006. **5**(8): pp. 2070–7.

[106] Geretti, E., A. Shimizu, and M. Klagsbrun, *Neuropilin structure governs VEGF and semaphorin binding and regulates angiogenesis*. Angiogenesis, 2008. **11**(1): pp. 31–9.

[107] Kitsukawa, T., et al., *Overexpression of a membrane protein, neuropilin, in chimeric mice causes anomalies in the cardiovascular system, nervous system and limbs*. Development, 1995. **121**(12): pp. 4309–18.

[108] Miao, H.Q., et al., *Neuropilin-1 expression by tumor cells promotes tumor angiogenesis and progression*. FASEB J, 2000. **14**(15): pp. 2532–9.

[109] Banerjee, S.K., et al., *Overexpression of vascular endothelial growth factor164 and its co-receptor neuropilin-1 in estrogen-induced rat pituitary tumors and GH3 rat pituitary tumor cells*. Int J Oncol, 2000. **16**(2): pp. 253–60.

[110] Han, F., et al., *MicroRNA-30b promotes axon outgrowth of retinal ganglion cells by inhibiting Semaphorin3A expression*. Brain Res, 2015. **1611**: pp. 65–73.

[111] Loginov, V.I., et al., *Tumor suppressor function of the SEMA3B gene in human lung and renal cancers*. PLoS One, 2015. **10**(5): pp. e0123369.

[112] Cai, G., S. Qiao, and K. Chen, *Suppression of miR-221 inhibits glioma cells proliferation and invasion via targeting SEMA3B*. Biol Res, 2015. **48**: p. 37.

[113] Mumblat, Y., et al., *Full-length semaphorin-3C is an inhibitor of tumor lymphangiogenesis and metastasis*. Cancer Res, 2015. **75**(11): pp. 2177–86.

[114] Meert, A.P., et al., *[Difficulties and limitations in conducting translational research in thoracic oncology. A practical example]*. Rev Mal Respir, 2016. **33**(7): pp. 594–9.

[115] Foley, K., et al., *Semaphorin 3D autocrine signaling mediates the metastatic role of annexin A2 in pancreatic cancer*. Sci Signal, 2015. **8**(388): p. ra77.

[116] Christensen, C., et al., *Proteolytic processing converts the repelling signal Sema3E into an inducer of invasive growth and lung metastasis*. Cancer Res, 2005. **65**(14): pp. 6167–77.

[117] Nasarre, P., et al., *Neuropilin-2 Is upregulated in lung cancer cells during TGF-beta1-induced epithelial-mesenchymal transition*. Cancer Res, 2013. **73**(23): pp. 7111–21.

[118] Clarhaut, J., et al., *ZEB-1, a repressor of the semaphorin 3F tumor suppressor gene in lung cancer cells*. Neoplasia, 2009. **11**(2): pp. 157–66.

[119] Jian, H., et al., *SEMA4B inhibits growth of non-small cell lung cancer in vitro and in vivo*. Cell Signal, 2015. **27**(6): pp. 1208–13.

[120] Jian, H., B. Liu, and J. Zhang, *Hypoxia and hypoxia-inducible factor 1 repress SEMA4B expression to promote non-small cell lung cancer invasion*. Tumour Biol, 2014. **35**(5): pp. 4949–55.

[121] Jian, H., et al., *SEMA4b inhibits MMP9 to prevent metastasis of non-small cell lung cancer*. Tumour Biol, 2014. **35**(11): pp. 11051–6.

[122] Li, J., Q. Wang, R. Wen, J. Liang, X. Zhong, W. Yang, et al. *MiR-138 inhibits cell proliferation and reverses epithelial-mesenchymal transition in non-small cell lung cancer cells by targeting GIT1 and SEMA4C*. J Cell Mol Med, 2015. **19**(12): pp. 2793–805.

[123] Gu, A., J. Lu, W. Wang, C. Shi, B. Han, M. Yao. *Role of miR-497 in VEGF-A-mediated cancer cell growth and invasion in non-small cell lung cancer*. Int J Biochem Cell Biol, 2016. **70**: pp. 118–25.

[124] Ruan, S.S., et al., *Expression and clinical significance of Semaphorin4D in non-small cell lung cancer and its impact on malignant behaviors of A549 lung cancer cells*. J Huazhong Univ Sci Technolog Med Sci, 2014. **34**(4): pp. 491–6.

[125] Liu, Y., et al., *MiR-214 suppressed ovarian cancer and negatively regulated semaphorin 4D*. Tumour Biol, 2016. **37**(6): pp. 8239–48.

[126] Fazzari, P., et al., *Plexin-B1 plays a redundant role during mouse development and in tumour angiogenesis*. BMC Dev Biol, 2007. **7**: p. 55.

[127] Lu, T.P., et al., *Identification of a novel biomarker, SEMA5A, for non-small cell lung carcinoma in nonsmoking women*. Cancer Epidemiol Biomarkers Prev, 2010. **19**(10): pp. 2590–7.

[128] Veliceasa, D., et al., *Therapeutic manipulation of angiogenesis with miR-27b*. Vasc Cell, 2015. **7**: p. 6.

[129] Urbich, C., et al., *MicroRNA-27a/b controls endothelial cell repulsion and angiogenesis by targeting semaphorin 6A*. Blood, 2012. **119**(6): pp. 1607–16.

[130] Ma, B., et al., *Role of chitinase 3-like-1 and semaphorin 7a in pulmonary melanoma metastasis*. Cancer Res, 2015. **75**(3): pp. 487–96.

[131] Narazaki, M., M. Segarra, and G. Tosato, *Sulfated polysaccharides identified as inducers of neuropilin-1 internalization and functional inhibition of VEGF165 and semaphorin3A*. Blood, 2008. **111**(8): pp. 4126-36.

[132] Wiggins, J.F., et al., *Development of a lung cancer therapeutic based on the tumor suppressor microRNA-34*. Cancer Res, 2010. **70**(14): pp. 5923–30.

[133] AUSTIN, Texas, BUSINESS WIRE - *Mirna Therapeutics*, Inc. (Nasdaq:MIRN) September 20, 2016

[134] Potente, M., et al., *Involvement of Foxo transcription factors in angiogenesis and postnatal neovascularization*. J Clin Invest, 2005. **115**(9): pp. 2382–92.

[135] Krug, S., et al., *Knock-down of Pdcd4 stimulates angiogenesis via up-regulation of angiopoietin-2*. Biochim Biophys Acta, 2012. **1823**(4): pp. 789–99.

[136] Wang, F., A.J. Nazarali, and S. Ji, *Circular RNAs as potential biomarkers for cancer diagnosis and therapy*. Am J Cancer Res, 2016. **6**(6): pp. 1167–76.

[137] Ricciuti, B., et al., *Long noncoding RNAs: new insights into non-small cell lung cancer biology, diagnosis and therapy*. Med Oncol, 2016. **33**(2): p. 18.

[138] Liu, Z., M. Sun, K. Lu, J. Liu, M. Zhang, W. Wu, et al. *The long noncoding RNA HOTAIR contributes to cisplatin resistance of human lung adenocarcinoma cells via downregualtion of p21(WAF1/CIP1) expression*. PLoS One, 2013. **8**(10): p. e77293.

[139] Li, Z. and T.M. Rana. *Therapeutic targeting of microRNAs: current status and future challenges*. Nat Rev Drug Discov, 2014. **13**(8): pp. 622–38.

[140] Roberts, T.C. and M.J. Wood. *Therapeutic targeting of non-coding RNAs*. Essays Biochem, 2013. **54**: pp. 127–45.

[141] Krutzfeldt, J., N. Rajewsky, R. Braich, K.G. Rajeev, T. Tuschl, M. Manoharan, et al. *Silencing of microRNAs in vivo with 'antagomirs'*. Nature, 2005. **438**(7068): pp. 685–9.

[142] Bagga, S., J. Bracht, S. Hunter, K. Massirer, J. Holtz, R. Eachus, et al. *Regulation by let-7 and lin-4 miRNAs results in target mRNA degradation*. Cell, 2005. **122**(4): pp. 553–63.

[143] Morrissey, D.V., J.A. Lockridge, L. Shaw, K. Blanchard, K. Jensen, W. Breen, et al. *Potent and persistent in vivo anti-HBV activity of chemically modified siRNAs*. Nat Biotechnol, 2005. **23**(8): pp. 1002–7.

[144] Akinc, A., et al., *A combinatorial library of lipid-like materials for delivery of RNAi therapeutics*. Nat Biotechnol, 2008. **26**(5): pp. 561–9.

[145] Peer, D., et al., *Systemic leukocyte-directed siRNA delivery revealing cyclin D1 as an anti-inflammatory target*. Science, 2008. **319**(5863): pp. 627–30.

[146] Palliser, D., et al., *An siRNA-based microbicide protects mice from lethal herpes simplex virus 2 infection*. Nature, 2006. **439**(7072): pp. 89–94.

[147] Kumar, P., et al., *A single siRNA suppresses fatal encephalitis induced by two different flaviviruses*. PLoS Med, 2006. **3**(4): pp. e96.

[148] Hu-Lieskovan, S., et al., *Sequence-specific knockdown of EWS-FLI1 by targeted, nonviral delivery of small interfering RNA inhibits tumor growth in a murine model of metastatic Ewing's sarcoma*. Cancer Res, 2005. **65**(19): pp. 8984–92.

[149] Song, E., et al., *Antibody mediated in vivo delivery of small interfering RNAs via cell-surface receptors*. Nat Biotechnol, 2005. **23**(6): pp. 709–17.

[150] Yao, Y.D., et al., *Targeted delivery of PLK1-siRNA by ScFv suppresses Her2+ breast cancer growth and metastasis*. Sci Transl Med, 2012. **4**(130): p. 130ra48.

[151] Gutschner, T., et al., *The noncoding RNA MALAT1 is a critical regulator of the metastasis phenotype of lung cancer cells*. Cancer Res, 2013. **73**(3): pp. 1180–9.

Section 4

Novel Methods in Angiogenesis Research

Chapter 15

Recent Advances in Angiogenesis Assessment Methods and their Clinical Applications

Imran Shahid, Waleed H. AlMalki,
Mohammed W. AlRabia, Muhammad Ahmed,
Mohammad T. Imam, Muhammed K. Saifullah and
Muhammad H. Hafeez

Additional information is available at the end of the chapter

http://dx.doi.org/10.5772/66504

Abstract

Angiogenesis, a natural phenomenon of developing new blood vessels, is an integral part of normal developmental processes as well as numerous pathological states in humans. The angiogenic assays are reliable predictors of certain pathologies in particular tumor growth, metastasis, inflammation, wound healing, tissue regeneration, ischemia, cardiovascular, and ocular diseases. The angiogenic inducer and inhibitor studies rely on both in vivo and in vitro angiogenesis methods, and various animal models are also standardized to assess qualitative and quantitative angiogenesis. Analogously, the discovery and development of anti-angiogenic agents are also based on the choice of suitable angiogenic assays and potential drug targeted sites within the angiogenic process. Similarly, the selection of cell types and compatible experimental conditions resembling the angiogenic disease being studied are also potential challenging tasks in recent angiogenesis studies. The imaging analysis systems for data acquisition from in vivo, in vitro, and in ova angiogenesis assay to preclinic, and clinical research also requires novel but easy-to-use tools and well-established protocols. The proposition of this pragmatic book chapter overviews the recent advances in angiogenesis assessment methods and discusses their applications in numerous disease pathogenesis.

Keywords: angiogenesis techniques, *in vitro* angiogenesis, angiogenic mouse models, quantitative angiogenesis, transgenic animal models, angiogenesis in clinical practice, angiogenic inhibitors

1. Introduction

The growth of new microvessels from the parent ones is an integral part of new tissue growth in growing organisms. It plays an essential part in human health while playing key roles in wound healing and tissue development [1]. Similarly, the phenomenon is regularly triggered in certain pathological conditions including rheumatoid arthritis, endometriosis, diabetic retinopathy, macular degeneration, tumor growth, and inflammatory conditions in response to certain antigens and toxins [2]. However, almost every normal tissues lack this phenomenon in adulthood, except cyclical events in the female reproductive organs [3]. Physiological angiogenesis in tissues contains a natural balance between endogenous pro- and anti-angiogenic factors [3]. When this balance gets disturbed and shifts more toward the pro-angiogenic side in certain pathological states (inflammation, ischemia, hypoxia, and cancer), microvascular endothelial cells (ECs) initiate a cascade of angiogenic reactions which may be retracted or progressive and turn microvessels to an angiogenic phenotype [4]. A considerable diversity exists among microvascular endothelial cells in different tissues and organs, and species heterogeneity cannot be ignored in this scenario [4].

Where angiogenesis is useful for tissue growth and development, excessive vessel growth is really problematic and a hallmark to propagate many diseases while contributing to turning tumor cells into cancer, tumor metastasis, psoriasis, arthritis, diabetic retinopathy, and predominantly metabolic disease such as obesity, atherosclerosis, and certain infectious diseases [5]. Conversely, insufficient angiogenesis or neovascularization may cause ischemic tissue states in heart, brain, and peripheral muscles which may lead to high blood pressure, preeclampsia, neurodegeneration, and osteoporosis [5]. In such pathological states, pro-angiogenic therapies which promote compensatory angiogenesis show promise to treat such pathologies [6]. In parallel to that, angiogenic inhibitors found highly effective in clinical trials as successful strategic treatment approaches with or without conventional chemotherapy for the treatment of solid tumors and metastasis [7]. The potential beneficiary of such novel treatment strategies are patients with aberrant ocular angiogenesis and cancer patients, where defective sight and cancer progression are entirely angiogenesis-dependent [7]. Such treatment paradigms are also heralding a new era of the treatment for other commonly occurring angiogenesis-related diseases.

The formation of new vessels involves many different cell types, and an intricate interplay of various endogenous vascular growth factors, receptors, extracellular matrix (ECM) proteins and the humoral factors [8]. To design and develop potentially effective pro- and anti-angiogenic treatments and to understand molecular mechanisms involved in angiogenesis and neovascularization, numerous in vivo and in vitro assays and animal models of angiogenesis have been developed [9]. Similarly, preclinical angiogenesis assays have also used for drug screening, molecular structure activities, and dosage effects of certain approved anti-angiogenic compounds although such assays are not equivalent and relevant to human disease regarding efficacy [10]. The prime objective of this book chapter is to overview current major and newly introduced angiogenic assays with regard to major advantages and limitations from biological, technical, ethical, and economic perspectives. The major assays which we discuss here include corneal micropocket assay, CAM (chick chorioallantoic membrane) assay, rodent mesentery, Matrigel plug assays, whole-animal assays (zebrafish), and animal models of angiogenesis in the context of cardiovascular, ocular, and adipose tissue diseases. A precise note on genetically engineered animal models for vascular endogenous genes and their spatial, temporal, and conditional expression is also included [9]. It is beyond the scope of this chapter to cover every angiogenesis assays in details, so we briefly overview quantitative techniques and/or methods to assess/evaluate neovascularization in tissues. We also briefly discuss molecular mechanisms and cell signaling pathways involved in angiogenesis and potential anti-angiogenic therapies, their clinical impact, limitations, and future prospects.

2. Prerequisite for good angiogenesis assays

Before to choose an ideal assay for angiogenesis studies, the investigators and researchers must know the assay kinetics in terms of operating procedures, handling the environment, ethical justification, and assay economy [8]. In vivo angiogenic studies are more informative than in vitro due to complex cellular and molecular activities of angiogenic reactions while providing biology of the assay and showing experimental design are relevant [9]. Similarly, in trauma-based assays (either physical or chemical), where cell damage triggers inflammatory reactions which mimic the release of several pro-angiogenic cytokines, the sensitivity and specificity of the assay are reduced [10]. For such assays, specific precautions must be taken to avoid any inflammatory reaction or to minimize the traumatic tissue state. In parallel to that, the test substance/compound should be designed as being angiogenic in a noninflammatory state. A near to physiological dose of the test compound should be administered for inducing an angiogenic response while to modulate angiogenic assay conditions and dosage response, a dose range of the clinical use must be chosen [10].

Vehicles carrying the test compound in many assays may also affect the pharmacokinetics of the tested drug and alter the dose-response curves among different experimental animals within one group. For such circumstances, the best solution is to compare test animals/samples with vehicle-exposed counterparts [9]. However, for data interpretation, one must be fully acquainted with the fact that how the vehicle-administered tested animals differ from the untreated controls [10]. Spatial and temporal distributions of the tested compounds are also necessary and vital because failure to do so may produce or hinder to generate reliable and rigorous dose-response curves [10]. As in different pathological states newly formed, vessels are delicate in quality and poorly functional, the selection of angiogenic assessment methods (either qualitative or quantitative) also matters to evaluate the morphology and physiology of the neovascularization in diseased tissues [9]. For in vivo angiogenesis assays, histological microscopy provides the detailed information precisely. Mammalian systems adopted for in vivo angiogenesis assays and mouse models for certain cardiovascular, ocular, and cerebral diseases are comparatively more close to relating human pathophysiology than the embryonic CAM assay, embryonic zebrafish (*Xenopus laevis*), and invertebrate (*Hirudo medicinalis*) angiogenic assays [9, 10].

3. Key components of an ideal angiogenesis assay

It would be interesting to describe that despite the much progress in the field of angiogenesis research, there is no single angiogenic model available which may fully elucidate the entire process and molecular mechanisms of the angiogenic and neovascularization process. Some exogenous and endogenous factors hinder the efforts to develop such an ideal system. Due to cell diversity among different tissues where angiogenesis takes place and intricate interplay among different cell signaling pathways of angiogenic reactions, it is an uphill task to develop and validate a unique assay that is optimal for all situations. However, different modalities and ingenious ways with the passage of time in a particular assay facilitate and provide optimisms for better measurements of angiogenesis than the past. In this context, Vallee et al. [11] conclude that "The design and verification of [new] specific, reliable, repeatable, and precise methodology to measure angiogenesis are considered an imperative of high priority in the field of angiogenesis research." Similarly, Auerbach et al. [10] state "Perhaps the most consistent limitation in all these studies and approaches has been the availability of simple, reliable, reproducible, quantitative assays of the angiogenic response." Moreover, it is challenging although not impossible in several angiogenic assays that the quantification of newly formed vessels regarding numbers and lengths. Similarly, the spatial and temporal distribution of tested compound is also necessary to get strong dose-response curves. Performing an assay in a blinded manner may helpful in this prospect and also to alleviate the influence of any preconceived notions. Analogously, the technical skills to perform any angiogenesis assay are of utmost importance to ensure maximum success.

Despite all these qualms as described above, an ideal angiogenesis assay for quantification of newly formed vessels must feature the following characteristics; first [12], "the release rate [R] and the spatial and temporal concentration distribution [C] of tested compounds should be known to evaluate dose-response curves; second, if tumor cells are used as a source of angiogenic factors, oncogene expression and production of growth factors (either stimulants or inhibitors) must be genetically well defined before the assay proceeding; third, the assay must be designed in a way ensure to provide quantitative measuring parameters of the newly formed vessels (e.g., vascular length [L], surface area [A], volume [V], number of vessels in the network [N], fractal dimensions of the network [Df], and extent of basement membrane [BM]); fourth, the assay should be designed in a way to weigh quantitative measure of morphological characteristics of new vessels (e.g., endothelial cell migration [MR], proliferation rate [PR], canalization rate [CR], blood flow rate [F], and vascular permeability [P]); fifth, a clear demarcation must exist between new and parent vessels; sixth, tissue trauma must be minimized to prevent the formation of new vessels; seventh, in vitro assessment should be verified by in vivo procedures; eighth, angiogenesis assay for long term and with noninvasive monitoring should be preferred; last, the selected assay should be economical, ethically justifiable, robust, and reliable." [12].

4. Process of angiogenesis

Endothelial cell activation, proliferation, and directed migration to form new microvasculature (capillaries) from the parent ones should be a complex process involving many molecular and cell signaling pathway events [2]. Some key regulators to switch on or off gene expression are also participating and influence by positive and negative feedbacks of cellular processes. The normal physiological angiogenesis initiates by sprouting of capillaries under the effect of vascular endothelial growth factors (VEGFs) from parent vessels [13]. It continuous during embryonic development and transiently during female reproductive cycle but almost stops in adult tissues except for some wound healing states [13]. Pathologic angiogenesis remains persistent with the continuous proliferation of ECs in different tissue pathologies and particularly in cancer [3]. Many tumor cells are capable of attracting adjacent blood vasculature from nearby tissues [2]. It was evident by the fact that for solid tumors to grow a certain size, neovascularization is necessary otherwise such tumors rarely metastasize as found in thin melanomas which reside on the avascular basement membrane [2, 13]. Also, for tumor growth, the nutrient supply, oxygen, and waste removal are also essential. The new vasculature fulfills this task while providing immune cells, macrophages, and humoral factors to the vicinity of the tumor cells [2].

The parent vessel wall comprises endothelial cell lining, basement membrane, and pericytic cells. Pro-angiogenic growth factors (VEGF, TGF-α, TNF-α) from tumor cells bind to the receptors of ECs and initiate a cascade of cell signaling pathways and angiogenic reactions [2]. Activation and resolution of ECs are two key steps of the angiogenic cascade reactions. When ECs activate and stimulate to grow, the cells secrete proteases, heparanase, and other digestive enzymes that degrade the extracellular matrix (ECM) [13]. ECM degradation allows the secretion of many pro-angiogenic factors from the endothelial cell matrix, and the junctions between ECs become leaky; new microvessel sprouts grow in the direct toward the stimulus [2] (**Figure 1**). For further ECs to grow, proliferate, and migrate, hematopoietic-endothelial progenitor cells (HEPC) also play an essential role [13]. In resolution phase, the new microvasculature tends to mature with the help of pericytic cell adhesion, reconstitution of basement membrane, and

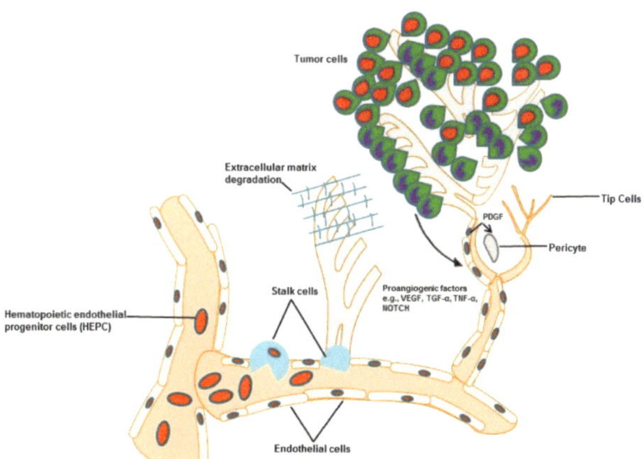

Figure 1. Process of angiogenesis from parent vessels: Angiogenesis sprouting initiates when vascular endothelial growth factors (e.g., VEGF-A) bind to VEGFR-2 receptors located on endothelial cells (ECs). ECs release matrix metalloproteinase (MMP) which degrades extracellular matrix (ECM) from which endothelial tip cells migrate. Vascular endothelial growth factors also regulate Notch cell signaling to inhibit proliferation of endothelial stalk cells. Platelet-derived growth factor (PDGF) released from ECs recruits smooth muscle cells (e.g., pericyte) to stabilize the neovasculature. TGF-α = transforming growth factor, TNF-α = tumor necrosis factor.

formation of cell junctions [14]. Interestingly, the resolution phase in tumor surrounding capillary network remains incomplete which results in irregular and tortuous microvasculature with partial ECs, increased cell permeability, and fragmentary basement membrane [15]. Tumor vasculature is disorganized with poor microcirculation, and vessel diameter changes without any differentiation into arterioles, capillaries, and venules [13]. Similarly, tumor vasculature is sprouting type, so assays which quantify sprouting angiogenesis are very useful to study the kinetics of tumor angiogenesis [15].

In the following section, we present the major and currently used preclinical angiogenesis assays in approximate chronological order of their first publication like chick chorioallantoic membrane (CAM), Matrigel plug, and corneal micropocket assays, while the others described in brief. [10]. CAM, Matrigel plug, and zebrafish assays are very useful for new angiogenic inhibitors screening. For a particular research focus, we provide advantages and disadvantages between different assays in a tabular form feasible for the readers (**Table 1**).

Assay name	Advantages	Disadvantages
***In vivo* angiogenesis assays**		
Corneal micropocket assay	(a) Easy-to-identify newly formed vessels	(a) Atypical assay due to avascular tissue nature
	(b) Easy to perform in animals (e.g., mice, rat, and rabbit)	(b) Induction of nonspecific inflammation to test substance
	(c) Qualitatively permits noninvasive and long-term monitoring	(c) Inaccessible to endogenous blood-borne angiogenic factors
	(d) Immunologically, cross reaction is minimized	(d) Ethical problems as using a major sensory organ for angiogenic assay
	(e) New vessel formation by sprouting	(e) Oxygen exposure may affect angiogenesis
		(f) Not a suitable site for tumor growth
		(g) Tested compounds are few
Chick chorioallantoic membrane assay	(a) Simple to perform and low in cost	(a) Inflammation-mediated angiogenic reactions
	(b) Suitable to study pro- and anti-angiogenic compounds	(b) Very sensitive to change in O_2 tension
	(c) Tumor angiogenesis may assess	(c) Not suitable for metabolically activated compounds
		(d) Embryonic nonmammalian procedure
		(e) Newly formed vessels are difficult to identify
Rodent mesentery assays	(a) Natively sparsely vascularized	(a) Less significant for quantitative angiogenesis in mice than rats
	(b) Lacks physiological angiogenesis	(b) Real-time observation is limited

Assay name	Advantages	Disadvantages
	(c) Angiogenesis induction with little or no trauma	(c) Technically require skills and time consuming
	(d) Suitable for quantitative measurement of microvessel variables (e.g., spatial extension, density, vessel number and length)	
	(e) Suitable to study tumor angiogenesis	
	(f) Sprouting type of angiogenesis	
Sponge/matrix implant assay	(a) Simple and inexpensive to proceed	(a) Nonspecific inflammatory host responses
	(b) Replicate in hypoxic tumor microenvironment so convenient for tumor angiogenesis studies	(b) Implant/sponge composition may vary
	(c) Reproducible and continuous assessment of angiogenesis	(c) s.c is not a reliable route for tumor growth
		(d) Variable drug retention within implant
Disk angiogenesis assay	(a) Inexpensive and easy to perform	(a) Continuous or kinetic observation is limited
	(b) Quantitative assessment of angiogenesis	(b) Encapsulated by granulation tissue
	(c) Wound healing may access	
	(d) Multiple disks can be used at one time	
Matrigel plug assay	(a) Rapid screening of pro- and anti-angiogenic compounds	(a) Matrigel chemical composition is not defined
	(b) An experimental model for tissue regeneration	(b) Three-dimensional plugs are difficult to generate
	(c) Simple to proceed and rapid screening in chambers	(c) Avascular test tissue
Whole-animal models for angiogenic assays		
***Xenopus* laevis (Zebrafish)**	(a) Embryonic and organogenic angiogenesis is assessed	(a) Expensive in breeding condition
	(b) Useful animal model for functional genomic analysis	(b) Non-mammalian and embryonic in nature
	(c) Simple to proceed and relatively fast	
	(d) Easy animal maintenance and significant number of tested animals per statistical analysis	
	(e) Single-drug dosing and small quantities of drugs are required	

Assay name	Advantages	Disadvantages
Mouse models of angiogenesis		
Adipose angiogenesis models		
1. ob/ob mice	(a) Deficient in leptin	(a) Expensive in terms of handling and treatment
	(b) Suitable to study angiogenesis in adipose tissue expansion	(b) Time consuming to assess angiogenesis
	(c) Helpful to test compounds related to metabolic disorders and obesity	
2. Db/db mice	(a) Excellent for role of angiogenesis in insulin resistance and obesity-related diabetes	(a) Difficult to handle and time consuming
Cardiovascular angiogenesis mouse models		
1. Hindlimb ischemic model	(a) Suitable to study arteries growth in tissue hypoxia	(a) Hind limb surgery is complicated
	(b) Can be performed in mice or rat	(b) Skilled and experienced person is required
	(c) Suitable to use for therapeutic agents which augment perfusion to ischemic limb	(c) Degree of tissue hypoxia may vary within experimental animals group
		(d) Residual blood flow may slightly differ in limb after surgery
2. Heart ischemic model	(a) Suitable for pathological and drug evaluation studies	(a) Inflammatory response–mediated angiogenesis
	(b) Efficient neovascularization	
Wound healing assays	(a) Suitable for vascular maturation/ remodelling studies	(a) Inflammatory responsemediated angiogenesis
	(b) Surgery is very simple	(b) limited to skin regeneration
	(c) Pro- or anti-angiogenic compounds can be tested for vessel morphology or regenerative angiogenesis	(c) Regeneration through new tissue formation instead repairing and replacing damaged tissue
	(d) Very easy and robust assay	
Transgenic animal models		
1. Transgenic choroidal neovascularization model	(a) Controlling transgene conditional expression and evaluation of spatial and temporal vascular gene expression	(a) Ethically questionable
2. Transgenic zebrafish model	(b) Knock-down vascular endogenous gene expression	(b) Time consuming
		(c) Differential gene expression may observed within same animal

Table 1. The advantages and disadvantages of major *in vivo, in vitro* and animal models angiogenesis assays.

5. In vivo angiogenesis models

5.1. The corneal micropocket assay

The firm foundation of systematic angiogenesis research was initiated by Folkman and associates who introduced first time the corneal micropocket assay and chick chorioallantoic membrane (CAM assay) in 1974 [16, 17]. The corneal micropocket assay allows the growth of newly formed blood vessels in vivo, and the techniques were first time applied in rabbits and after that in mice and rat [16]. In this assay, a micropocket is made in the stroma where a pellet containing the growth factors is placed inside the micropocket on the corneal surface of the eye. The growth factors induce a reproducible angiogenic response, and by implanting multiple pellets of different growth factors into parallel micropockets, the various stimuli of angiogenic response may be assessed. The angiogenic response in this assay is entirely due to direct stimulation of blood vessels instead to indirect induction of inflammation reaction. The assay shows minimal inflammatory cellular activity. However, the tested compounds are slowly released from the polymer of the micropocket, and such formulations may cause irritation and ultimately lead to inflammatory reactions which may alter angiogenesis quantification. The micropocket itself is inaccessible to certain blood borne growth factors and blood progenitor cells which may influence angiogenesis. The new vasculature mainly forms through the sprouting from the adjacent limbal area. Being avascular in nature, the corneal assay is useful in visibility and accessibility of new vessel formation and topical application of test drugs and biomicroscopic grading of new vasculature. However, it makes the assay atypical because normal tissues are vascular with few exceptions [16].

5.2. Chick chorioallantoic membrane (CAM) assay

The assay was introduced by Folkman and associates, but embryologists used this method to evaluate embryonic tissue grafts for their developmental potential [17]. The assay is useful to study tumor angiogenesis as well as pro- and anti-angiogenesis compound screening [18]. Fertilized hen's egg incubated at 37°C for 3 days is prepared for grafting by removing enough egg albumin to reduce shell membrane adhesion. Carriers containing the tested compound are placed directly onto the CAM by making a rectangular opening in the eggshell. Slow-release polymer pellets, air-dried disks, and gelatin sponges can be used as tested compound carriers; however, Elvax 40 and Hydron which are used to form sponges and membranes remain inert when applied to the CAM [19]. The quantification of angiogenesis can be made 3–4 days after grafting [18–20]. The in ovo CAM assay is relatively simple to perform as described above. However, a complementary in vitro method has also been described during which the chicken embryos grow in Petri dishes after 3 days of incubation. The assay is technically in vitro, but strictly speaking, it presents a whole-animal assay. After three to six days' extra incubation, the CAM develops, and grafts can be assessed for subsequent development. In vitro CAM allows the quantification of blood vessels over a wider area than in ovo CAM assay. Similarly, a large number of samples can be evaluated at one time, and response occurs within a short period of time (i.e., 2–3 days). Furthermore, the test compound can be placed on the underside of the coverslips. Generally, in ovo CAM assay is performed more than in vitro CAM. The calculated time for CAM angiogenesis response is very critical as between day five and twelve, the experimentally induced acceleration or suppression of embryonic organogenic angiogenesis can be determined. From day 12 onward, endogenous organogenic angiogenesis under the influence of undefined growth factor may initiate, and identification of newly formed vessels under the effect of tested compound becomes vague [18].

5.3. Rodent mesentery assay

The rodent mesentery assay was introduced by K. Norrby and associates in 1986 and refined later on [21, 22]. The peculiarity of the assay is to use the small gut mesentery of small rodents which is considered ideal for the physiological measurement of angiogenesis. It can be exteriorized from the abdominal cavity, and it's "window" like thin membranous parts make it an ideal angiogenic test tissue by using intravital microscopy. Other potential advantage is that the intestinal mesentery of mouse, rat, guinea pig, rabbit, cat, and dog is almost identical. The test tissue is a 5–10 μm thin membrane which is covered by a single layer of mesothelial cells covered on both sides bordering onto a delicate basal membrane. The thin membrane sandwiches a tissue space that contains mast cells, histiocytes, fibroblasts, and some lymphocytes. It is the thinnest tissue found in the body of Sprague-Dawley (SD) rats. Avascular part of the test tissue contains predominantly 52% fibroblasts and 48% of the mesothelial cells in adult male SD rats. The connective tissue elements of varying size including collagen, elastin, and elastic fiber are also a part of mesentery test tissue [21].

A microscopic analysis clearly shows the cellular and vascular components of the mesenteric windows [22]. The microvessel number per mm circumference is increased in the 15-week-old male rat as compared to 5.5-week-old which demonstrates a slow progression of physiological angiogenesis to the peripheral part of the windows. The same phenomenon is noticed in female SD rats with an age increase; however, the increase in microvessel length, density, and vascularization is not seen in untreated male SD rats at the age of 7 weeks. The distal part of the mesentery (i.e., standard test tissue) of these rats shows no significant angiogenesis for 2–3 weeks which is the usual duration of angiogenesis assay. The test compound usually in the form of an intraperitoneal injection (i.p.) reaches all targeted microvessel of the test tissue because the mesothelial cell lining is highly permeable to a wide range of the molecular weight of the test compounds. The test tissue is unaffected by inflammation mediated angiogenesis as it is untouched mechanically, and no surgery is involved. The assay was tested for the first time for mast cell-induced angiogenesis and later on inflammatory cytokines, and humoral growth factors were also tested almost near to physiologic level doses [22].

The quantitative assessment of angiogenesis is performed by immunohistochemically using a specific primary monoclonal antibody against the rat endothelium. The assay allows clear cut identification of even the smallest newly formed vessels in the test tissue. Thus, the quantitative vessel parameters (as discussed on page 4) can be measured easily which are very vital to determine molecular activity, the effect of low molecular weight heparinized preparations, and dose-response curves. Computer imaging and microscopic morphometry may be used to further validate the immunohistochemistry findings in a blinded fashion [22].

http://dx.doi.org/10.5772/66504

5.4. The sponge implant assays

The assay was introduced by Andrade and associates by which tested compound is directly injected into a sponge which is implanted subcutaneously in the rat [23]. The assay is used for continuous assessment of the angiogenesis as sterile polyester sponge implants become vascularized, and the measurement of blood flow in sponge by using Xe^{133} clearance technique produces reproducible and objective angiogenesis. The exudate fluid for biochemical analysis may be extracted after local injection of angiogenic stimulator or inhibitors. The assay is useful to study tumor angiogenesis as the sponge implant may replicate the hypoxic tumor microenvironment although the composition of sponge implant may vary [9]. The potential disadvantage of the assay is a nonspecific inflammatory response to sponge implant which may infiltrate the sponge substance as the subcutaneous implant becomes encapsulate due to granulation tissue. A variable composition of sponge sometimes makes inter-experimental comparison difficult, and use of Xe^{133} becomes complicated [23].

5.5. Disk angiogenesis system (DAS)

The assay was introduced to study wound healing and solid tumor angiogenesis as well as the angiogenic response of soluble substances in mice [24]. A synthetic foam disk composed of polyvinyl alcohol foam and covered on both flat sides by filters is inserted into mice abdomen or thorax which is well tolerated. The disk is easy to assemble, and the tested compound or tumor cells suspension is placed at the center of the disk. The slow release of the tested drug or tumor cell suspension is managed by the use of agarose or ethylene-vinyl acetate copolymer. The disk is removed within a period of 7–21 days, during which microvascular growth occurs centripetally into the disc. Paraffin-prepared sections of the disk are used to microscopically view the vascular growth as well as fibroblasts and connective tissue components. The quantitative vessel parameters can be determined by point counting on histological sections, intravascular volume, and so on. The disadvantage of the assay is inflammation-mediated angiogenesis as the disk is always surrounded by fibroblasts whenever vascular growth occurs. Similarly, the kinetic observation of newly formed vessels is difficult because one disk provides information for only one point in time [9].

5.6. The Matrigel plug assay

The Matrigel plug assay was introduced by Passaniti and coworkers in 1992 [25]. The Matrigel was extracted from Engelberth-Holm-Swarm (EHS) tumor, which is rich in ECM proteins. It is a solubilized basement membrane preparation which liquefies at 4°C but reconstitutes into a gel at 37°C when injected subcutaneously into mice where it is slowly surrounded by granulation tissue. The gel induces highly vascularized response under the influence of angiogenic growth factors in particular bFGF [25]. The assay is noninvasive and easy to administer but time-consuming to handle.

The Matrigel composition is not fully defined. However, the major components include epidermal, transforming, platelet, nerve, and insulin-like growth factors (e.g., PDGF, TGF, and bFGF) laminin, collagen, heparin sulfate proteoglycans, and entactin [26]. For this reason, care should be taken while using Matrigel assay for the cellular activity studies. It was observed that when Matrigel with reduced growth factors is implanted, few cells invade the plug or gel. However, with known angiogenic growth factors (e.g., bFGF), mixed with Matrigel and injected subcutaneously, endothelial cells migrate into the gel and constitute vessel-like structures. A fine network of endothelial cell tubes enlarged by micro- and macro-vessel endothelial cells slowly progress to capillary networks in vivo [26].

For the quantitative assessment of angiogenesis, Matrigel and surrounded granulation tissue are removed after 1–3 weeks, and immunohistochemistry and histological sections are measured [27]. However, determining the profiles of capillary-like vessels is difficult. Similarly, the hemoglobin (Hb) test does not differentiate the blood flow in newly formed blood vessels and large parent vessels. Fluorochrome-labeled high molecular weight dextran and quantitative vascular specific indicators are alternative methods to assess neovascularization [27].

The assay is suitable for tissue regeneration experiment model where neovascularization is coupled with organogenesis, fibrosis, and monocytes/macrophages play a pivotal structural role. A possible drawback of the assay is that Matrigel plug contains only capillary network rather than no tissue without any pro- and anti-angiogenic factors to influence angiogenic reactions [28].

A variation of the Matrigel plug assay is the combination of Matrigel and sponge techniques. Five-hundred microliters of Matrigel is injected subcutaneously into mice and solidify for 20–30 min [27]. After that, the mice are anesthetized, skin overlying Matrigel is shaved, and a small nick is made. A similar nick is made to Matrigel plug, and a sterile polyvinyl sponge with the test compound is introduced into the center of the Matrigel plug with the help of tweezers. The same procedure may use for angiogenic growth factors or test tissue to be implanted in the Matrigel plug. By this modification, neovascularization is directional, and assay sensitivity is increased to measure direct angiogenesis as compared to standard Matrigel plug assay. However, the sponge/Matrigel combined assay is time-consuming, and the total number of assayed animals become limited [27].

5.7. Whole-animal angiogenesis model

Zebrafish was introduced in 1999 as a whole small angiogenesis model for the screening of pro-angiogenic compounds which directly influence the newly formed vessels [29]. The choice of the whole animal as a tested tissue was based on the remarkable similarity of zebrafish organs to those of a human at the physiological, anatomical, and molecular levels [30]. Moreover, the short generation time (approx. 3 months) and easy to house in small space and relatively large numbers also facilitate to evaluate many tested animals in one assay [31]. The external development of zebrafish embryos and optical transparency during embryonic stage assists continuous microscopic evaluations of different developmental processes from gastrulation to organogenesis [30]. Furthermore, external mode of fertilization also permits easy access to experiment design and assessment. Small tested compounds dissolve to water diffuse directly to fish embryo and induce distinct and dose-dependent angiogenic effects. Both pro- and anti-angiogenic compounds exhibit similar effects in zebrafish as exerted in mammals [31].

6. Animal models of angiogenesis

In biomedical research, mouse models are of utmost importance for a wide variety of medical tests including gene expression, gene knockout, and medical genetic analysis [32]. For this purpose, SCID, transgenic, and genetically engineered mouse models are of particular interests which allow sophisticated investigations for genetically induced pathological states and molecular pathogenesis of certain genetic disorders. Furthermore, such mouse models are useful to study genes essential for angiogenesis and vascular biology [32]. In parallel to that mice with conditional, global knockouts, over-expressing angiogenic factors are also considerable in this prospect [33]. As remarkable similarity exists between human and murine vasculatures, such tools are valuable to search possible molecular interactions among distinct angiogenic factors in the onset and progression of various human diseases [32, 33]. In the following section, we shed light on some practically used mouse models in the context of pathological angiogenesis which directly plays a part in human diseases.

6.1. Mouse model of angiogenesis in adipose tissue

Genetically engineered mouse model for adipose tissue angiogenesis is highly reproducible and produces robust results because the mice are inbred and share a highly similar genetic background. This approach is irrelevant to humans because high caloric intake and little physical exercise are the predisposing factors for developing obesity instead a little genetics involved. Thus, mice fed on high-fat diet present an ideal animal model to study non-genetically related obesity [34].

6.1.1. Ob/ob mice

The mouse carrying the obese mutation (ob) was first described in 1950, and later on, it was shown that the mutation located in the gene coding for a hormone leptin, which regulates appetite and food intake [35]. The hormone binds to leptin receptor (Ob-R) in the hypothalamus and subsequent cell signaling regulates food uptake, energy expenditure as well as fat and glucose metabolism. Ob/ob mice are deficient in leptin exhibit uncontrolled and continuous food intake which results in a gain of body weight. Consequently, mutated mice weight is three times higher, and body fat content elevates up to fivefold as compared to wild-type species. The mutated mice also show decreased physical activity and energy expenditure, infertility, and immune deficiencies. The mutation is recessive, so the heterozygotes do not display such phenotype [35]. Ob/ob mice can be used as an outstanding model to explore the role of angiogenesis in adipose tissue expansion, and with specific angiogenic inhibitors, obesity may be prevented in such mice [36]. As the leptin kinetics in mice to regulate food intake and obesity are homologous to human, such angiogenic model can be used to search novel therapeutic targets to treat obesity and metabolic disorders [37].

6.1.2. Db/db mice

The mouse strain C57BL/KsJ was first described with an autosomal recessive mutation diabetes (db) in 1966 [38]. Homozygous mice with such mutation are deficient for the leptin receptor and exhibit a phenotype that resembles human diabetes mellitus. The mice with such mutations are also characterized as an obese phenotype. Furthermore, such mice exhibit infertility and hyperglycemia while heterozygotes are typically lived as wild type. Db/db mice can be used to study molecular mechanisms involved in obesity-related diabetes and insulin insensitivity, and the role of angiogenesis and neovascularization can be elucidated in this regard [38].

6.2. Hindlimb ischemic model of angiogenesis

Most of the angiogenic models described above are very useful to study pathological angiogenesis and search for novel anti-angiogenic treatment in the form of angiogenic inhibitors. However, certain pathological states (e.g., myocardial infarction, stroke, and wound healing/regeneration) in human body require accelerated blood vessel growth to reinstate the proper function of such vital organs [39]. In myocardial infarction, an occluded coronary artery obstructs blood flow to a part of the cardiac muscle tissue which leads to severe tissue hypoxia (ischemia). The cardiac muscle requires a regular supply of oxygen and glucose levels for normal function. To overcome tissue hypoxia, the growth of highly functional arteries is eagerly awaited in such situations. Hind limb ischemia in rat or mice presents an excellent model to study and manipulate newly formed vessels in particular arteries in response to tissue hypoxia [39].

In this assay, the arteries supply blood to one back limb of the mice is ligated to stop the blood circulation in the entire limb [40]. The occlusion of arteries leads to tissue ischemia and the initiation of arteriogenesis from collateral arteries. Pro-angiogenic factors and even anti-angiogenic compounds under investigation can be administered to the limb musculature to modulate the arteriogenic response. Doppler angiography is used to evaluate the blood circulation in the hind limb, and the procedure can be repeated in the same animal to know that how the blood flow improves over time. To study newly formed microvessels, the tissue can be excised and stained, and morphology of the blood vessels is elucidated [40].

The assay is the first in class to present therapeutic angiogenesis and widely used in fundamental discoveries to demonstrate that how to generate highly functional and stable arteries therapeutically [39]. On the other side, the potential disadvantage of the assay is very complicated hind limb surgery and requires highly skilled professionals and experienced surgeons. Similarly, the proportion of blood flow in a hind limb may vary after surgery, and it may affect the degrees of tissue hypoxia which ultimately influence on the therapeutic activity of pro- and anti-angiogenic compounds under investigation [39].

6.3. Wound healing assays

The wound healing assay allows to study and evaluate both angiogenesis and vascular maturation/remodeling in injured or damaged tissues [41]. The assay is usually performed on the skin of mice because other accessible tissues (e.g., tail and ears) do not regenerate well. Two circular holes (approx. 5mm in diameter) are punched through the dorsal skin of anesthetized wild-type C57B16 mice. One hole would serve as control while drugs under investigation can be administered on the other. No bandages or sponge is required as no major blood vessels exist in this region of the skin and wound formation allows very little bleeding in the surrounding area. Wound sealing starts within two weeks, and complete wound healing occurs within a month [41].

Photography and measuring of wound area with calipers provide information about wound size, scar formation, and re-epithelization of the wound [41]. The drugs under investigation (either pro- or anti-angiogenic compounds) in this model may be administered either systemically by oral administration, injection, or topically. The drug effects can be determined by excision of the skin tissue, fixed, and stained with specific dyes. The tested compounds may influence regenerative angiogenesis, vessel morphology, and function. The assay is easy to setup, and surgery is very simple. The wound size remains uniform and homogenous for all animals used in one experiment [41].

The potential disadvantage of the assay is that angiogenesis is inflammation-dependent involving blood clotting phenomenon and other complex biological processes and occurs only in the skin [41]. Similarly, skin tissue regeneration is entirely different as compared to other highly vascular tissues such as the heart and nervous system and does not provide an adequate understanding of the role of angiogenesis in tissue regeneration. Furthermore, tissue regeneration is mainly due to reconstitute new tissue rather than repairing or replacing, which is hard to replace in ischemic insults which produce large patches of dead tissue [41].

6.4. Genetically engineered animal model for angiogenesis

Gene expression analysis and gene function studies are contributing widely to almost every research in life sciences, biomedical research, biotechnology, molecular pathology, and human health [42]. In vivo applied and functional genomic studies are particularly considered by overexpressing a candidate gene or suppressing the gene expression for the purpose of gene knockout [43]. Such approaches are achieved and applicable by genome manipulation of wild-type animals [43]. Similarly, the generation of transgenic animals by injecting desired DNA constructs to fertilized eggs also presents some standard technology in gene expression studies [44]. Transgenic animal models and DNA constructs (e.g., gene expression plasmids and vectors) with desired gene expression are widely used to study gene function and molecular pathogenesis of diseases, and it create models to demonstrate the complex, intricate interplay between gene overexpression or suppression for the molecular epidemiology of human diseases [44]. In the following section, we briefly overview such novel approaches to be involved in the context of vascular angiogenesis.

The control of target gene expression in vascular cells of transgenic animals by cell or tissue expression plasmid with specific promoters is very helpful to study developmental and pathological gene function in the vasculature [42]. It was found that the promoters derived from the sequences of VEGFR-1, ICAM-2, vWF, or endoglin efficiently work in mouse endothelial cells both in vivo and in vitro with specific intensity and specificity [42]. Similarly, lacZ selective transgene expression was seen in ECs cells under the control of promoters derived from Tie 2 (angiopoietin receptor), ICAM-2, or VE-Cadherin [42]. However, the expression of a transgene in smooth muscle cells (SMCs) is difficult to achieve because most SMC markers are expressed differentially, and SMC growth and cell differentiation are an exclusive process [42]. In contrast, transgenic mice may obtain using selective promoters expressing smooth muscle myosin heavy chain (SM-MHC), smooth muscle α-actin, and SM22α [42]. Such models provide valuable information about the function of a specific gene in a particular tissue, and controlling the expression of such genes may use as a therapeutic approach to certain disease and also for angiogenesis and cancer [42]. However, the transgene expression depends on promoter's characteristics to be used while constructing cell or tissue expression plasmids with the gene of interests including; promoters is constitutively active, capable to express and replicate gene of interest or to express in embryonic or in the adulthood stage [45]. Failure to do so may limit studies in molecular pathogenesis, leads to nonviable transgenic animals or compensatory responses. More powerful tools are being developed based on conditional transgene expression systems [45].

The inhibition of endogenous gene expression is also a potential method to suppress the gene function involved in the molecular pathogenesis of many genetic disorders and infectious diseases [46]. Many studies show that sequence-specific mRNA degradation by double-strand RNA strongly inhibits the function of that gene involved in pathogenesis or propagation of a particular disease [47]. The technique is known as RNA interference (RNAi) and may be used in certain genetic disorders, in cancer, HIV, and other harder to treat infections. Recent publish data indicate that mammalian expression vectors expressing short hairpin RNA (shRNA) under the control of specific vascular promoters inhibit gene expression through an RNAi effect [47].

7. Angiogenesis and cancer

The phenomenon of angiogenesis is fundamental in tumor growth, progression, and metastasis [48]. Angiogenesis itself is the result of a highly orchestrated series of molecular and cellular events including a plethora of genes, signal cascades, and transcription factors which are highly organized and work in a systematic way to generate microvessels in normal physiological angiogenesis [49]. However, the tumor angiogenesis is disorganized, irregular, and not systematic at the level of molecular and cellular events and ultimately propagates many tumors into cancers [48]. The cancer cells contain the ability to stimulate angiogenesis by producing a lot of angiogenic factors including cell growth factors, cytokines, and numerous other molecules [48, 49].

Many pro- and anti-angiogenic molecules involved in the induction of angiogenesis and neovascularization, their receptor ligands, and intracellular signaling pathways have been identified within last 30 years [50]. Much work has been done to develop anti-angiogenic treatment strategies for cancer patients [51]. However, numerous preclinical trials show no promise regarding high efficacy and tolerability with classical anti-angiogenic drugs as monotherapy [51]. It spurred the researchers and investigators to design and develop novel anti-angiogenic compounds to be used in combination with classical cytotoxic agents and radiotherapy [52]. FDA-approved angiogenesis inhibitors in combination with chemotherapy have proven their clinical worth regarding improved patient survival time and patient tolerability in certain cancers [52].

In the coming section, we briefly overview molecular mechanisms of major cell signaling pathways involved in the induction of angiogenesis, and at the end, some brief glimpse about the clinical impacts of newly developed angiogenic inhibitors will be described. The cellular events in the regeneration and propagation of tumor angiogenesis are already explained briefly at page 5 and depicted in **Figure 1**.

7.1. VEGF intracellular signaling

Vascular endothelial-derived growth factor (VEGF) is one of the most important and potent angiogenic molecules which play an integral role in tumor angiogenesis [50]. It presents the first in a class of cytokines which induce vascular leakage and therefore also known as vascular permeability factor. Until now, six members (VEGF-A to VEGF-F) of this unique family of cytokines have been discovered [53]. VEGF-A is mainly involved in angiogenesis and vasculogenesis whereas VEGF-B is a survival factor for ECs, SMCs, and pericytes [54]. VEGF-C and VEGF-D are essential for lymphangiogenesis, and PGF also acts as a survival factor for ECs and modulates VEGF cell signaling [55].

Vascular endothelial growth factors activate ECs by binding to a family of class III transmembrane receptor tyrosine kinases (RTKs) expressing at high levels in endothelial cell lineage [53]. VEGF-R1 and VEGF-R2 are located on ECs and activate during angiogenesis while VEGF-R3 induces intracellular signaling in lymphatic cells. VEGF-R1 acts as a decoy receptor as it is RTK defective and acts as a negative regulator of angiogenesis (**Figure 2**) [54]. The angiogenic multiple cell signaling pathways are initiated as VEGF-A binds to VEGF-R2, and the receptor dimerizes and intracellular receptor domains are phosphorylated in ECs and induce overexpression of growth factors, cell proliferation, mitogenesis, chemotaxis, and prosurvival signaling (**Figure 2**) [55]. VEGF-C binds to VEGFR-3 and initiates mitogenesis in lymphatic cells and stimulates hyperplasia in parent lymphatic vessels [53–55]. The production of VEGF is regulated by several growth factors produced by the tumor cells including, endothelial growth factor (EGF), transforming growth factor (TGF-α & β), fibroblast growth factor (FGF), and platelet-derived growth factor (PDGF) [54]. Some hormones (e.g., estrogen, thyroid-stimulating hormone (TSH)) and interleukins (e.g., IL-1 & 6) also stimulate VEGF-induced intracellular events in other types of cells [56].

7.2. Notch signaling pathways

The Notch receptors are located on stromal cells and expressed as a heterodimeric complex of two domains, that is, the Notch extracellular domain (NECD) and Notch intracellular domain (NICD) which are associated with each other via noncovalent interactions (**Figure 3a**) [57]. The Notch cell signaling may mimic direct tumor angiogenesis however actively involved to trigger dormant tumors [1]. Notch ligand Delta-like 4 (DLL4) induces cell signaling pathways to improve vascular functions by endocytosis and nonenzymatic dissociation of Notch heterodimer in host stromal cells (**Figure 3a**) [1]. DLL4 inhibition may promote cell proliferation response in ECs which ultimately increase angiogenic sprouting and vessel branching [58]. Despite increased endothelial cell vascularity, the tumor cells perfuse poorly, which reduces cell oxygen concentrations (i.e., increased hypoxia), and consequently, tumor growth is inhibited [59].

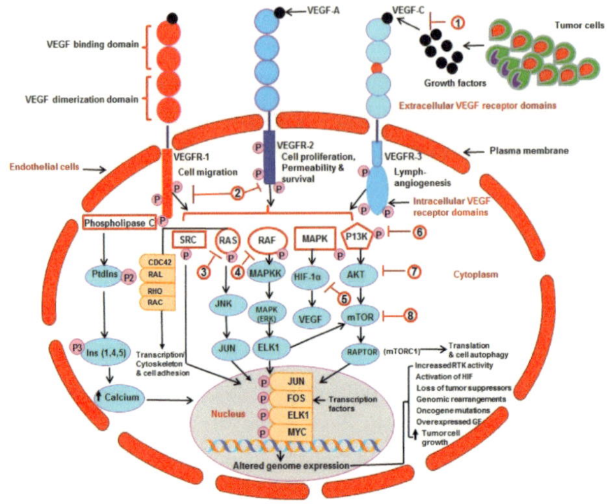

Figure 2. VEGF-induced intracellular signaling in tumor angiogenesis and angiogenic inhibitors with targeted active sites: The binding of vascular endothelial growth factors (VEGF) to respective transmembrane receptors stimulates a plethora of intracellular signaling pathways which regulate nuclear transcription factors for altered gene expressions of normal cell responses including loss of tumor suppression, activation of hypoxia inducible factor (HIF-α), increased receptor tyrosine kinase activity, increased tumor cell growth, and repression of oncogene mutations. Angiogenic inhibitors to their targeted active sites are also shown with numerical circles in the figure. Only anti-angiogenic compounds approved by the US Food and Drug Administration (FDA) for the treatment of numerous solid tumors and carcinomas are depicted where circle 1 represents growth factor inhibitors (bevacizumab, aflibercept); circle 2, growth factor receptor inhibitors (sunitinib, sorafenib); circle 3, RAS inhibitors (tipifarnib, lonafarnib); circle 4, RAF inhibitors (sorafenib); circle 5, HIF-1α inhibitors (geldanamycin, chetomin, echinomycin, 2ME2); circle 6, PI3K inhibitors (wortmannin, LY294002); circle 7, AKT inhibitors (FARA-A); and circle 8, mTOR inhibitors (rapamycin and analogues). JNK = JUN N-terminal kinase; MAPK = mitogen-activated protein serine/threonine kinase, MAPKK = MAPK kinase, PDK1 = phosphoinositide-dependent protein kinase-1; PLC = phospholipase C; PtdInP2 = phosphatidylinositol 4,5-bisphosphate, Ins (1,4,5) = inositol 1,4,5-triphosphates.

In contrast, DLL4 expressed in ECs stimulates Notch 3 receptors located on adjacent cells (e.g., colorectal cancer or T-cell acute lymphoblastic leukemia cells) to activate tumor progression from dormant to active phase [60]. Such findings consider Notch pathways a potential therapeutic target for the design and development of novel anti-angiogenic compounds, although the Notch cell signaling shows a mixed behavior of tumor progression and inhibition in clinical assays [58, 59].

7.3. Transforming growth factor-β (TGF-β)

Transforming growth factor is a ubiquitously expressed paracrine polypeptide of approximately 25 kDa molecular weight [61]. TGF 1 to TGF 3 are three highly homologous isoforms of the polypeptide and discovered in humans and mammals [62]. TGF-β is initially synthesized as a zymogen, and after secretion, an associated peptide is proteolytically sliced to release active form of the growth factor [63].

Active TGF-β binds to constitutively active serine/threonine kinase TGFBR2 receptors to activate TGFBR1 in a heterodimer complex which controls transcription via activation of canonical signal pathways mediated by a family of SMAD proteins (SMAD1-5) (**Figure 3b**) [64]. The

http://dx.doi.org/10.5772/66504

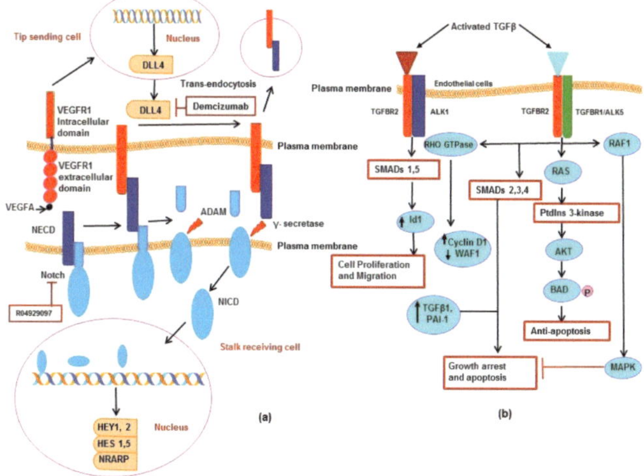

Figure 3. A schematic diagram of Notch and TGF-β induced cell signaling pathways in tumor angiogenesis: (a) Notch cell signaling pathways: The ligand DLL4 dissociates Notch heterodimers by nonenzymatic degradation and cell endocytosis. Notch extracellular domain exposes Notch to ADAM metalloproteases and γ-secretase in sending cells (tip cells) for proteolytic cleavage and the release of Notch intracellular domain which translocates to the nucleus of receiving cells (stalk cells) for the transcriptional activation of Notch target genes (shown in the nucleus of the stalk cells). The DLL4 ligand and Notch inhibitors are also depicted in the red rectangular boxes. (b) Transforming growth factor (TGF-β) induced intracellular signaling pathway: In normal cells, the binding of TGF-β to transmembrane TGFBR2 receptors activates TGFBR1 receptors which upregulate the expression of a series of SMAD proteins (SMAD 2, 3, and 4) and cause cell cycle arrest and apoptosis. However, TGF-β stimulates other molecular pathways in transformed cells to inhibit cell apoptosis and accelerates cell migration and metastasis. In contrast, a second type 1 receptor (ALK1) is expressed in ECs which stimulates cell proliferation and migration via activating SMADs 1 and 5 genes.

activation of SMAD 1 and 5 proteins in transformed cells inhibits apoptosis and mediates cell proliferation and migration via the activation of other cell signaling pathways [65]. However, in normal cells, the stimulation of SMAD 2, 3, and 4 exhibits cell cycle arrests and apoptosis [66]. Similarly, the SMAD 2, 3, and 4 proteins increase the expression of PAI-1which is essential for vessel maturation in angiogenesis (**Figure 3b**) [66].

8. Clinical impact of angiogenic inhibitors

The discovery and development of angiogenic inhibitors have raised the hopes to treat a lot of tumors and carcinomas and ultimately to reduce the morbidity and mortality related to tumors and cancers [67]. Five classes of anti-angiogenic compounds have established and are still under investigation on the basis of potential antitumor drug targeted sites including proteases inhibitors (MMP synthesis inhibitors), ECs proliferation and migration inhibitors, vascular endothelial growth factor inhibitors, cell matrix protein inhibitors, and angiogenic inhibitors with unique mechanisms (**Figure 2**) [68, 69].

Although the anti-angiogenic compounds approved by the FDA show therapeutic efficacy in some categories of cancer as monotherapy, however, sufficient published data recently reveal this fact that angiogenic inhibitors are best therapeutic choices for tumors when used in combination with traditional chemotherapies [70, 71]. However, one would not expect in the first instance that angiogenic inhibitors might reduce the intratumoral delivery of cytotoxic agents (traditional chemotherapy) by decreasing perfused blood vessels with impaired blood flow and decrease drug transport in treated tumor cells [48, 72]. It would also increase tissue hypoxia and inhibit tumor cell proliferation although proliferating cells are an easy target for chemotherapy [48, 72].

To overcome such hurdles and to enhance synergistic therapeutic potential of chemo and anti-angiogenic drugs when used in combination, Kerbel proposed three mechanistic approaches in this scenario to be adopted; first, normalization of tumor microvessels by anti-angiogenic compounds [73, 74]; second, maximum tolerated dose chemotherapy during the break periods of successive courses [72, 75], and third, use of known chemotherapeutic agents having anti-angiogenic effects [72]. The additional advantages of chemotherapy while improving their anti-angiogenic effects may be grabbed by adopting "metronomic chemotherapy" which states that "the administration of chemotherapeutic agents at relatively low, minimally toxic doses on a frequent schedule of administration at regular close intervals, with no prolonged drug-free breaks [76, 77]." By such approaches, endothelial cells are directly killed, and progenitor ECs are suppressed in circulation. Furthermore, minimal use of toxic doses lowers the frequency of adverse events in treated patients [72, 76, 77]. Such treatment strategies may be adopted for a prolonged period of time with angiogenic inhibitors in the treatment of advanced solid tumors with little side effects as validated by phase II clinical trials; however, phase III clinical studies are extensively demanded in this direction [70, 71].

9. Conclusions

In vivo, in vitro, and in ova assays for angiogenesis assessment are the reliable approaches in basic research and to some extent in real-world clinical practices. However, in vivo systems are difficult to perform and time consumable, and the process of quantification is much complicated than in vitro assays. Conversely, these are relatively better due to complex nature of the vascular response to the test compound. In vitro angiogenesis assays may perform in a short period and provide the accurate and reliable outcome of angiogenic processes. Mouse models based angiogenesis assays have also standardized to an improved understanding of tumor angiogenesis and lymphangiogenesis. Similarly, such models are also used to assess vasculogenesis and arteriogenesis in ischemic heart diseases, blindness, psoriasis, and arthritis. Angiogenesis assessment always plays a focal role to determine the pathogenesis and progression of certain challenging diseases in human populations in particular human cancer. An ample understanding of angiogenesis research in tumor progression, by knowing the molecular mechanisms and cellular pathways, also opens the ways to design and develop effective anti-angiogenic inhibitors. The manipulation of the human genome in a precise and predictable manner due to recently developed molecular techniques has opened new gates for the generation of more reliable models for angiogenesis studies and the testing of new therapeutic strategies.

http://dx.doi.org/10.5772/66504

Author details

Imran Shahid[1,2*], Waleed H. AlMalki[1], Mohammed W. AlRabia[3], Muhammad Ahmed[1], Mohammad T. Imam[4], Muhammed K. Saifullah[5] and Muhammad H. Hafeez[6]

*Address all correspondence to: iyshahid@uqu.edu.sa

1 Department of Pharmacology and Toxicology, College of Pharmacy, Umm Al-Qura University, Makkah, Saudi Arabia

2 Applied and Functional Genomics Laboratory, Center of Excellence in Molecular Biology (CEMB), University of the Punjab, Lahore, Pakistan

3 Department of Medical Microbiology, College of Medicine, King Abdul Aziz University, Jeddah, Saudi Arabia

4 Department of Clinical Pharmacy, College of Pharmacy, Umm Al-Qura University, Makkah, Saudi Arabia

5 Department of Pharmaceutical Chemistry, College of Pharmacy, Umm Al-Qura University, Makkah, Saudi Arabia

6 Department of Gastroenterology and Hepatology, Fatima Memorial College of Medicine and Dentistry, Shadman, Lahore, Pakistan

References

[1] Herbert SP, Huisken J, Kim TN, et al. Arterial-venous segregation by selective cell sprouting: an alternative mode of blood vessel formation. *Science* 2009; 326:294–298.

[2] Fidler IJ, Ellis LM. The implications of angiogenesis for the biology and therapy of cancer metastasis. *Cell* 1994; 79:185–188.

[3] Carmeliet P, Jain RK. Angiogenesis in cancer and other diseases. *Nature* 2000; 407:249–257.

[4] Kerbel RS. Tumor angiogenesis: past, present and the near future. *Carcinogenesis* 2000; 21:505–515.

[5] Carmeliet P. Angiogenesis in health and disease. *Nat Med* 2003; 9:653–660.

[6] Adams RH, Alitalo K. Molecular regulation of angiogenesis and lymphangiogenesis. *Nat Rev Mol Cell Biol* 2007; 8:464–478.

[7] Staton CA, Brown NJ, Reed MW. Current status and future prospects for antiangiogenic therapies in cancer. *Expert Opin Drug Discov* 2009; 4:961–979.

[8] Rouslahti E, Rajotte D. An address system in the vasculature of normal tissues and tumors. *Annu Rev Immunol* 2000; 18:813–27.

[9] Hasan J, Shnyder SD, Bibby et al. Quantitative angiogenesis assays *in vivo*—a review. *Angiogenesis* 2004; 7:1–16.

[10] Auerbach R, Auerbach W, Polakowski I. Assays for angiogenesis: a review. *Pharmacol Ther* 1991; 51:1–11.

[11] Vallee BL, Riordan JF, Lobb RR, et al. Tumor-derived angiogenesis factors from rat Walker 256 carcinoma: an experimental investigation and review. *Experientia* 1985; 41:1–15.

[12] Jain RK, Schlenger K, Höckel M, et al. Quantitative angiogenesis assays: progress and problems. *Nat Med* 1997; 3:1203–8.

[13] Fregene TA, Khanuja PS, Noto AC, et al. Tumor-associated angiogenesis in prostate cancer. *Anticancer Res* 1993; 13:2377–2381.

[14] Weidner N, Carroll PR, Flax J, et al. Tumor angiogenesis correlates with metastasis in invasive prostate carcinoma. *Am J Pathol* 1993; 143:401–409.

[15] Craft PS, Harris AL. Clinical prognostic significance of tumour angiogenesis. *Ann Oncol* 1994; 5:305–311.

[16] Gimbrone MA, Cotran RS, Leapman SB, et al. Tumor growth and neovascularization: an experimental model using the rabbit cornea. *J Natl Cancer Inst* 1974; 52:413–27.

[17] Auerbach R, Kubai L, Knighton D, et al. A simple procedure for the long-term cultivation of chicken embryos. *Dev Biol* 1974; 41:391–4.

[18] Ausprunk DH, Knighton DR, Folkman J. Differentiation of vascular endothelium in the chick choriallantois: a structural and autoradiographic atudy. *Dev Biol* 1974; 38:237–48.

[19] Ausprunk DH, Knighton DR, Folkman J. Vascularization of normal and neoplastic tissues grafted to the chick chorioallantois. Role of host and pre-existing graft blood vessels. *Am J Pathol* 1975; 79:597–628.

[20] Folkman J. Tumor angiogenesis. *Adv Cancer Res* 1974; 19:331–9.

[21] Norrby K, Jakbsson A, Sörbo J. Mast-cell-mediated angiogenesis: a novel experimental model using the rat mesentery. *Virchows Arch. [Cell Pathol.]* 1986; 52:195–206.

[22] Norrby K, Jakobsson A, Sörbo J. Quantitative angiogenesis in spreads of intact rat mesenteric windows. *Microvasc Res* 1990; 39:341–8.

[23] Andrade SP, Fan TP, Lewis GP. Quantitative in-vivo studies on angiogenesis in a rat sponge model. *Br J Exp Pathol* 1987; 68:755–66.

[24] Fajardo L-F, Kowalski J, Kwan HH, et al. The disc angiogenesis system. *Lab Invest* 1988; 58:718–24.

[25] Passaniti A, Taylor RM, Pili R, et al. A simple, quantitative method for assessing angiogenesis and antiangiogenic agents using reconstituted basement membrane, heparin, and fibroblast growth factor. *Lab Invest* 1992;67:519–28.

[26] Anghelina M, Krishnan P, Moldovan L, et al. Monocytes/macrophages cooperate with progenitor cells during neovascularization and tissue repair: conversion of cell columns into fibrovascular bundles. *Am J Pathol* 2006; 168:529–41.

[27] Kragh M, Hjarnaa PJ, Bramm E, et al. *In vivo* chamber angiogenesis assay: an optimized Matrigel plug assay for fast assessment of anti-angiogenic activity. *Int J Oncol* 2003; 22:305–11.

[28] Ley CD, Olsen MW, Lund EL, et al. Angiogenic synergy of bFGF and VEGF is antagonized by angiopoietin-2 in a modified *in vivo* Matrigel assay. *Microvasc Res* 2004; 68:161–8.

[29] Serbedzija GN, Flynn E, Willett CE. Zebrafish angiogenesis: a new model for drug screening. *Angiogenesis* 1999; 3:353–9.

[30] Isogai S, Horiguchi M, Weinstein BM. The vascular anatomy of the developing zebrafish: an atlas of embryonic and early larval development. *Dev Biol* 2001; 230:278–301.

[31] Lawson ND, Weinstein BM. *In vivo* imaging of embryonic vascular development using transgenic zebrafish. *Dev Biol* 2002; 248:307–18.

[32] Jensen LD, Cao R, Cao Y. In vivo angiogenesis and lymphangiogenesis models. *Curr Mol Med* 2009; 8:982–91.

[33] Houdebine L M. The methods to generate transgenic animals and to control transgene expression. *J Biotechnol* 2002; 98:145160.

[34] Emanueli CA, Caporali N, Krankel B, et al. Type-2 diabetic Lepr(db/db) mice show a defective microvascular phenotype under basal conditions and an impaired response to angiogenesis gene therapy in the setting of limb ischemia. *Front Biosci* 2007; 12:3–12.

[35] Ingalls JM, Dickie MM, Snell GD. Obese, a new mutation in the house mouse. *J Hered* 1950; 41:17–18.

[36] Brakenhielm E, Cao R, Gao B, et al. Angiogenesis inhibitor, TNP-470, prevents diet induced and genetic obesity in mice. *Circ Res* 2004; 94:79–88.

[37] Friedman JM, Halaas JL. Leptin and the regulation of body weight in mammals. *Nature* 1998;395:63–70.

[38] Hummel KP, Dickie MM, Coleman DL. Diabetes, a new mutation in the mouse. *Science* 1966; 153:1127–8.

[39] Cao Y. Therapeutic angiogenesis for ischemic disorders: what is missing for clinical benefits? *Discov Med* 2010; 9:179–84.

[40] Lundberg G, Luo F, Blegen H, et al. A rat model for severe limb ischemia at rest. *Eur Surg Res* 2002; 35:430–8.

[41] Xue Y, Religa P, Cao R, et al. Anti-VEGF agent confer survival advantages to tumor-bearing mice by improving cancer-associated systemic syndrome. *Proc Natl Acad Sci U S A*, 2008;105:18513–8.

[42] Melo LG, Gnecchi, AS, Pachori D, et al. Endothelium-targeted gene and cell-based therapies for cardiovascular disease. *Arterioscler Thromb Vasc Biol* 2004;24:1761–1774.

[43] Nagy A. Cre recombinase: the universal reagent for genome tailoring. *Genesis* 2000; 26:99–109.

[44] Mallo M. Controlled gene activation and inactivation in the mouse. *Front Biosci* 2006; 11:313–327.

[45] Houdebine L M. Animal transgenesis: recent data and perspectives. *Biochimie* 2002; 84:1137–1141.

[46] Ryding AD, Sharp MG, Mullins JJ. Conditional transgenic technologies. *J Endocrinol* 2001; 171:1–14.

[47] Brummelkamp TR, Bernards R, Agami R. Stable suppression of tumorigenicity by virus-mediated RNA interference. *Cancer Cell* 2002; 3:243–7.

[48] Folkman J. What is the evidence that tumors are angiogenesis dependent? *J Natl Cancer Inst* 1990; 82:4–6.

[49] Folkman J. Tumor angiogenesis: therapeutic implications. *N Engl J Med*. 1971; 285:1182–1186.

[50] Ohta M, Konno H, Tanaka T, et al. The significance of circulating vascular endothelial growth factor (VEGF) protein in gastric cancer. *Cancer Lett* 2003; 192:215–225.

[51] Mauriz JL, Gonzalez-Gallego J. Antiangiogenic drugs: current knowledge and new approaches to cancer therapy. *J Pharm Sci* 2008; 97:4129–4154.

[52] Benny O, Fainaru O, Adini A, et al. An orally delivered small-molecule formulation with antiangiogenic and anticancer activity. *Nat Biotechnol* 2008; 26:799–807.

[53] Yokoyama Y, Charnock-Jones DS, Licence D, et al. Expression of vascular endothelial growth factor (VEGF)- D and its receptor, VEGF receptor 3, as a prognostic factor in endometrial carcinoma. *Clin Cancer Res* 2003; 9:1361–1369.

[54] Kurahara H, Takao S, Maemura K, et al. Impact of vascular endothelial growth factor-C and -D expression in human pancreatic cancer: its relationship to lymph node metastasis. *Clin Cancer Res* 2004; 10:8413–8420.

[55] Adini A, Kornaga T, Firoozbakht F, et al. Placental growth factor is a survival factor for tumor endothelial cells and macrophages. *Cancer Res* 2002; 62:2749–2752.

[56] Carmeliet P, Ferreira V, Breier G, et al. Abnormal blood vessel development and lethality in embryos lacking a single VEGF allele. *Nature* 1996; 380:435–439.

[57] Li JL, Sainson RC, Shi W, et al. Delta-like 4 Notch ligand regulates tumor angiogenesis, improves tumor vascular function, and promotes tumor growth in vivo. *Cancer Res* 2007; 67:11244–11253.

[58] Noguera-Troise I, Daly C, Papadopoulos NJ, et al. Blockade of Dll4 inhibits tumour growth by promoting non-productive angiogenesis. *Nature* 2006; 444:1032–1037.

[59] Ridgway J, Zhang G, Wu Y, et al. Inhibition of Dll4 signalling inhibits tumour growth by deregulating angiogenesis. *Nature* 2006; 444:1083–1087.

[60] Indraccolo S, Minuzzo S, Masiero M, et al. Cross-talk between tumor and endothelial cells involving the Notch3-Dll4 interaction marks escape from tumor dormancy. *Cancer Res* 2009; 69:1314–1323.

[61] de Larco JE, Todaro GJ. Growth factors from murine sarcoma virus transformed cells. *Proc Natl Acad Sci U S A* 1978; 75:4001–4005.

[62] Laiho M, DeCaprio JA, Ludlow JW, et al. Growth inhibition by TGF-beta linked to suppression of retinoblastoma protein phosphorylation. *Cell* 1990; 62:175–185.

[63] Niles RM, Thompson NL, Fenton F. Expression of TGF-beta during in vitro differentiation of hamster tracheal epithelial cells. *In Vitro Cell Dev Biol Anim* 1994; 30A:256–262.

[64] Filvaroff EH, Ebner R, Derynck R. Inhibition of myogenic differentiation in myoblasts expressing a truncated type II TGF-beta receptor. *Development* 1994; 120:1085–1095.

[65] Le Roy C, Leduque P, Dubois PM, et al. Repression of transforming growth factor beta 1protein by antisense oligonucleotide induced increase of adrenal cell differentiated functions. *J Biol Chem* 1996; 271:11027–11033.

[66] Goumans MJ, Valdimarsdottir G, Itoh S, et al. Balancing the activation state of the endothelium via two distinct TGF beta type I receptors. *EMBO J* 2002; 21:1743–1753.

[67] Cobleigh MA, Langmuir VK, Sledge GW, et al. A phase I/II dose escalation trial of bevacizumab in previously treated metastatic breast cancer. *Semin Oncol* 2003; 30:117–24.

[68] Majima M, Hayashi I, Muramatsu M, et al. Cyclo-oxygenase-2 enhances basic fibrobrast growth factor-induced angiogenesis through induction o vascular endothelial growth factor in rat sponge implants. *Br J Pharmacol* 2000; 268:641–9.

[69] Yang JC, Haworth L, Sherry RM, et al. A randomized trial of bevacizumab, an anti–vascular endothelial growth factor antibody, for metastatic renal cancer. *N Engl J Med* 2003; 349:427–34.

[70] Hurwitz H, Fehrenbacher L, Novotny W, et al. Bevacizumab plus irinotecan, fluorouracil, and leucovorin for metastatic colorectal cancer. *N Engl J Med* 2004; 350:2335–2342.

[71] Giantonio B, Catalano PJ, Meropol NJ, et al. High-dose bevacizumab in combination with FOLFOX-4 improves survival in patients with previously treated advanced colorectal cancer: results from the Eastern Cooperative Group (ECOG) study E2300. *J Clin Oncol* 2005; 23(16S):2.

[72] Kerbel RS. Antiangiogenic therapy: a universal chemosensitization strategy for cancer? *Science* 2006 312:1171–1175.

[73] Jain RK. Normalizing tumor vasculature with antiangiogenic therapy: a new paradigm for combination therapy. *Nat Med* 2001; 7:987–989.

[74] Jain RK. Normalization of tumor vasculature: an emerging concept in antiangiogenic therapy. *Science* 2005; 307:58–62.

[75] Hudis CA. Clinical implications of antiangiogenic therapies. *Oncology* (Willits Park NY) 2005; 19:26–31.

[76] Kerbel RS, Kamen BA. The anti-angiogenic basis of metronomic chemotherapy. *Nat Rev Cancer* 2004; 4:423–436.

[77] Kerbel RS, Klement G, Pritchard KI, et al. Continuous low-dose anti-angiogenic/metronomic chemotherapy: from the research laboratory into the oncology clinic. *Ann Oncol* 2002; 13:12–15.

Chapter 16

Novel Methods to Study Angiogenesis Using Tissue Explants

Tomoko Takahashi, Keiko Fujita and Masumi Akita

Additional information is available at the end of the chapter

http://dx.doi.org/10.5772/66400

Abstract

Tissue explants of skeletal muscles, brain, kidney, liver and spleen from mice were cultured using collagen gel. Electron microscopic observation revealed that formation of capillary tubes with pericyte-like cells occurred only from the tissue explant of skeletal muscles. The capillary tubes formed in the collagen gel were positive for tomato lectin and platelet/endothelial cell adhesion molecule (PCAM)-1 antibody. Formation of capillary tubes in the rat was more predominant than in the mouse. Plasmalemmal vesicles were clearly observed in the capillary tubes from rat tissue explant. Muscle fiber-type differences were also observed. In the soleus muscle, the formation of capillary tubes was predominant than the tibialis anterior muscle. Using this culture model from the rat soleus muscle, effects of α-isoproterenol (β-adrenergic receptor agonist) and low-frequency electrical stimulation were examined on the formation of capillary tubes and fine structures of skeletal muscle explant. The formation of capillary tubes was promoted by α-isoproterenol administration. At low-frequency electrical stimulation, the formation of capillary tubes was inhibited. Both α-isoproterenol and electrical stimulation reduced the degeneration of skeletal muscles. This culture method of skeletal muscles may provide a useful model that can examine the effects of various drugs and physical stimulations.

Keywords: angiogenesis, skeletal muscles, collagen gel culture, α-isoproterenol, low-frequency electrical stimulation

1. Introduction

To study the process of angiogenesis and test new agents with angiogenic or anti-angiogenic potential, suitable assays are essential [1]. For in vitro studies of angiogenesis, several culture techniques have been developed. The most commonly used in vivo assays are the chorioallantoic membrane (CAM) assay, the corneal micropocket assay and the dorsal skin-fold assay [2–5]. The corneal micropocket assay, an analysis conducted within an avascular environment, is often used to study the efficacy of angiogenic compounds. The efficacy of anti-angiogenic compounds in inhibiting growth factor-induced vascularization and spontaneous vascularization is usually studied in vascular environments such as the CAM assay or the dorsal skin-fold assay. These assays have proven useful and have dramatically advanced our knowledge of angiogenesis. However, they are also limited in several respects (for a detailed review see Refs. [6, 7]) : (a) complicated surgical techniques are required; (b) only a limited number of test compounds can be assayed (e.g., in the case of the micropocket assay); and (c) simultaneous assessment of both angiogenic and anti-angiogenic compounds in the same assay is not feasible without the addition of exogenous growth factors. Fortunately, the method using collagen gel is free from these limitations. Collagen gel culture has been widely used for analyzing the biological process of angiogenesis [8–11]. Using the collagen gel culture, we have conducted electron microscopic studies and immunohistochemical studies during angiogenesis. In the collagen gel culture of aortic explants, capillary tubes with pericyte-like cells were observed [12]. As a source of angiogenesis, however, aortic explants were generally used in the collagen gel culture. Capillary permeability varies greatly among tissues, and this can be correlated partly with the type of endothelium. For simulation of angiogenesis, establishment of suitable in vitro model of capillaries might be effective. The endothelial cells of some capillaries have fenestrations or pores. For instance, fenestrated capillaries occur in renal glomeruli. Capillaries without fenestrations in the brain and skeletal muscle are known as continuous capillaries. As discontinuous capillaries, there are sinusoids. Sinusoids occur in large numbers in the liver and spleen [13].

In this study, we report the formation of capillary tubes from tissue explants of skeletal muscle, brain, kidney, liver and spleen from mice was cultured using collagen gel. Electron microscopic observation revealed that the formation of capillary tubes with pericyte-like cells occurred only from the skeletal muscle explant. Lectin and immunohistochemical studies showed that the capillary tubes formed in the collagen gel have architecture of capillary in vivo. There were some differences regarding the formation of capillary tubes among animal species and fiber types. We demonstrated that the soleus muscle from rats was most suitable model to study angiogenesis. Using tissue explant from the rat soleus muscle, effects of α-isoproterenol and low-frequency electrical stimulation were examined.

2. Materials and methods

2.1. Collagen gel culture

This collagen culture technique is a modification of our previous works [14, 15]. Samples (soleus muscles, cerebral cortex of frontal lobe, liver, cortex of kidney and spleen) were obtained from 1-month-old ICR male mice (n = 5). The samples were cut into small pieces (2 × 2 × 2 mm) under a stereoscopic microscope. The small pieces were placed at the bottom of tissue culture dish (35 mm; n = 25). Each tissue culture dish consists four pieces. An even layer of reconstituted collagen solution (0.3% Cellmatrix type IA, Nitta Gelatin, Tokyo, Japan) was

http://dx.doi.org/10.5772/66400

overlaid and gelled at 37°C for about 10 min. After gelation, Ham's F-12 medium (Invitrogen Corp., Carlsbad, CA, USA) containing 20% fetal bovine serum (FBS), 1% nonessential amino acids, 100 units/ml of penicillin and 100 mg/ml of streptomycin (Invitrogen Corp., Carlsbad, CA, USA) was added. Cultures were performed for 14 days in an incubator (95% air/5% CO_2). During the culture period, a phase contrast microscope was used to observe the capillary tube formation. These experiments were made three times. To examine the differences in animal species and fiber type, explants from skeletal muscles (soleus and tibialis anterior muscles) from rats were cultured as described above. All animal experiments were approved by the Committee on Animal Experimentation, Saitama Medical University (Permission No. 851 for mice and No. 934 for rats) and carried out in accordance with the "Guidelines for Animal Experimentation at Saitama Medical University."

2.2. Electron microscopy

The cultured materials were fixed with 2.5% glutaraldehyde in 0.1 M phosphate buffer (pH 7.2) for 1 h and then fixed with 1% OsO_4 in 0.1 M phosphate buffer (pH 7.2) for another hour. After dehydration with ethanol, samples were embedded in epoxy resin. After preparation of ultrathin sections, ultrathin sections were stained with uranyl acetate and lead citrate. Kajikawa's tannic acid stain was also used for demonstrating of elastic fibers [16]. The stained ultrathin sections were observed under a transmission electron microscope (JEOL JEM-1010, Tokyo, Japan). When capillary-like structures were observed, following lectin and immunohistochemistry were performed.

2.3. Lectin and immunohistochemistry

After fixation with cold 80% ethanol, capillary tubes were observed with FITC-conjugated endothelial cell-specific tomato lectin (*Lycopersicon esculentum*; EY Labo, CA, USA), a lectin that selectively binds to fucose residues on the endothelial cell surface [17]. Cold 80% ethanol-fixed, collagen gel-embedded specimens were stained by streptavidin/peroxidase immunohistochemistry technique for intercellular adhesion molecule-1 (ICAM-1), platelet/endothelial cell adhesion molecule-1 (PCAM-1) and integrin β_2 detection. The specimens were treated with 0.3% H_2O_2 in methanol to block endogenous peroxide activity and then incubated with the polyclonal rabbit anti-rat ICAM-1, PCAM-1 or integrin β_2 antibody (Santa Cruz Biotechnology, Inc. California, USA). Biotinylated anti-rabbit immunoglobulin was added as a secondary antibody. The horseradish peroxidase labeled streptavidin-biotin complex was then used to detect the second antibody. Finally, the specimens were stained with 3,3'-diaminobenzidine, which was used as a chromogen. The brown or dark brown stained cells were considered as positive. Some specimens were stained with Giemsa before being examined under a light microscope.

2.4. Effects of α-isoproterenol and low-frequency electrical stimulation

Excised material was divided into three groups as follows:

a. α-isoproterenol administration group (n = 48): To the culture medium, 10 μM α- isoproterenol was added [18].

b. low-frequency electrical stimulation group (n = 24): Using C-Dish (ION Optix, Milton, MA, USA), electrical stimulation (50 Hz, 2 h at 1.0 V; [19]) was performed by Ohm Pulser LFP-4000 A (Zen Iryoki corp, Fukuoka, Japan).

c. control group (n = 48): without α-isoproterenol and low-frequency electrical stimulation.

2.5. Semiquantitative enzyme-linked immunosorbent assay (ELISA)

Eight different cytokines involved in angiogenesis in the culture medium were semiquantified by ELISA (Signosis; Angiogenesis ELISA Strip, Santa Clara, CA, USA). Tumor necrosis factor (TNF)-α, vascular endothelial growth factor (VEGF), interleukin (IL)-6, fibroblast growth factor (FGF)-2, interferon (IFN)-γ, leptin, insulin-like growth factor (IGF)-1 and epidermal growth factor (EGF) were tested. ELISA was carried out according to the manufacturer's instructions. Outline is as follows. Eight wells were coated with eight different primary antibodies against a specific angiogenesis cytokine. The test sample was sandwiched between the primary antibody and enzyme-linked antibody. After incubation, unbound-labeled antibodies were washed out. TMB (3,3′,5,5′-tetramethylbenzidine) is added, and the color developed. After addition of stop solution, absorbance is measured spectrophotometrically at 450 nm. The concentrations of the test samples are directly proportional to the color intensity. Data were shown as fold change relative control group.

2.6. Measurement of the length of the capillary tubes

Digital photography equipment (FUJIX DIGITAL CAMERA HC-2500, 3CCD, FUJI PHOTO FILM, Tokyo, Japan) was used with an optical microscope (objective lens ×5). Because capillary tubes were overlapped in the vicinity of the explant, it is impossible to identify each other. Length of capillary tubes was measured from a distance of 200 μm of the outer edge of the explant. Using six culture dishes (four pieces of the explant per dish), capillary tubes captured by the objective lens ×5 (1262 × 991 pixel). It was taken four places of one explant.

2.7. Statistical analysis

Tube formation from the soleus and tibialis anterior muscles of rats is quantified by measuring the length of these capillary tubes in two-dimensional microscope images of six culture dishes. Data were shown as means ± standard error of the mean. Statistical analysis for the data represented was conducted using two samples, with Mann–Whitney U test. A particular result was considered significant if the p value was <0.01 for a two-tailed test.

3. Results

3.1. Collagen gel culture

3.1.1. Skeletal muscles

After 2 days, some cells were migrating in the collagen gel in the vicinity of the explants (**Figure 1a**). Spindle-shaped cells were orientated radially to the explant. After 6–7 days, the cell strands were recognized. At this time, lumen formation could not be clearly demonstrated

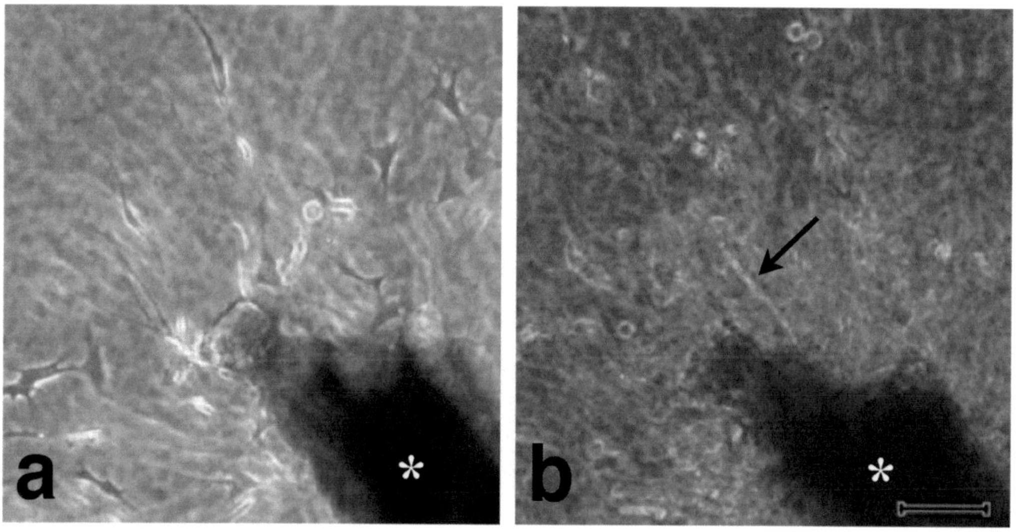

Figure 1. Mouse soleus muscle. (a) After 2 days of cultivation, phase-contrast microscopy reveals fibroblastic cells outgrown from a mouse skeletal muscle explant (*) into a three-dimensional collagen gel. (b) After 6 days of cultivation, phase-contrast microscopy shows a tubular structure protruding (arrow) from a mouse skeletal muscle explant (*) into a three-dimensional collagen gel. Scale bar:90 μm.

(**Figure 1b**). After 10 days, the capillary tube formation with lumen was well demonstrated by electron microscopic observation. As revealed by cross section, several endothelial cells with pericyte-like cells were involved in the composition of capillary tubes (**Figure 2a, b**). The structure as capillary tubes was maintained at least 2 weeks. When the culture was continued, degradation of the capillary tubes was observed.

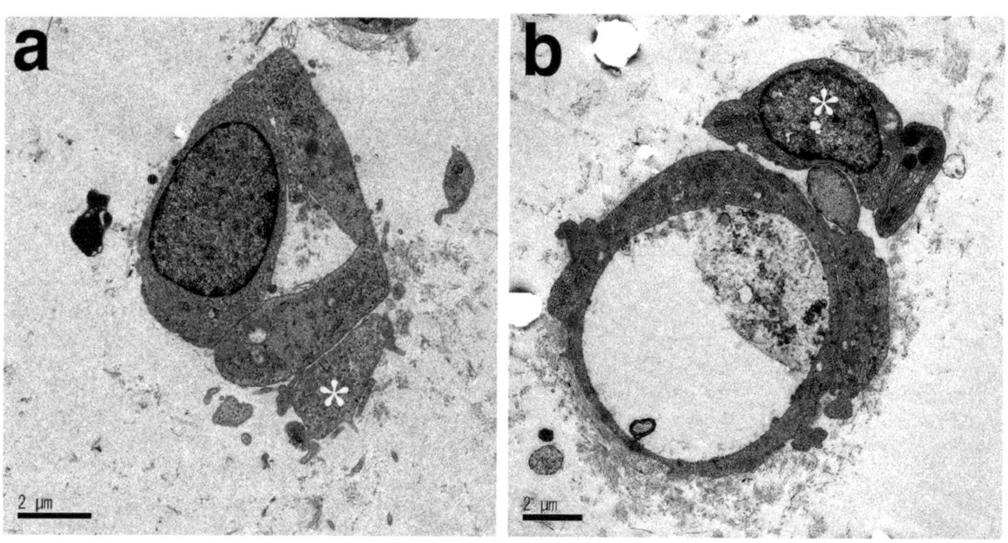

Figure 2. Mouse soleus muscle. (a, b) Electron micrographs of capillary tubes. In a cross section of capillary tube, the lumen is surrounded by two to three cells. Pericyte-like cells (*) are associated with the capillary tube. Scale bar: 2 μm.

3.1.2. Cerebral cortex of frontal lobe

After 3–4 days, spindle-shaped cells were migrated from the explants. The number was quite few. The strand of spindle-shaped cells was elongated (**Figure 3a**). The longitudinal axis was orientated radially to the stump. As revealed by cross section, several cells surrounded a cell with elastic membrane-like structure. Tube formation with lumen was not recognized (**Figure 3b**).

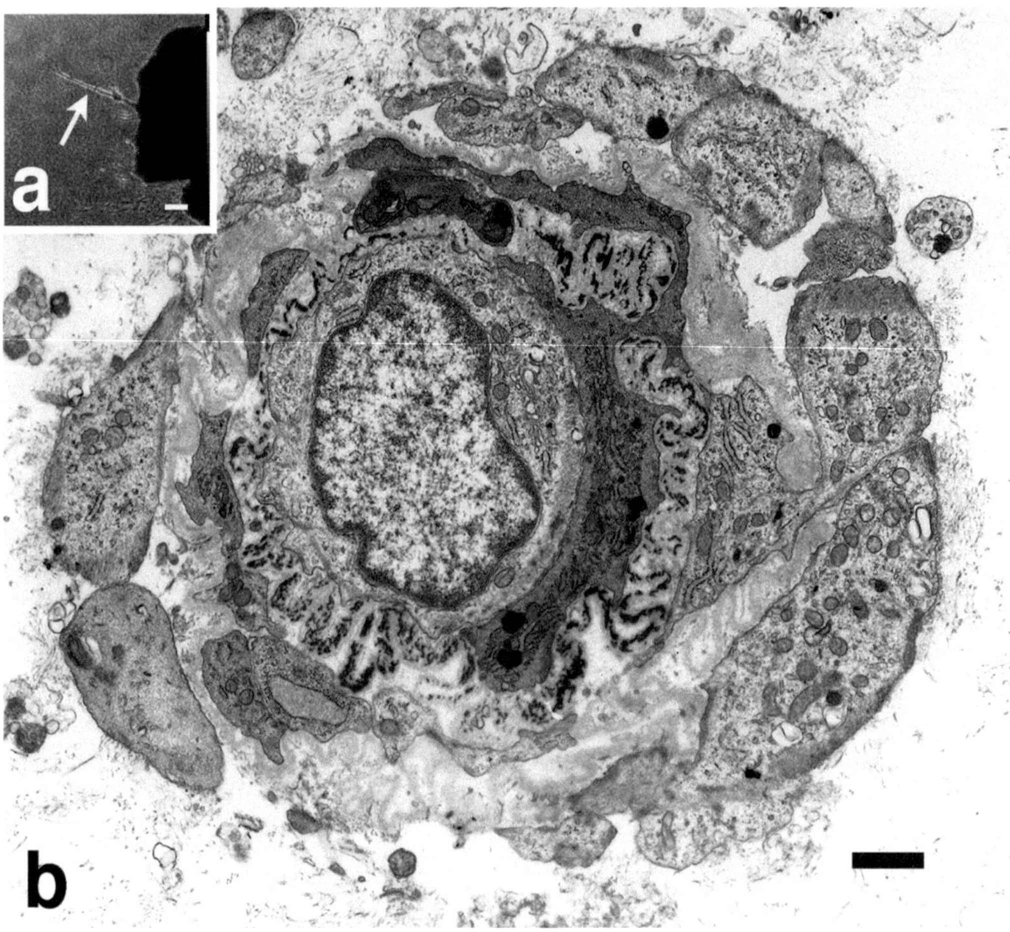

Figure 3. Mouse brain. (a) After 12 days of cultivation, a phase-contrast microphotograph shows tube formation (arrow) from mouse cortex of brain into a three-dimensional collagen gel. Scale bar: 50 μm. (b) An electron microphotograph of the collagen gel-induced tube formation. A cross section shows no lumen. Kajikawa's tannic acid stain for elastic fibers. Electron dense materials are defined among cells. Scale bar:1 μm.

3.1.3. Cortex of kidney

After 3–4 days, spindle- and cobblestone-shaped cells were migrated from the explants. The strands of spindle-shaped cells were elongated (**Figure 4a**). As revealed by cross section, several cells were attached each other and formed cellular mass (**Figure 4b**). Some area, a single cell, formed the outline of a tube with a lumen. A cell of the wall was consisted of microvilli (**Figure 4c**).

http://dx.doi.org/10.5772/66400

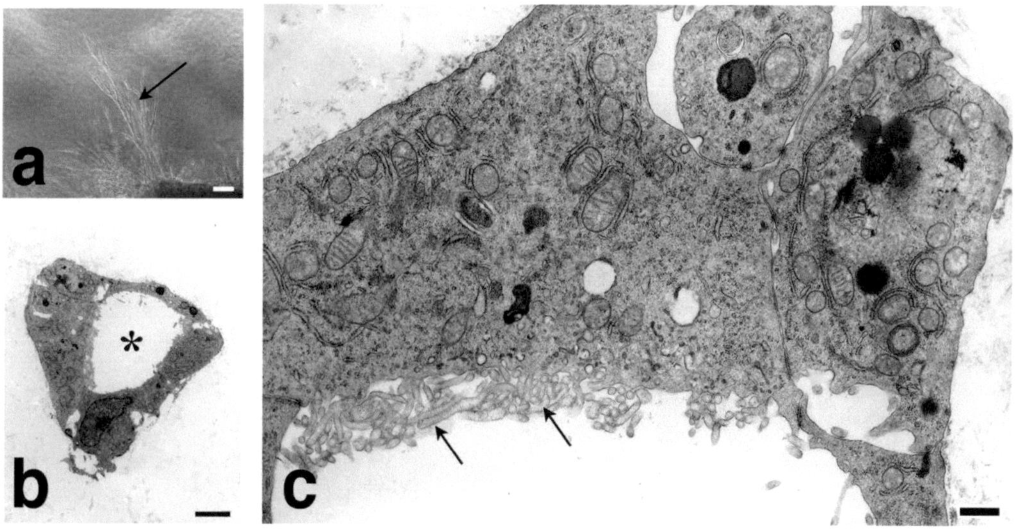

Figure 4. Mouse kidney. (a) After 7 days of cultivation, a phase-contrast microphotograph shows tube-like structure (arrow) from mouse cortex of kidney into a three-dimensional collagen gel. Scale bar: 50 μm. (b) An electron microphotograph of the collagen gel-induced tube-like structure. A cross section shows lumen (*). Scale bar: 2 μm. (c) Enlarged electron microphotograph of the cells showed in (b). Arrows indicate microvilli. Scale bar: 500 nm.

3.1.4. Liver

After 3–4 days, spindle-shaped cells were migrated from the explants. The strands of spindle-shaped cells were elongated (**Figure 5a**). As revealed by cross section, several cells were attached each other and formed cellular mass (**Figure 5b**).

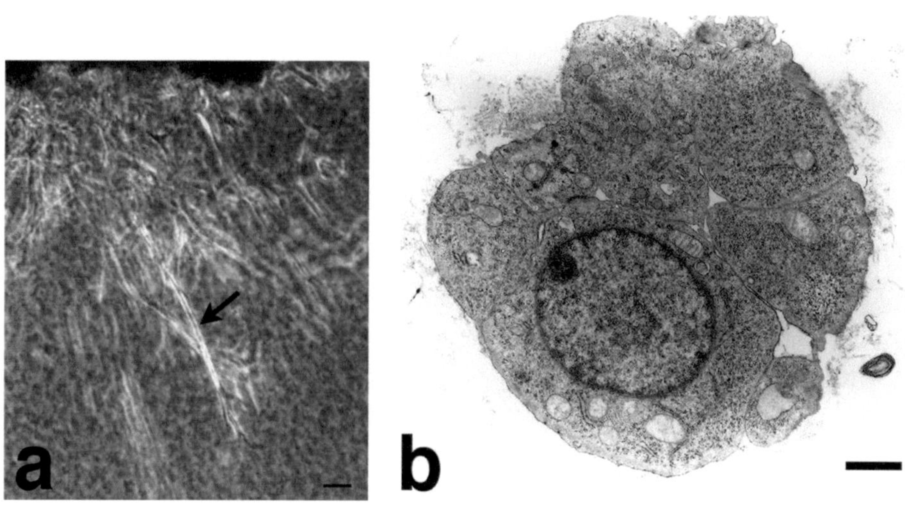

Figure 5. Mouse liver. (a) After 10 days of cultivation, a phase-contrast microphotograph shows tube-like structure (arrow) from mouse liver into a three-dimensional collagen gel. Scale bar: 50 μm. (b) An electron microphotograph of the collagen gel-induced tube-like structure. A cross section shows tightly connected cells. Scale bar: 1 μm.

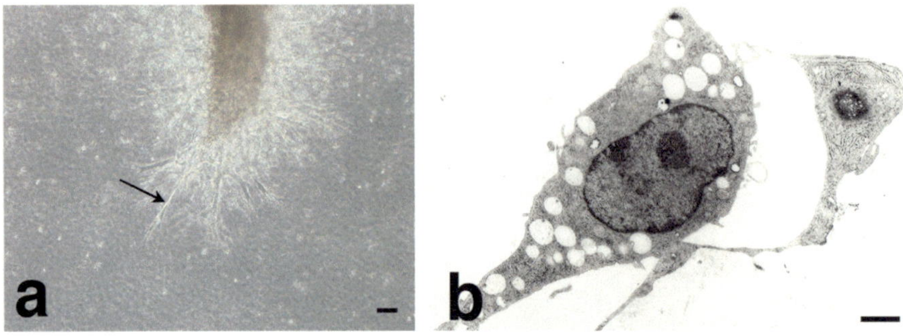

Figure 6. Mouse spleen. (a) After 7 days of cultivation, a phase-contrast microphotograph shows tube-like structure (arrow) from mouse spleen into a three-dimensional collagen gel. Scale bar: 50 μm. (b) An electron microphotograph of the collagen gel-induced tube-like structure. A cross section shows loosely contacted cells. Scale bar: 1 μm.

3.1.5. Spleen

After 2 days, numerous cells were migrated from the explants. Numerous cell strands of spindle-shaped cells were elongated (**Figure 6a**). Some cells were partly contacted, but distinct lumen was not observed (**Figure 6b**).

3.2. Lectin and immunohistochemistry

Since capillary tubes were observed only from the skeletal muscle explants, lectin and immunohistochemistry with antibodies were performed only for the cultured materials from skeletal muscle explants. Capillary tubes formed in the collagen gel were strongly positive for tomato lectin (**Figure 7**). Capillary tubes formed from the explants of muscles showed clearly

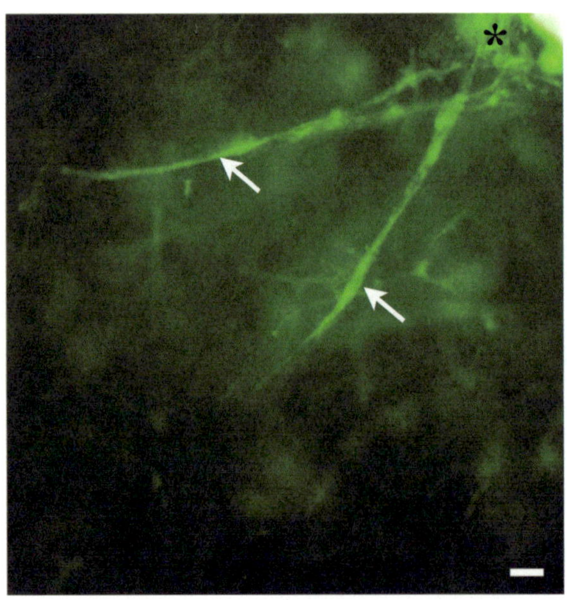

Figure 7. Mouse soleus muscle. After 11 days of cultivation, a fluorescent microphotograph of capillary tube (arrows). Capillary tube is strongly positive for FITC-conjugated endothelial cell-specific tomato lectin. Asterisk shows a muscle tissue explant. Scale bar: 50 μm.

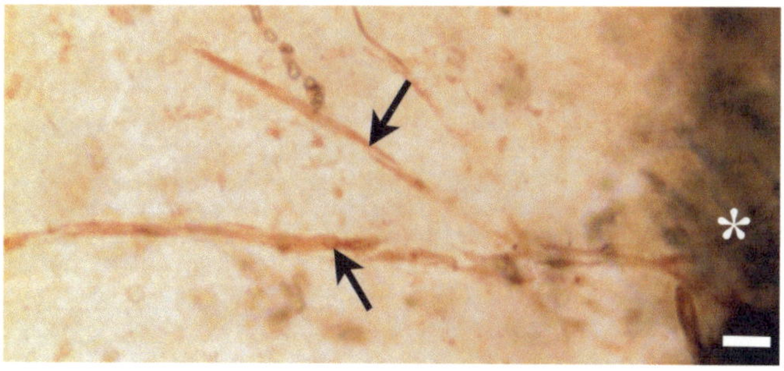

Figure 8. Mouse soleus muscle. Capillary tubes (arrows) showed clearly immunoreactivity of PCAM-1. Asterisk shows a muscle tissue explant. Scale bar: 50 μm.

immunoreactivity of PCAM-1 (**Figure 8**). ICAM-1 and integrin β_2 positive cells were sparsely distributed, but capillary tubes were almost negative (figure not shown).

3.3. Species difference in capillary tube formation from the skeletal muscle explant

In rats, numerous and long capillary tubes were observed from an explant. In mice, capillary tubes were few in number and short. Even without the statistical analysis, the difference is apparent (**Figure 9a, b**). Capillary tubes from rats were also positive for tomato lectin (**Figure 9c**) and PCAM-1 antibody (figure not shown). By electron microscopic observation, plasmalemmal vesicles or caveolae were clearly observed (**Figure 10a, b**). Typical gap junctions and tight junctions were not observed. Larger capillary tubes were also observed (**Figure 11**).

3.4. Difference in capillary tube formation between the soleus and tibialis anterior muscles

In the soleus muscle containing a large amount of red muscle fibers, the formation of capillary tube was predominant than the tibialis anterior muscle containing a large amount of white muscle fibers (**Figure 12a, b**). **Figure 13** indicates the results of statistical analysis.

3.5. Effects of α-isoproterenol and low-frequency electrical stimulation

3.5.1. α-Isoproterenol

Fine structures of explant: compared with the control group, the α-isoproterenol administration group was kept striated pattern (**Figure 14a, b**).

Formation of capillary tubes: in the α-isoproterenol administration group was seen promoting effect on the formation of capillary tubes (**Figure 15a, b**).

3.5.2. Low-frequency electrical stimulation

Fine structures of explant: compared with the control group, the low-frequency electrical stimulation group was kept striated pattern (**Figure 14a, c**).

Formation of capillary tubes: compared with the control group, the formation of capillary tubes was suppressed. Also, it appeared to have led to damage to the migratory cells (**Figure 15a, c**). **Figure 16** indicates the results of statistical analysis.

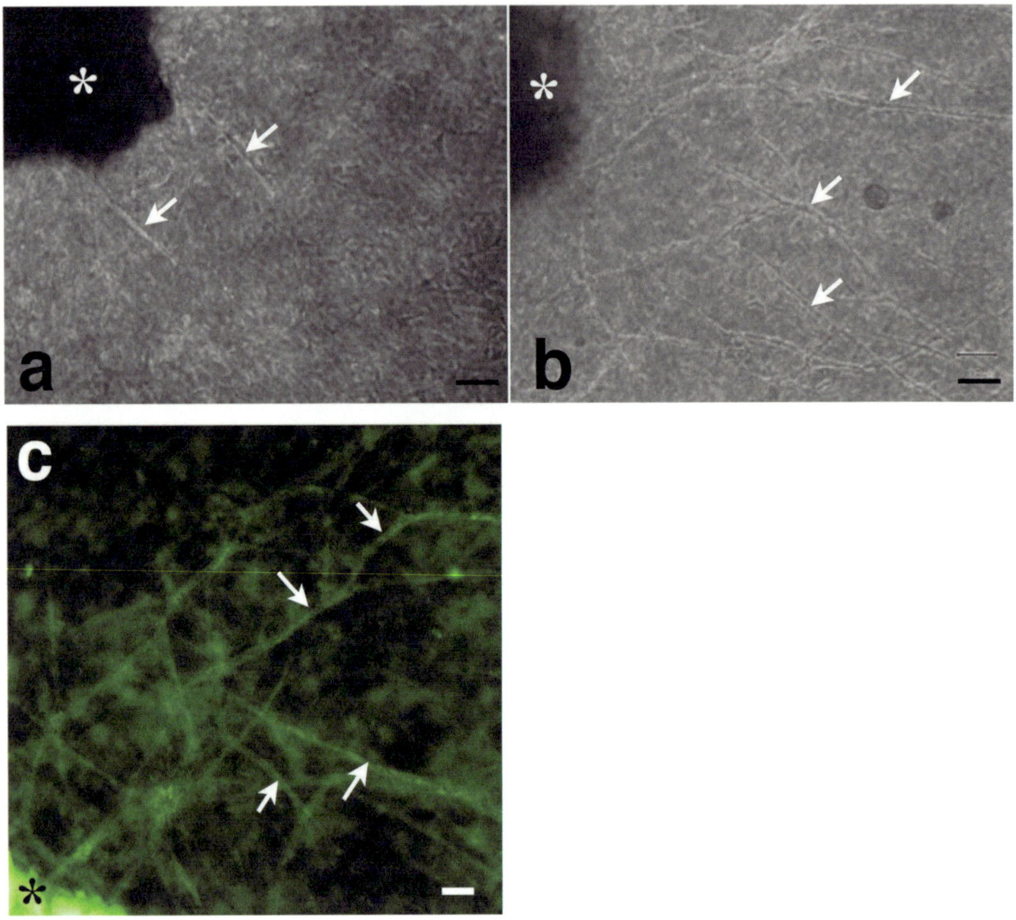

Figure 9. After 10 days of cultivation of soleus muscles. (a) Mouse soleus muscle, (b) rat soleus muscle. Phase-contrast microphotographs. Arrows indicate numerous and long capillary tubes. Scale bar: 90 μm. (c) Rat soleus muscle, tomato lectin staining. Arrows indicate numerous and long capillary tubes (cf. **Figure 7**). Scale bar: 50 μm. Asterisks show a muscle tissue explant.

3.6. ELISA

Compared with the culture medium, significant difference ($p < 0.01$) was observed only in the concentration of FGF-2 in the culture medium of the mouse soleus muscle. In the rat, no significant difference was observed. No significant difference in the concentration of eight kinds of angiogenic factor was observed between the soleus and tibialis anterior muscles from the rat and mouse (data not shown). In the α-isoproterenol administration group, increase in leptin was observed in the rat soleus muscle. However, no significant difference was observed. In the electrical stimulation group, increase in angiogenic factors except for the TNF-alpha was observed. Significant difference ($p < 0.01$) was seen in the concentration of the VEGF, FGF-2 and EGF (**Table 1**).

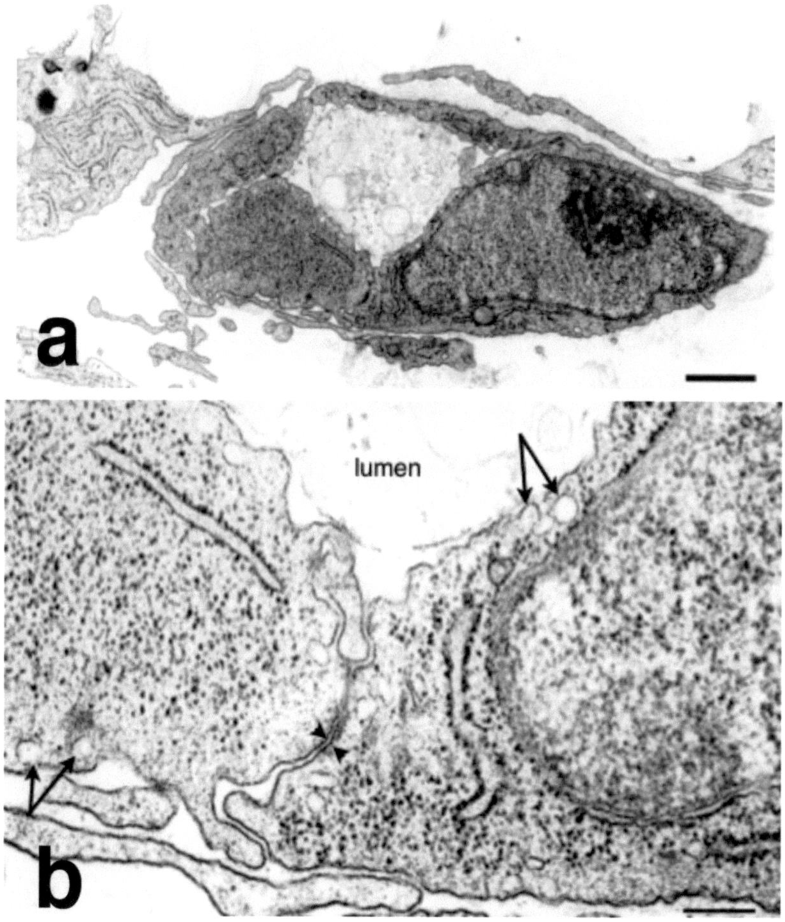

Figure 10. Rat soleus muscle. (a) Electron micrograph of capillary tube from rat soleus muscle. In a cross section of capillary tube, the lumen is surrounded by two to three cells. Scale bar: 1 μm. (b) Higher magnification of a part of (a). Arrowheads indicate a focal adhesion or an adherens junction. Arrows indicate plasmalemmal vesicles or caveolae. Scale bar: 200 nm.

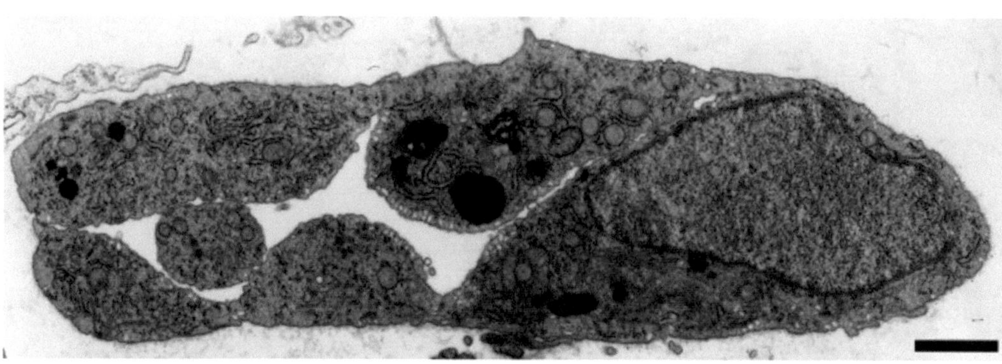

Figure 11. Rat soleus muscle. Electron micrograph of a large capillary tube. The wall is made up by five cells. Scale bar: 1 μm.

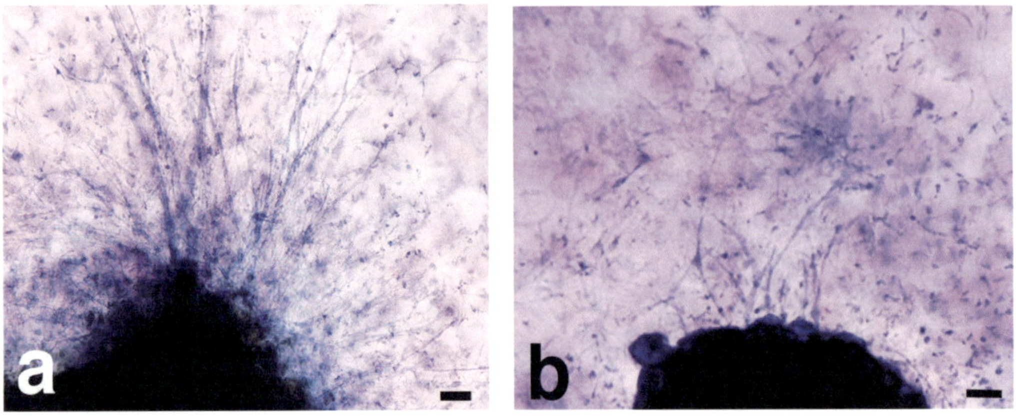

Figur 12. Capillary density of rat soleus and tibialis anterior muscles. (a) Rat soleus muscle, (b) rat tibialis anterior muscle. Capillary tubes were stained by Giemsa solution. Scale bar: 50 μm.

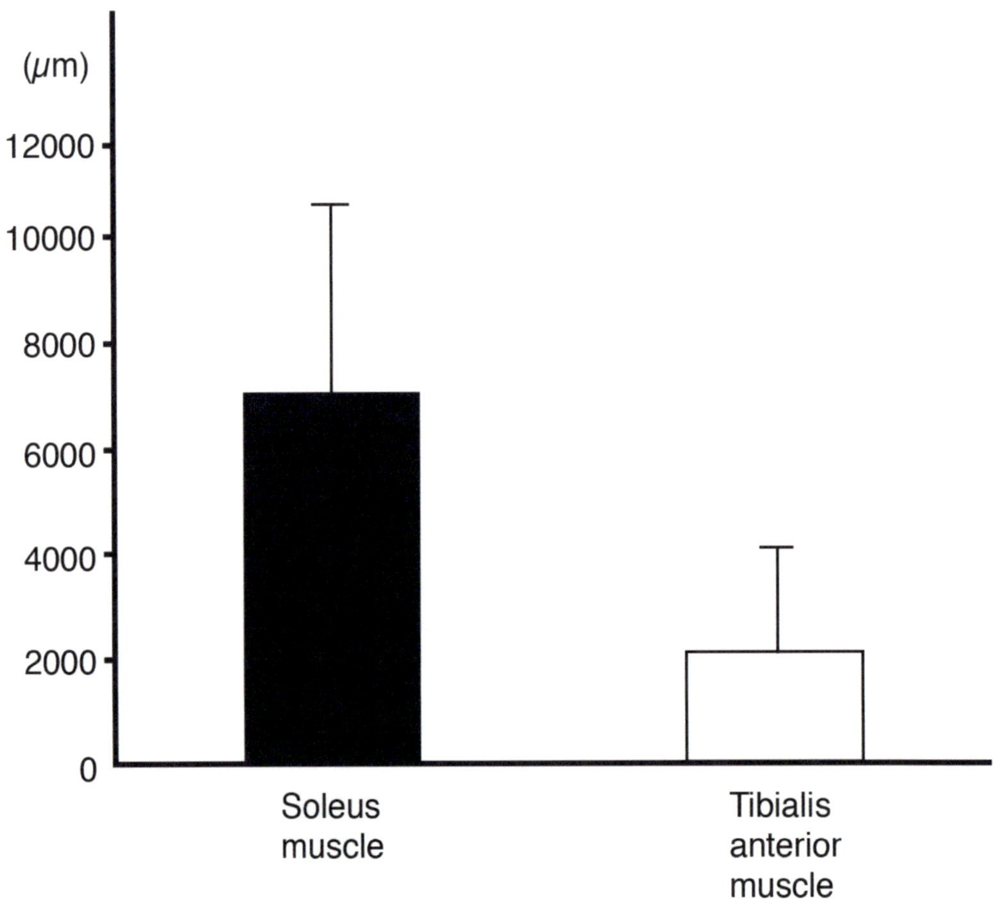

Figure 13. Statistical analysis of length of capillary tubes. Capillary density of soleus muscles had significantly greater than tibialis anterior muscles at $p < 0.01$.

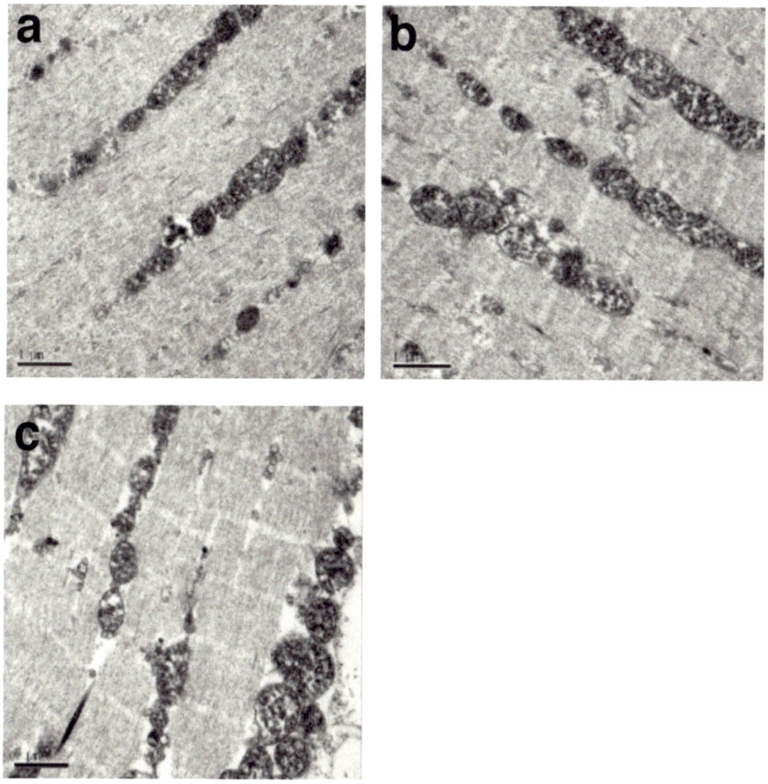

Figure 14. Electron micrographs of tissue explants of rat soleus muscle. (a) Control, (b) α-isoproterenol administration, (c) electrical stimulation. Both α-isoproterenol and electrical stimulation reduced the degeneration of skeletal muscles. Banding pattern of skeletal muscles is maintained when compared to the control. Scale bar: 1 μm.

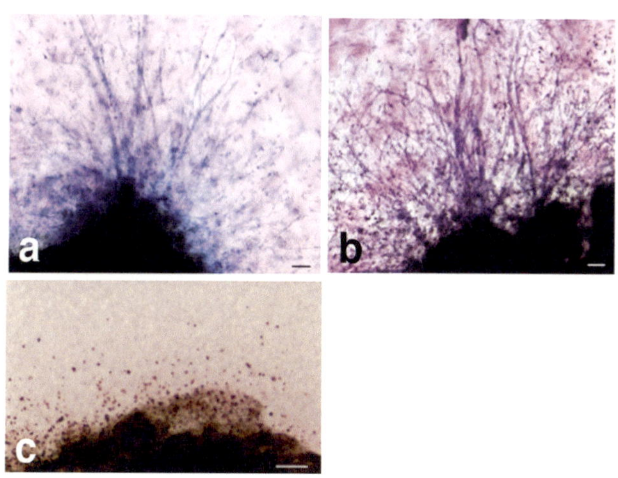

Figure 15. Rat soleus muscle. Effects of α-isoproterenol administration and electrical stimulation. Numerous capillary tubes were observed both control and α-isoproterenol administration groups. No capillary tubes were observed in the electrical stimulation group. (a) Control, rat soleus muscle. (b) α-Isoproterenol administration. (c) Electrical stimulation. Capillary tubes were stained by Giemsa solution. Numerous capillary tubes were observed both control and α-isoproterenol administration groups. No capillary tubes were observed in the electrical stimulation group. Scale bar: 100 μm.

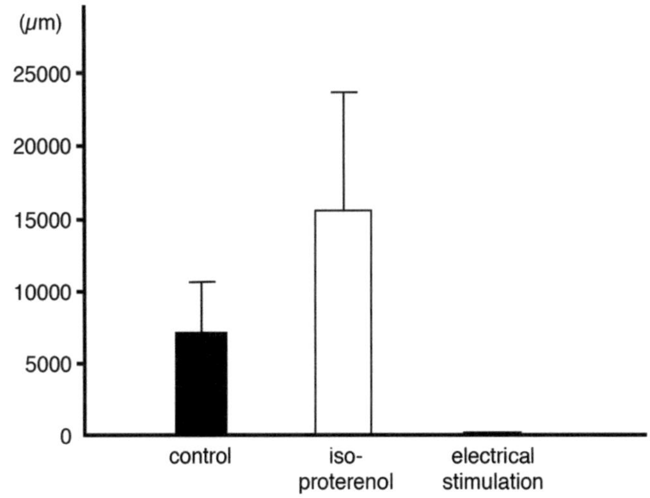

Figure 16. Statistical analysis of length of capillary tubes. Control: rat soleus muscle. The formation of capillary tubes was promoted by α-isoproterenol administration. At low-frequency electrical stimulation, the formation of capillary tubes was inhibited. Capillary density of α-isoproterenol administration group had significantly greater than control group at $p < 0.01$.

	Control	α-Isoproterenol	Electric stimulation
TNF-α	1	1.040	1.016
VEGF	1	0.843	1.542*
IL-6	1	0.980	1.350
FGF-2	1	0.912	1.335*
IFN-γ	1	0.969	1.286
Leptin	1	1.232	1.446
IGF-1	1	0.913	1.003
EGF	1	1.027	1.313*

Data were shown as fold change relative control. In the α-isoproterenol administration group, no significant difference was observed. In the electrical stimulation group, significant difference (*$p < 0.01$) was seen in the concentration of the VEGF, FGF-2 and EGF.

Table 1. ELISA of eight angiogenic factors.

4. Discussion

4.1. Formation of capillary tube from tissue explant of skeletal muscles

In this study, we tested tissue explants of skeletal muscles, brain, kidney, liver and spleen. In the light microscopic level, tubular structures are newly formed from all tissue explants tested. By electron microscopic observation, tubular structures with a lumen were observed only from the tissue explant of skeletal muscles and kidney cortex. By further detail electron microscopic observation, tubular structures from the kidney cortex have microvilli. The capillary tubes had quite similar architecture observed in the collagen gel culture of aortic explant [12]. Plasmalemmal vesicles or caveolae were also observed. Plasmalemmal vesicles are plasma membrane invaginations. They are particularly numerous in the continuous endothelium of microvascular beds such as skeletal muscles in which they have been identified as transcytotic vesicular carriers [20, 21].

In the present study, we demonstrated that capillary tubes have architecture of capillary by tomato lectin, as we have previously shown [22]. Cell adhesion molecules are a family of closely related cell surface glycoproteins involved in cell-cell interactions during growth and are thought to play an important role in embryogenesis and development. PECAM-1, also referred to as CD31, is a glycoprotein expressed on the cell surfaces of endothelial cells, as well as platelets and mononuclear cells. PECAM-1 positive cells were clearly demonstrated as a capillary-like structure. ICAM-1, also referred to as CD54, is an integral membrane protein of the immunoglobulin superfamily and recognizes the $\beta 2\alpha 1$ and $\beta 2\alpha M$ integrins. In the present study, ICAM-1 positive cells were sparse. It may accord with $\beta 2$ integrin which was not detected. We have reported that pericyte-like cells were observed in the aortic explant culture (for a detailed review see Ref. [12]). Pericyte-like cells were positive for actin [12, 23]. In this study, pericyte-like cells were also observed around the capillary tubes, as shown in the aortic explant culture. Pericytes were reported to stimulate angiogenesis through the secretion of growth factors such as fibroblast growth factor (FGF) [24], VEGF and placenta growth factor [25]. In addition, pericytes appear to promote endothelial cell (EC) survival [26] and affect EC behavior such as sprouting [27]. It is strongly suggested that pericytes play an important role in angiogenesis. VEGF is a key promoter of angiogenesis. VEGF acts as a chemoattractant and directs capillary growth. VEGF concentration gradients are important for activation and chemotactic guidance of capillary sprouting [28, 29]. Zhang et al. [30] reported that a variety of cells in the body, including myocyte (skeletal muscle fibers), secrete VEGF at different rates. Ji et al. [31] also reported that VEGF is secreted by myocytes and binds VEGF receptors and neuropilin-1 on endothelial cell surface. Further studies are needed to understand the angiogenic factors.

It should be noted that, when compared with mice and rats, capillary tubes formation was predominant in rats than mice. We could not demonstrate the difference in angiogenic factors between rats and mice. It is widely accepted that endothelial cells derived from different species display different morphological, biochemical and phenotypical heterogeneity [32, 33]. For instance, FGF1 or collagen-coated dish is not required for culturing endothelial cells from the bovine and pig, unlike the rabbit and rat [34]. Difference in the properties of endothelial cells by species is considered in angiogenesis. It should be also noted that there is difference between red and white muscles. The number of capillaries in the soleus muscle of rat is 2.8/muscle fiber. The corresponding value for the tibialis anterior muscle is 1.2–2.0 [35]. The density of capillaries in the soleus muscle is greater than the tibialis anterior muscle. The difference in the capillary density may relate the formation of capillary tubes.

4.2. Effects of α-isoproterenol

Isoproterenol (β-adrenergic receptor agonist) promotes skeletal muscle hypertrophy in several animals, including rats and mice [36, 37]. The hypertrophy by isoproterenol induces through the stimulation of β_2-adrenergic receptor [38], and β-adrenergic receptor is involved in skeletal muscle growth and regeneration [39]. Expression of β-adrenergic receptor and its coupling to cAMP are important components of the signaling mechanism that controls atrophy and hypertrophy of skeletal muscle [40]. We have reported that α-isoproterenol reduced the degeneration of muscle after the facial nerve crush [41]. In this study, the direct effect of α-isoproterenol was confirmed even in vitro.

There are a number of reports about the increase in skeletal muscle capillary density with exercise. Exercise such as endurance training increases the capillary network to adapt to oxygen demand, particularly arteriolar portion of capillaries to favor the oxygen supply [42, 43]. When the endurance training was loaded in normal rats, angiogenesis of the soleus muscle is promoted, and arteriolar portion of capillaries is increased significantly [44]. Increase in arteriolar portion of capillaries is believed to be caused by "arteriolarization of capillaries" promoted by an increase in wall tension [44–46]. From the fact that circulating catecholamines (adrenalin and noradrenalin) are concerned with contraction/expansion of the blood vessels, catecholamines are expected to be associated with an increase in capillary density. Circulating catecholamines, which are adrenergic receptor agonist, are the main hormones whose concentrations increase markedly during exercise [47]. Many researchers have worked on the effect of exercise on these catecholamines and reported 1.5 to >20 times basal concentrations depending on exercise characteristics (e.g., duration and intensity) [48]. The increase in circulating catecholamines results in stimulating of β-adrenergic receptor activity and, consequently, increased intercellular concentration of cyclic AMP [49]. However, we have no direct effect that catecholamines associate with an increase in capillary density. Although an experiment in culture, in the brown fat precursor cells, noradrenalin encourages the growth of capillaries [50]. In the soleus muscle in the present study, α-isoproterenol, which is also an adrenergic receptor agonist, encourages the growth of capillary tubes. Although we could not detect the angiogenic factors, it has become possible to study the direct effect of α-isoproterenol on the skeletal muscle and formation of capillary tubes.

4.3. Effects of low-frequency electrical stimulation

From the results of the electrical stimulation, the effect of suppressing the denaturation of the muscle was observed. Young et al. [39] reported that electrical stimulation increased the number of β-receptors and promoted the synthesis of cAMP.

In this study, we could demonstrate that electrical stimulation also reduced the degeneration of skeletal muscles.

For angiogenesis in skeletal muscle in vivo, Cotter et al. [51] showed an increase in capillary density by the low-frequency electrical stimulation. After that, angiogenesis by skeletal muscle has been made under the various conditions of electrical stimulation [52–54].

For electrical stimulation in vitro, studies using myoblast cell line have been reported [55–57]. However, in vitro study of skeletal muscles capillaries is very few. Endothelial cells isolated from skeletal muscle capillaries are studied to make physical and chemical stress to the cells [58]. A number of angiogenic factors involve in angiogenesis by electrical stimulation [59, 60]. VEGF can be mentioned as the most important proteins. VEGF encourages the growth of vascular endothelial cells. VEGF played a central role in angiogenesis [59, 60].

As the mechanism, skeletal muscle contraction due to electrical stimulation has been considered to induce hypoxia [61, 62] and shear stress [63]. However, Kanno et al. [19] applied the electrical stimulation (50 Hz) without muscle contraction to the skeletal muscle and showed the increase in VEGF protein in vitro, and they showed the increased in capillary density in the rat model of hindlimb ischemia. In this study, the condition (50 Hz) according to the report of Kanno et al. [19] was adopted.

Electrical stimulation upregulated FGF-2 and EGF protein levels in the brains of stroke rats [64]. In this study, VEGF, FGF-2 and EGF protein levels are increased. However, under the condition used in this study, it was harmful to the migrating cells. The effect of promoting angiogenesis was not observed. On the contrary, angiogenesis was inhibited. Further studies including the setting of the condition are necessary.

4.4. The usefulness of this in vitro model

Endothelial progenitor cells derived from bone marrow are present in the peripheral blood. These cells reach the ischemic site, and angiogenesis occurs by proliferation and differentiation. However, it is difficult to collect a large amount of bone marrow stem cells for treatment of ischemia. Transplantation of CD133-positive endothelial precursor cells to the damaged muscle tissue has been studied [65]. In this report, angiogenesis is promoted, and the damaged muscle tissue is expected to recover. Recently, cardiac tissue sheets from human iPS cells have been shown to be effective in engraftment and transplantation in the rat model of myocardial infarction [66]. This cardiac tissue sheets include vascular cells (vascular endothelial cells and pericytes), in addition to the cardiomyocytes. Higher survival rate than the sheet of only cardiomyocytes has been shown. Transplantation including vascular cells may become research to increase the possibility of therapeutic angiogenesis.

In this study, we propose the possibility of autologous transplantation using tissue explants of skeletal muscle in cardiovascular disease including critical hind limb ischemia.

4.5. The drawback of this in vitro model

Clearly, those capillary tubes that emanate from the muscle explants are very similar to capillaries in vivo. However, the capillary tubes are not filled with flowing blood. Although the structure as capillary tubes is maintained at least 2 weeks, further studies are needed for long-term culture.

Author details

Tomoko Takahashi[1], Keiko Fujita[1] and Masumi Akita[2,*]

*Address all correspondence to: makita@saitama-med.ac.jp

1 Department of Anatomy, Saitama Medical University, Saitama, Japan

2 Division of Morphological Science, Biomedical Research Center, Saitama Medical University, Saitama, Japan

References

[1] Deckers M, van der Pluijm G, Dooijewaard S, Kroon M, van Hinsbergh V, Papapoulos S, Lowik C: Effect of angiogenic and antiangiogenic compounds on the outgrowth of capillary structures from fetal mouse bone explants. Lab Invest. 2001; 81:5–15.

[2] Jakob W, Jentzsch KD, Mauersberger B, Heder G: The chick embryo choriallantoic membrane as a bioassay for angiogenesis factors: reactions induced by carrier materials. Exp Pathol (Jena). 1978; 15:241–249.

[3] Fournier GA, Lutty GA, Watt S, Fenselau A, Patz A: A corneal micropocket assay for angiogenesis in the rat eye. Invest Ophthalmol Vis Sci. 1981; 21:351–354.

[4] Kenyon BM, Voest EE, Chen CC, Flynn E, Folkman J, D'Amato RJ: A model of angiogenesis in the mouse cornea. Invest Ophthalmol Vis Sci. 1996; 37:1625–1632.

[5] Lehr HA, Leunig M, Menger MD, Nolte D, Messmer K: Dorsal skinfold chamber technique for intravital microscopy in nude mice. Am J Pathol. 1993; 143:1055–1062.

[6] Jain RK, Schlenger K, Hockel M, Yuan F: Quantitative angiogenesis assays: progress and problems. Nat Med. 1997; 3:1203–1208.

[7] Staton CA, Stribbling SM, Tazzyman S, Hughes R, Brown NJ, Lewis CE: Current methods for assaying angiogenesis in vitro and in vivo. Int J Exp Pathol. 2004; 85:233–248.

[8] Montesano R, Mouron P, Orci L: Vascular outgrowths from tissue explants embedded in fibrin or collagen gels: a simple in vitro model of angiogenesis. Cell Biol Int Rep. 1985; 9:869–875.

[9] Mori M, Sadahira Y, Kawasaki S, Hayashi T, Notohara K, Awai M: Capillary growth from reversed rat aortic segments cultured in collagen gel. Acta Pathol Jpn. 1988; 38:1503–1512.

[10] Nicosia RF, Ottinetti A: Growth of microvessels in serum-free matrix culture of rat aorta. A quantitative assay of angiogenesis in vitro. Lab Invest. 1990; 63:115–122.

[11] Artym VV, Matsumoto K: Imaging Cells in Three-Dimensional Collagen Matrix. Curr Protoc Cell Biol. 2010; Chapter 10: Unit–10.1820. doi:10.1002/0471143030.cb1018s48.

[12] Akita M: Development of in vitro method for assaying anti angiogenic effect of drugs. In: Atta-ur-Rahman, M.Iqbal Choudhary, editors. Anti-Angiogenesis Drug Discovery and Development, Vol. 2. Sharjah: Bentham Science Publishers; 2014, pp. 63-111. doi:10 .2174/97816080586621140201

[13] Standring S: Smooth muscle and the cardiovascular and lymphatic systems. In: Standring S, editor-in-chief. Gray's Anatomy 39th ed. Churchill Livingstone, London: Elsevier; 2005. p.143.

[14] Akita M, Murata E, Merker HJ, Kaneko K: Formation of new capillary-like tubes in a three-dimensional in vitro model (aorta/collagen gel). Ann Anat. 1997; 179:137–147.

[15] Akita M, Murata E, Merker HJ, Kaneko K: Morphology of capillary-like structures in a three-dimensional aorta/collagen gel culture. Ann Anat. 1997; 179:127–136.

[16] Kajikawa K, Yamaguchi T, Katsuda S, Miwa A: An improved electron stain for elastic fibers using tannic acid. J Electron Microsc (Tokyo). 1975; 24:287–289.

[17] Hoffmann S, Spee C, Murata T, Cui JZ, Ryan SJ, Hinton DR: Rapid isolation of choriocapillary endothelial cells by Lycopersicon esculentum-coated Dynabeads. Graefes Arch Clin Exp Ophthalmol. 1998; 236:779–784.

[18] Inomata T, Murata E, Akita M: Effects of α-isoproterenol on the atrophy of soleus and tibialis anterior muscles after sciatic nerve crush injury, and on microstructure of submandibular gland. J Saitama Medical University. 2001; 28:171–178.

[19] Kanno S, Oda N, Abe M, Saito S, Hori K, Handa Y, Tabayashi K, Sato Y: Establishment of a simple and practical procedure applicable to therapeutic angiogenesis. Circulation. 1999; 99:2682–2687.

[20] Fawcett DW: Surface specializations of absorbing cells. J Histochem Cytochem. 1965; 13:75–91.

[21] Stan RV, Roberts WG, Predescu D, Ihida K, Saucan L, Ghitescu L, Palade GE: Immunoisolation and partial characterization of endothelial plasmalemmal vesicles (caveolae). Mol Biol Cell. 1997; 8:595–605.

[22] Fujita K, Komatsu K, Tanaka K, Ohshima S, Asami Y, Murata E, Akita M: An in vitro model for studying vascular injury after laser microdissection. Histochem Cell Biol. 2006; 125:509–514.

[23] Fujita K, Asami Y, Tanaka K, Akita M, Merker HJ: Anti-angiogenic effects of thalidomide: expression of apoptosis-inducible active-caspase-3 in a three-dimensional collagen gel culture of aorta. Histochem Cell Biol. 2004; 122:27–33.

[24] Watanabe S, Morisaki N, Tezuka M, Fukuda K, Ueda S, Koyama N, Yokote K, Kanzaki T, Yoshida S, Saito Y: Cultured retinal pericytes stimulate in vitro angiogenesis of endothelial cells through secretion of a fibroblast growth factor-like molecule. Atherosclerosis. 1997; 130:101–107.

[25] Yonekura H, Sakurai S, Liu X, Migita H, Wang H, Yamagishi S, Nomura M, Abedin MJ, Unoki H, Yamamoto Y, Yamamoto H: Placenta growth factor and vascular endothelial growth factor B and C expression in microvascular endothelial cells and pericytes. Implication in autocrine and paracrine regulation of angiogenesis. J Biol Chem. 1999; 274:35172–35178.

[26] Benjamin LE, Hemo I, Keshet E: A plasticity window for blood vessel remodeling is defined by pericyte coverage of the preformed endothelial network and is regulated by PDGF-B and VEGF. Development. 1998; 125:1591–1598.

[27] Nehls V, Denzer K, Drenckhahn D: Pericyte involvement in capillary sprouting during angiogenesis in situ. Cell Tissue Res. 1992. 270:469–474.

[28] Gerhardt H, Golding M, Fruttiger M, Ruhrberg C, Lundkvist A, Abramsson A, Jeltsch M, Mitchell C, Alitalo K, Shima D, Betsholtz C: VEGF guides angiogenic sprouting utilizing endothelial tip cell filopodia. J Cell Biol. 2003; 161:1163–1177.

[29] Helm CL, Fleury ME, Zisch AH, Boschetti F, Swartz MA: Synergy between interstitial flow and VEGF directs capillary morphogenesis in vitro through a gradient amplification mechanism. Proc Natl Acad Sci USA. 2005; 102:15779–15784.

[30] Zhang QX, Magovern CJ, Mack CA, Budenbender KT, Ko W, Rosengart TK: Vascular endothelial growth factor is the major angiogenic factor in omentum: mechanism of the omentum-mediated angiogenesis. J Surg Res. 1997; 67:147–154.

[31] Ji JW, Mac Gabhann F, Popel AS: Skeletal muscle VEGF gradients in peripheral arterial disease: simulations of rest and exercise. Am J Physiol Heart Circ Physiol. 2007; doi:10.1152/ajpheart.00009.2007

[32] Fajardo LF. The complexity of endothelial cells. A review. Am J Clin Pathol. 1989; 92:241–250.

[33] Browning AC, Gray T, Amoaku WM: Isolation, culture, and characterisation of human macular inner choroidal microvascular endothelial cells. Br J Ophthalmol. 2005; 89:1343–1347. doi:10.1136/bjo.2004.063602

[34] Yamamoto K: Methods for long-term cultivation of endothelial cells (in Japanese). Murota S Editor. Modern Chemistry 16, Tokyo: Tokyo Kagaku Dojin; 1989, pp. 151–157.

[35] Schmalbruch H, Oksche A, Vollrath L: Skeletal muscle, v.II/6, Handbook of Microscopic Anatomy. Berlin, Tokyo: Springer-Verlag; 1985. pp. 22–30.

[36] Deshaies Y, Willemot J, Leblanc J: Protein synthesis, amino acid uptake, and pools during isoproterenol-induced hypertrophy of the rat heart and tibialis muscle. Can J Physiol Pharmacol. 1981; 59:113–121.

[37] Mersmann HJ: Species variation in mechanisms for modulation of growth by beta-adrenergic receptors. J Nutr. 1995; 125:1777S–1782S.

[38] Hinkle RT, Hodge KM, Cody DB, Sheldon RJ, Kobilka BK, Isfort RJ: Skeletal muscle hypertrophy and anti-atrophy effects of clenbuterol are mediated by the 2-Adrenergic receptor. Muscle Nerve. 2002; 25:729–734.

[39] Beitzel F, Gregorevic P, Ryall JG, Plant DR, Sillence MN, Lynch GS: 2-Adrenoceptor agonist fenoterol enhances functional repair of regenerating rat skeletal muscle after injury. J Appl Physiol. 2004; 96:1385–1392.

[40] Young RB, Bridge KY, Strietzel CJ: Effect of electrical stimulation on beta-adrenergic receptor population and cyclic amp production in chicken and rat skeletal muscle cell cultures. In Vitro Cell Dev Biol Anim. 2000; 36:167–173.

[41] Ishii K, Sowa K, Zhai WG, Akita M. Effects of α-isoproterenol on denervation atrophy in orbicularis oculi muscle fibers. Histol Histopathol. 1998; 13:1015–1018.

[42] Suzuki J, Gao M, Batra S, Koyama T: Effects of treadmill training on the arteriolar and venular portions of capillary in soleus muscle of young and middle-aged rats. Acta Physiol Scand. 1997; 159:113–121.

[43] Suzuki J, Kobayashi T, Uruma T, Koyama T: Time-course changes in arteriolar and venular portions of capillary in young treadmill trained rats. Acta Physiol Scand. 2001; 171:77–86.

[44] Suzuki J: Effects of endurance training on skeletal muscle capillarity in IDDM model rats. 2004; 7:1–7. http://s-ir.sap.hokkyodai.ac.jp/dspace/handle/123456789/6776

[45] Price RJ, Owens GK, Skalak TC: Immunohistochemical identification of arteriolar development using markers of smooth muscle differentiation. Evidence that capillary arterialization proceeds from terminal arterioles. Circ Res. 1994; 75:520–527.

[46] Price RJ, Skalak TC: A circumferential stress-growth rule predicts arcade arteriole formation in a network model. Microcirculation. 1995; 2:41–51.

[47] Paroo Z, Noble EG: Isoproterenol potentiates exercise-induction of Hsp70 in cardiac and skeletal muscle. Cell Stress & Chaperones. 1999; 4:199–204.

[48] Zouhal H, Jacob C, Delamarche P, Gratas-Delamarche A: Catecholamines and the effects of exercise, training and gender. Sports Med. 2008; 38:401–423.

[49] Hoffman BB, Lefkowitz RL: Catecholamines and sympathomimeric drugs. In: Gilman AG, Rall TW, Taylor AS, editors. The Pharmacological Basis of Therapeutic drugs. New York: Pergamon Press; 1990. pp.187–219.

[50] Yamashita H, Sato N, Kizaki T, Oh-ishi S, Segawa M, Saitoh D, Ohira Y, Ohno H: Norepinephrine stimulates the expression of fibroblast growth factor 2 in rat brown adipocyte primary culture. Cell Growth Differ. 1995; 6:1457–1462.

[51] Cotter M, Hudlická O, Pette D, Staudte H, Vrbová G: Changes of capillary density and enzyme pattern in fast rabbit muscles during long-term stimulation. J Physiol. 1973; 230:34P–35P.

[52] Brown MD, Cotter MA, Hudlická O, Vrbová G: The effects of different patterns of muscle activity on capillary density, mechanical properties and structure of slow and fast rabbit muscles. Pflugers Arch. 1976; 361:241–250.

[53] Hudlicka O, Tyler KR: The effect of long-term high-frequency stimulation on capillary density and fibre types in rabbit fast muscles. J Physiol. 1984; 353:435–445.

[54] Hudlicka O: Growth of capillaries in skeletal and cardiac muscle. Circ Res. 1982; 50:451–461.

[55] Ohno Y, Yamada S, Sugiura T, Ohira Y, Yoshioka T, Goto K: Possible role of NF-κB signals in heat stress-associated increase in protein content of cultured C2C12 cells. Cells Tissues Organs. 2011; 194:363–370.

[56] Goto K, Okuyama R, Sugiyama H, Honda M, Kobayashi T, Uehara K, Akema T, Sugiura T, Yamada S, Ohira Y, Yoshioka T: Effects of heat stress and mechanical stretch on

protein expression in cultured skeletal muscle cells. Pflugers Arch. 2003; 447:247–253. doi:10.1007/s00424-003-1177-x

[57] Iwata M, Nishihama K, Tsuchida W, Suzuki S: The hypertrophic effect of electrical pulse stimulation on cultured skeletal muscle cells. J Health Sci, Nihon Fukushi Univ. 2013; 16:1–7.

[58] Milkiewicz M, Doyle JL, Fudalewski T, Ispanovic E, Aghasi M, T Haas TL: HIF-1α and HIF-2α play a central role in stretch-induced but not shear-stress-induced angiogenesis in rat skeletal muscle. J Physiol. 2007; 583:753–766.

[59] Hang J, Kong L, Gu JW, Adair TH: VEGF gene expression is upregulated in electrically stimulated rat skeletal muscle. Am J Physiol. 1995; 269(5 Pt2):H1827–1831.

[60] Annex BH, Torgan CE, Lin P, Taylor DA, Thompson MA, Peters KG, Kraus WE: Induction and maintenance of increased VEGF protein by chronic motor nerve stimulation in skeletal muscle. Am J Physiol. 1998; 274(3 Pt2):H860–867.

[61] Hudlicka O: Is physiological angiogenesis in skeletal muscle regulated by changes in microcirculation? Microcirculation. 1998; 5:7–23.

[62] Forsythe JA, Jiang BH, Iyer NV, Agani F, Leung SW, Koos RD, Semenza GL: Activation of vascular endothelial growth factor gene transcription by hypoxia-inducible factor 1. Mol Cell Biol. 1996; 16:4604–4613.

[63] Hudlicka O, Price S: The role of blood flow and muscle hypoxia in capillary growth in chronically stimulated fast muscles. Pflugers Arch. 1990; 417:67–72.

[64] Xiang Y, Liu H, Yan T, Zhuang Z, Jin D, Peng Y: Functional electrical stimulation-facilitated proliferation and regeneration of neural precursor cells in the brains of rats with cerebral infarction. Neural Regen Res. 2014; 9:243–251. doi:10.4103/1673-5374.128215

[65] Shi M, Ishikawa M, Kamei N, Nakasa T, Adachi N, Deie M, Asahara T, Ochi M: Acceleration of skeletal muscle regeneration in a rat skeletal muscle injury model by local injection of human peripheral blood-derived CD133-positive cells. Stem Cells. 2009; 27:949–960. doi:10.1002/stem.4.

[66] Masumoto H, Ikuno T, Takeda M, Fukushima H, Marui A, Katayama S, Shimizu T, Ikeda T, Okano T, Sakata R, Yamashita JK: Human iPS cell-engineered cardiac tissue sheets with cardiomyocytes and vascular cells for cardiac regeneration. Sci Rep. 2014; 4:6716. doi:10.1038/srep06716.

Section 5

Pro-angiogenic and Anti-angiogenic Therapies

Chapter 17

Therapeutic Angiogenesis: Foundations and Practical Application

Pavel Igorevich Makarevich and
Yelena Viktorovna Parfyonova

Additional information is available at the end of the chapter

http://dx.doi.org/10.5772/66411

Abstract

Angiogenesis as therapeutic target has emerged since early works by Judah Folkman, yet his "holy grail" was inhibiting vascular growth to block tumor nutrition. However, in modern biomedicine, "therapeutic angiogenesis" became a large field focusing on stimulation of blood vessel growth for ischemia relief to reduce its detrimental effects in the tissues. In this review, we introduce basic principles of tissue vascularization in response to ischemia exploited in this field. An overview of recent status in therapeutic angiogenesis is given with introduction to emerging technologies, including gene therapy, genetic modification of cells ex vivo and tissue engineering.

Keywords: therapeutic angiogenesis, growth factors, cytokines, gene therapy, cell therapy, plasmid, viral vector

1. Introduction

Blood vessel growth is a natural process driven by multiple stimuli of which hypoxia is one of the strongest inducing potent response until O_2 pressure is normalized by the blood coming through de novo formed vasculature. However, a large group of diseases is caused by hypoxic or ischemic state of tissue. These include peripheral artery disease (PAD) and intermittent claudication (IC), coronary heart disease (CHD), myocardial infarction (MI) and ischemic stroke. Accompanied by endothelial dysfunction and age-related reduction of angiogenic response, they result in disabilities and mortality rate of 25–25% annually. Existing strategies for surgical bypass or endovascular interventions have limited efficacy as far as a cohort of non-option patients expands reaching 25–50% after certain extent of disease progression. Moreover, long-term prognosis after most interventions is negative as grafts undergo restenosis and vascular biocompatible prosthetics are yet to come for wide application. This drew attention of physicians and researchers to the concept of angiogenic therapy to stimulate body's own resource and form new blood vessels to relieve ischemia. During recent decade the field of biomedicine known as *therapeutic angiogenesis* evolved rapidly using protein delivery, gene therapy, cell therapy and tissue engineering for induction of vessel growth and overview of its basic concepts and recent achievements will be presented to the reader in chapters below.

2. Biological foundations of therapeutic angiogenesis

Postnatal growth of blood vessels is mediated by three mechanisms: vasculogenesis, angiogenesis and arteriogenesis [1]. Vasculogenesis is de novo formation of vasculature from specific progenitor or stem cells; however, it is attributed to prenatal period and after birth its role is unclear [2] and major extent of blood vessel formation involves two other mechanisms focusing our attention on them. Molecular and cellular basics underlying these processes became the cornerstones of therapeutic angiogenesis and become the source of novel objects for applied researchers and translational medicine.

2.1. Angiogenesis: hypoxia-driven growth of blood vessels

Angiogenesis is the formation of a blood vessel de novo, yet in contrast to vasculogenesis, it relies on migration, proliferation and sprouting of existing endothelial cells (EC) comprising capillaries. The latter are small (8–15 μm) vessels lacking tunica media responsible for majority of tissue blood supply and O_2/CO_2 exchange [3]. Reduction of tissue O_2 induces angiogenesis response in health (intense exercise, tissue growth, etc.) and in disease: in the case of interrupted or declining supply due to atherosclerotic lesions or anemia [4]. Under normal condition, capillaries are stabilized by autocrine and paracrine stimuli (Notch1 axis, angiopoietins, thrombospondin, angiostatin, transforming growth factor (TGF)-β, etc.) that balance influence of pro-angiogenic cytokines within blood vessels' vicinity (vascular endothelial growth factors (VEGFs), fibroblast growth factors (FGFs), hepatocyte growth factor (HGF), platelet-derived growth factor (PDGF)). Hypoxia dislodges this balance toward angiogenic events and this is mediated by O_2-sensitive system existing in a variety of cells including EC themselves, smooth muscle cells (SMC), pericytes and fibroblasts. Cells respond to hypoxia via a system of hypoxia-induced factors (HIFs) [5]—a group of heterodimeric transcription regulators controlled by O_2-sensitive prolyl hydroxylases. Briefly, stability of HIFs is increased drastically in hypoxic environment resulting in their binding to hypoxia-responsive elements within promoter regions of genes increasing their expression [6]. HIF-dependent genes include a vast array of cytokines stimulating EC proliferation, blood vessel sprouting and, thus, labeled "angiogenic growth factors" [7, 8]. The latter include soluble growth factors associated with EC proliferation and differentiation (acidic FGF (aFGF), basic FGF (bFGF), HGF, VEGFs) [9, 10] and cytokines bound to extracellular matrix (ECM) and released during its cleavage [11]. These changes induce EC proliferation and migration forming a vascular sprout guided by a "tip cell." This cell follows a gradient of concentration and produces matrix metalloproteinases (MMPs) and urokinase (uPA) to cleave the ECM [12], releasing growth factors and basically tunneling ECM followed by "stalk cells" that form a new capillary [13]. After lumen

http://dx.doi.org/10.5772/66411

formation occurs normalized blood supply switches off hypoxic stimuli, "tip cells" lose their phenotype and proteolytic potential [14] commencing microenvironment stabilization. Expression of tissue metalloproteinase inhibitors and Dll4-Notch1 axis [15] induction in EC is followed by reestablishment of a balanced state between pro- and antiangiogenic molecules in the tissue leaving a new capillary-sized blood vessel [16]. However, it should be mentioned that this sequence of events never occurs as a perfectly tuned mechanism. "Stub" branches are formed and must be removed, certain "tip cells" fail to form a sprout and maturation of vascular network includes dissociation of certain anastomoses [16], which overall describes angiogenesis as a dynamic process modulated by multiple stimuli [17]. Finally, under influence of stabilizing signals from surrounding EC, pericytes and stromal cells, the vascular bed returns to normal steady state.

2.2. Arteriogenesis: shear stress-induced vascular remodeling

Arteriogenesis is triggered by rise of shear stress after an occlusion and induces collateral vessel remodeling forming a bypass 20–100 μm in diameter with developed tunica media. Arteriogenesis may occur gradually (e.g., in increasing stenosis of a large-caliber artery) or can be triggered by a rapidly developed occlusion with both situations are to result in effective blood flow delivery "around an obstacle" to distal portions of the limb or organ [18]. Certain studies show that collateral remodeling can be reversible till certain point of this process in case shear stress drops to normal after thrombolysis or surgical thrombectomy [19]. Effective arteriogenesis may bypass up to 30–40% of basal blood flow in critical stenosis and thrombosis, which is sufficient for tissue survival. However, its efficacy is drastically reduced in disease and with aging [20]. Smoking-related hypercoagulation, hypertension and diabetes also limit arteriogenic response resulting in critical level of ischemia and tissue loss [21].

After pressure rise in collaterals above the site of thrombosis, shear stress induces EC membrane deformation and flow-sensitive ion channels activate downstream MAP-kinase (ERK1/2, Rho, etc.) phosphorylation and expression of, growth factors, adhesion molecules and chemokines (interleukin-8, macrophage chemoattractant proteins, etc.) [20]. Eventually leukocytes begin to "roll" on EC surface resembling inflammatory changes of vascular function and infiltrate the collateral's wall [22]. Pivotal role in wall thickening is played by monocytes and their differentiated forms—macrophages and dendritic cells. Their function is not limited to ECM and basal lamina cleavage by MMP and uPA production to destabilize the collateral and make it "flexible" [23], but they seem to profoundly change the properties of the blood vessel by induction of SMC proliferation and hypertrophy [24]. Under these influences, media thickness may increase 3- to 4-fold and collateral vessel's volume can enlarge up to 20-fold [25]. Moreover, monocytes produce a wide spectrum of angiogenic and mitogenic cytokines, some of which have antiapoptotic properties required for tissue protection [26]. The role of monocytes and macrophages has been especially emphasized in cardiac arteriogenesis where immunosuppressive steroid hormones [27], anti-inflammatory therapies and even aspirin [28] have been shown to negatively impact the outcomes and collateral remodeling. Toxic depletion of monocytes by clodronate reduced arteriogenesis in cryo-injured myocardium and led to decreased ventricular function and higher mortality [29]. As collaterals increase shear stress stimulus is relieved and EC reduce production of chemokines and lose their "adhesive" phenotype. Macrophages limit production of proteolytic enzymes and start

ECM reconstruction producing collagens, laminin and elastin and forming adventitial and medial portions of a new arterial vessel.

Typically, we mention "therapeutic angiogenesis" referring gene or cell therapy to relieve ischemia. Nevertheless, one may see that angiogenesis and arteriogenesis share common mediators—namely growth factors and enzymes, ECM components, EC activation, etc. Eventually, for adequate function therapeutic angiogenesis has to rebuild both—medium/large-caliber arteries providing influx of blood and capillary-sized vessels that deliver it to the cells.

3. Therapeutic angiogenesis: methods and approaches

3.1. Protein-based therapeutics

After the discovery of proteins with angiogenic effects, the concept of their therapeutic application was introduced by the 1990s and a vast array of animal studies was published to demonstrate angiogenic efficacy of recombinant protein delivery. Going beyond the VEGF family, experimental works showed induction of angiogenesis by FGFs, HGF, PDGF and placental growth factor (PlGF) in small rodents and rabbits [30, 31]. Injection of these cytokines to ischemic tissue or blood vessels increased perfusion and vascular density. However, promise of this method was questioned as far as achievement of local pharmacological concentration by injection was extremely expensive (especially for human body mass) and half-life of most cytokines was too low to render potent effects [32]. Furthermore, little was known on pharmacokinetics of recombinant proteins delivered intravascularly and their potential involvement in tumor growth and chance of "washout" to systemic blood flow raised safety concerns.

In 2000, the first clinical trials of recombinant human bFGF were initiated in PAD/IC patients after a pilot study showing safety and tolerance of intra-arterial delivery of bFGF solution. Unfortunately, it was halted prior to completion of protocol due to urinalysis data revealing proteinuria in bFGF-treated subjects and no positive changes of endpoints at the moment when the trial was put to a premature end [33]. The final attempt to achieve success in the field was the Therapeutic angiogenesis with recombinant fibroblast growth Factor-2 for intermittent claudication (TRAFFIC) randomized placebo-controlled trial in patients with PAD showing significant improvement in walking time and ankle-brachial index (ABI) in bFGF group. However, safety profile was compromised and yet no cardiac adverse effects or evidence for tumor formation was found in recurrent cases of proteinuria and signs of nephrotoxicity were an issue [34].

These results were as disappointing as valuable for the field and suggested that gene therapy with its local sustained expression of desired protein is the best alternative possible [32]. Recently, no further attempts to implicate protein delivery for therapeutic angiogenesis were made in clinics and advantages of other methods are exploited to patients' benefit.

3.2. Gene therapy for angiogenesis

Gene therapy relies on delivery of genetic information by introduction of nucleic acids to target cells/tissues using vector systems. This results in local expression and production of desired protein over a certain period depending on vector used and properties of tissue. First

http://dx.doi.org/10.5772/66411

experiments indicating possibility of in vivo gene delivery using simple injection of a recombinant plasmid DNA (pDNA) opened the gate for hundreds of studies published within the last two decades [35].

As far as the "cornerstone" of gene therapy is the vector system, a brief overview of existing options is required. General concept in the field is that all vectors can be divided into "viral" and "nonviral" subgroups covering nearly any possible way of genetic material delivery. Among nonviral vectors, pDNA is the most widely used due to its long-studied safety profile, ease of production and low immunogenicity allowing repetitive administration [31, 36]. Moreover, plasmids are feasible for combined delivery of several growth factors by mixing them in a formulation or generating a multicistronic vector. However, low transfection efficacy (0.5–2.0% in various tissues) in large mammals including human is an efficacy-limiting issue for pDNA [37]. Viral delivery systems comprise a broad spectrum of recombinant or chimeric viruses of different capacity having a great potential. The latter is due to high transduction efficacy and long expression period accompanied by tissue tropism in certain viruses. However, disadvantages are safety issues: immune reactions and risk of carcinogenesis due to integration to host genome. The most widely spread vectors include adeno- [38], adeno-associated [39] and retroviruses, yet in therapeutic angiogenesis, the latter have limited application due to high risk of insertional mutagenesis [40]. Recent progress of molecular engineering allowed development of optimized viral systems exploiting their advantages as well as novel more effective pDNA systems [41, 42].

Period of growth factor-based gene delivery dates back to the seminal study by Dr. J. Isner [43] who used injection of pDNA encoding VEGF-A 165 (VEGF165) isoform to succeed in treatment of a non-option patient with critical limb ischemia. "First in-human" data were supported by Baumgartner et al. who found increased collateral formation after intramuscular delivery of VEGF165 and EC proliferation in amputation material providing proof of mechanism [44]. Later a number of vectors using VEGF-A and its isoforms were evaluated in experimental and clinical trials making it the most intensively studied object in therapeutic angiogenesis.

Among numerous clinical examples, one may highlight the first "head-to-head" comparison of adenovirus with VEGF165 (Ad-VEGF165) and liposome-packed pDNA-VEGF165 in PAD patients undergoing angioplasty. The trial showed low clinical efficacy of both approaches—Rutherford severity class stayed comparable to control group yet vascular density was increased after treatment [45]. This and other studies using catheter delivery hinted that this method lacks site specificity and intramuscular injection technique was generally adopted. However, initial Groningen double-blind placebo-controlled trial intramuscular injection of pDNA-VEGF165 in PAD patients with diabetes mellitus failed the primary endpoint (amputation rate), yet improvements in ulcer healing, TcO_2 and ABI were observed [46].

Later, Regional angiogenesis with VEGF (RAVE) trial was the first double-blind placebo-controlled trial of VEGF-A 121 isoform (VEGF121). This cytokine is considered to have better solubility than VEGF165 isoform as it lacks a heparin-binding domain [47]. Key feature of this study was an attempt to perform dose optimization of Ad-VEGF121 dividing 105 patients with PAD/IC into three subgroups that received a single session of 20 intramuscular injections of AdVEGF165 delivering low dose (4×10^9 particles), high dose (4×10^{10} particles), or placebo. Final assessment after 12 weeks revealed no significant differences in endpoints between control and treatment subgroups, yet dose-dependent increase of edema adverse effect was observed. Indeed, since first studies delivery of VEGF-A isoforms was haunted by evidence of edema formation due to its influence on endothelial permeability [48] with certain authors claiming this was a putative reason for low efficacy of therapy [49].

Trials in MI patients were initiated as early as in 1998 using a pDNA-VEGF165 showing good safety profile and no positive changes [50]. It was followed by Kuopio Angiogenesis Trial [51] using a comparative design with Ad-VEGF165 or pDNA-VEGF165 delivery by intramyocardial injection during transcutaneous angioplasty. In this trial, no differences between control and treatment groups were found, yet at 6 months after injection of Ad-VEGF165, myocardium perfusion was higher than pDNA-VEGF165, which was attributed to its high transduction efficacy. EuroInject One trial gave similar results showing no significant improvement of myocardial perfusion after injection of pDNA-VEGF165, yet local contractility was higher than control [52].

Trials using delivery of HGF were initiated and conducted by Dr. Morishita's group aiming to treat PAD by intramuscular injection of pDNA-HGF. Encouraging results in animal models [31, 53] promoted clinical translation and after safety assessment a Phase II trial was initiated comparing single and repeated dose of pDNA-HGF in favor of multiple injections: only this dosing regimen showed improvement of TcO_2 compared to control [54]. Further results in a placebo-controlled I/IIa phase trial showed good safety with no traces of secreted HGF in peripheral blood and repeated injection of 8 mg pDNA-HGF showed significant improvements of secondary endpoints (ulcer size, ABI and pain reduction) [55]. Similar results were obtained in a placebo-controlled trial in PAD patients where by the end of week 12, 70% decrease of ulcer size was observed [56]. Further attempts to increase efficacy included the use of a bicistronic plasmid encoding two forms of HGF named dHGF and cHGF. They were evaluated in animal models showing better perfusion after expression of dHGF + cHGF than each one alone [57]. Clinical trial of this approach in PAD patients showed that multifocal intramuscular injections of 4–16 mg of pDNA-dHGF/cHGF resulted in improvement within 3 months independently of dose: rest and walking pains reduced and a trend toward ulcer healing and increase of TcO_2 was observed [58].

Overall, we may expect HGF-based drugs to become the first widely marketed for PAD—in Japan it has been registered under "Collategene" name and now undergoes stage III clinical trial in PAD cohort. Furthermore, despite HGF has never been tested for MI treatment in clinical settings, preclinical assessments indicate that it may be effective as it has antifibrotic and angiogenic mode of action that can be a good option for this disease or subsequent ventricular failure due to tissue scarring [53, 59].

Fibroblast growth factor has been the first used in protein delivery and gene therapy studies were to follow as soon as it gained attention. Therapeutic angiogenesis leg ischemia study for the management of arteriopathy and non-healing ulcer (TALISMAN-201) have evaluated pDNA-FGF-1 in no-option PAD patients [60] and showed improvements as decreased amputation rate within 1 year after treatment [61] and its prospective part showed reduced general mortality in treated subjects [62]. However, phase III placebo-controlled "TAMARIS" (n = 525) trial drew disappointing results and all primary endpoints including amputation events failed to improve after treatment by pDNA-FGF-1 [62, 63]. Similar results obtained in OPTIMIST and

EuroOPTIMIST trials indicated safety and lack of efficacy after treatment and lead to wrapping up of this prospective drug testing. Nevertheless, in a follow-up stage, important safety data showing no increased cancer, stroke, or MI in FGF-treated patients was obtained and positively impacted new proceedings in the field [64].

In MI patients, FGF-4 was delivered using an intracoronary injection of an adenovirus with this gene (Ad-FGF-4) in an Angiogenic gene therapy (AGENT) trial. Result evaluation showed that the only subgroup with reduced size of ischemic myocardium after treatment was female patients when compared to male subgroup. The authors speculated that it may be attributed to higher extent of microcirculatory disorders in females [65, 66] accompanied by fewer critical stenosis typical in men [67]. As far as FGF-4 is known to positively influence endothelial function, this might have been the mechanism for observed changes in the trial. Among other therapeutic factors used for stimulation of angiogenesis, HIF-1α and development endothelial locus-1 (DEL) are both worth a mention as far as they made it to the bedside in recent years using adenovirus or pDNA vectors. However, trials showed minimal improvement in PAD patients and further evaluations were ceased up to date [68, 69].

Overall despite failure to show expected efficacy in clinic, gene therapy is safe and well tolerated by patients showing little evidence although long-term evaluations are yet to be completed. Key obstacle in pDNA-mediated gene therapy relates to transfection efficacy and thus protein production levels after administration [70]. Viral vectors show some promise in solving the problem, yet optimization of dosage regimen, delivery routes and administration protocols also provide a field for further development.

From the point of translational potential, pDNA-based gene therapy has the best safety profile and the best results are definitely yet to come in the following years yet points for improvement are obvious. Efficacy improvement in gene therapy can be achieved by combined approaches basing on the point that angiogenesis is a dynamic process controlled by numerous cytokines, each playing its party in initiation/cessation of different stages. This puts the basis for combined gene therapy to treat ischemia with higher efficacy and it has been supported by experimental findings using VEGF165 combined with another pro-angiogenic growth factor: bFGF [71], PDGF [72], angiopoietin-1 [73], or Stromal cell-derived factor-1α (SDF-1α) [74]. Our previous experience in mouse hind limb ischemia model showed that combination of VEGF165 and uPA [75] or HGF [76] induced angiogenic response more effectively than each factor alone or allowed to reduce pDNA dose for combined delivery [75]. A crucial transcription factor in angiogenesis, HIF-1α, was also used for combined gene therapy with VEGF165 showing good results in animal model [77] as well as bFGF + heme oxygenase-1 (HO-1) [78]. Regarding the latter, it is known that HO-1 is an important regulator of endothelial function with protective function. Its expression is known to induce angiogenesis in ischemic tissues and blockade or knockout reduces EC proliferation and motility and thus capillary growth [79].

Triple combined gene therapy has not been evaluated for angiogenesis, yet a study was published where controlled release scaffolds containing a mix of VEGF165, HGF and angiopoietin-1 or their double combinations were evaluated for enhancing efficacy of endothelial progenitor cell (EPC) therapy. Triple combinations resulted in significantly higher

SMC counts indicating more efficient vessel stabilization due to angiopoietin-1 effects on perivascular cell chemotaxis [80].

Authors claimed that the use of VEGF165 + another cytokine typically leads to decreased edema and vascular permeability: this has been shown for a well-known stabilizing cytokines—angiopoietin-1 [73] and HGF [81]. Thus, another rationale for combined therapy is decrease of certain "side effects" observed in "monotherapy" by VEGF as a key player in gene therapy. The latter point is not limited to reduction of adverse reactions, but also arises from a large spectrum of pleiotropic effects of cytokines. For example, VEGF may act as a pro-inflammatory cytokine by induction of nuclear factor κ-B, while HGF [82] or angiopoietin-1 shows antagonistic effects leading to reduction of VEGF-driven cell adhesion and inflammation [83]. Indeed, this has been confirmed in a number of in vitro tests and skin inflammation model indicating that these properties may be utilized for development of next-generation gene therapy drugs for angiogenesis exploiting pleiotropy of cytokines besides their main angiogenic effect. Another approach is delivery of growth factors in two sessions apart in time: for example, pre-treatment by angiopoietin-1 pDNA resulted in better angiogenic response after subsequent pDNA-VEGF165 injection in mouse hind limb ischemia model hinting time of administration as an important factor for efficacy [84].

3.3. Cell therapy and *ex vivo* modified cells

Cell therapy is a promising tool for regenerative medicine and therapeutic angiogenesis using progenitor or stem cells' ability to self-renew and mediate tissue repair. For potential use of cell therapy for vascular repair, one of the most intriguing findings was the discovery of endothelial progenitor cells (EPC) in circulating blood which hinted involvement of postnatal vasculogenesis in perfusion restoration [85]. However, further works sparkled controversy about EPC phenotype, origin [86], role in recovery from disease and even existence. Report by Prokopi et al. [87] claimed that EPC can be false-detected as endothelium-like (CD31/vWF+) monocytes in cultures due to phagocytosis of residual platelets rich with these protein markers.

Clinical trials up to date focus on delivery of bone marrow (BM) cells for induction of angiogenesis. These studies evaluated effects of BM mesenchymal stem cells (BM-MSC) or mononuclear cells (BM-MNC) delivered by intramuscular or intravascular injection in PAD patients. Most studies supported efficacy and indicated improvement in evaluated endpoints: ABI, pain-free walking distance, TcO_2, ulcer healing, or amputation-free period. However, some pivotal trials are to be mentioned in detail for better understanding of the field's status.

First set of crucial data was obtained during "head-to-head" comparison of different cell types to identify the optimal cell source. In a double-blind randomized study, administration of BM-MSC to diabetic PAD patients with foot ulcerations showed efficacy superior to BM-MNC [88]. Subjects that received BM-MSC showed complete ulcer healing 4 weeks earlier than BM-MNC; perfusion assessment, pain-free walking time, ABI and angiography data also spoke in favor of BM-MSC as a more effective cellular angiogenic agent [88].

However, limitation of BM-based treatment is invasive procedure to obtain material and alternative approach was proposed using peripheral blood mononuclear cells (PB-MNC) mobilized by granulocyte colony-stimulating factor (G-CSF) pre-administration. Feasibility of this

http://dx.doi.org/10.5772/66411

approach was obvious and a trial was initiated to confirm its efficacy compared to BM-MNC enrolling a total of 150 patients split in two groups. After 12 weeks of observation, PB-MNC patients showed significantly higher limb temperature, ABI and reduced rest pains than BM-MNC. Yet no difference was found in TcO_2, ulcer healing rate and amputation frequency hinting that two methods showed comparable efficacy profile with a trend to PB-MNC application due to feasibility and endpoint improvements [89]. Interestingly, a trial of conventional therapy + G-CSF monotherapy was compared to BM cells and in these groups, improvements in ABI and TcO_2 were comparable and significantly better than in conventional drug therapy control. This was an intriguing finding which showed that mobilization of endogenous mononuclear cells (MNC) was sufficient to replace BM grafting and injection [90].

Another source of cells for therapeutic angiogenesis is adipose-derived mesenchymal stromal cells (AD-MSC). Despite sources of mesenchymal stem cells (MSC) are not limited to adipose tissue, these adult stromal cells can be isolated from samples obtained during lipoaspiration or surgery. Taken together with ease of expansion, well-established phenotype and abundance in healthy individuals, it makes AD-MSC an excellent object for autologous and allogeneic use for angiogenesis stimulation [91]. Published experimental studies show that AD-MSC use their paracrine potential for induction of angiogenesis and support of collateral remodeling [92]. This is referred as "bystander effect" to emphasize that AD-MSC render their effects by paracrine mechanism in contrast to previously existing opinion about their significant ability to differentiate into specific vascular cells and EC in particular [93].

These cells have not been evaluated in PAD or MI clinical trials yet and considered to be a very attractive option to complement existing strategies. Certain factors limiting potency of AD-MSC exist including donors' age [94], comorbidities and effects of *ex vivo* culture [95]. However, improvement can be achieved by manipulation of cells' paracrine activity, e.g., by viral transduction to increase expression of cytokines forming an "alliance of gene and cell therapy" for higher efficacy [96]. This approach has become possible after development of effective viral gene delivery systems as far as pDNA transfection in primary human cultures was extremely low or at the level of toxicity exerted by transfection reagents [97]. Modification of cells intended for therapy use in performed *ex vivo* after sufficient amount of material is obtained in appropriate culture condition. Selection of a viral vector depends on safety precautions and vector capacity for genetic material; however, cDNA of most angiogenic cytokines "fit" into commonly used adenoviruses or adeno-associated virus (AAV).

This method has been tested in animal models of ischemia using exogenous delivery of VEGF165 [98], insulin-like growth factor-1 [99], HO-1 [100], or other genes to different types of cells: AD-MSC, EC, BM-MSC, etc. In majority of reports, modification resulted in improvement of response after delivery to ischemic tissue. In our experience, administration of human VEGF165-expressing AD-MSC to ischemic limb of immunodeficient mice resulted in enhanced perfusion and vascular density superior to control cells. Furthermore, muscle necrosis was minimal in this group indicating enhanced blood supply and antiapoptotic effects of VEGF165 as mode of action [98].

Application of modified stem cells for induction of angiogenesis may be limited in coming years unless safety of modification and full extent of its influence on biological properties of cells is understood. *Ex vivo* modified cells are widely used for treatment of oncology and hereditary disease where benefit for patient overwhelms existing risks [101]; however, for treatment of PAD and MI, additional measures of precaution will be required prior to active clinical trials. Nevertheless, recently a group led by Dr. J. Laird began a phase I trial to evaluate the use of VEGF-expressing MSC in patients with critical limb ischemia. The trial is now ongoing with expected completion in 2017 and preclinical data indicated good safety profile with long-term expression of VEGF in MSC after viral modification [102]. Recent progress in virus biology and gene engineering allowed development of safer vector systems with controlled expression, integration, or directed insertion to genomic "safe harbors" where they induce minimal to none disturbances [103]. Preclinical evaluation of these systems is expected to give more data on long-term impact of modification and facilitate translation.

4. Cell sheets: minimal tissue-engineered constructs

Cell sheets (CS) were first introduced by Dr. Okano's group and occupied a niche between 3D tissue engineering and 2D cell cultures used to obtain therapeutic cellular materials [104]. Briefly, CS is an attached mono- or multilayered xeno-free construct that consists of viable cells with ECM produced by these cells. Application of this method allowed to circumvent a crucial setback observed in a number of experimental works—poor survival of cells used for therapeutic interventions. One of main reasons for this is procedure of detachment by proteolytic enzymes leading to disruption of ECM (along with deposited cytokines) and loss of intercellular contacts resulting in anoikis and high prevalence of cell death aggravated by passage of cells through a catheter or needle causing mechanical damage. Loss of cells implanted to the tissue by injection in suspended form is estimated as 40–75% within the first 3 days [105], while CS limits this damage to minimum keeping the cells viable after delivery and enhancing their engraftment [106]. Furthermore, ECM proteins delivered as a part of the construct are known to have a beneficial impact on regeneration and do not have toxic or immunogenic features of chemical or xenogeneic scaffolds. Generation of CS is possible from MSC, fibroblasts, EC, skeletal myoblasts, induced pluripotent stem cells and cardiomyocytes derived from them, BM cells and cardiac progenitor cells [107]—literally, any adherent cell culture after it produces enough ECM to stand mechanical manipulation [108]. CS can be used to cover a significant surface making it a good technique for superficial lesions, cardiomyoplasty and ophthalmologic and microsurgical manipulations. Numerous clinical trials are being run in Japan these years to reveal their full potential in a wide array of disorders [109].

In relation to angiogenesis, this technique was evaluated in MI models using CS from skeletal myoblasts, AD-MSC, or cardiac progenitor cells showing their ability to generate vascularized additional layer of tissue and facilitate vascular growth in underlying tissue [110, 111]. This resulted in improved ventricular function, limited MI size and fibrosis and favorable outcomes in experimental animals. Comparative study of CS vs. injection of suspended cells showed CS to be superior in terms of most functional and histological endpoints analyzed and using a bioluminescent method, the authors reported higher survival of transplanted rat neonatal cardiomyocytes after CS delivery compared to injection [112]. Recently, clinical application of CS from autologous skeletal myoblasts has begun to treat severe heart failure patients with left ventricular assist devices. Delivery of multilayered constructs resulted in ejection fraction increase sufficient to remove the device and postpone heart transplant as well showing good potential of this approach [113].

In limb ischemia and diabetes, CS are generally considered to be a tool for ulcer treatment and indeed numerous clinical trials have been initiated within last years. However, our group has been extensively investigating application of CS as an angiogenic therapy in PAD. We have found that subcutaneous delivery of CS from AD-MSC to mice with limb ischemia resulted in robust angiogenic response and CS were superior to dispersed cells in terms of tissue perfusion and vessel density [114]. This piece of evidence provided basis for CS application in PAD indicating that their potential is not limited to cutaneous healing but that paracrine factors are capable to induce angiogenic response in ischemic muscle. Our data were supported almost at the same time in a study by Bak et al. who used mixed CS from SMC and EC for successful treatment of experimental limb ischemia in mice by subcutaneous delivery [115].

Further improvement of CS potential is possible by application of *ex vivo* modification to express growth factors and discussed above. Our group's experience with viral vectors expressing VEGF165 suggested robust increase of angiogenesis in MI and limb ischemia after delivery of sheets from AD-MSC expressing VEGF165 after viral transduction [114, 116]. Effect of these constructs was superior to control CS and we observed no changes in immune response to genetically modified sheets or cell proliferation/viability within them [114].

Overall, application of CS for therapeutic angiogenesis is a new field and its expansion is expected within next years. These constructs are feasible from a translational point of view as far as they do not contain xenogeneic, artificial, or cadaveric materials circumventing many ethical and safety problems in translation.

5. Concluding remarks

Overall, therapeutic angiogenesis has accumulated a "critical mass" of evidence and approaches that would allow its application in practice within the next 10–15 years expanding the capabilities of treatment. However, possibility to shift from initially used non-option or critical patients may lead to better results in clinical trials, especially in gene therapy, where numerous failures put the whole concept under question several years ago. Development of cell therapy was accompanied by a large framework of regulatory, legal, ethical and industrial work to ensure safety and patients' benefit. Number of clinical trials is growing every year and fortunately no serious evidence for adverse events or other risks for subjects' health and well-being was found up-to-date.

Therapeutic angiogenesis has become one of the pioneer methods in translational medicine and its full potential is yet to be unleashed especially in the field of *ex vivo* modification and tissue-engineered approaches to increase efficacy and ensure safety.

Funding

Study and publication was supported by a grant from Russian Scientific Foundation (RSF) №16-45-03007.

Abbreviations

AAV	adeno-associated virus
(a/b)FGF	(acidic/basic) fibroblast growth factor
ABI	ankle-brachial (pressure) index
AD-MSC	adipose-derived mesenchymal stem cells
BM-MNC	bone marrow mononuclear cell(s)
BM-MSC	bone marrow mesenchymal stem cell(s)
CHD	coronary heart disease
CS	cell sheet
EC	endothelial cell(s)
ECM	extracellular matrix
G-CSD	granulocyte colony-stimulating factor
HGF	hepatocyte growth factor
HIFs	hypoxia-induced factors
HO-1	heme oxygenase-1
IC	intermittent claudication
MI	myocardial infarction
MMP	matrix metalloproteinase
MSC	mesenchymal stem cell(s)
PAD	peripheral artery disease
PB-MNC	peripheral blood mononuclear cell(s)
pDNA	plasmid DNA
PlGF	placental growth factor
SDF-1α	Stromal cell-derived factor-1α
SMC	smooth muscle cell(s)
TcO_2	transcutaneous O_2 pressure
TGF	transforming growth factor
uPA	urokinase plasminogen activator
VEGF	vascular endothelial growth factor
vWF	von Willebrand factor
PDGF	platelet-derived growth factor

http://dx.doi.org/10.5772/66411

Author details

Pavel Igorevich Makarevich[1-3*] and Yelena Viktorovna Parfyonova[1, 3]

*Address all correspondence to: pmakarevich@mc.msu.ru

1 Institute of Regenerative Medicine, Lomonosov Moscow State University, Moscow, Russia

2 Faculty of Medicine, Lomonosov Moscow State University, Moscow, Russia

3 Institute of Experimental Cardiology, Russian Cardiology Research and Production Complex, Russia

References

[1] Carmeliet P, Jain RK. Molecular mechanisms and clinical applications of angiogenesis. Nature. 2011;473(7347):298–307.

[2] Beck H, Voswinckel R, Wagner S, Ziegelhoeffer T, Heil M, Helisch A, et al. Participation of bone marrow-derived cells in long-term repair processes after experimental stroke. Journal of cerebral blood flow and metabolism: official journal of the International Society of Cerebral Blood Flow and Metabolism. 2003;23(6):709–17.

[3] Folkman J. Angiogenesis in cancer, vascular, rheumatoid and other disease. Nature medicine. 1995;1(1):27–31.

[4] Fong GH. Regulation of angiogenesis by oxygen sensing mechanisms. Journal of molecular medicine (Berlin). 2009;87(6):549–60.

[5] Deveza L, Choi J, Yang F. Therapeutic angiogenesis for treating cardiovascular diseases. Theranostics. 2012;2(8):801–14.

[6] Semenza GL. Oxygen sensing, hypoxia-inducible factors and disease pathophysiology. Annual review of pathology. 2014;9:47–71.

[7] Murakami M, Simons M. Fibroblast growth factor regulation of neovascularization. Current opinion in hematology. 2008;15(3):215–20.

[8] Taimeh Z, Loughran J, Birks EJ, Bolli R. Vascular endothelial growth factor in heart failure. Nature reviews cardiology. 2013;10(9):519–30.

[9] Ferrara N, Gerber HP, LeCouter J. The biology of VEGF and its receptors. Nature medicine. 2003;9(6):669–76.

[10] Xin X, Yang S, Ingle G, Zlot C, Rangell L, Kowalski J, et al. Hepatocyte growth factor enhances vascular endothelial growth factor-induced angiogenesis in vitro and in vivo. The American journal of pathology. 2001;158(3):1111–20.

[11] Menshikov M, Torosyan N, Elizarova E, Plakida K, Vorotnikov A, Parfyonova Y, et al. Urokinase induces matrix metalloproteinase-9/gelatinase B expression in THP-1

monocytes via ERK1/2 and cytosolic phospholipase A2 activation and eicosanoid production. Journal of vascular research. 2006;43(5):482–90.

[12] Adams RH, Alitalo K. Molecular regulation of angiogenesis and lymphangiogenesis. Nature reviews molecular cell biology. 2007;8(6):464–78.

[13] Gerhardt H, Golding M, Fruttiger M, Ruhrberg C, Lundkvist A, Abramsson A, et al. VEGF guides angiogenic sprouting utilizing endothelial tip cell filopodia. The journal of cell biology. 2003;161(6):1163–77.

[14] Fischer C, Schneider M, Carmeliet P. Principles and Therapeutic Implications of Angiogenesis, Vasculogenesis and Arteriogenesis. In: Moncada S, Higgs A, editors. The Vascular Endothelium II. Berlin, Heidelberg: Springer Berlin Heidelberg; 2006. p. 157–212.

[15] Hellstrom M, Phng LK, Hofmann JJ, Wallgard E, Coultas L, Lindblom P, et al. Dll4 signalling through Notch1 regulates formation of tip cells during angiogenesis. Nature. 2007;445(7129):776–80.

[16] Chung AS, Lee J, Ferrara N. Targeting the tumour vasculature: insights from physiological angiogenesis. Nature reviews cancer. 2010;10(7):505–14.

[17] Jain RK. Molecular regulation of vessel maturation. Nature medicine. 2003;9(6):685–93.

[18] Persson AB, Buschmann IR. Vascular growth in health and disease. Frontiers in molecular neuroscience. 2011;4:14.

[19] Heil M, Eitenmuller I, Schmitz-Rixen T, Schaper W. Arteriogenesis versus angiogenesis: similarities and differences. Journal of cellular and molecular medicine. 2006;10(1):45–55.

[20] Schaper W. Collateral circulation: past and present. Basic research in cardiology. 2009;104(1):5–21.

[21] de Groot D, Pasterkamp G, Hoefer IE. Cardiovascular risk factors and collateral artery formation. European journal of clinical investigation. 2009;39(12):1036–47.

[22] Hillmeister P, Lehmann KE, Bondke A, Witt H, Duelsner A, Gruber C, et al. Induction of cerebral arteriogenesis leads to early-phase expression of protease inhibitors in growing collaterals of the brain. Journal of cerebral blood flow and metabolism: official journal of the International Society of Cerebral Blood Flow and Metabolism. 2008;28(11):1811–23.

[23] Tkachuk V, Stepanova V, Little PJ, Bobik A. Regulation and role of urokinase plasminogen activator in vascular remodelling. Clinical and experimental pharmacology & physiology. 1996;23(9):759–65.

[24] Parfyonova YV, Plekhanova OS, Tkachuk VA. Plasminogen activators in vascular remodeling and angiogenesis. Biochemistry Biokhimiia. 2002;67(1):119–34.

[25] Scholz D, Ito W, Fleming I, Deindl E, Sauer A, Wiesnet M, et al. Ultrastructure and molecular histology of rabbit hind-limb collateral artery growth (arteriogenesis). Virchows Archiv: an international journal of pathology. 2000;436(3):257–70.

[26] Jaipersad AS, Lip GY, Silverman S, Shantsila E. The role of monocytes in angiogenesis and atherosclerosis. Journal of the American College of Cardiology. 2014;63(1):1–11.

[27] Roberts R, DeMello V, Sobel BE. Deleterious effects of methylprednisolone in patients with myocardial infarction. Circulation. 1976;53(3 Suppl):I204–6.

[28] Duelsner A, Gatzke N, Glaser J, Hillmeister P, Li M, Lee EJ, et al. Acetylsalicylic acid, but not clopidogrel, inhibits therapeutically induced cerebral arteriogenesis in the hypoperfused rat brain. Journal of cerebral blood flow and metabolism: official journal of the International Society of Cerebral Blood Flow and Metabolism. 2012;32(1):105–14.

[29] van Amerongen MJ, Harmsen MC, van Rooijen N, Petersen AH, van Luyn MJ. Macrophage depletion impairs wound healing and increases left ventricular remodeling after myocardial injury in mice. The American journal of pathology. 2007;170(3):818–29.

[30] Baffour R, Berman J, Garb JL, Rhee SW, Kaufman J, Friedmann P. Enhanced angiogenesis and growth of collaterals by in vivo administration of recombinant basic fibroblast growth factor in a rabbit model of acute lower limb ischemia: dose–response effect of basic fibroblast growth factor. Journal of vascular surgery: official publication, the Society for Vascular Surgery [and] International Society for Cardiovascular Surgery, North American Chapter. 1992;16(2):181–91.

[31] Morishita R, Nakamura S, Hayashi S, Taniyama Y, Moriguchi A, Nagano T, et al. Therapeutic angiogenesis induced by human recombinant hepatocyte growth factor in rabbit hind limb ischemia model as cytokine supplement therapy. Hypertension. 1999;33(6):1379–84.

[32] Grochot-Przeczek A, Dulak J, Jozkowicz A. Therapeutic angiogenesis for revascularization in peripheral artery disease. Gene. 2013;525(2):220–8.

[33] Lazarous DF, Unger EF, Epstein SE, Stine A, Arevalo JL, Chew EY, et al. Basic fibroblast growth factor in patients with intermittent claudication: results of a phase I trial. Journal of the American College of Cardiology. 2000;36(4):1239–44.

[34] Lederman RJ, Mendelsohn FO, Anderson RD, Saucedo JF, Tenaglia AN, Hermiller JB, et al. Therapeutic angiogenesis with recombinant fibroblast growth factor-2 for intermittent claudication (the TRAFFIC study): a randomised trial. Lancet. 2002;359(9323):2053–8.

[35] Wolff JA, Malone RW, Williams P, Chong W, Acsadi G, Jani A, et al. Direct gene transfer into mouse muscle in vivo. Science. 1990;247(4949 Pt 1):1465–8.

[36] Morishita R, Aoki M, Hashiya N, Makino H, Yamasaki K, Azuma J, et al. Safety evaluation of clinical gene therapy using hepatocyte growth factor to treat peripheral arterial disease. Hypertension. 2004;44(2):203–9.

[37] van Gaal EV, Hennink WE, Crommelin DJ, Mastrobattista E. Plasmid engineering for controlled and sustained gene expression for nonviral gene therapy. Pharmaceutical research. 2006;23(6):1053–74.

[38] Khare R, Chen CY, Weaver EA, Barry MA. Advances and future challenges in adenoviral vector pharmacology and targeting. Current gene therapy. 2011;11(4):241–58.

[39] Dismuke DJ, Tenenbaum L, Samulski RJ. Biosafety of recombinant adeno-associated virus vectors. Current gene therapy. 2013;13(6):434–52.

[40] Verma IM, Weitzman MD. Gene therapy: twenty-first century medicine. Annual review of biochemistry. 2005;74:711–38.

[41] MacColl GS, Novo FJ, Marshall NJ, Waters M, Goldspink G, Bouloux PM. Optimisation of growth hormone production by muscle cells using plasmid DNA. Journal of endocrinology. 2000;165(2):329–36.

[42] Makarevich PI, Rubina KA, Diykanov DT, Tkachuk VA, Parfyonova YV. Therapeutic angiogenesis using growth factors: current state and prospects for development. Kardiologiia. 2015;55(9):59–71.

[43] Takeshita S, Zheng LP, Brogi E, Kearney M, Pu LQ, Bunting S, et al. Therapeutic angiogenesis. A single intraarterial bolus of vascular endothelial growth factor augments revascularization in a rabbit ischemic hind limb model. The journal of clinical investigation. 1994;93(2):662–70.

[44] Baumgartner I, Pieczek A, Manor O, Blair R, Kearney M, Walsh K, et al. Constitutive expression of phVEGF165 after intramuscular gene transfer promotes collateral vessel development in patients with critical limb ischemia. Circulation. 1998;97(12):1114–23.

[45] Makinen K, Manninen H, Hedman M, Matsi P, Mussalo H, Alhava E, et al. Increased vascularity detected by digital subtraction angiography after VEGF gene transfer to human lower limb artery: a randomized, placebo-controlled, double-blinded phase II study. Molecular therapy: the journal of the American Society of Gene Therapy. 2002;6(1):127–33.

[46] Kusumanto YH, van Weel V, Mulder NH, Smit AJ, van den Dungen JJ, Hooymans JM, et al. Treatment with intramuscular vascular endothelial growth factor gene compared with placebo for patients with diabetes mellitus and critical limb ischemia: a double-blind randomized trial. Human gene therapy. 2006;17(6):683–91.

[47] Rajagopalan S, Mohler ER, 3rd, Lederman RJ, Mendelsohn FO, Saucedo JF, Goldman CK, et al. Regional angiogenesis with vascular endothelial growth factor in peripheral arterial disease: a phase II randomized, double-blind, controlled study of adenoviral delivery of vascular endothelial growth factor 121 in patients with disabling intermittent claudication. Circulation. 2003;108(16):1933–8.

[48] Vajanto I, Rissanen TT, Rutanen J, Hiltunen MO, Tuomisto TT, Arve K, et al. Evaluation of angiogenesis and side effects in ischemic rabbit hindlimbs after intramuscular injection of adenoviral vectors encoding VEGF and LacZ. The journal of gene medicine. 2002;4(4):371–80.

[49] Shimamura M, Nakagami H, Koriyama H, Morishita R. Gene therapy and cell-based therapies for therapeutic angiogenesis in peripheral artery disease. BioMed research international. 2013;2013:186215.

http://dx.doi.org/10.5772/66411

[50] Losordo DW, Vale PR, Symes JF, Dunnington CH, Esakof DD, Maysky M, et al. Gene therapy for myocardial angiogenesis: initial clinical results with direct myocardial injection of phVEGF165 as sole therapy for myocardial ischemia. Circulation. 1998;98(25):2800–4.

[51] Hedman M, Hartikainen J, Syvanne M, Stjernvall J, Hedman A, Kivela A, et al. Safety and feasibility of catheter-based local intracoronary vascular endothelial growth factor gene transfer in the prevention of postangioplasty and in-stent restenosis and in the treatment of chronic myocardial ischemia: phase II results of the Kuopio Angiogenesis Trial (KAT). Circulation. 2003;107(21):2677–83.

[52] Gyongyosi M, Khorsand A, Zamini S, Sperker W, Strehblow C, Kastrup J, et al. NOGA-guided analysis of regional myocardial perfusion abnormalities treated with intramyocardial injections of plasmid encoding vascular endothelial growth factor A-165 in patients with chronic myocardial ischemia: subanalysis of the EUROINJECT-ONE multicenter double-blind randomized study. Circulation. 2005;112(9 Suppl):I157–65.

[53] Aoki M, Morishita R, Taniyama Y, Kida I, Moriguchi A, Matsumoto K, et al. Angiogenesis induced by hepatocyte growth factor in non-infarcted myocardium and infarcted myocardium: up-regulation of essential transcription factor for angiogenesis, ets. Gene therapy. 2000;7(5):417–27.

[54] Morishita R, Aoki M, Hashiya N, Yamasaki K, Kurinami H, Shimizu S, et al. Therapeutic angiogenesis using hepatocyte growth factor (HGF). Current gene therapy. 2004;4(2):199–206.

[55] Morishita R, Makino H, Aoki M, Hashiya N, Yamasaki K, Azuma J, et al. Phase I/IIa clinical trial of therapeutic angiogenesis using hepatocyte growth factor gene transfer to treat critical limb ischemia. Arteriosclerosis, thrombosis and vascular biology. 2011;31(3):713–20.

[56] Shigematsu H, Yasuda K, Iwai T, Sasajima T, Ishimaru S, Ohashi Y, et al. Randomized, double-blind, placebo-controlled clinical trial of hepatocyte growth factor plasmid for critical limb ischemia. Gene therapy. 2010;17(9):1152–61.

[57] Pyun WB, Hahn W, Kim DS, Yoo WS, Lee SD, Won JH, et al. Naked DNA expressing two isoforms of hepatocyte growth factor induces collateral artery augmentation in a rabbit model of limb ischemia. Gene therapy. 2010;17(12):1442–52.

[58] Gu Y, Zhang J, Guo L, Cui S, Li X, Ding D, et al. A phase I clinical study of naked DNA expressing two isoforms of hepatocyte growth factor to treat patients with critical limb ischemia. The journal of gene medicine. 2011;13(11):602–10.

[59] Taniyama Y, Morishita R, Nakagami H, Moriguchi A, Sakonjo H, Shokei K, et al. Potential contribution of a novel antifibrotic factor, hepatocyte growth factor, to prevention of myocardial fibrosis by angiotensin II blockade in cardiomyopathic hamsters. Circulation. 2000;102(2):246–52.

[60] Nikol S, Baumgartner I, Van Belle E, Diehm C, Visona A, Capogrossi MC, et al. Therapeutic angiogenesis with intramuscular NV1FGF improves amputation-free

survival in patients with critical limb ischemia. Molecular therapy: the journal of the American Society of Gene Therapy. 2008;16(5):972–8.

[61] Comerota AJ, Throm RC, Miller KA, Henry T, Chronos N, Laird J, et al. Naked plasmid DNA encoding fibroblast growth factor type 1 for the treatment of end-stage unreconstructible lower extremity ischemia: preliminary results of a phase I trial. Journal of vascular surgery: official publication, the Society for Vascular Surgery [and] International Society for Cardiovascular Surgery, North American Chapter. 2002;35(5):930–6.

[62] Fowkes FG, Price JF. Gene therapy for critical limb ischaemia: the TAMARIS trial. Lancet. 2011;377(9781):1894–6.

[63] Belch J, Hiatt WR, Baumgartner I, Driver IV, Nikol S, Norgren L, et al. Effect of fibroblast growth factor NV1FGF on amputation and death: a randomised placebo-controlled trial of gene therapy in critical limb ischaemia. Lancet. 2011;377(9781):1929–37.

[64] Niebuhr A, Henry T, Goldman J, Baumgartner I, van Belle E, Gerss J, et al. Long-term safety of intramuscular gene transfer of non-viral FGF1 for peripheral artery disease. Gene therapy. 2012;19(3):264–70.

[65] Reis SE, Holubkov R, Conrad Smith AJ, Kelsey SF, Sharaf BL, Reichek N, et al. Coronary microvascular dysfunction is highly prevalent in women with chest pain in the absence of coronary artery disease: results from the NHLBI WISE study. American heart journal. 2001;141(5):735–41.

[66] Handberg E, Johnson BD, Arant CB, Wessel TR, Kerensky RA, von Mering G, et al. Impaired coronary vascular reactivity and functional capacity in women: results from the NHLBI Women's Ischemia Syndrome Evaluation (WISE) Study. Journal of the American College of Cardiology. 2006;47(3 Suppl):S44–9.

[67] Hochman JS, Tamis JE, Thompson TD, Weaver WD, White HD, Van de Werf F, et al. Sex, clinical presentation and outcome in patients with acute coronary syndromes. Global Use of Strategies to Open Occluded Coronary Arteries in Acute Coronary Syndromes IIb Investigators. The New England journal of medicine. 1999;341(4):226–32.

[68] Yonemitsu Y, Matsumoto T, Itoh H, Okazaki J, Uchiyama M, Yoshida K, et al. DVC1-0101 to treat peripheral arterial disease: a Phase I/IIa open-label dose-escalation clinical trial. Molecular therapy: the journal of the American Society of Gene Therapy. 2013;21(3):707–14.

[69] Creager MA, Olin JW, Belch JJ, Moneta GL, Henry TD, Rajagopalan S, et al. Effect of hypoxia-inducible factor-1 alpha gene therapy on walking performance in patients with intermittent claudication. Circulation. 2011;124(16):1765–73.

[70] Yla-Herttuala S, Markkanen JE, Rissanen TT. Gene therapy for ischemic cardiovascular diseases: some lessons learned from the first clinical trials. Trends in cardiovascular medicine. 2004;14(8):295–300.

[71] Spanholtz TA, Theodorou P, Holzbach T, Wutzler S, Giunta RE, Machens HG. Vascular endothelial growth factor (VEGF165) plus basic fibroblast growth factor (bFGF) producing cells induce a mature and stable vascular network--a future therapy for ischemically challenged tissue. The journal of surgical research. 2011;171(1):329–38.

[72] Kupatt C, Hinkel R, Pfosser A, El-Aouni C, Wuchrer A, Fritz A, et al. Cotransfection of vascular endothelial growth factor-A and platelet-derived growth factor-B via recombinant adeno-associated virus resolves chronic ischemic malperfusion role of vessel maturation. Journal of the American College of Cardiology. 2010;56(5):414–22.

[73] Arsic N, Zentilin L, Zacchigna S, Santoro D, Stanta G, Salvi A, et al. Induction of functional neovascularization by combined VEGF and angiopoietin-1 gene transfer using AAV vectors. Molecular therapy: the journal of the American Society of Gene Therapy. 2003;7(4):450–9.

[74] Yu JX, Huang XF, Lv WM, Ye CS, Peng XZ, Zhang H, et al. Combination of stromal-derived factor-1 alpha and vascular endothelial growth factor gene-modified endothelial progenitor cells is more effective for ischemic neovascularization. Journal of vascular surgery: official publication, the Society for Vascular Surgery [and] International Society for Cardiovascular Surgery, North American Chapter. 2009;50(3):608–16.

[75] Traktuev DO, Tsokolaeva ZI, Shevelev AA, Talitskiy KA, Stepanova VV, Johnstone BH, et al. Urokinase gene transfer augments angiogenesis in ischemic skeletal and myocardial muscle. Molecular therapy: the journal of the American Society of Gene Therapy. 2007;15(11):1939–46.

[76] Makarevich P, Tsokolaeva Z, Shevelev A, Rybalkin I, Shevchenko E, Beloglazova I, et al. Combined transfer of human VEGF165 and HGF genes renders potent angiogenic effect in ischemic skeletal muscle. PLoS one. 2012;7(6):e38776.

[77] Lee S, Kim K, Kim HA, Kim SW, Lee M. Augmentation of erythropoietin enhancer-mediated hypoxia-inducible gene expression by co-transfection of a plasmid encoding hypoxia-inducible factor 1 alpha for ischemic tissue targeting gene therapy. Journal of drug targeting. 2008;16(1):43–50.

[78] Bhang SH, Kim JH, Yang HS, La WG, Lee TJ, Sun AY, et al. Combined delivery of heme oxygenase-1 gene and fibroblast growth factor-2 protein for therapeutic angiogenesis. Biomaterials. 2009;30(31):6247–56.

[79] Dulak J, Jozkowicz A, Foresti R, Kasza A, Frick M, Huk I, et al. Heme oxygenase activity modulates vascular endothelial growth factor synthesis in vascular smooth muscle cells. Antioxidants & redox signaling. 2002;4(2):229–40.

[80] Saif J, Schwarz TM, Chau DY, Henstock J, Sami P, Leicht SF, et al. Combination of injectable multiple growth factor-releasing scaffolds and cell therapy as an advanced modality to enhance tissue neovascularization. Arteriosclerosis, thrombosis and vascular biology. 2010;30(10):1897–904.

[81] Yang Y, Chen QH, Liu AR, Xu XP, Han JB, Qiu HB. Synergism of MSC-secreted HGF and VEGF in stabilising endothelial barrier function upon lipopolysaccharide stimulation via the Rac1 pathway. Stem cell research & therapy. 2015;6:250.

[82] Min JK, Lee YM, Kim JH, Kim YM, Kim SW, Lee SY, et al. Hepatocyte growth factor suppresses vascular endothelial growth factor-induced expression of endothelial ICAM-1 and VCAM-1 by inhibiting the nuclear factor-kappaB pathway. Circulation research. 2005;96(3):300–7.

[83] Kim I, Moon SO, Park SK, Chae SW, Koh GY. Angiopoietin-1 reduces VEGF-stimulated leukocyte adhesion to endothelial cells by reducing ICAM-1, VCAM-1 and E-selectin expression. Circulation research. 2001;89(6):477–9.

[84] Yamauchi A, Ito Y, Morikawa M, Kobune M, Huang J, Sasaki K, et al. Pre-administration of angiopoietin-1 followed by VEGF induces functional and mature vascular formation in a rabbit ischemic model. The journal of gene medicine. 2003;5(11):994–1004.

[85] Asahara T, Murohara T, Sullivan A, Silver M, van der Zee R, Li T, et al. Isolation of putative progenitor endothelial cells for angiogenesis. Science. 1997;275(5302):964–7.

[86] Rohde E, Malischnik C, Thaler D, Maierhofer T, Linkesch W, Lanzer G, et al. Blood monocytes mimic endothelial progenitor cells. Stem cells. 2006;24(2):357–67.

[87] Prokopi M, Pula G, Mayr U, Devue C, Gallagher J, Xiao Q, et al. Proteomic analysis reveals presence of platelet microparticles in endothelial progenitor cell cultures. Blood. 2009;114(3):723–32.

[88] Lu D, Chen B, Liang Z, Deng W, Jiang Y, Li S, et al. Comparison of bone marrow mesenchymal stem cells with bone marrow-derived mononuclear cells for treatment of diabetic critical limb ischemia and foot ulcer: a double-blind, randomized, controlled trial. Diabetes research and clinical practice. 2011;92(1):26–36.

[89] Huang PP, Yang XF, Li SZ, Wen JC, Zhang Y, Han ZC. Randomised comparison of G-CSF-mobilized peripheral blood mononuclear cells versus bone marrow-mononuclear cells for the treatment of patients with lower limb arteriosclerosis obliterans. Thrombosis and haemostasis. 2007;98(6):1335–42.

[90] Arai M, Misao Y, Nagai H, Kawasaki M, Nagashima K, Suzuki K, et al. Granulocyte colony-stimulating factor: a noninvasive regeneration therapy for treating atherosclerotic peripheral artery disease. Circulation journal: official journal of the Japanese Circulation Society. 2006;70(9):1093–8.

[91] Bourin P, Bunnell BA, Casteilla L, Dominici M, Katz AJ, March KL, et al. Stromal cells from the adipose tissue-derived stromal vascular fraction and culture expanded adipose tissue-derived stromal/stem cells: a joint statement of the International Federation for Adipose Therapeutics and Science (IFATS) and the International Society for Cellular Therapy (ISCT). Cytotherapy. 2013;15(6):641–8.

[92] Rubina K, Kalinina N, Efimenko A, Lopatina T, Melikhova V, Tsokolaeva Z, et al. Adipose stromal cells stimulate angiogenesis via promoting progenitor cell differentia-

tion, secretion of angiogenic factors and enhancing vessel maturation. Tissue engineering Part A. 2009;15(8):2039–50.

[93] Yang D, Wang W, Li L, Peng Y, Chen P, Huang H, et al. The relative contribution of paracrine effect versus direct differentiation on adipose-derived stem cell transplantation mediated cardiac repair. PLoS one. 2013;8(3):e59020.

[94] Efimenko A, Starostina E, Kalinina N, Stolzing A. Angiogenic properties of aged adipose derived mesenchymal stem cells after hypoxic conditioning. Journal of translational medicine. 2011;9:10.

[95] Efimenko A, Dzhoyashvili N, Kalinina N, Kochegura T, Akchurin R, Tkachuk V, et al. Adipose-derived mesenchymal stromal cells from aged patients with coronary artery disease keep mesenchymal stromal cell properties but exhibit characteristics of aging and have impaired angiogenic potential. Stem cells translational medicine. 2014;3(1):32–41.

[96] Makarevich PI, Dergilev KV, Tsokolaeva ZI, Efimenko AY, Gluhanuk EV, Gallinger JO, et al. Delivery of genetically engineered adipose-derived cell sheets for treatment of ischemic disorders-development of application in animal models. Molecular therapy; Nature Publishing Group: New York, NY, USA; 2015. p. S262-S.

[97] Merdan T, Kopecek J, Kissel T. Prospects for cationic polymers in gene and oligonucleotide therapy against cancer. Advanced drug delivery reviews. 2002;54(5):715–58.

[98] Shevchenko EK, Makarevich PI, Tsokolaeva ZI, Boldyreva MA, Sysoeva VY, Tkachuk VA, et al. Transplantation of modified human adipose derived stromal cells expressing VEGF165 results in more efficient angiogenic response in ischemic skeletal muscle. Journal of translational medicine. 2013;11:138.

[99] Sen S, Merchan J, Dean J, Ii M, Gavin M, Silver M, et al. Autologous transplantation of endothelial progenitor cells genetically modified by adeno-associated viral vector delivering insulin-like growth factor-1 gene after myocardial infarction. Human gene therapy. 2010;21(10):1327–34.

[100] Suzuki M, Iso-o N, Takeshita S, Tsukamoto K, Mori I, Sato T, et al. Facilitated angiogenesis induced by heme oxygenase-1 gene transfer in a rat model of hindlimb ischemia. Biochemical and biophysical research communications. 2003;302(1):138–43.

[101] Holzinger A, Barden M, Abken H. The growing world of CAR T cell trials: a systematic review. Cancer Immunol Immunother. 2016;65(12):1433–50.

[102] Phase I study of IM injection of VEGF-producing MSC for the treatment of critical limb ischemia [Available from: https://www.cirm.ca.gov/our-progress/awards/phase-i-study-im-injection-vegf-producing-msc-treatment-critical-limb-ischemia-0.

[103] Papapetrou EP, Lee G, Malani N, Setty M, Riviere I, Tirunagari LM, et al. Genomic safe harbors permit high beta-globin transgene expression in thalassemia induced pluripotent stem cells. Nature biotechnology. 2011;29(1):73–8.

[104] Kumashiro Y, Fukumori K, Takahashi H, Nakayama M, Akiyama Y, Yamato M, et al. Modulation of cell adhesion and detachment on thermo-responsive polymeric surfaces through the observation of surface dynamics. Colloids and surfaces B: biointerfaces. 2013;106:198–207.

[105] Aguado BA, Mulyasasmita W, Su J, Lampe KJ, Heilshorn SC. Improving viability of stem cells during syringe needle flow through the design of hydrogel cell carriers. Tissue engineering Part A. 2012;18(7–8):806–15.

[106] Lin CY, Lin KJ, Li KC, Sung LY, Hsueh S, Lu CH, et al. Immune responses during healing of massive segmental femoral bone defects mediated by hybrid baculovirus-engineered ASCs. Biomaterials. 2012;33(30):7422–34.

[107] Dergilev K, Tsokolaeva Z, Rubina K, Sysoeva V, Makarevich P, Boldyreva M, et al. Isolation and characterization of cardiac progenitor cells from myocardial right atrial appendage tissue. Cell and tissue biology. 2016;10(5):349–56.

[108] Elloumi-Hannachi I, Yamato M, Okano T. Cell sheet engineering: a unique nanotechnology for scaffold-free tissue reconstruction with clinical applications in regenerative medicine. Journal of internal medicine. 2010;267(1):54–70.

[109] Matsuura K, Utoh R, Nagase K, Okano T. Cell sheet approach for tissue engineering and regenerative medicine. Journal of controlled release: official journal of the Controlled Release Society. 2014;190:228–39.

[110] Yang J, Yamato M, Shimizu T, Sekine H, Ohashi K, Kanzaki M, et al. Reconstruction of functional tissues with cell sheet engineering. Biomaterials. 2007;28(34):5033–43.

[111] Yang J, Yamato M, Kohno C, Nishimoto A, Sekine H, Fukai F, et al. Cell sheet engineering: recreating tissues without biodegradable scaffolds. Biomaterials. 2005;26(33):6415–22.

[112] Sekine H, Shimizu T, Dobashi I, Matsuura K, Hagiwara N, Takahashi M, et al. Cardiac cell sheet transplantation improves damaged heart function via superior cell survival in comparison with dissociated cell injection. Tissue engineering Part A. 2011;17(23–24):2973–80.

[113] Mitamura Y. Current status of left ventricular assist devices and cell sheet engineering for treatment of severe heart disease in Japan. Artificial organs. 2015;39(7):543–9.

[114] Makarevich P, Boldyreva M, Dergilev K, Gluhanyuk E, Gallinger J, Efimenko A, et al. Transplantation of cell sheets from adipose-derived mesenchymal stromal cells effectively induces angiogenesis in ischemic skeletal muscle. Genes and cells. 2015;10(3):68–77.

[115] Bak S, Ahmad T, Lee YB, Lee JY, Kim EM, Shin H. Delivery of a cell patch of cocultured endothelial cells and smooth muscle cells using thermoresponsive hydrogels for enhanced angiogenesis. Tissue engineering Part A. 2016;22(1–2):182–93.

[116] Yeh TS, Fang YH, Lu CH, Chiu SC, Yeh CL, Yen TC, et al. Baculovirus-transduced, VEGF-expressing adipose-derived stem cell sheet for the treatment of myocardium infarction. Biomaterials. 2014;35(1):174–84.

Chapter 18

Platelet Lysate to Promote Angiogenic Cell Therapies

Scott T. Robinson and Luke P. Brewster

Additional information is available at the end of the chapter

http://dx.doi.org/10.5772/66934

Abstract

Cellular therapies for patients with ischemic muscle have been limited by poor cell retention and survivability. Platelets are a robust source of growth factors and structural proteins, and extracts from this peripheral blood component may be manipulated to improve both cell retention and survivability in percutaneous delivery methods. Human platelet lysate is generated from pooled human platelets and contains a growth factor milieu that promotes robust human mesenchymal stem cell (MSC) proliferation without risk of xenogenic contamination. As such, platelet lysate is a practical alternative to animal serum for MSC culture and, with minor adjustments to the production process, can also be used as a scaffold for cell delivery. Human platelet lysate is a promising substrate that can provide nutritive delivery both in vitro and during cell implantation, potentially improving retention and survivability of MSCs that may improve angiogenic function for cell therapy in *treatment* of ischemic tissues.

Keywords: critical limb ischemia, mesenchymal stromal cells, platelet lysate, angiogenic cell therapy

1. Introduction

The legs are a site of ischemic muscle that are particularly attractive to application of angiogenic therapies. Decreased perfusion of the legs is known as peripheral arterial disease (PAD), and PAD is pandemic with extreme costs to society. In its most severe form, it is called critical limb ischemia (CLI). CLI patients do not have adequate perfusion to their resting nutritional needs resulting in rest pain or even tissue loss. While only 1–2% of PAD patients will develop CLI, CLI affects 1 million individuals annually [1]. Surgical revascularization of CLI patients can prevent major amputation. Current treatment for limb salvage includes endovascular therapy (angioplasty or stent placement) and surgical bypass. However, despite improvements in medical and surgical therapies, successful management of CLI is difficult with ~0.5

of patients with CLI dying or undergoing major amputation within 1 year [2]. Since many patients with CLI either fail revascularization therapy or are not candidates for these procedures, amputation is commonly performed. In addition to the impaired quality of life that results from lower limb amputation, historically mortality rates for this procedure have been reported to approach 40% [3]. New and innovative therapies are imperative to improve mortality and quality of life in patients with CLI and provide an alternative to limb amputation.

Cell therapy is a promising new treatment strategy for patient with CLI. The concept of cell therapy for treatment of critical limb ischemia coincided with the discovery of a circulating endothelial progenitor cell (EPC) in 1997, which described a population of circulating peripheral blood mononuclear cells that presumably arise from the bone marrow yet is also capable of displaying characteristics of a mature endothelium [4]. This discovery challenged the prevailing paradigm of postnatal neovascularization [5] in which blood vessel growth was the result of angiogenesis (the formation of new blood vessels from the existing endothelium through sprouting or intussusception) and arteriogenesis (the expansion of preexisting collateral vessels due to an increase in blood flow in response to changes in shear stress [6]). The work by Asahara et al. was significant for two reasons. First, it introduced the concept of postnatal vasculogenesis, suggesting that bone marrow-derived cells could contribute to the formation of new blood vessels in the adult similar to the process of vasculogenesis seen in embryogenesis, where primitive hemangioblasts give rise to de novo blood vessels in the developing fetus. Second, it pioneered the idea of cell therapy, through experiments in which the ischemic limbs of nude mice were injected with a population of human peripheral blood mononuclear cells enriched for CD34+ and Flk-1 (VEGFR-2), and found that the transplanted cells incorporated into the blood vessel endothelium at sites of neovascularization.

The notion that bone marrow-derived cells incorporate directly into native endothelium is controversial. Despite several initial reports suggesting differentiation of bone marrow cells into endothelial cells [7–9], several subsequent studies demonstrated that endogenous and transplanted bone marrow cells did not directly incorporate into the endothelium but instead support neovascularization through a paracrine mechanism [10–13]. Numerous stem and progenitor cell populations derived from the bone marrow, adipose tissue, and embryonic stem cells and induced pluripotent stem cells have been shown to enhance blood vessel growth in animal models of hind limb ischemia, suggesting a role for cell therapy in therapeutic neovascularization [4, 14–16]. Mesenchymal stromal cells (MSCs) are a potential cell source that can be easily isolated, rapidly expanded ex vivo, and have potent proangiogenic qualities [17] mediated through paracrine stimulation of endogenous tissues [18]. The use of MSCs for cell therapy is advantageous over other cell types because they can be derived from an autologous source, thereby avoiding the immunogenicity and loss of tolerance observed when allogeneic MSCs are exposed to an inflammatory environment [19, 20].

Despite numerous animal studies and small clinical pilot trials demonstrating the ability of MSCs to promote angiogenesis [17, 21, 22], the biology and clinical benefit of this approach has not yet been demonstrated in patients with CLI. Two major limitations have prevented the translation of MSC therapy from the laboratory to the clinical arena. First, the use of an autologous cell source in this demographic is complicated by the fact that progenitor cell populations

http://dx.doi.org/10.5772/66934

are depleted or functionally impaired in patients with coronary artery disease [23], stroke [24], and diabetes mellitus [25–27] and who are smokers [28]; all risk factors or comorbidities are highly prevalent in patients with CLI. A second major limitation of stem cell therapy thus far has been maintaining a clinically significant cell number in target tissues, as direct intramuscular injection or intra-arterial infusion alone typically does not enable adequate cell delivery [29–31]. In order to fully realize the potential of cell therapy, these limitations must be addressed before successful clinical deployment of MSC therapy can be achieved.

As cell therapy is translated from preclinical animal studies to human clinical trials, strict cell culture techniques must be employed to ensure human safety. The vast majority of clinical trials to date have utilized fetal bovine serum (FBS) for ex vivo expansion and growth of MSCs. However, FBS has considerable xenogenic potential and transplanted autologous MSCs can be rapidly rejected after culture in FBS [32]. Therefore, new human-derived alternatives have been evaluated as possible cell culture supplements to ensure that growth and expansion of MSCs are complain with current good manufacturing processes (GMPs).

Platelets are small enucleated cell fragments derived from megakaryocytes in the bone marrow and play a critical role in initiating hemostasis by binding and adhering to extracellular matrix components after endothelial injury, which in turns leads to platelet activation. Activated platelets then subsequently aggregate and become crosslinked with fibrin through activation of the coagulation cascade, thereby generating a platelet plug capable of blocking the flow of the blood. Platelets normally represent 0.1–0.25% of the blood and typically circulate for 5–9 days. Platelets are also an abundant source of growth factors, accounting for the majority of growth factors found in serum [33, 34]. As a result, various platelet extracts have been used for regenerative medicine applications. Platelet lysate (PL) is one such supplement that has been utilized as a supplement for culture of MSCs and has been shown to be superior to FBS [35, 36]. We and several collaborators have performed extensive characterization of platelet lysate as a cell culture supplement for expansion of human MSCs suitable for cell therapy trials. More recently, we have modified the PL production process such that PL may be used to form a 3D scaffold for MSC growth and invasion. In this chapter, we elaborate on our experience with PL as it pertains to culture of MSCs as well as describe a novel scaffold for cell delivery derived from PL extract.

2. Platelet lysate

2.1. Soluble platelet lysate for expansion of human MSCs

2.1.1. Generation of fibrinogen-depleted platelet lysate

The platelet lysate supplement for cell culture used by our group and our collaborators is manufactured through the Emory Personal Immunotherapy Center (EPIC). The specific production strategy was initially optimized and described by Copland et al. The current protocol employed by EPIC emphasizes good manufacturing process (GMP) technique and results in a fibrinogen-depleted form of platelet lysate (dPL) that is a soluble media supplement for ex vivo expansion of human MSCs. EPIC has provided numerous research groups with dPL and has received FDA approved for use of dPL for human cell therapy trials using MSCs for treatment of Crohn's disease (NCT01659762) and graft vs. host disease following allogenic bone marrow transplantation (NCT02359929). The production process utilizes outdated plateletpheresis products obtained from the Emory University Hospital blood bank. For each lot of dPL, five plateletpheresis products are exposed to sequential freeze-thaw cycles to ensure adequate membrane fracturing. The platelet products are first stored at -20°C, then thawed at 4°C, and aliquoted into smaller volumes of 20–25 mL. The aliquots are then refrozen at -80°C and filtered through a 40 μm filter. The filtered PL is then centrifuged at 4000×g for 20 min at room temperature and refiltered in 40 μm filters. The PL is then mixed with $CaCl_2$ and heparin solution and stored at 4°C overnight to allow formation of a fibrin clot. Following this, the dPL samples are centrifuged again at 4000×g at room temperature, filtered at 0.2 μm, and then stored at -80°C [37]. These final aliquots are then thawed and immediately ready for use in cell culture.

The standard plateletpheresis process employed by the American Red Cross involves the addition of 10% v/v acid citrate dextrose (ACD) to platelet products, which serves as a calcium chelator to disrupt the coagulation cascade and prevent clot formation. In order to generate fibrin clot for depletion of the fibrinogen from the platelet lysate supplement, 20 mM $CaCl_2$ is added to the platelet lysate, which enables the protease-driven conversion of fibrinogen to fibrin, thus leading to spontaneous clot formation. The addition of heparin at a concentration of 2 U/mL also stabilizes clot formation and increases yield of the soluble fraction of the platelet lysate. Under these conditions, over 85% of the platelet lysate is recovered with a final fibrinogen concentration of less than 5 μg/mL (compared to a fibrinogen concentration of ~120 μg/mL in the unfractionated platelet lysate) [37].

The growth factor content of dPL has been well characterized and contains numerous abundant mitogens for cell culture. Specifically, dPL contains ample amounts of PDG-BB, TFG-β1, VEGF, EGF, and BDNF. These growth factors exist in levels significantly higher than standard serum and are preserved in both unfractionated and fibrinogen-depleted PL preparations. Furthermore, dPL is remarkably stable, with room temperature preparations of PL capable of maintaining consistent levels of PDGF-BB and EGF for up to 3 weeks [37]. The stability of dPL and low interlot variability are extremely desirable qualities in a cell culture supplement and therefore are well suited for ex vivo growth and expansion of human therapeutic cell lines.

2.1.2. Immunomodulatory effect of PL fibrinogen depletion on MSCs

The use of dPL as a cell culture supplement is advantageous because it not only decreases the risk of xenogenic contamination but dPL also induces a robust proliferative response in human MSCs. When compared to cells grown in FBS, low passage MSCs cultured in equivalent concentrations of dPL had significantly decreased doubling times and decreased cell volumes. Despite the increase in proliferation, cells grown in dPL maintained expression of typical MSC markers including CD44, CD90, CD73, HLA-I, and CD105 and lacked expression of CD45 and CD34 [37].

In addition to impacting proliferative capacity of MSCs, platelet lysate composition may also affect the immunomodulatory properties of MSCs. MSCs can have a profound immunosuppressive effect on various inflammatory processes. Exposure of MSCs to fibrinogen upregulates integrin and non-integrin fibrinogen-binding complexes. Furthermore, the analysis of the secretome of MSCs exposed to fibrinogen in vitro demonstrated a significant increase in pro-inflammatory cytokines IL-8, MCP-1, and IL-6 [37]. The impact of fibrinogen content in various PL formulations on T-cell activation and proliferation has also been examined. Recently, upregulation of indoleamine 2,3-dioxygenase (IDO) in MSCs has been shown to correlate with suppression of T-cell proliferation [38]. MSCs cultured in unfractionated PL had decreased IDO expression compared to cells cultured in FBS; however, the IDO response was restored when dPL was used as a culture supplement. This functional effect of MSCs on T-cell proliferation was also examined through a coculture assay where MSCs were cocultured with PBMCs exposed to CD3/CD8. T-cell proliferation was noted to be higher in the unfractionated PL compared to dPL and standard FBS. These data suggest that an increased fibrinogen content promotes a pro-inflammatory phenotype of MSCs in vitro, and conversely fibrinogen depletion of PL preserves the immunosuppressive properties of MSCs.

2.1.3. *Ex vivo enhancement of MSCs with dPL*

The ex vivo expansion for MSCs is essential for cell therapy, as a large number of cells are needed to achieve a desired therapeutic effect. Bone marrow aspirates and peripheral blood cultures provide a relatively low yield of MSCs, and this necessitates prolonged in vitro expansion in order to obtain an adequate number of cells for autologous cell therapy. An unfortunate consequence of this process is that prolonged culture leads to MSC senescence, loss of plasticity, and loss of self-renewal capacity. Typically, human MSCs grown in media supplemented with FBS begin to show signs of senescence after 10 passages, so either increasing proliferation at early passages or delaying the effect of senescence would improve the yield of MSCs for treatment of CLI.

The enriched milieu of growth factors contained within dPL can potentially overcome the senescence associated with long-term MSC culture. Griffith et al. demonstrated that proliferation in senescent MSCs (passage 13 or greater) could be reversed with culture in dPL. MSCs cultured in 5% dPL showed reduction in cell size and a decrease in doubling time while maintaining MSC markers and reducing β-gal production compared to control MSCs cultured in FBS. These effects were short-lived, however, and by passage 16, MSCs failed to proliferate adequately regardless of culture conditions. The transient increase in proliferative response was also evident in *late* passage MSCs (passages 10–11). Culturing in dPL led to a marked decrease in doubling time, but by passage 16, MSCs showed severe signs of senescence in both dPL and FBS treatment groups. Consistent with these results, no changes in telomerase activity were noted between groups [39]. This study clearly established that poor-quality MSCs could be rescued and restored to a robust proliferative state using dPL, even if the effect was only temporary.

2.1.4. *Expansion of MSCs from patients with CLI*

Expanding on the research of our collaborators, we have worked to exploit the benefits of dPL for cell therapy in patients with CLI. By generating patient-specific MSC cell lines from individuals with CLI, we were able to test the feasibility of expanding MSCs with dPL for future cell therapy trials. In our initial series, we isolated MSCs from bone marrow of amputated limbs of four patients with critical limb ischemia and four patients with critical limb ischemia and concomitant diabetes mellitus. This cohort of patients had no further surgical or endovascular revascularization options and therefore is representative of the population of patients who would benefit from new cell therapy strategies. Additionally, we obtained MSCs from four healthy donors through EPIC. All MSCs were initially plated in media containing FBS; however, at passage 4 they were transitioned to either media containing FBS or dPL. As demonstrated in previous studies, MSCs grown in dPL maintained a similar phenotype based on cell surface markers compared to cells grown in FBS (**Figure 1**), with no notable differences detected across all patient groups. Additionally, differentiation capacity was preserved in MSCs from all patient groups and culture conditions, with all cells differentiating toward osteogenic or adipogenic lineage under appropriate assay conditions [40].

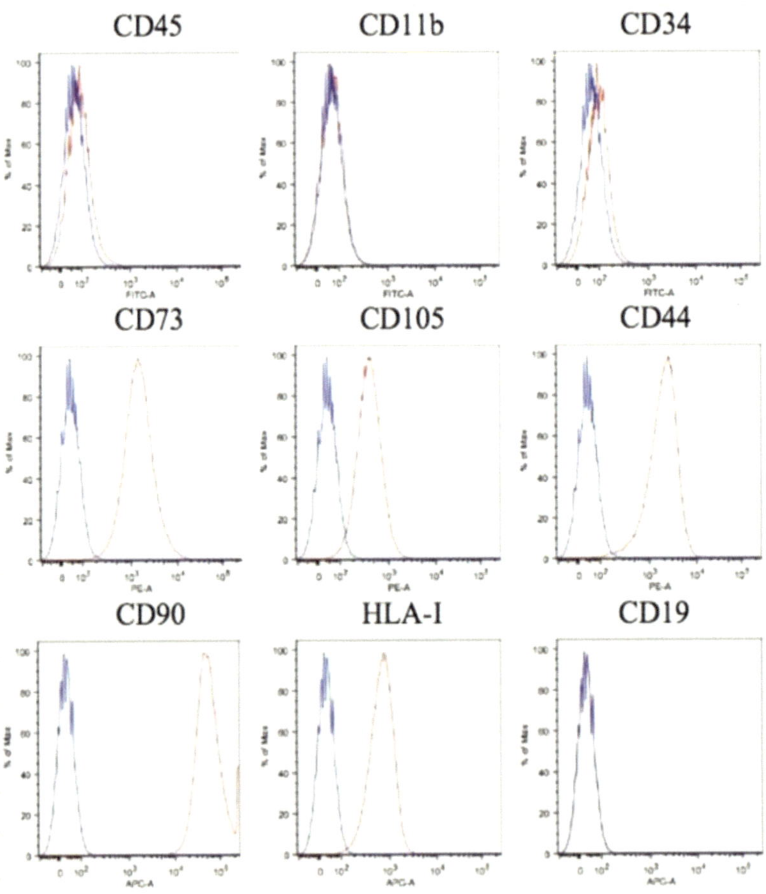

Figure 1. Representative flow cytometry of human MSCs cultured in dPL expresses typical MSC markers. Reprinted from Brewster et al. [40] with permission from Elsevier.

The proliferative response of MSCs from all patient groups and in culture conditions containing both FBS and dPL was examined by quantifying population doublings over multiple passages. For these experiments, a direct comparison of FBS and PL was performed, such that cells were cultured in either 5% FBS or 5% dPL. Cell counts were recorded at 7-day intervals, at which point MSCs were replated up to passage 11. We found that when all patient groups were analyzed together, the number of mean population doublings was increased in the dPL group at earlier passages, but by mid to late passage, the benefit of culturing cells in dPL had disappeared (**Figure 2**). When stratified according to disease state, cells cultured in dPL were non-inferior to cells cultured in FBS, and at early passage, cells cultured in dPL had increased number of population doublings across all groups. At early passage, there was also no difference when disease states were compared, suggesting that proliferative capacity of MSCs was preserved regardless of patient characteristics. From a practical standpoint, it should be noted that MSCs grown in dPL grew so rapidly at early passages that they quickly became confluent prior to subculturing, and thus proliferation was likely impaired by contact inhibition, so our experimental design may not have captured the full proliferative effect of dPL [40].

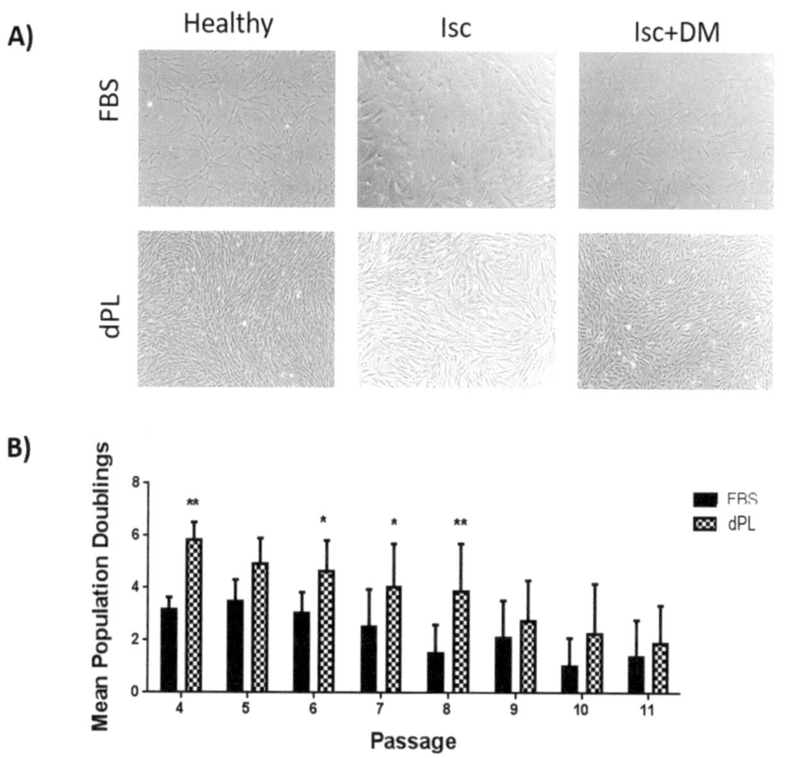

Figure 2. Cell culture with dPL leads to robust proliferation of human MSCs. In (A), MSCs from healthy controls are shown in comparison to MSCs isolated from the bone marrow of patients with CLI or CLI with concomitant diabetes mellitus. In (B), quantification of population doublings in MSCs across all patient groups was higher when grown in dPL than FBS at early passages, but by later passages, there was no difference between culture conditions. Reprinted from Brewster et al. [40] with permission from Elsevier.

We also characterized the functional capacity of MSCs across the different patient groups in vitro, in order to predict potential efficacy of MSCs for therapeutic angiogenesis in future human trials. A colony-forming unit (CFU) assay was performed on MSCs from each patient group. The number of CFUs in MSCS from patients with critical limb ischemia was similar to healthy control donors, suggesting that clonal capacity was independent of patient characteristics. A robust secretome analysis was also performed for all patient groups on MSCs that were cultured in either FBS or dPL. We specifically examined MSC production of bFGF, VEGF, HGF, and MCP-1. The secretome profiles were similar across all patient groups and culture conditions, with only minor differences noted. Furthermore, there were no obvious functional differences when conditioned media from the different treatment and patient groups were used to stimulate endothelial cell migration or proliferation. In order to assess the proangiogenic function of MSCs from patients with fibrinogen-rich platelet lysate (frPL), a coculture assay was used where MSCs from each patient mixed with a human endothelial cell line and embedded as cell pellets in 3D fibrin hydrogels. In this model the two cell types form sprouts which invade the fibrin hydrogel. Sprout length was quantified as a surrogate for angiogenic potential and was noted to be similar among all patient groups when MSCs were precultured in dPL. When MSCs were precultured in FBS, sprout length in the CLI group (without diabetes) was significantly lower than the CLI group with diabetes and the health controls. Despite any residual impairment within MSCs from patients with CLI that may result from epigenetic changes to the cells, the functional quality of MSCs from patients with CLI cultured with dPL appears to be equivalent of that healthy controls. These data support the use of dPL for expansion of MSCs and suggest that autologous cell therapy with MSCs for augmentation of neovascularization is a viable treatment strategy in patients with CLI.

Our study was the first in vitro testing of the proangiogenic characteristics of the bone marrow from amputated limbs in patients with CLI, but it is notably limited by the small sample size for each group. However, two important conclusions can be drawn from this study. First, we provide compelling data that, despite numerous reports that progenitor cell populations are impaired in patients with cardiovascular disease or associated risk factors, at least early-passage MSCs from patients with CLI are similar in quality to healthy controls when expanded ex vivo. Diabetes specifically has been shown to impair mesenchymal stem cell (MSC) function [41], at least partially due the effect of oxidative stress from Nox4 upregulation. Diabetes has also been shown to induce epigenetic changes in the promoter of IL-12 in bone marrow cells, such that cell fate is predisposed toward a pro-inflammatory phenotype. This raises the possibility that MSCs in patients with diabetes mellitus may have irreversible changes to the epigenetic signature. However, our study is consistent with other reports that demonstrate functional capacity of MSCs in patients with CLI is equivalent to healthy controls after short-term culture [42] and that ex vivo expansion in either FBS or PL may at least transiently overcome the epigenetic changes induced by patient comorbidities.

2.2. Platelet lysate as a scaffold for MSC delivery

2.2.1. Generation of fibrinogen-rich platelet lysate

Poor cell retention and viability at targeted sites of delivery have impaired advancement of cell therapies, as the number of functioning cells in the desired tissue appears to be critical for therapeutic efficacy [31, 43, 44]. Numerous biologic materials have been developed to promote cell retention and viability including encapsulation with alginate [45, 46], prefabrication of a tissue engineered patch [47, 48], and seeding of elongated fibrin strands [49]. While these approaches demonstrate that scaffold-mediated cell delivery improves the functional impact of cell therapy, the scaffold designs fail to incorporate any nutritive support for MSCs. In contrast to the fibrinogen-depleted form of platelet lysate used as a cell culture supplement for MSC growth, modifying the production process to retain clotting factors within platelet lysate (fibrinogen-rich platelet lysate or frPL) permits thrombin-induced self-assembly of a hydrogel with incorporated growth factors.

In order to generate platelet lysate that can spontaneously polymerize into 3D hydrogels, we modified the production process of dPL to maximize fibrinogen content of the platelet lysate. This was achieved by eliminating the step in which fibrin clot is formed and extracted from the solution. Our protocol again involves obtaining human platelets from Emory University blood bank in collaboration with EPIC. The platelets are then pooled and exposed to two sequential freeze-thaw cycles [freezing at -80°C for 48 h, then rapidly thawing at 37°C for 8 h] followed by centrifugation at 1500×g for 10 min. The rapid thawing phase is essential to prevent the formation of cryoprecipitate, which will deplete the solution of soluble clotting factors. The supernatant is then collected and stored at -20°C until ready for use. For hydrogel formation, the frPL is rapidly thawed at 37°C immediately prior to use and then centrifuged at 10,000×g for 10 min in 1.5 mL microcentrifuge tubes and sequentially filtered through 0.45 and 0.2 μm syringe tip filters.

Using this processing technique, we generated frPL with a fibrinogen concentration of 450 μg/mL which rapidly self-assembled into a 3D hydrogel with the addition of thrombin [50]. The hydrogel production process was refined for optimal durability and seeding with MSCs. For most applications, a 50% frPL hydrogel has preferential mechanical properties and provides appropriate MSC support. For hydrogel formation, an activating solution is prepared containing αMEM media with calcium chloride and thrombin so that the final concentrations are 5 mM and 2 U/mL, respectively, in a 50% PL gel. MSCs are then added to the activating solution at the desired cell density. The complete activating solution is then quickly mixed in a 1:1 ratio with frPL and cast in a cell culture plate and stored at 37°C for 1 h.

2.2.2. Structural composition of frPL

Microstructural analysis of [50] frPL indicates that fibrin is an essential component of frPL hydrogels. To evaluate the contribution to the frPL scaffold, frPL hydrogels and fibrin controls were loaded with 5% fluorescein isothiocyanate (FITC)-labeled fibrinogen and imaged with confocal microscopy to visualize the fibrin microstructure. The resulting images reveal an organized fibrin network within the frPL hydrogels that is more dense than control fibrin hydrogels but lacks clear elongated fibers (**Figure 3**). Additional imaging with scanning electron microscopy shows that the morphology of the frPL consists of thin, highly interconnected branched networks that are distinct from the fibrin hydrogels, which formed more distinct elongated fibrils (**Figure 3**) [50]. This was surprising since the 50% frPL contained only 225 μg/mL of fibrinogen, compared to the 1 mg/mL concentration of the fibrin-only controls. The proteolytic activity of thrombin rapidly initiates the polymerization for liquid frPL into a 3D scaffold. The conversion of fibrinogen to fibrin clearly plays an important role in hydrogel formation, but other structural components are also likely. At present, it is unclear which specific proteins contribute to the mesh network visualized with microscopy, although we speculate that there are additional clotting factors and retained membrane and cytoskeletal elements from platelets that incorporate into the scaffold.

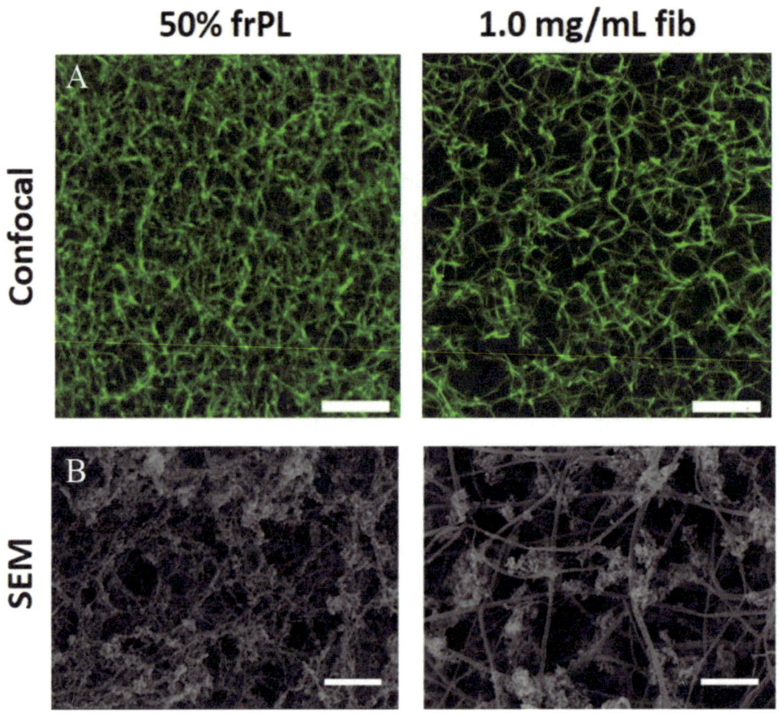

Figure 3. Microstructure of frPL and fibrin hydrogels is visualized in (A) with confocal microscopy after spiking with 5% FITC-labeled fibrinogen (scale bar equal to 20 μm) and (B) with scanning electron microscopy (SEM, scale bar equal to 1.0 μm). Reprinted from Robinson et al. [50], with permission from Elsevier.

The functional attributes of frPL hydrogels are also unique when compared to gels containing only fibrin. Mechanical testing on frPL revealed that these hydrogels behave as a viscoelastic solid with a storage and loss modulus equivalent to fibrin hydrogels with four times greater fibrin content [50]. The specific etiology of this property is unclear, but it may be the result of enhanced fibrin crosslinking due to the presence of additional components of the coagulation cascade, including Factor XIII. Additionally, numerous extracellular proteins (i.e., fibronectin, collagen), proteoglycans, and adhesion proteins such as Von Willebrand factor within the PL may reinforce the underlying fibrin network. Under experimental conditions, composite hydrogels containing additional elements such as collagen have improved mechanical strength over their homogenous control hydrogels without a change in total protein content [51, 52]. Therefore, the presence of these additional proteins may essentially act to form composite fibrin hydrogels with improved mechanical properties. The improved mechanical properties of frPL may also result from thrombin-induced polymerization of alternative macromolecules within the frPL that either alter fibrin binding sites or function as molecular crowders, thereby enhancing the viscoelastic behavior of the gel at relatively low fibrin concentrations [53, 54].

The microstructural differences between frPL and standard fibrin hydrogels extend beyond the microscopic appearance of the scaffold. Diffusion of FITC-labeled dextran molecules from 20 to 150 kDa that were embedded in hydrogels and diffusion of labeled dextran were significantly decreased. However, these differences between diffusion rates within hydrogels were due, at least in part, to the resistance of frPL hydrogels to proteolytic degradation [50]. This was supported by the fact that inclusion of aprotinin (a protease inhibitor) in culture media abrogated the differences between frPL and fibrin hydrogels. Additionally, frPL hydrogels containing 5% FITC-labeled fibrinogen retained labeled fibrin for up to 7 days, while fibrin-only gels rapidly degraded. Again, degradation rates were significantly decreased in fibrin gels with the addition of aprotinin, indicating that frPL is highly resistant to protease degradation compared to pure fibrin hydrogels [50]. Although the specific mechanism by which frPL hydrogels are stabilized has not been explored, it is likely due to the presence of serine protease inhibitors within frPL such as α2-antiplasmin or plasminogen activator inhibitor-1 (PAI-1), which are abundant in platelets and plasma and significantly impair fibrinolysis.

During hydrogel polymerization, the abundant growth factors present in soluble PL become entrapped within the frPL scaffold. We found that frPL hydrogels are enriched in PDGF-BB, which is released over 20 days in vitro, and ~45% of PDGF-BB persisted within the frPL gel at completion of that time course [50]. The retention of PDGF-BB in frPL hydrogels is superior to that seen in optimized formulations of fibrin-only hydrogels in vitro [55, 56], where greater than 90% of PDGF-BB is released after 7 days [57]. In addition to serving as a proangiogenic growth factor [58], PDGF-BB is also a critical mediator of MSC engraftment into tissue [59]; therefore, frPL can serve to both enhance engraftment of MSCs delivered within the scaffold and also exert a proangiogenic effect on native endothelial cells. The unique microstructure of frPL and resistance to degradation permit sustained release of these growth factors, such that the therapeutic window of MSCs embedded within the frPL scaffold is prolonged.

2.2.3. *Impact of frPL on MSC function*

The enriched milieu of growth factors and cytokines contained within frPL hydrogel has numerous beneficial effects on both MSCs and endothelial cells in vitro. Seeding of MSCs in frPL hydrogels leads to extensive proliferation of MSCs when quantified with MTS assay. In fact, cell number was higher in an frPL gel than fibrin-only gels when quantified over 7 days and also higher than in cells grown in a monolayer with dPL supplemented media. The frPL does not appear to have the same mitogenic effect on endothelial cells, as HUVECs grown in frPL hydrogels showed very little proliferative activity compared to controls [50].

The frPL hydrogel also has a significant impact on cell invasion. Sprout length from MSC/EC coculture pellets embedded in hydrogels was significantly longer than sprout length in fibrin controls (**Figure 4**) [50]. When MSCs or ECs alone were embedded in frPL, there was a notable difference in effect between the two different cell types. MSC sprouting appeared to be dependent on fibrin content, as sprout invasion was greater in low concentration fibrin hydrogels in addition to frPL. In contrast to its effect on MSCs, the frPL scaffold led to superior invasion of HUVECs compared to both high and low fibrin controls. Cells with the frPL scaffold receive both biochemical and biomechanical cues, which have a variable effect on different cell types. The frPL induces endothelial migration through biochemical signaling, but does not impact proliferation. On the other hand, growth factor signaling within the frPL causes substantial proliferation in MSCs, while the soft substrate of the scaffold provides mechanical cues to stimulate cell migration of MSCs. Based on this in vitro data, we can infer that frPL hydrogels embedded with MSCs have the ability to recruit remote endothelial cells, as demonstrated in the transwell migration assay. These data support the proposed clinical treatment strategy, whereby PL gel embedded with MSCs recruits host ECs for neovascularization following implantation in ischemic tissues.

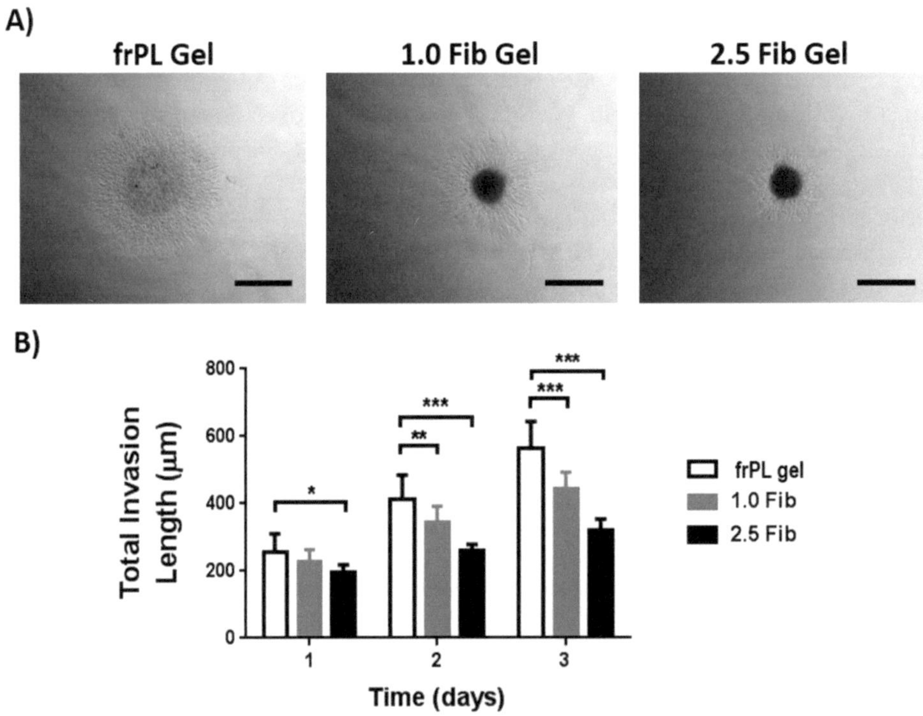

Figure 4. Cell sprouting of hydrogels. Human MSCs and HUVECs were mixed in a 1:1 ratio and embedded in frPL, 1.0 mg/mL fibrin, or 2.4 mg/mL fibrin hydrogels. Sprout length was assessed over 3 days in culture. Representative bright field images of each group at day 3 are shown in (A). Sprout length is quantified in (B). Reprinted from Robinson et al. [50], with permission from Elsevier.

http://dx.doi.org/10.5772/66934

Preliminary testing in a mouse model of hind limb ischemia supports this treatment strategy. Implantation of MSCs embedded in PL into ischemic limbs in a mouse model of HLI led to rapid neovascularization of ischemic tissues by 8 days when assessed with LDPI. Rapid and complete neovascularization of gastrocnemius muscle occurred in 8 days, which was increased significantly when compared to PL gel alone and MSCs alone (**Figure 5**) [50].

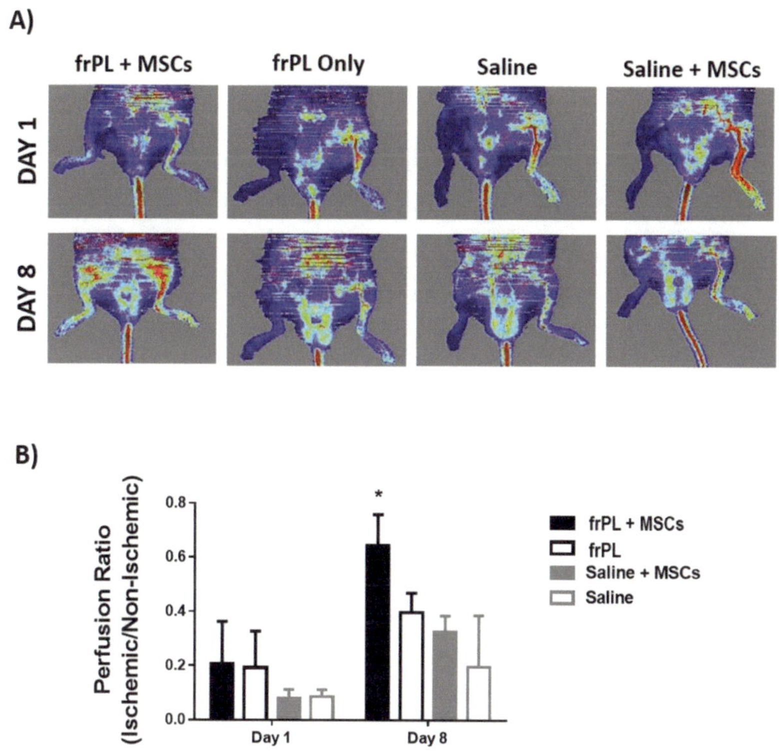

Figure 5. MSCs in saline or frPL were injected into the ischemic hind limb of mice, and perfusion with LDPI was assessed after 8 days. (A) Representative LDPI images are shown of the different groups. (B) Perfusion ratio of the ischemic to nonischemic limb is quantified for each group. Reprinted from Robinson et al. [50] with permission from Elsevier.

2.2.4. *Encapsulation of MSCs with frPL*

More recently, we have identified an additional novel application of frPL that results from its unique effect on MSCs. For most experiments hydrogels are cast in sterile, tissue culture treated polystyrene wells. In most cases the hydrogel will adhere to the walls and floor of the dish. However, when tissue culture plates are preincubated with a solution containing 2% albumin, hydrogels are no longer tethered to the plastic. When MSCs are embedded in fibrin gels, they exert a modest contractile effect on the scaffold that results in ~75% reduction in gel volume. However, when MSCs are embedded in an untethered frPL, hydrogel gel volume is reduced to 1–2% of the initial volume over 3 days (**Figure 6**). Cells were stained with CellTracker Red, and labeled fibrinogen was added to the frPL, and the reorganization of fibrin strands can clearly be seen with rounding of the cell bodies with loss of extending processes (**Figure 6**). Cell viability is preserved in cells encapsulated within frPL pellets. The pellets can be degraded and MSCs can be released with dispase treatment. Viability of MSCs within the frPL pellets is preserved for up to 3 days in vitro, as determined with a live/dead assay. The ability of frPL to form dense cell spheroids containing MSCs provides yet another practical application of platelet lysate. The frPL MSC spheroids could serve as an additional mechanism of cell delivery, by encapsulating MSCs in a thin fibrin shell.

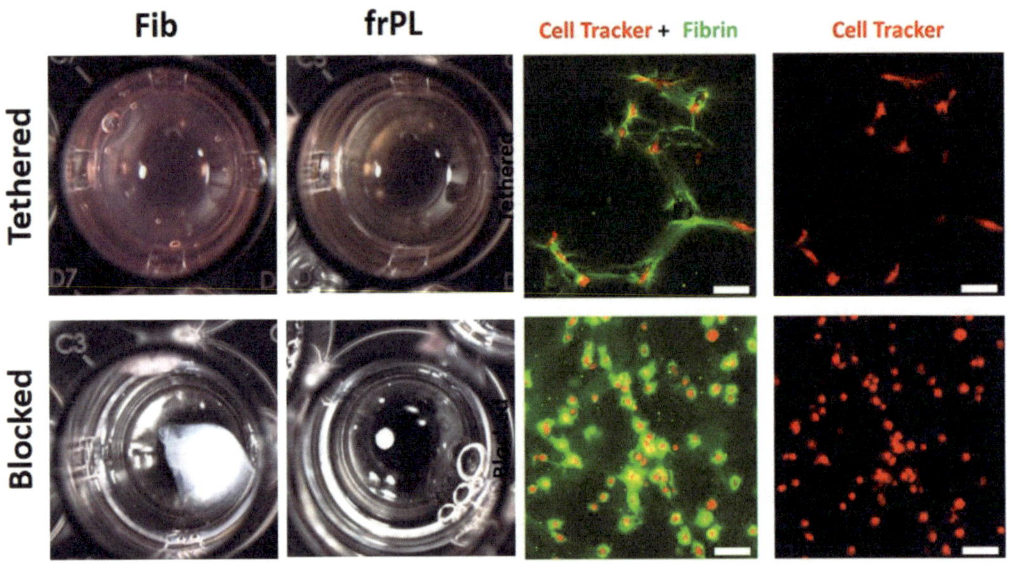

Figure 6. MSCs embedded in untethered frPL form cell spheroids. 2×10^5 MSCs/mL were embedded in frPL or fibrin hydrogels in six well tissue culture dishes with (untethered) and without (tethered) preblocking the plate with 2% albumin solution. MSCs within the frPL formed dense spheroids. Hydrogels were labeled with 5% FITC-dextran and seeded with CellTracker Red-labeled MSCs in tethered and untethered culture conditions. Scale bars represent 20 μm (original figure).

3. Conclusion

Innovative strategies are needed for enhancing quality of MSCs in patients with CLI while also improving delivery and retention of MSCs for cell-based therapy. Here we discuss the dual use of human platelet lysate as both a cell culture supplement and a scaffold for cell delivery. When bereft of clotting factors, depleted form of platelet lysate (dPL) supplemented media enables rapid expansion of MSCs without diminishing their angiogenic activity. In contrast, with preservation of clotting factors, frPL forms a rapidly assembling hydrogel with desirable structural properties and biological activity on MSC and ECs. In both soluble and hydrogel form, PL augments the proangiogenic qualities of MSCs and is readily derived from human source materials that have been tested for safe delivery to patients. As a result of these unique traits, PL hydrogel is ideally suited to serve as a cell culture supplement for MSC growth and as a vector for delivery of MSCs to ischemic tissues.

Author details

Scott T. Robinson[1] and Luke P. Brewster[2, 3*]

*Address all correspondence to: lbrewst@emory.edu

1 Department of Surgery, University of Michigan School of Medicine, Ann Arbor, MI, USA

2 Department of Surgery, Emory University of Medicine, Atlanta, GA, USA

3 Atlanta VA Medical Center, Surgical and Research Services, Decatur, GA, USA

References

[1] Hirsch, A. T. *et al.* Peripheral arterial disease detection, awareness, and treatment in primary care. *JAMA* **286**, 1317–24 (2001).

[2] Norgren, L. *et al.* Inter-society consensus for the management of peripheral arterial disease (TASC II). *J. Vasc. Surg.* **45 Suppl S**, S5–67 (2007).

[3] Otteman, M. G. & Stahlgren, L. H. Evaluation of factors which influence mortality and morbidity following major lower extremity amputations for arteriosclerosis. *Surg. Gynecol. Obstet.* **120**, 1217–20 (1965).

[4] Asahara, T. *et al.* Isolation of putative progenitor endothelial cells for angiogenesis. *Science (80-.).* **275**, 964–966 (1997).

[5] Risau, W. Mechanisms of angiogenesis. *Nature* **386**, 671–4 (1997).

[6] Heil, M., Eitenmüller, I., Schmitz-Rixen, T. & Schaper, W. Arteriogenesis versus angiogenesis: similarities and differences. *J. Cell. Mol. Med.* **10**, 45–55 (2006).

[7] Asahara, T. *et al.* Bone marrow origin of endothelial progenitor cells responsible for postnatal vasculogenesis in physiological and pathological neovascularization. *Circ. Res.* **85**, 221 (1999).

[8] Takahashi, T. *et al.* Ischemia- and cytokine-induced mobilization of bone marrow-derived endothelial progenitor cells for neovascularization. *Nat. Med.* **5**, 434–8 (1999).

[9] Shi, Q. *et al.* Evidence for circulating bone marrow-derived endothelial cells. *Blood* **92**, 362 (1998).

[10] Rajantie, I. *et al.* Adult bone marrow-derived cells recruited during angiogenesis comprise precursors for periendothelial vascular mural cells. *Blood* **104**, 2084 (2004).

[11] Ziegelhoeffer, T. *et al.* Bone marrow-derived cells do not incorporate into the adult growing vasculature. *Circ. Res.* **94**, 230–8 (2004).

[12] O'Neill, T. J., Wamhoff, B. R., Owens, G. K. & Skalak, T. C. Mobilization of bone marrow-derived cells enhances the angiogenic response to hypoxia without transdifferentiation into endothelial cells. *Circ. Res.* **97**, 1027–35 (2005).

[13] Purhonen, S. *et al.* Bone marrow-derived circulating endothelial precursors do not contribute to vascular endothelium and are not needed for tumor growth. *Proc. Natl. Acad. Sci.* **105**, 6620 (2008).

[14] Planat-Benard, V. *et al.* Plasticity of human adipose lineage cells toward endothelial cells: physiological and therapeutic perspectives. *Circulation* **109**, 656–63 (2004).

[15] Cho, S. W. *et al.* Improvement of postnatal neovascularization by human embryonic stem cell derived endothelial-like cell transplantation in a mouse model of hindlimb ischemia. *Circulation* **116**, 2409–19 (2007).

[16] Lian, Q. *et al.* Functional mesenchymal stem cells derived from human induced pluripotent stem cells attenuate limb ischemia in mice. *Circulation* **121**, 1113–23 (2010).

[17] Al-Khaldi, A., Al-Sabti, H., Galipeau, J. & Lachapelle, K. Therapeutic angiogenesis using autologous bone marrow stromal cells: improved blood flow in a chronic limb ischemia model. *Ann. Thorac. Surg.* **75**, 204–209 (2003).

[18] Gnecchi, M., Zhang, Z., Ni, A. & Dzau, V. J. Paracrine mechanisms in adult stem cell signaling and therapy. *Circ. Res.* **103**, 1204–19 (2008).

[19] Eliopoulos, N., Stagg, J., Lejeune, L., Pommey, S. & Galipeau, J. Allogeneic marrow stromal cells are immune rejected by MHC class I- and class II-mismatched recipient mice. *Blood* **106**, 4057–65 (2005).

[20] Nauta, A. J. *et al.* Donor-derived mesenchymal stem cells are immunogenic in an allogeneic host and stimulate donor graft rejection in a nonmyeloablative setting. *Blood* **108**, 2114–20 (2006).

[21] Kinnaird, T. *et al.* Local delivery of marrow-derived stromal cells augments collateral perfusion through paracrine mechanisms. *Circulation* **109**, 1543–9 (2004).

[22] Moon, M. H. *et al.* Human adipose tissue-derived mesenchymal stem cells improve postnatal neovascularization in a mouse model of hindlimb ischemia. *Cell. Physiol. Biochem.* **17**, 279–90 (2006).

[23] Heeschen, C. *et al.* Profoundly reduced neovascularization capacity of bone marrow mononuclear cells derived from patients with chronic ischemic heart disease. *Circulation* **109**, 1615–22 (2004).

[24] Ghani, U. *et al.* Endothelial progenitor cells during cerebrovascular disease. *Stroke.* **36**, 151–3 (2005).

[25] Loomans, C. J. M. *et al.* Endothelial progenitor cell dysfunction: a novel concept in the pathogenesis of vascular complications of type 1 diabetes. *Diabetes* **53**, 195–9 (2004).

[26] Pistrosch, F. *et al.* PPARgamma-agonist rosiglitazone increases number and migratory activity of cultured endothelial progenitor cells. *Atherosclerosis* **183**, 163–7 (2005).

[27] Tepper, O. M. Human endothelial progenitor cells from type II diabetics exhibit impaired proliferation, adhesion, and incorporation into vascular structures. *Circulation* **106**, 2781–2786 (2002).

[28] Kondo, T. *et al.* Smoking cessation rapidly increases circulating progenitor cells in peripheral blood in chronic smokers. *Arterioscler. Thromb. Vasc. Biol.* **24**, 1442–7 (2004).

[29] Fan, W. *et al.* Adipose stromal cells amplify angiogenic signaling via the VEGF/mTOR/Akt pathway in a murine hindlimb ischemia model: a 3D multimodality imaging study. *PLoS One* **7**, e45621 (2012).

[30] van der Bogt, K. E. A. *et al.* Comparison of different adult stem cell types for treatment of myocardial ischemia. *Circulation* **118**, S121–9 (2008).

[31] Sheikh, A. Y. *et al.* In vivo functional and transcriptional profiling of bone marrow stem cells after transplantation into ischemic myocardium. *Arterioscler. Thromb. Vasc. Biol.* **32**, 92–102 (2012).

[32] Spees, J. L. *et al.* Internalized antigens must be removed to prepare hypoimmunogenic mesenchymal stem cells for cell and gene therapy. *Mol. Ther.* **9**, 747–56 (2004).

[33] Sporn, M. B. & Roberts, A. B. Transforming growth factor-beta. Multiple actions and potential clinical applications. *JAMA* **262**, 938–41 (1989).

[34] Ross, R., Bowen-Pope, D. F. & Raines, E. W. Platelet-derived growth factor and its role in health and disease. *Philos. Trans. R. Soc. Lond. B. Biol. Sci.* **327**, 155–69 (1990).

[35] Bieback, K. *et al.* Human alternatives to fetal bovine serum for the expansion of mesenchymal stromal cells from bone marrow. *Stem Cells* **27**, 2331–41 (2009).

[36] Schallmoser, K. *et al.* Human platelet lysate can replace fetal bovine serum for clinical-scale expansion of functional mesenchymal stromal cells. *Transfusion* **47**, 1436–46 (2007).

[37] Copland, I. B., Garcia, M. A., Waller, E. K., Roback, J. D. & Galipeau, J. The effect of platelet lysate fibrinogen on the functionality of MSCs in immunotherapy. *Biomaterials* **34**, 7840–50 (2013).

[38] François, M., Romieu-Mourez, R., Li, M. & Galipeau, J. Human MSC suppression correlates with cytokine induction of indoleamine 2,3-dioxygenase and bystander M2 macrophage differentiation. *Mol. Ther.* **20**, 187–95 (2012).

[39] Griffiths, S., Baraniak, P. R., Copland, I. B., Nerem, R. M. & McDevitt, T. C. Human platelet lysate stimulates high-passage and senescent human multipotent mesenchymal stromal cell growth and rejuvenation in vitro. *Cytotherapy* **15**, 1469–83 (2013).

[40] Brewster, L. L. *et al.* Expansion and angiogenic potential of mesenchymal stem cells from patients with critical limb ischemia. *J. Vasc. Surg.* 2016 Feb 24. pii: S0741-5214(16)00222-6. doi: 10.1016/j.jvs.2015.02.061. [Epub ahead of print] PMID:26921003.

[41] Yan, J. *et al.* Type 2 diabetes restricts multipotency of mesenchymal stem cells and impairs their capacity to augment postischemic neovascularization in db/db mice. *J. Am. Heart Assoc.* **1**, e002238 (2012).

[42] Gremmels, H. *et al.* Neovascularization capacity of mesenchymal stromal cells from critical limb ischemia patients is equivalent to healthy controls. *Mol. Ther.* **22**, 1960–70 (2014).

[43] Swijnenburg, R. J. J. *et al.* Timing of bone marrow cell delivery has minimal effects on cell viability and cardiac recovery after myocardial infarction. *Circ. Cardiovasc. Imaging* **3**, 77–85 (2010).

[44] Hong, K. U. *et al.* C-Kit+ cardiac stem cells alleviate post-myocardial infarction left ventricular dysfunction despite poor engraftment and negligible retention in the recipient heart. *PLoS One* **9**, 1–7 (2014).

[45] Landázuri, N. & Levit, R. Alginate microencapsulation of human mesenchymal stem cells as a strategy to enhance paracrine-mediated vascular recovery after hindlimb ischaemia. *J Tissue Eng Regen Med.* 2016 Mar; 10(3):222–32. doi: 10.1002/term.1680. Epub 2012 Dec 21.

[46] Levit, R. D. *et al.* Cellular encapsulation enhances cardiac repair. *J. Am. Heart Assoc.* **2**, e000367 (2013).

[47] Simpson, D. L., Boyd, N. L., Kaushal, S., Stice, S. L. & Dudley, S. C. Use of human embryonic stem cell derived-mesenchymal cells for cardiac repair. *Biotechnol. Bioeng.* **109**, 274–83 (2012).

[48] Wei, H. J. *et al.* Bioengineered cardiac patch constructed from multilayered mesenchymal stem cells for myocardial repair. *Biomaterials* **29**, 3547–3556 (2008).

[49] Guyette, J. P. *et al.* A novel suture-based method for efficient transplantation of stem cells. *J. Biomed. Mater. Res.–Part A* **101 A**, 809–818 (2013).

[50] Robinson, S. T. *et al.* A novel platelet lysate hydrogel for endothelial cell and mesenchymal stem cell-directed neovascularization. *Acta Biomater.* **36**, 86–98 (2016).

[51] Rowe, S. L. & Stegemann, J. P. Microstructure and mechanics of collagen-fibrin matrices polymerized using ancrod snake venom enzyme. *J. Biomech. Eng.* **131**, 61012 (2009).

[52] Rowe, S. L. & Stegemann, J. P. Interpenetrating collagen-fibrin composite matrices with varying protein contents and ratios. *Biomacromolecules* **7**, 2942–8 (2006).

[53] Stabenfeldt, S. E., Gourley, M., Krishnan, L., Hoying, J. B. & Barker, T. H. Engineering fibrin polymers through engagement of alternative polymerization mechanisms. *Biomaterials* **33**, 535–44 (2012).

[54] Barker, T. H., Fuller, G. M., Klinger, M. M., Feldman, D. S. & Hagood, J. S. Modification of fibrinogen with poly(ethylene glycol) and its effects on fibrin clot characteristics. *J. Biomed. Mater. Res.* **56**, 529–35 (2001).

[55] Thomopoulos, S. & Zaegel, M. PDGF-BB released in tendon repair using a novel delivery system promotes cell proliferation and collagen remodeling. *J Orthopaedic Res.* 1358–1368 (2007). doi:10.1002/jor

[56] Sakiyama-Elbert, S. & Das, R. Controlled-release kinetics and biologic activity of platelet-derived growth factor-BB for use in flexor tendon repair. *J Hand Sur.* **33**, 1548–1557 (2008).

[57] Greisler, H. P. *et al.* Enhanced endothelialization of expanded polytetrafluoroethylene grafts by fibroblast growth factor type 1 pretreatment. *Surgery* **112**, 244-54–5 (1992).

[58] B-receptors, P. *et al.* PDGF-BB modulates endothelial proliferation and angiogenesis in vitro. **125**, 917–928 (1994).

[59] Lin, R.-Z. *et al.* Human endothelial colony-forming cells serve as trophic mediators for mesenchymal stem cell engraftment via paracrine signaling. *Proc. Natl. Acad. Sci. U. S. A.* **111**, 10137–42 (2014).

Chapter 19

Anti-VEGF Therapy in Cancer: A Double-Edged Sword

Victor Gardner, Chikezie O. Madu and Yi Lu

Additional information is available at the end of the chapter

http://dx.doi.org/10.5772/66763

Abstract

Vascular endothelial growth factor (VEGF) is a mitogen that plays a crucial role in angiogenesis and lymphangiogenesis. It is involved in tumor survival through inducing tumor angiogenesis and by increasing chemoresistance through autocrine signaling. Because of its importance in tumor formation and survival, several medications have been developed to inhibit VEGF and reduce blood vessel formation in cancer. Although these medications have proven to be effective for late-stage and metastatic cancers, they have been shown to cause side effects such as hypertension, artery clots, complications in wound healing, and, more rarely, gastrointestinal perforation and fistulas. Current research in using anti-VEGF medication as a part of cancer treatments is focusing on elucidating the mechanisms of tumor resistance to VEGF medication, developing predictive biomarkers that assess whether a patient will respond to VEGF therapy and creating novel treatments and techniques that increase the efficacy of antiangiogenic medication. This chapter aims to review the role of VEGF in tumor angiogenesis and metastasis, the structure and function of VEGF and its receptors, and VEGF's role in cancer are discussed. Furthermore, tumor therapies targeting VEGF along with their side effects are presented and, finally, new directions in anti-VEGF therapy are considered along with the challenges.

Keywords: VEGF, angiogenesis, side effect, medication

1. Introduction

Oxygen and nutrients are critical to the functioning and survival of cells in the body. This need is met through the creation of an extensive vascular system, which is maintained through the process of angiogenesis, and the creation of blood vessels from the existing vasculature [1]. In the angiogenesis process, endothelial cells initially respond to changes in the local environment and migrate toward the growing tumor. The endothelial cells then migrate together forming tubular structures that are ultimately encapsulated by recruiting periendothelial support cells to establish a vascular network that facilitates tumor growth and metastasis. Angiogenesis is subject to a complex regulatory system of both pro- and antiangiogenic factors after a tissue is fashioned [1–3] and deregulating angiogenesis–a classic trademark of cancer–leads to an aberrant microenvironment and promotion of tumor progression. Angiogenesis is initiated by the binding actions of vascular endothelial growth factor (VEGF) and fibroblast growth factors (FGF1/2) [4].

VEGF is an essential proangiogenic factor whose production is itself extensively regulated by a plethora of growth factors, cytokines, and other extracellular molecules produced in response to the various metabolic and mechanical conditions present in the cell's environment [2–6]. VEGF plays a pivotal role in tumor angiogenesis. The overexpression of VEGF is one of the central factors that leads to the onset and progression of cancer. In order to sustain their growth beyond any current size, tumors require an increased supply of blood, and this is achieved through the expression and secretion of VEGF, which stimulates the induction of new blood vessels around the tumor. Furthermore, the cancer cells, through the action of this subfamily of growth factors, invade other organs and areas of the body (metastasis) [4]. Consequently, VEGF and the resulting tumor angiogenesis present an attractive therapeutic target in the treatment of cancer. Inhibitors of VEGF/angiogenesis have been garnering interest and studied for their therapeutic application in most solid tumors [7, 8]. Moreover, a series of preclinical studies have revealed that anti-VEGF compounds increase the efficacy of ensuing antitumor treatment, although the mechanism of this effect is unclear [9].

2. Structure and function of VEGF and VEGFRs

VEGF is a dimeric glycoprotein secreted by cells that is able to induce permeability of blood vessels and promotes angiogenesis. The VEGF family contains seven members, all part of the platelet-derived growth factor (PDGF) supergene family: VEGF-A, VEGF-B, VEGF-C, VEGF-D, VEGF-E, VEGF-F, and PlGF [10, 11]. All members contain a core region comprised of eight cysteine residues forming a cysteine knot motif. These residues are involved in both inter- and intramolecular disulfide bonds at one end of a central four-stranded β-sheet within each monomer, which dimerizes in antiparallel fashion [11]. VEGFs A–D and PlGF are all produced in humans, whereas VEGF-E is produced in the Orf virus, has a 25% amino acid homology to mammalian VEGF, and lacks a heparin-binding domain [12]. VEGF-F is produced in snake venom and varies its structure and function by species, helping to produce a variety of venom [13].

The VEGF-A gene contains eight different exons that create six different isoforms through alternative splicing. These isoforms have lengths (in amino acids) of 121, 145, 165, 183, 189, and 206 that are produced by the alternate splicing of a single gene containing eight exons, and they all contain exons 1–5 and 8. All forms of VEGF-A except for VEGF-A_{121} can bind to heparin [11]. $VEGF_{165}$ is the one most commonly secreted by tumor cells and acts most strongly

http://dx.doi.org/10.5772/66763

on endothelial cells to lead them to form new capillaries. VEGF-B exists as two isoforms of lengths 167 and 186 amino acids and has been shown to act as a cell survival factor while exhibiting little proangiogenic effect [14]. VEGF-C and VEGF-D are resealed proteolytically from their respective precursor proteins and play important roles in regulating lymphangiogenesis [10, 11]. PlGF upregulates angiogenesis through binding to VEGFR-1 (thereby freeing VEGF-A to bind to VEGFR-2) and exists in four isoforms of amino acid lengths 131, 152, 203, and 224 [15]. It has also been shown to induce a specific phosphorylation and activation of c-Jun N-terminal kinase (JNK) and p38 [16].

VEGF signaling pathway plays a major role in angiogenesis. VEGF receptors (VEGFRs) are type V receptor tyrosine kinases (RTKs) activated upon ligand-mediated dimerization [17]. Two high-affinity VEGF receptors, VEGFR-1 (Flt-1) and VEGFR-2 (Flk-1/KDR), have been identified in endothelial cells. Flk-1 (R2) has been shown to play a major role in tumor angiogenesis. In all, there are three types of receptors, with VEGFR-3 only binding to VEGFs –C and –D. Each of the three types of receptor (VEGFR-1, -2, and -3) is composed of seven immunoglobulin-like domains in the extracellular region, a transmembrane region, and a tyrosine kinase sequence with a kinase insert domain [11].

Signaling of VEGF is initiated via binding to its receptors, which are tyrosine kinases that are able to transphosphorylate tyrosine residues of SH2 domain-containing signaling molecules, thus activating kinase-dependent transcription factors known as STAT proteins, to modulate cell responses induced by VEGF. VEGFR-1 and -2 are both involved in endothelial cell function and angiogenesis [18], while VEGFR-3, to which only VEGFs –C and –D can bind, plays a critical role in lymphangiogenesis and primarily involved in normal embryonic development [11]. VEGF-1 has also been shown to be required in inducing the migration of monocytes and macrophages [19]. Neuropilins-1 and -2 are important coreceptors for VEGF signaling and increase the affinity of VEGF-A_{165} for its receptors [5]. Refer to **Figure 1** for a summary of how each VEGF pairs with each VEGF receptor.

VEGF is heavily involved in promoting angiogenesis and research suggests that it also plays a role in regulating intussusceptive angiogenesis as well. In sprouting angiogenesis, hypoxia induces parenchymal cells to release VEGF-A into the extracellular matrix (ECM). VEGF-A then causes tip cells to produce the Delta-like-4 (Dll4) ligand, which is a membrane-bound ligand that serves to activate the Notch receptor, a highly conserved transmembrane receptor that regulates cell proliferation, cell fate, and cell death in metazoans on neighboring cells through cell to cell contact [20]. Dll4 then inhibits migratory behavior through activating the Notch receptor on neighboring stalk cells. Tip cell filopodia, actin-rich protrusions on the cell membrane that serve as a mechanism for a cell to explore its environment, sense a gradient in VEGF-A and align their sprouting to this gradient. The tip cell then anchors itself onto the substratum while actin microfilaments in the filopodia contract, pulling the tip cell toward the VEGF-A source while stalk cells proliferate. When the tip cells from different sprouts meet, they fuse to become a functional capillary through which blood can flow [1]. The function of VEGF in sprouting angiogenesis is less well understood, although it is suspected that VEGF cooperating with angiopoietin-1 (Ang-1) plays a role in stimulating the process [21, 22].

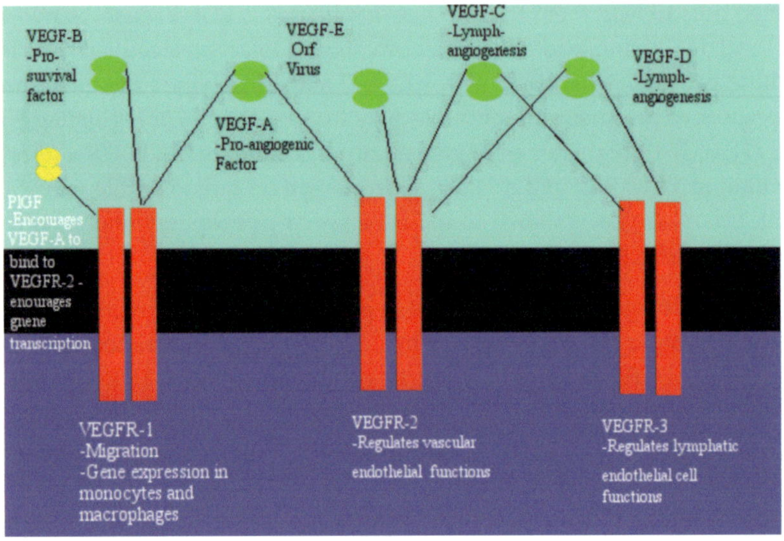

Figure 1. A summary of the functions of each form of VEGF and PlGF and each VEGF receptor. VEGFR-1 regulates cell migration and gene expression in monocytes and macrophages; VEGFR-2 regulates vascular endothelial functions; and VEGFR-3 regulates lymphatic endothelial functions. VEGF-A is a proangiogenic factor; VEGF-B is a prosurvival factor; VEGF-C and –D regulate lymphangiogenesis; VEGF-E is found in the Orf virus; and PlGF encourages VEGF-A to bind to VEGFR-2, thereby stimulating angiogenesis, and encourages the transcription of JNK and p38.

3. The role of VEGF in cancer

Tumors need oxygen to survive. At first, they are able to obtain enough oxygen by coopting the surrounding vasculature, altering its morphology, physiology, and response to therapy in the process. However, when a tumor becomes too large to be sufficiently supplied by existing vasculature, an "angiogenic switch" is turned on, and the tumor begins the process of tumor angiogenesis, thereby creating its own vasculature for an oxygen supply [23–26].

The angiogenic switch is triggered by hypoxia occurring when the tumor becomes too large for oxygen to diffuse from existing vasculature to tumor cells [27]. Hypoxia induces the production of VEGF in tumor cells through hypoxia-inducible factor-1α (HIF-1α) [25, 27], a master transcriptional factor that regulates a group of downstream genes including VEGF that promote angiogenesis and metastasis, while inhibitors of angiogenesis such as angiostatin and interferon are downregulated [23]. A suite of other proangiogenic genes (such as Ang-1 and -2) and regulatory mechanisms (such as micro-RNAs) are also regulated by the hypoxia-induced HIF pathway [25]. Tumor cells then release VEGF into the surrounding extracellular space, which binds to VEGF R of surrounding or nearby endothelial cells, promoting local angiogenesis and forming tumor-associated microvessels in order to delivering oxygen-carrying blood to the tumor.

Compared with normal vasculature, tumor vessels are highly irregular and inefficient at delivering nutrients. They branch irregularly, follow a tortuous path, are far larger than their normal counterparts, are unusually permeable to large molecules, have a high interstitial pressure, and are inefficient at carrying blood [26, 28]; these abnormalities of the tumor vasculature result in poor delivery of nutrients, causing certain areas of the tumor to be chronically hypoxic, stabilizing the HIF/VEGF signaling pathway described above and therefore resulting in even more tumor vasculature [25]. The overproduction of VEGF-A results in an abundance of tip cells from the Dll4 signaling pathway, which in part causes the malformed vasculature associated with tumors through excessive branching of these tip cells [25, 29].

Tumor blood vessel can be divided into six general classes: (1) mother vessels, which are enlarged, tortuous, thin-walled, lacking in pericytes, and highly permeable; (2) capillaries, which are similar to normal capillaries; (3) glomeruloid microvascular proliferations, which are tangles of vessels situated within a mixture of disordered pericytes; (4) vascular malformations, which are large vessels with an irregular coat of smooth muscle cells; (5) feeder arteries; and (6) draining vessels, which are enlarged, serpentine smooth muscle cell-coated vessels that supply and drain the blood vessels within the tumor [30]. The irregular pericyte and smooth muscle cell formations on these vessels, which in normal vasculature serve to enhance tight junctions and decrease leakiness, serve to decrease vessel efficacy in tumor angiogenesis [31].

Oncogenes play a prominent role in triggering the angiogenic switch. Expression of the H-Ras oncogene in the immortalized rat intestinal epithelial cell line IEC-18 led to the upregulation of VEGF and a significant increase of *in vivo* vascularization [32]. Ras signaling also results in the stabilization of the resulting mRNAs and possible enhancement of their transcription [33]. The p53 suppressor gene normally serves to downregulate VEGF while upregulating thrombospondin-1, an antiangiogenic factor; mutations in these genes serve to increase the activity of VEGF [34, 35]. p53 acts as a foil to C-Myc, a gene that triggers the expression of VEGF while downregulating thrombospondin-1. In tumors, mutations in p53 serve to increase the activity of c-Myc, thereby increasing the activity of VEGF [34].

Compared to VEGF-A, VEGF-B plays an insignificant role in angiogenesis. Rather, it acts as a potent survival factor, inhibiting the production of several proapoptotic factors such as BH-3-related proteins. The prosurvival effects of VEGF-B are mediated by both VEGFR-1 and the coreceptor NP-1 [36, 37]. More recent research suggests that VEGF-B may trigger tumor angiogenesis through a VEGF-A-independent pathway and that it may even be a prognostic marker for cancer metastasis [38].

VEGF-C and VEGF-D are both heavily involved in lymphangiogenesis. In tumors, these two forms of VEGF are overexpressed and activate VEGFR-3 by means of a paracrine signaling loop, thereby encouraging lymphatic growth within the tumor [39, 40]. Lymphatic vessels created through tumor angiogenesis tend to be larger than normal, enhancing the delivery of tumor cells to the lymph nodes, from which metastasis can occur (while VEGFR-3 activation causes lymphatic vessels to sprout, it should be noted that VEGFR-2 causes the vessels to become dilated) [41]. For example, metastasis of breast cancer occurs primarily through the lymphatic system, and VEGF-C has been shown to enhance tumor metastasis in this disease [42]. Because both lymphatic vessels and blood vessels provide nutrients and a metastatic pathway for a tumor, vascular density (lymphatic vessels density or blood vessel density) within the tumor may be a prognostic factor of metastatic potential [41, 43].

4. Anti-VEGF medications

Because of tumor dependence on VEGF for growth and survival, much work has been put into developing VEGF inhibitors for use in the clinic. Most of these inhibitors fall under two broad categories that differ in structure and mechanism of action: small-molecule inhibitors (SMIs) and monoclonal antibodies (mAbs). **Table 1** contains a list of the anti-VEGF medications mentioned in this chapter, their types, FDA approval dates, the forms of cancer they are approved to treat, and some common side effects associated with their use.

Some SMIs targeting VEGF signaling pathway are able to pass through the cellular membrane and interact with the cytoplasmic domain of receptor tyrosine kinases (RTKs) [44, 45]. Most act as competitive inhibitors with ATP. As the ATP binding site is common to all RTKs, specificity in the SMI is created by engineering the part of the molecule not similar to ATP [44]. Small molecule tyrosine kinase inhibitors (SMTKIs) can be divided into three broad categories: those that hydrogen bond with the ATP binding site of the enzyme's active conformation (type I), those that hydrogen bond with the hydrophobic pocket directly next to the ATP binding site in the enzyme's inactive conformation (type II), and those that bond covalently and irreversibly with specific cysteine residues on the kinase (type III) [44].

Sunitinib is a type I SMTKI [44] that is able to inhibit RTKs containing a split-kinase domain, such as VEGFRs -1, -2, and -3; PDGFRs –A and –B; cKIT; FLT3; CSF-1R; and RET [46]. The inhibition of the RTKs blocks signal transduction, thereby preventing tumor growth and angiogenesis among other processes. Sunitinib is administered orally in a recommended dose of 50 mg once daily for 4 weeks followed by a 2-week rest [47]. The medicine is currently FDA approved for use in progressive well-differentiated pancreatic neuroendocrine tumors in patients with unresectable, locally advanced, or metastatic disease; metastatic renal cell carcinoma; and gastrointestinal stromal tumors after intolerance to imatinib mesylate [46].

Sorafenib is a type II SMTKI [45]. Sorafenib inhibits VEGFR-2, VEGFR-3, PDGFR-β, and Kit; therefore, it operates through a dual mechanism of action, inhibiting both tumor growth and angiogenesis [48]. Sorafenib is administered in a recommended dose of 400 mg twice daily around mealtimes [47]. The medicine is FDA approved for use in recurrent or metastatic progressive differentiated thyroid carcinoma, advanced renal cell carcinoma, and unresectable hepatocellular carcinoma [49].

Vandetanib is a type III SMTKI [44]. It inhibits VEGFR-2, EGFR, and RET, blocking several signal transduction pathways that control tumor growth and angiogenesis [50]. Vandetanib was approved in 2011 for use against unresectable, locally advanced, or metastatic medullary thyroid cancer. The recommended daily dose of the medicine is 300 mg per day, administered orally [51].

In contrast to small molecule inhibitors, monoclonal antibodies (mAbs) cannot translocate through the plasma membrane to interact with the cytoplasmic domains of RTKs; they are, however, more specific in action than SMIs [45]. mAbs used in antiangiogenic therapies can be divided into two broad categories: those that bind to VEGF and inhibit VEGF's ability to bind with its receptors, and those that bind to VEGFRs and inhibit ligand-receptor interaction and activate immune responses.

http://dx.doi.org/10.5772/66763

Medicine	Type of medication	FDA approval date	Types of cancers approved for to date	Common Grade 3-4 side effects
Apatinib [114]	SMI	N/A	N/A	N/A
Bevacizumab [125]	mAb	26-Feb-04	Metastatic colorectal cancer, nonsmall cell lung cancer, glioblastoma, metastatic renal cell carcinoma, cervical cancer (in combination with chemotherapy), platinum-resistant recurrent epithelial ovarian, fallopian tube, or primary peritoneal cancer in combination with chemotherapy FDA approval for the use of bevacizumab in metastatic HER2-negative breast cancer was revoked on 18 Nov. 2011 on account of potentially life-threatening side effects and the few benefits associated with its use	Sensory neuropathy, hypertension, fatigue, neutropenia, vomiting, diarrhea
Cabozantinib [116]	SMI	25-Apr-16	Renal cell carcinoma in patients who have received prior antiangiogenic therapy	Abdominal pain, pleural effusion, diarrhea, and nausea
Pazopanib [126]	SMI	Oct-09	Advanced renal cell carcinoma, advanced soft tissue sarcoma	Diarrhea, hypertension, and proteinuria
Ramucirumab [96]	mAb	21-Apr-14	Gastric/gastroesophageal junction adenocarcinoma (with and without paclitaxel), with docetaxel for platinum-resistant metastatic nonsmall cell lung cancer, with FOLFIRI for metastatic colorectal cancer	Hypertension, hyponatremia, neutropenia, pneumonia
Sorafenib [50]	SMI	20-Dec-05	Advanced renal cell carcinoma, unresectable hepatocellular carcinoma, progressive differentiated thyroid carcinoma	Diarrhea, hand-foot syndrome
Sunitinib [46]	SMI	26-Jan-06	Gastrointestinal stromal tumor, advanced kidney cancer, pancreatic neuroendocrine tumors	Hypertension, diarrhea, nausea, vomiting
Vandetanib [52]	SMI	6-Apr-11	Medullary thyroid cancer in patients with unresectable, locally advanced, or metastatic disease	Diarrhea/colitis, hypertension and hypertensive crisis, QT prolongation, fatigue, and rash
Zif-Aflibercept [127]	VEGF-Trap (hybrid of VEGFR-1 binding domain and VEGFR-2 domain 3)	3-Aug-12	Metastatic colorectal cancer that is resistant to an oxaliplatin-containing regimen	Neutropenia, diarrhea, hypertension, leukopenia, stomatitis, fatigue, proteinuria, and asthenia
33C3 [57]	mAb	N/A	N/A	N/A

Table 1. FDA approvals for antiangiogenic drugs.

Perhaps the most well-known mAb targeting VEGF is bevacizumab, first approved in the EU in January 2005 [52]. The medicine targets all forms of VEGF-A, thereby inhibiting its ability to activate angiogenesis [53]. 2C3 is another mAb that binds to VEGF, preventing it from interacting with VEGFR-2, but not VEGFR-1; it blocks the growth of blood vessels in tumors and inhibits increases in vascular permeability [54]. IMC1121B (ramucirumab) binds to the ligand binding site of VEGFR-2 [55]. 33C3 is an antibody that binds to Ig domains 4-7 of VEGFR-2 and therefore, on account of binding to VEGFR-2 as opposed to a VEGF molecule, has the potential to act independently of VEGF concentration [56].

A type of VEGF inhibitor that defies simple classification into one of these two categories was developed recently as VGEF-trap, otherwise known as aflibercept. Aflibercept is a fusion protein consisting of the VEGFR-1 and VEGFR-2 binding domains and the Fc region of the IgG1 antibody [57, 58]. The protein binds to VEGF-A, VEGF-B, and PlGF, inhibiting activation of VEGFR-1 and VEGFR-2 and thereby inhibiting angiogenesis [57, 58]. Aflibercept was approved as Zaltrap on 3 August 2012 for use in combination with a FOLFIRI (folinic acid, fluorouracil, and irinotecan) chemotherapy regimen in adults with colorectal cancer [59], and has been shown to provide significant benefits in OS and PFS [60].

5. Side effects of anti-VEGF medications

No metabolically active tissue in the human body is more than a few hundred micrometers away from a capillary vesicle. The extensive nature of the vascular system in humans is produced and maintained through angiogenesis; changes in metabolic activity lead to changes in demand for oxygen which in turn regulate angiogenesis [1]. Therefore, angiogenesis inhibitors are bound to have adverse side effects. These side effects are generally less severe than those encountered from chemotherapy, although they can still be life-threatening [61]. Common side effects include hypertension, arterial thromboembolic events (ATEs), cardiotoxicity, and problems with bleeding, gastrointestinal perforation, and wound healing. See **Table 2** for a description of grades of adverse events.

Perhaps the most well documented side effect of angiogenesis inhibitors is hypertension. VEGF has been shown to decrease blood pressure; for example, in a phase I clinical trial (the VIVA trial, a double-blind placebo-controlled study), recombinant VEGF was shown to decrease systolic blood pressure by as much as 22% [62]. This decrease in blood pressure is caused by the generation of blood capillaries, which increases the total cross-sectional surface area available for blood to flow and thereby reduces blood pressure, and VEGF-induced vasodilation, which occurs when VEGF induces the production of nitric oxide and PGI_2 as part of its signal transduction pathway [63]. VEGF inhibitors therefore cause hypertension by inhibiting the production of nitric oxide and PGI_2, leading to vasoconstriction and an increase in blood pressure [64, 65]. Hypertension caused from VEGF inhibition can be managed using standard therapies, such as angiotensin-converting enzyme inhibitors, beta blockers, calcium channel blockers, diuretics, and angiotensin II receptor blockers [66].

VEGF-dependent interactions between the glomeruli and endothelial cells are also inhibited through anti-VEGF therapies (such as bevacizumab, sunitinib, and sorafenib [67]), leading to proteinuria, a common side effect in anti-VEGF treatment [65, 68]. Inhibition of the VEGF signaling pathway leads to the suppression of nephrin, which in turn leads to a decrease in maintenance of the glomerular slit diaphragm [68]. Luckily, most instances of proteinuria are mild, presenting as only grades I and II, although more severe proteinuria has been reported in a share of cases [67, 68].

Treatment with VGEF inhibitors is also associated with an increased risk of arterial thromboembolic events (ATEs) [65, 69, 70]. This increased risk is caused by a reduction in the regenerative capacity of endothelial cells and can diminish antiapoptotic factors while encouraging procoagulant changes in the blood vessels [70]. The rate of venous thromboembolic events does not seem to be affected by VEGF inhibition, at least when comparing bevacizumab with chemotherapy and chemotherapy alone [69]. It is recommended that patients on anti-VEGF therapy who develop an ATE be taken off the therapy immediately [65]. The use of aspirin during therapy has been shown to increase the likelihood of grade 3 and 4 bleeding events, although no significant difference has been found between aspirin users in control and bevacizumab-treated groups [69]. Patients with a history of ATEs and older patients are at greater risk in developing a thromboembolic event when using VEGF inhibitors such as bevacizumab [69].

Cardiotoxicity is also a common side effect of VEGF inhibition, and has been observed in patients on bevacizumab, sunitinib, and sorafenib. The exact mechanisms of this toxicity are often unclear, and they may either have to do with inhibition of VEGF, inhibition of other signaling pathways concomitantly with VEGF, or both. Cardiomyopathy has been observed in sunitinib monotherapy in a phase I/II trial in which 11% of all participants (8/75) had a cardiovascular event [71]. Another study found evidence that sunitinib induces cardiotoxocity through the inhibition of the AMPK signal transduction pathway [72]. Moreover, bevacizumab given after acute myelogenous leukemia chemotherapy resulted in an increase in cardiovascular toxicity, although the mechanisms for this toxicity remain unknown [73]. Sorafenib has also been demonstrated to cause cardiotoxicity in mice due to myocyte necrosis [74].

Grade	Description	Example with gastric fistula
I	Mild with few or no symptoms; no interventions required	Asymptomatic; clinical or diagnostic observations only; intervention not indicated
II	Moderate, with minimal intervention needed; some limitation of activities	Symptomatic; altered GI function
III	Severe but not life threatening; hospitalization required; limitation of patient's ability to care for him or herself	Severely altered GI function; bowel rest tube feeding; TPN or hospitalization indicated
IV	Life threatening; urgent intervention required	Life-threatening consequences; urgent operative intervention indicated
V	Death related to adverse event	death

Table 2. Explanation of grades of adverse events [76].

Some side effects are caused by the fact that VEGF impairment impairs wound healing on account of its antiangiogenic properties [65]. Gastrointestinal perforation has been known to occur in patients on anti-VEGF therapy. In the AVOREN trial, three patients receiving bevacizumab in combination with IFN-α experienced grade 4 gastrointestinal perforations, while one patient experienced grade 3 gastrointestinal perorations [66]. Sorafenib and sunitinib have also been shown to cause gastrointestinal perforations [65]. These perforations are caused by tumors, often metastatic, and the healing of these perforations is impaired because angiogenesis is itself prevented. Moreover, a significantly increased risk of hemorrhagic events of all grades is observed in patients on sorafenib, sunitinib, pazopanib, bevacizumab, and aflibercept [65, 75].

6. New directions

Although much progress has been made in angiogenesis inhibition therapy, research in the field is still ongoing. The following section reviews (i) how does tumor resistance against anti-VEGF mediation grow? (ii) what are the challenges in assessing biomarkers for the efficacy of antiangiogenic therapies in specific cases? and (iii) how can treatment methodologies and new treatments improve overall survival (OS)?

6.1. How does tumor resistance against anti-VEGF medication grow?

Tumor resistance to antiangiogenic therapies can be classified into two broad categories: intrinsic and acquired [65, 77]. Acquired antiangiogenic resistance, in contrast to normal methods of acquired drug resistance in which mutational alteration of the drug target prevent the drug from working, consists of tumors initiating alternative methods to cope with hypoxia [77]. There are at least four distinct mechanisms through which this acquired resistance operates: (1) through the activation and upregulation of alternative proangiogenic pathways; (2) through the recruitment of bone marrow-derived proangiogenic cells including increased pericyte coverage of tumor vasculature; (3) through increased tumor aggressiveness resulting in metastasis to provide vasculature through widespread vessel cooption as opposed to tumor angiogenesis; and (4) through the adoption of alternative angiogenic mechanisms [77].

6.1.1. *Proangiogenic pathways not involving VEGF*

Several proangiogenic molecular pathways are upregulated when the VEGF/VEGFR pathway is inhibited. This often results in a return of tumor vascularization after a period of refractoriness [65, 78]. Some examples of alternative proangiogenic pathways include fibroblast growth factors (FGFs), platelet-derived growth factors (PDGFs), tumor necrosis factor-α (TNF-α), placenta growth factor (PlGF), angiogenin, stromal-derived factor 1α (SDF-1α), and interleukins-1α and -1β (IL-1α, IL-1β) [79–81]. Several of these molecules are regulated through HIF-1 expression, which in turn is controlled by hypoxia [79]. Therefore, through inducing the regression of tumor vasculature, anti-VEGF therapies can induce the expression of other proangiogenic pathways that reduce their own efficacy.

Several therapies are being developed that target both VEGF and alternative angiogenic pathways at the same time. For example, blockage of both VEGF and bFGF with brivanib resulted in prolonged tumor stasis following previous angiogenic inhibition in mouse neuroendocrine tumors [82]. Another study reported that inhibiting SDF-1α after irradiating mice with implanted human U251 GBM tumors prevented the revascularization of irradiated tumors more effectively than inhibiting VEGF, thereby suggesting that SDF-1α may be involved in acquired resistance to anti-VEGF therapies as well [81]. It has also been suggested that synergism between FGF-2 and PDGF-bb could induce angiogenesis, even if they are only present at low concentrations within the cytoplasm [79]. Taken together, these results suggest that inhibition of alternative angiogenic pathways in addition to inhibiting VEGF could increase the efficacy of antiangiogenic therapy.

6.1.2. BMDCs

Bone marrow–derived cells (BMDCs) such as pericytes and macrophages play important roles in both normal and pathological angiogenesis [1, 83, 84]. Tumor-associated macrophages (TAMs) are attracted to hypoxic regions of tumors through the upregulation of chemoattractants caused by hypoxia. Following extravasation into the tumor region, monocytes migrate into hypoxic areas of the tumor, following a chemoattractant gradient [85]. Monocyte chemoattractant protein-1 (MCP-1) has been shown to be an important chemoattractant in this process [86]. Once in the hypoxic region of the tumor, macrophages will promote tumor progression and metastasis through their trophic role (breaking down the ECM and encouraging tumor cell motility) and through excreting compound such as mutagenic oxygen, nitrogen radicals, and several proangiogenic factors such as VEGF and angiopoietin-2 [83, 87].

The process through which pericytes contribute to cancer progression and metastasis is poorly understood. Normally, pericytes are associated with newly formed blood vessels, creating a single, often discontinuous, layer around the endothelial cell tube that serves to support a mature vessel. However, in tumor angiogenesis, pericyte coverage can be greater than, or less than normal tissue vasculature depending on the tumor type; for example, glioblastoma exhibits lower than normal pericytes coverage, while islet carcinomas exhibit higher than normal coverage. This aberrant pericyte coverage can result in tumor growth and metastasis [88]. Current pericytes-targeted cancer therapies aim to reach a balance between pro-and anti-angiogenic factors, encouraging vascular normalization [89].

6.1.3. Increased tumor aggressiveness

In most cancers, the appearance of a proinvasive phenotype following antiangiogenic therapy is in question; however, in glioblastoma it is relatively undisputed [78], and there is evidence suggesting its occurrence in pancreatic cancer [90]. The proinvasive phenotype allows tumors from these cancers to circumvent the need for a blood supply, obviating the necessity of tumor angiogenesis. The mechanisms underlying this increased tumor aggressiveness are not fully known. HIFs have been widely accepted as playing a role in increased tumor aggressiveness and metastasis [90]. Moreover, increased collagen signaling in the presence of VEGF inhibition, including activation of discoidin domain receptor 1, protein tyrosine kinase 2, and pseudopodium-enriched atypical kinase 1, has been shown to increase tumor progression and aggressiveness in murine models of pancreatic ductal adenocarcinoma [91]. In glioblastoma, VEGF inhibition creates hypoxic conditions in the tumor, which in turn causes increased expression of c-Met, an HGF receptor tyrosine kinase, through HIF-1α; this increase in c-Met expression correlates with increased invasion and poorer survival [80]. When both VEGF and c-Met are blocked, the increased tumor invasiveness and aggressiveness associated with anti-VEGF medications is suppressed in murine GBM and PNET, suggesting new routes for research in antiangiogenic therapies [80, 92].

6.1.4. Alternative angiogenic mechanisms

Another method through which tumors can circumvent angiogenic inhibition is though alternative angiogenic mechanisms such as intussusceptive angiogenesis, glomeruloid angiogenesis, vasculogenic mimicry, looping angiogenesis, and vessel cooption [78, 83]. These forms of angiogenesis occur through other signaling pathways that do not involve VEGF, and are upregulated when VEGF signaling is inhibited. One such alternative angiogenic pathway is vasculogenic mimicry (VM), which may be encouraged when anti-VEGF medications provide selective pressure for stem-like cancer cells that participate in the process. This phenomenon highlights the need for novel therapeutic methods that target the signaling pathways that control VM in addition to VEGF [93]. Similar combination therapies could be used to increase the efficacy of antiangiogenic medication in general by restricting the tumor's ability to acquire resistance to antiangiogenic therapies.

6.2. Challenges in biomarkers

Unfortunately, no validated biomarkers are currently available for determining which patients will respond best to antiangiogenic therapy [93, 94]. An array of biomarkers has been studied in hope to find effective biomarkers, including systemic measurements, gene analysis, circulating biomarkers, tissue markers, and imaging parameters [95]. Various challenges stand in the way of establishing effective biomarkers, such as the inability to perform repeated biopsies (inhibiting researchers' ability to assess dynamic biomarkers), the unpredictability of response and toxicity, the expensive and complex nature of human trials, the unpredictability of toxicity and response to therapies, and the specificity of each biomarker to disease [95].

The degree of hypertension experienced by a patient has been proposed as a potential systemic biomarker of tumor response, although more research is needed to establish the validity of this measurement [95, 96, 97]. Because hypertension is dependent on the VEGF-signaling pathway, it is possible that patients who do not develop hypertension are not responding to VEGF treatment at the current dose. In fact, the degree of hypertension correlates with survival, with patients who develop more severe hypertension experiencing better cancer remission than patients who develop no hypertension [97]. Interestingly, VEGF polymorphisms may play a role in determining the degree of hypertension, of anti-VEGF medications, which certain polymorphisms being more susceptible to inhibition than others. For example, VEGF-634 SNP (single nucleotide polymorphism) G/G is correlated with higher hypertension in suninitib-treated patients with mRCC than either VEGF-634 C/G or VEGF-634 C/C [98].

Several circulating biomarkers have been proposed that circulate in the bloodstream of patients. For example, high levels of soluble VEGF-R1 (sVEGFR1) correlate with decreased efficacy of bevacizumab in GBM, rectal carcinoma, breast cancer, hepatocellular carcinoma, and metastatic colorectal carcinoma. This correlation is probably caused by sVEGFR1 acting as an endogenous VEGF-trap, so adding a VEGF-specific monoclonal antibody does little to further inhibit VEGF signaling pathways [94]. Another potential circulating biomarker is SDF1α, as levels of this chemokine correlate with evasion of anti-VEGF therapies, although further study is needed to assess this potential biomarker [94]. Pretreatment levels of circulating VEGF-A has been shown to be prognostic in metastatic colorectal, lung, and renal cell cancers, but it is not predictive for bevacizumab treatment [99]. Moreover, a phase II study presented evidence that plasma concentrations of VEGF-A and IL-8 are prognostic for OS in MRCC, with high levels being unfavorable, while low plasma levels or sVEGFR-3 are may be predictive for a positive outcome in patients with mRCC receiving sunitinib [100]. Another phase II trial found that serum levels of Ang-2 and MMP-2, along with tumor levels of HIF-1α, are potential baseline efficacy biomarkers for sunitinib in advanced RCC [101]. Finally, low circulating endothelial cell levels (<65 CEC/4 mL blood) have been found to correlate with longer median PFS and OS in patients with colorectal cancer receiving bevacizumab [102].

Imaging techniques provide potential of imaging parameters as biomarkers as well. For example, MRI- and CT-based tissue vascular measured such as blood flow, blood volume, and permeability have been shown to occur after bevacizumab administration, although more research is needed to assess the efficacy of these measures as biomarkers [95]. Moreover, pretreatment ADC histogram analysis has been shown to be a possible predictive biomarker for bevacizumab treatment in recurrent glioblastoma [103]. Imaging studies can also be used to augment other biomarker studies, and can be used in cooperation with systems pharmacology to create multilevel computational models that predict the efficacy of treatment in patients, as well as suggesting dosing schedules that could be more efficacious than current practices [104]. Another potential biomarker could be patient genotype. As discussed above, some VEGF SNPs may be more receptive to treatment than others. However, some genes show little or no correlation with the efficacy of antiangiogenic therapies. For example, the mutation status of KRAS, a common oncogene, does not correlate with VEGF therapy efficacy [105]. More research must be done to establish which genes can and cannot be considered biomarkers.

6.3. Treatment methodologies and new treatments

According to the normalization hypothesis, during the course of antiangiogenic therapy, there is a dose-dependent window of time during which aberrant tumor vasculature is normalized. In this state, it is easier to deliver cytotoxic drugs from conventional chemotherapy to the tumor in a treatment schedule that takes advantage of the window presented by antiangiogenic agents given in low doses [106]. However, there are two important considerations to take into account when scheduling chemotherapy with antiangiogenic agents: first, the dose of antiangiogenic agents affects the normalization window during which chemotherapy can be delivered effectively. Second, the size of the chemotherapeutic agents matters, as vascular normalization causes the pores in aberrant tumor vessels to shrink, limiting the ability of large molecules to pass through to the tumor [94]. Vascular normalization has also been shown to improve the outcome of immunotherapy, making delivery of immune cells to the tumor easier, and can even decrease the intravasation of cancer cells, limiting the possibility of metastasis [94].

Most of the time, resistance to chemotherapy occurs through heritable changes in the tumor genotype. However, because resistance to VEGF inhibitors does not occur through natural selection, as discussed above, it is possible that rechallenging after disease progression following an intervening interval of time during which VEGF therapy is suspended may allow for a return of efficacy in antiangiogenic VEGF inhibitors. For example, patients with metastatic renal cell carcinoma (mRCC) who experience disease progression after initial response to sunitinib can eventually respond to the drug upon rechallenge after an intervening period on alternative therapies, such as sorafenib (patients with more than 6 months off sunitinib experienced greater PFS than patients with less than 6 months off sunitinib, although in each case the second PFS was shorter than the original) [99]. Moreover, in a randomized phase III trial, patients with unresectable metastatic colorectal cancer progressing up to 3 months after discontinuing bevacizumab plus chemotherapy experienced moderate survival benefits when bevacizumab plus chemotherapy was given as a second line treatment as compared to chemotherapy alone [107].

More research must be done to assess the efficacy of antiangiogenic agents in the adjuvant and neoadjuvant settings. In the neoadjuvant setting, VEGF inhibition may cause tumor regression, converting an unresectable tumor to a resectable one [82], with 12 of 30 patients in one single-arm phase II study who received oxaliplatin plus bevacizumab having initial nonsynchronous unresectable CLM become resectable [108]. However, antiangiogenic neoadjuvant treatment in mouse models of metastatic disease has been shown not to correlate with postsurgical survival [109]. In the adjuvant setting, it is possible that antiangiogenic therapies may prevent relapse by preventing the reestablishment of tumor vasculature. However, bevacizumab has delivered poor results in OS when used in combination with chemotherapy for adjuvant colorectal cancer, although PFS is improved [78].

Some work is also being put into developing novel VEGF and VEGFR inhibitors. For example, ramucirumab, a monoclonal antibody that inhibits VEGFR-2, was given FDA approval in 2014 for use as a single agent in the treatment of patients with gastroesophageal carcinoma; it has since been given approval for use in combination with paclitaxel, docetaxel, and FOLFIRI [110]. Ramucirumab is the first biological treatment to show moderate survival benefits as a single agent after gatroesophageal adenocarcinoma progression following first-line chemotherapy in a phase 3 trial (ramucirumab vs. placebo, OS = 5.2 months vs. 3.8 months, respectively) [111]. The drug has also shown moderate OS benefits when used in combination with docetaxel for second-line treatment of stage IV NNSCLS compared with docetaxel alone after progression on platinum-based chemotherapy (10.5 months vs. 9.1 months, ramucirumab plus docetaxel vs. docetaxel alone, respectively) [112]. Apatinib is another novel VEGFR-2 inhibitor, a small molecule not yet given FDA approval (although it is approved for use in China in treating metastatic gastric or gastroesophageal adenocarcinoma after second-line chemotherapy) [113]. The drug thus far has shown only moderate survival benefits of 1.8 months, and several trials are ongoing to assess its efficacy in different settings [114].

Yet another new small molecule VEGF inhibitor, cabozantinib (Cabometyx, Exelixis, Inc.) was given FDA approval on 25 April, 2016, for the treatment of renal cell carcinoma in patients who have received prior antiangiogenic therapy. Approval was given based on improved progression-free survival (7.4 months vs. 3.8 months in the cabozantinib and everolimus arms, respectively), improved overall survival (21.4 months vs. 16.5 months) and improved confirmed response rate (17 vs. 3%). The drug exhibits the standard side effects associated with VEGF inhibition; 40% of patients who received cabozantinib experienced a serious adverse event such as abdominal pain, pleural effusion, diarrhea, and nausea [115].

Another potential target for anticancer therapy has also been found in lymphangiogenesis. Several studies are examining the potential of inhibiting the VEGFR-3/VEGF-C/VEGF-D signaling axis in preventing lymph-node-mediated metastasis and disease progression. Inhibition of VEGF-C/-D with soluble VEGFR-3 has been shown to reduce tumor metastasis in mouse models, as has blocking VEGF-C/-D proteolysis or blocking VEGF-C from binding with the Nrp-2 receptor [116]. Moreover, foretinib, a multiple kinase inhibitor currently undergoing clinical trials, has shown promise in inhibiting the activity of VEGFR-3 and lymphangiogenesis and could potentially be used to inhibit lymph-node-mediated metastasis [117]. Corosolic acid has also been shown to induce apoptosis in CT-26 colon carcinoma in a mouse model, in addition to inhibiting lymphangiogenesis, but more study is needed before this substance becomes useable as a cancer therapy [118].

PlGF inhibition is another potential novel therapeutic approach in the fight against cancer, and preclinical studies have shown that inhibiting PlGF using genetic inhibition or anti-PlGF antibodies slows tumor growth and metastasis, and can even induce tumor regression in preexisting medulloblastoma [119]. However, the efficacy of inhibiting PlGF in tumors has come under question, with some preclinical studies showing that inhibiting PlGF does not significantly inhibit tumor grows [120, 121]. More research is needed to assess whether PlGF inhibition could be an efficacious cancer therapy.

7. Conclusion

Ever since its discovery, VEGF has been at the center of attention in new and developing cancer therapies. Since its early successes, however, antiangiogenic therapy has often presented only modest improvements in overall survival and progression-free survival [122]. Researchers have not given up hope that this therapeutic technique contains promise in the arsenal against cancer. Therefore, much recent research has been done in pushing the frontier of antiangiogenic therapies, trying to improve patient outcome.

Because the biology of VEGF and its receptors is well understood, current research focuses on why some tumors become resistant to antiangiogenic therapies and others are intrinsically resistant, how to circumvent this intrinsic or acquired resistance, and how to best utilize these expensive therapies by developing predictive biomarkers for treatment outcome. More research is also being done to develop novel VEGF inhibition techniques, and in characterizing the rare yet serious toxicities associated with these drugs.

As they stand now, antiangiogenic therapies face a set of limitations that severally impacts their efficacy. Tumors can acquire resistance to the drugs (if they do not already have intrinsic resistance) and demonstrate an increase in aggressiveness. Moreover, antiangiogenic therapies may cause a decrease in chemotherapy perfusion, lowering the efficacy of chemotherapies given in combination with antiangiogenic medicine [123]. These difficulties suggest that, at least when given alone, antiangiogenic therapies may face severe limitations in survival benefits. Therefore, future research should focus on more than simply inhibiting VEGF on a continuous schedule. Rather, it should focus on increasing the efficacy of chemotherapy through utilizing antiangiogenic therapy to induce vascular normalization, allowing for more efficient delivery of chemotherapeutic agents [123, 124]. Moreover, research should also find ways to decrease resistance to these therapies through inhibiting proangiogenic factors that are upregulated in response to the inhibition of VEGF and through developing predictive biomarkers for the efficacy of these expensive treatments [123, 124].

Author details

Victor Gardner[1], Chikezie O. Madu[1, 2] and Yi Lu[2*]

*Address all correspondence to: ylu@uthsc.edu

1 White Station High School, Memphis, TN, USA

2 Department of Pathology and Laboratory Medicine, University of Tennessee Health Science Center, Memphis, TN, USA

References

[1] Adair TH, Montani JP. Angiogenesis. San Rafael (CA): Morgan & Claypool Life Sciences; 2010. Chapter 1, Overview of Angiogenesis. Available from: http://www.ncbi.nlm.nih.gov/books/NBK53238/

[2] Adair TH, Montani JP. Angiogenesis. San Rafael (CA): Morgan & Claypool Life Sciences; 2010. Chapter 3, Regulation: Metabolic Factors. Available from: http://www.ncbi.nlm.nih.gov/books/NBK53243/

[3] Adair TH, Montani JP. Angiogenesis. San Rafael (CA): Morgan & Claypool Life Sciences; 2010. Chapter 4, Regulation: Mechanical Factors. Available from: http://www.ncbi.nlm.nih.gov/books/NBK53240/

[4] Hanahan D, Weinberg RA. Hallmarks of cancer: the next generation. Cell. 2011;**144**(5):646–74. DOI: 10.1016/j.cell.2011.02.013

[5] Neufeld G, Cohen TG, Poltorak Z. Vascular endothelial growth factor (VEGF) and its receptors. The FASEB Journal. 1999;**13**(1):9–22. DOI: 10.1016/j.cell.2011.02.013

[6] Groothuis A, DudaGN, Wilson CJ, Thompson, MS, Hunter MR, Simon P, Bail HJ, van Scherpenzeel KM, Kasper G. Mechanical stimulation of the pro-angiogenic capacity

of human fracture haematoma: involvement of VEGF mechano-regulation. Bone. 2010;**47**(2):438–44. DOI: 10.1016/j.bone.2010.05.026

[7] Heath VL, Bicknell R. Anticancer strategies involving the vasculature. Nature Reviews Clinical Oncology. 2009;**6**(7):395–404. DOI: 10.1038/nrclinonc.2009.52

[8] Cesca M, Bizzaro F, Zucchetti M, Giavazzi R. Tumor delivery of chemotherapy combined with inhibitors of angiogenesis and vascular targeting agents. Frontiers in Oncology. 2013;**3**:259. DOI: 10.3389/fonc.2013.00259

[9] Fuso Nerini I, Cesca M, Bizzaro F, Giavazzi R. Combination therapy in cancer: effects of angiogenesis inhibitors on drug pharmacokinetics and pharmacodynamics. Chinese Journal of Cancer. 2016;**35**:61. DOI:10.1186/s40880-016-0123-1

[10] Shibuya M. Vascular endothelial growth factor (VEGF) and its receptor (VEGFR) signaling in angiogenesis: a crucial target for anti- and pro-angiogenic therapies. Genes & Cancer 2011;**2**(12):1097–105. DOI: 10.1177/1947601911423031

[11] Hoeben A, Landuyt B, Highley MS, Wildiers H, Van Oosterom AT, De Brujin EA. Vascular endothelial growth factor and angiogenesis. Pharmacological Reviews 2004;**56**(4):549–80. DOI: 10.1124/pr.56.4.3

[12] Ogawa S, Oku A, Sawano A, Yamaguchi S, Yazaki Y, Shibuya M. A novel type of vascular endothelial growth factor, VEGF-E (NZ-7 VEGF), preferentially utilizes KDR/Flk-1 receptor and carries a potent mitotic activity without heparin-binding domain. The Journal of Biological Chemistry. 1998;**273**(43):31273–82.

[13] Yamazaki Y, Matsunaga Y, Tokunaga Y, Obayashi S, Saito M, Morita T. Snake venom vascular endothelial growth factors (VEGF-Fs) exclusively vary their structures and functions among species. The Journal of Biological Chemistry. 2009;**284**(15):9885–91. DOI: 10.1074/jbc.M809071200

[14] Li X, Lee C, Tang Z, et al. VEGF-B: a survival, or an angiogenic factor? Cell Adhesion & Migration 2009;**3**(4):322–7.

[15] De Falco S. The discovery of placental growth factor and its biological activity. Experimental and Molecular Medicine 2012;**44**:1–9. DOI: 10.3858/emm.2012.44.1.025

[16] "The biochemistry and role of placenta growth factor (PlGF)" (Application Note), ParkinElmer, Inc., 2009. Available from: https://shop.perkinelmer.com/Content/ApplicationNotes/APP_BiochemistryAndRoleOfPlGF.pdf

[17] Stuttfeld E, Ballmer-Hofer K. Structure and function of VEGF receptors. IUBMB Life. 2009;**61**:915–22. DOI: 10.1002/iub.234

[18] Rahimi N. VEGFR-1 and VEGFR-2: two non-identical twins with a unique physiognomy. Frontiers in Bioscience?: A Journal and Virtual Library. 2006;**11**:818–29.

[19] Holmes K, Robert OL, Thomas AM, Cross MJ. Vascular endothelial growth factor receptor-2: structure, function, intracellular signaling and therapeutic inhibition. Cell Signal. 2007;**10**:2003–12. DOI: 10.1016/j.cellsig.2007.05.013

[20] Kopan R. Notch signaling. Cold Spring Harbor Perspectives in Biology. 2016;**8**(7). DOI: 10.1101/cshperspect.a011213

[21] Makanya AN, Hushchuk R, DjnovVG. Intussuseptive angiogenesis and its role in vascular morphogenesis, patterning, and remodeling. Angiogenesis. 2009;**12**(2):113–23. DOI: 10.1007/s10456-009-9129-5

[22] Burri PH, Hlushchuk R, Djonov V. Intussusceptive angiogenesis: its emergence, its characteristics, and its significance. Developmental Dynamucs. 2004;**231**:474–88. DOI: 10.1002/dvdy.20184

[23] Nishida N, Yano H, Nishida T, Kamura T, Kojiro M. Angiogenesis in cancer. Vascular Health and Risk Management. 2006;**2**(3):213–9.

[24] Carmeliet P. VEGF as a key mediator of angiogenesis in cancer. Oncology. 2005;**69**(31):4–10. DOI: 10.1159/000088478

[25] Krock BL, Skuli N, Simon MC. Hypoxia-induced angiogenesis: good and evil. Genes & Cancer. 2011;**2**(12):1117–33. DOI: 10.1177/1947601911423654

[26] Leendders WPJ, Kusters B, de Waal RMW. Vessel co-option: how tumors obtain blood suppl in the absence of sprouting angiogenesis. Endothelium: Journal of Endothelial Cell Research. 2002;**9**(2):83–7.

[27] Cavallaro U, Christofori G. Molecular mechanisms of tumor angiogenesis and tumor progression. Journal of Neuro-Oncology. 2000;**50**(1):63–70.

[28] Nagy JA, Chang S-H, Shih S-C, Dvorak AM, Dvorak HF. Heterogeneity of the tumor vasculature. Seminars in Thrombosis and Hemostasis. 2010;**36**(3):321–31. DOI: 10.1055/s-0030-1253454

[29] Dudley AC. Tumor endothelial cells. Cold Spring Harbor Perspectives in Medicine. 2012;**2**(3): a006536. DOI: 10.1101/cshperspect.a006536.

[30] Nagy JA, Chang S-H, Dvorak AM, Dvorak HF. Why are tumour blood vessels abnormal and why is it important to know? British Journal of Cancer. 2009;**100**:865–9. DOI: 10.1038/sj.bjc.6604929

[31] Bergers G, Song S. The role of pericytes in blood-vessel formation and maintenance. Neuro-Oncology. 2005;**7**:452–64. DOI: 10.1215/S1152851705000232

[32] Rak J. Oncogenes and angiogenesis: signaling three-dimensional tumor growth. Journal of Investigative Dermatology Symposium Proceedings. 2000;**5**(1):24–33. DOI: 10.1046/j.1087-0024.2000.00012.x

[33] Onno K, Martijn F.B.G, Emile EV. Stimulation of angiogenesis by Ras proteins. Biochimica et Biophysica Acta (BBA) – Reviews on Cancer. 2004;**1654**(1):23–37. DOI: 10.1016/j.bbcan.2003.09.004

[34] Bottos A, Bardelli A. Oncogenes and angiogenesis: a way to personalize anti-angiogenic therapy? Cellular and Molecular Life Sciences. 2013;**70**(21):4131–40. DOI: 10.1007/s00018-013-1331-3

[35] Rak J, Filmus J, Finkenzeller G, Grugel S, Marme D, Kerbel RS. Oncogenes as indicators of tumor angiogenesis. Cancer and Metastasis Reviews. 1995;**14**(4):263–77. DOI: 10.1007/BF00690598

[36] Zhang F, Tang Z, Hou X, et al. VEGF-B is dispensable for blood vessel growth but critical for their survival, and VEGF-B targeting inhibits pathological angiogenesis. Proceedings of the National Academy of Sciences of the United States of America. 2009;**106**(15):6152–7. DOI: 10.1073/pnas.0813061106

[37] Li Y, et al. VEGF-B inhibits apoptosis via VEGFR-1–mediated suppression of the expression of BH3-only protein genes in mice and rats. Journal of Clinical Investigation. 2008;**118**(3):913–23. DOI: 10.1172/JCI33673

[38] Yang X, Zhang Y, Hosaka K, Andersson P, et al. VEGF-B promotes cancer metastasis through a VEGF-A-independent mechanism and serves as a marker of poor prognosis for cancer patients. Proceedings of the National Academy of Sciences of the United States of America. 2015;**112**(22):E2900–9. DOI: 10.1073/pnas.1503500112

[39] Yonemura Y, Endo Y, Tabata K, Kawamura T, Yun HY, Bandou E, Sasaki T, Miura M. Role of VEGF-C and VEGF-D in lymphangiogenesis in gastric cancer. International Journal of Clinical Oncology 2005;**10**(5):316–27. DOI: 10.1007/s10147-005-0508-7

[40] Achen MG, Williams RA, Baldwin ME, Lai P, Roufail S, Alitalo K, Stacker SA. The angiogenic and lymphangiogenic factor vascular endothelial growth factor-D exhibits a paracrine mode of action in cancer. Growth Factors 2002;**20**(2):99–107.

[41] Christiansen A, Detmar M. Lymphangiogenesis and cancer. Genes and Cancer. 2011;**2**(12):1146–58. DOI: 10.1177/1947601911423028

[42] Skobe M, Hawighorst T, Jackson DG, et al. Induction of tumor lymphangiogenesis by VEGF-C promotes breast cancer metastasis. Nature Medicine. 2001;**7**:192–8. DOI: 10.1038/84643

[43] Liu W, Xu J, Wang M, Wang Q, Bi Y, Han M. Tumor-derived vascular endothelial growth factor (VEGF)-a facilitates tumor metastasis through the VEGF-VEGFR1 signaling pathway. International Journal of Oncology. 2011;**39**:1213–20. DOI: 10.3892/ijo.2011.1138

[44] Gotink KJ, Verheul HMW. Anti-angiogenic tyrosine kinase inhibitors: what is their mechanism of action? Angiogenesis. 2010;**13**(1):1–14. DOI: 10.1007/s10456-009-9160-6

[45] Imai K, Takaoka A. Comparing antibody and small-molecule therapies for cancer. Nature Reviews Cancer 2006;**6**:714–27. DOI 10.1007/s10456-009-9160-6

[46] National Cancer Institute: FDA Approval for Sunitinib Malate [Internet]. 2011. http://www.cancer.gov/about-cancer/treatment/drugs/fda-sunitinib-malate [Accessed 2016-06-22].

[47] Kim A, Balis FM, Widemann BC. Sorafenib and sunitinib. Oncologist. 2009;**8**:800–5. DOI: 10.1634/theoncologist.2009-0088

[48] Adnane L, Trail PA, Taylor I, Wilhelm SM. Sorafenib (BAY 43-9006, Nexavar), a dual-action inhibitor that targets RAF/MEK/ERK pathway in tumor cells and tyrosine kinases

VEGFR/PDGFR in tumor vasculature. Methods Enzymol. 2006;**407**:597–612. DOI: 10.1016/S0076-6879(05)07047-3

[49] National Cancer Institute: FDA Approval for Sorafenib Tosylate [Internet]. 2013. Available from: http://www.cancer.gov/about-cancer/treatment/drugs/fda-sorafenib-tosylate [Accessed 2016-06-23].

[50] Morabito A, Piccirillo MC, Falasconi F, De Feo G, Del Giudice A, Bryce J, Di Maio M, De Maio E, Normanno N, Perrone F. Vandetanib (ZD6474), a dual inhibitor of vascular endothelial growth factor receptor (VEGFR) and epidermal growth factor receptor (EGFR) tyrosine kinases: current status and future directions. Oncologist. 2009;**4**:378–90. DOI: 10.1634/theoncologist.2008-0261

[51] National Cancer Institute: FDA Approval for Vandetanib [Internet]. 2013. Available from: http://www.cancer.gov/about-cancer/treatment/drugs/fda-vandetanib [Accessed 2016-06-23].

[52] European Medicines Agency: Avastin [Internet]. 2016. Available from: http://www.ema.europa.eu/ema/index.jsp?curl=pages/medicines/human/medicines/000582/human_med_000663.jsp [Accessed 2016-06-26].

[53] Keating GM. Bevacizumab: a review of its role in advanced cancer. Drugs. 2014;**74**(16):1891–925. DOI: 10.1007/s40265-014-0302-9

[54] Sullivan LA, Brekken RA. The VEGF family in cancer and antibody-based strategies for their inhibition. mAbs. 2010;**2**(2):165–175.

[55] Lilly R. CYRAMZA is a human, monoclonal antibody that specifically blocks activation of vascular endothelial growth factor (VEGF) Receptor 2 [Internet]. 2015. Available from: http://www.cyramzahcp.com/lung/mechanism-of-action.html [Accessed 2016-06-25].

[56] Kendrew J, Eberlein C, Hedberg B, McDaid K, Smith NR, Weir HM, Wedge SR, Blakey DC, Foltz I, Zhou J, Kang JS, Barry ST. An antibody targeted to VEGFR-2 Ig domains 4-7 inhibits VEGFR-2 activation and VEGFR-2-dependent angiogenesis without affecting ligand binding. Molecular Cancer Therapeutics. 2011;**10**(5):770–83. DOI: 10.1158/1535-7163

[57] Regeneron Pharmaceuticals: Multiple Angiogenic Factor Trap [Internet]. 2016. Available from: http://www.zaltrap.com/hcp/about/mechanism-of-action [Accessed 2016-07-01].

[58] Holash J, Davis S, Papadopoulos N, et al. VEGF-trap: a VEGF blocker with potent anti-tumor effects. Proceedings of the National Academy of Sciences of the United States of America. 2002;**99**(17):11393–8. DOI: 10.1073/pnas.172398299

[59] U.S. Food and Drug Administration: FDA approves Zaltrap for metastatic colorectal cancer [Internet]. 2012. Available from: http://www.fda.gov/NewsEvents/Newsroom/PressAnnouncements/ucm314372.htm [Accessed 2016-03-04].

[60] Al-Husein B, Abdalla M, et al. Anti-angiogenic therapy for cancer: an update. Pharmacotherapy. 2012;**32**(12):1095–111. DOI: 10.1002/phar.1147

[61] "Anti-Angiogenesis Treatment", American Cancer Society [Internet]. 2009. Available from: http://www.cancer.org/acs/groups/cid/documents/webcontent/002988-pdf.pdf [Accessed 2016-03-15].

[62] Henry TD, Annex BH, McKendall GR, Azrin MA, Lopez JJ, Giordano FJ, Shah PK, Willerson JT, Benza RL, Berman DS, et al. The VIVA trial: vascular endothelial growth factor in Ischemia for Vascular Angiogenesis. Circulation. 2003;**107**:1359–65.

[63] Sane DC, Anton L, Brosnihan KB. Angiogenic growth factors and hypertension. Angiogenesis. 2004;**7**(3):193–201. DOI: 10.1007/s10456-004-2699-3

[64] van Heeckeren WJ, Ortiz J, Cooney MM, Remick SC. Hypertension, proteinuria, and antagonism of vascular endothelial growth factor signaling: clinical toxicity, therapeutic target, or novel biomarker? Journal of Clinical Oncology. 2007;**25**:2993–5. DOI: 10.1200/JCO.2007.11.5113

[65] Chen HX, Cleck JN: Adverse effects of anticancer agents that target the VEGF pathway. Nature Reviews Clinical Oncology. 2009;**6**(8):465–77. DOI: 10.1038/nrclinonc.2009.94

[66] Hutson T, Figlin R, Kuhn J, Motzer R. Targeted therapies for metastatic renal cell carcinoma: an overview of toxicity and dosing strategies. Oncologist. 2008;**13**:1084–96. DOI: 10.1634/theoncologist.2008-0120

[67] Tesarova P, Tesar V. Proteinuria and hypertension in patients treated with inhibitors of the VEGF signalling pathway–incidence, mechanisms and management. Folia Biol (Praha). 2013;**59**:15–25.

[68] Izzedine H, Massard C, Spano JP. VEGF signalling inhibition-induced proteinuria: mechanisms, significance and management. European Journal of Cancer. 2010;**46**:439–48. DOI: 10.1016/j.ejca.2009.11.001

[69] Scappaticci FA, Skillings JR, Holden SN, et al. Arterial thromboembolic events in patients with metastatic carcinoma treated with chemotherapy and bevacizumab. Journal of the National Cancer Institute. 2007;**99**:1232–9. DOI: 10.1093/jnci/djm086

[70] Kamba T, McDonald DM. Mechanisms of adverse effects of anti-VEGF therapy for cancer. British Journal of Cancer. 2007;**96**(12):1788–95. DOI: 10.1038/sj.bjc.6603813

[71] Chu TF, Jeffrey A, et al. Cardiotoxicity associated with tyrosine kinase inhibitor sunitinib. The Lancet 2007;**370**(9604):2011–9. DOI: 10.1016/S0140-6736(07)61865-0

[72] Kerkela R, Woulfe KC, Durand J-B, et al. Sunitinib-induced cardiotoxicity is mediated by off-target inhibition of AMP-activated protein kinase. Clinical and Translational Science. 2009;**2**(1):15–25. DOI: 10.1111/j.1752-8062.2008.00090.x

[73] Karp JE, Gojo I, Pili R, Gocke CD, Greer J, Guo C, et al. Targeting vascular endothelial growth factor for relapsed and refractory adult acute myelogenous leukemias: therapy with sequential 1-beta-d-arabinofuranosylcytosine, mitoxantrone, and bevacizumab. Clinical Cancer Research. 2004;**10**:3577–85. DOI: 10.1158/1078-0432.CCR-03-0627

[74] Duran JM, Makarewich CA, Trappanese D, et al. Sorafenib cardiotoxicity increases mortality after myocardial infarction. Circulation Research. 2014;**114**(11):1700–12. DOI: 10.1161/CIRCRESAHA.114.303200

[75] Qi WX, Tang LN, Sun YJ, et al. Incidence and risk of hemorrhagic events with vascular endothelial growth factor receptor tyrosine-kinase inhibitors: an up-to-date meta-analysis of 27 randomized controlled trials. Annals of Oncology. 2013;**24**(12):2943–52. DOI: 10.1093/annonc/mdt292

[76] Common Terminology Criteria for Adverse Events. Version 4.0, National Institutes of Health, National Cancer Institute, 14 June 2010. Available from: http://evs.nci.nih.gov/ftp1/CTCAE/CTCAE_4.03_2010-06-14_QuickReference_5x7.pdf

[77] Bergers G, Hanahan D. Modes of resistance to anti-angiogenic therapy. Nature Reviews Cancer. 2008;**8**(8):592–603. DOI: 10.1038/nrc2442

[78] Vasudev NS, Reynolds AR. Anti-angiogenic therapy for cancer: current progress, unresolved questions and future directions. Angiogenesis. 2014;**17**(3):471–94. DOI: 10.1007/s10456-014-9420-y

[79] Renaud G, Gilles P. Molecular mechanisms of resistance to tumour anti-angiogenic strategies. Journal of Oncology. 2010;2010:8 p. Article ID 835680, DOI:10.1155/2010/835680

[80] Lu KV, Bergers G. Mechanisms of evasive resistance to anti-VEGF therapy in glioblastoma. CNS Oncology. 2013;**2**(1):49–65. DOI: 10.2217/cns.12.36

[81] Kioi M, Vogel H, Schultz G, Hoffman RM, Harsh GR, Brown JM. Inhibition of vasculogenesis, but not angiogenesis, prevents the recurrence of glioblastoma after irradiation in mice. The Journal of Clinical Investigation. 2010;**120**(3):694–705. DOI: 10.1172/JCI40283

[82] Allen E, Walters IB, Hanahan D. Brivanib: a dual FGF/VEGF inhibitor, is active both 1st and 2nd line against mouse pancreatic neuroendocrine tumors (PNET) developing adaptive/evasive resistance to VEGF inhibition. Clinical Cancer Research: An Official Journal of the American Association for Cancer Research. 2011;**17**(16):5299–310. DOI: 10.1158/1078-0432

[83] Newman AC, Hughes CW. Macrophages and angiogenesis: a role for Wnt signaling. Vascular Cell. 2012;**4**(1):13. DOI: 10.1186/2045-824X-4-13

[84] Ding Y, Song N, Luo Y. Role of bone marrow-derived cells in angiogenesis: focus on macrophages and pericytes. Cancer Microenvironment. 2012;**5**(3):225–36. DOI: 10.1007/s12307-012-0106-y

[85] Murdoch C, Giannoudis A, Lewis CE. Mechanisms regulating the recruitment of macrophages into hypoxic areas of tumors and other ischemic tissues. Blood. 2004;**104**(8):2224–34. DOI: 10.1182/blood-2004-03-1109

[86] Deshmane SL, Kremlev S, Amini S, Sawaya BE. Monocyte chemoattractant protein-1 (MCP-1): an overview. Journal of Interferon & Cytokine Research. 2009;**29**(6):313–26 DOI: 10.1089/jir.2008.0027

[87] Lal A, Peters H, St Croix B, Haroon ZA, Dewhirst MW, Strausberg RL, et al. Transcriptional response to hypoxia in human tumors. Journal of National Cancer Institute. 2001;**93**:1337–43.

[88] Hall AP. Review of the pericyte during angiogenesis and its role in cancer and diabetic retinopathy. Toxicology Pathology. 2006;**34**(6):763–75. DOI: 10.1080/01926230600936290

[89] Meng MB, Zaorsky NG, Deng L, Wang HH, Chao J, Zhao LJ, Yuan ZY, Ping W. Pericytes: a double-edged sword in cancer therapy. Future Oncology. 2015;**11**(1):169–79. DOI: 10.2217/fon.14.123

[90] Bao B, et al. Hypoxia-induced aggressiveness of pancreatic cancer cells is due to increased expression of VEGF, IL-6 and miR-21, which can be attenuated by CDF treatment. PLoS One. 2012;**7**(12). DOI: 10.1371/journal.pone.0050165

[91] Aguilera KY, Rivera LB, Hur H, et al. Collagen signaling enhances tumor progression after anti-VEGF therapy in a murine model of pancreatic ductal adenocarcinoma. Cancer Research. 2014;**74**(4):1032–44. DOI: 10.1158/0008-5472

[92] Sennino B, Ishiguro-Oonuma T, Wei Y, et al. Suppression of tumor invasion and metastasis by concurrent inhibition of c-Met and VEGF signaling in pancreatic neuroendocrine tumors. Cancer Discovery. 2012;**2**(3):270–87. DOI: 10.1158/2159-8290.CD-11-0240

[93] Schnegg CI, Yang MH, Ghosh SK, Hsu M-Y. Induction of vasculogenic mimicry overrides VEGF-A silencing and enriches stem-like cancer cells in melanoma. Cancer Research. 2015;**75**(8):1682–90. DOI: 10.1158/0008-5472.CAN-14-1855

[94] Jain RK. Normalizing tumor microenvironment to treat cancer: bench to bedside to biomarkers. Journal of Clinical Oncology. 2013;**31**(17):2205–18. DOI: 10.1200/JCO.2012.46.3653

[95] Jain RK, Duda DG, Willett CG, et al. Biomarkers of response and resistance to antiangiogenic therapy. Nature Reviews Clinical Oncology. 2009;**6**(6):327–38. DOI: 10.1038/nrclinonc.2009.63

[96] Rini BI, et al. Association of diastolic blood pressure (dBP) ≥ 90 mmHg with overall survival (OS) in patients treated with axitinib (AG- 013736). Journal Clinical Oncology (Meeting Abstracts). 2008;**26**(90150):3543. DOI: 10.1200/jco.2008.26.90150.3543

[97] Robinson ES, Khankin EV, Karumanchi SA, Humphreys BD. Hypertension induced by VEGF signaling pathway inhibition: mechanisms and potential use as a biomarker. Seminars in Nephrology. 2010;**30**(6):591–601. DOI: 10.1016/j.semnephrol.2010.09.007

[98] Kim JJ. VEGF single nucleotide polymorphisms (SNPs) and correlation to sunitinib-induced hypertension (HTN) in metastatic renal cell carcinoma (mRCC) patients (pts). Journal of Clinical Oncology. 2009;**27**(15):15S 5005.

[99] Hegde PS, Jubb AM, Chen D, et al. Predictive impact of circulating vascular endothelial growth factor in four phase III trials evaluating bevacizumab. Clinical Cancer Research. 2013;**19**:929–37. DOI: 10.1158/1078-0432.CCR-12-2535

[100] Harmon CS, DePrimo SE, Figlin RA, et al. Circulating proteins as potential biomarkers of sunitinib and interferon-α efficacy in treatment-naïve patients with metastatic renal cell carcinoma. Cancer Chemotherapy and Pharmacology. 2014;**73**(1):151–61. DOI: 10.1007/s00280-013-2333-4

[101] Motzer RJ, Hutson TE, Hudes GR, et al. Investigation of novel circulating proteins, germ line single-nucleotide polymorphisms, and molecular tumor markers as potential efficacy biomarkers of first-line sunitinib therapy for advanced renal cell carcinoma. Cancer Chemotherapy and Pharmacology. 2014;**74**(4):739–750. DOI: 10.1007/s00280-014-2539-0

[102] Wehland M, Bauer J, Magnusson NE, Infanger M, Grimm D. Biomarkers for anti-angiogenic therapy in cancer. International Journal of Molecular Sciences. 2013;**14**(5):9338–64. DOI: 10.3390/ijms14059338

[103] Ellingson BM, Sahebjam S, Kim HJ, Pope WB, Harris RJ, Woodworth DC, Lai A, Nghiemphu PL, Mason WP, Cloughesy TF. Pretreatment ADC histogram analysis is a predictive imaging biomarker for bevacizumab treatment but not chemotherapy in recurrent glioblastoma. American Journal of Neuroradiology. 2014;**35**:673–9. DOI: 10.3174/ajnr.A3748

[104] Sharan S, Woo S. Systems pharmacology approaches for optimization of antiangiogenic therapies: challenges and opportunities. Frontiers in Pharmacology. 2015;**6**:33. DOI: 10.3389/fphar.2015.00033

[105] Kim ST, Park KH, Shin SW, Kim YH. Dose KRAS mutation status affect on the effect of VEGF therapy in metastatic colon cancer patients? Cancer Research and Treatment: Official Journal of Korean Cancer Association. 2014;**46**(1):48–54. DOI: 10.4143/crt.2014.46.1.48

[106] Goel S, Wong AH-K, Jain RK. Vascular normalization as a therapeutic strategy for malignant and nonmalignant disease. Cold Spring Harbor Perspectives in Medicine. 2012;**2**(3):a006486. DOI: 10.1101/cshperspect.a006486

[107] Bennouna J, Sastre J, Arnold D, et al. Continuation of bevacizumab after first progression in metastatic colorectal cancer (ML18147): a randomised phase 3 trial. *The Lancet Oncology*. 2013;**14**(1):29–37. DOI: 10.1016/S1470-2045(12)70477-1

[108] Wong R, Cunningham D, Barbachano Y, Saffery C, Valle J, Hickish T. A multicentre study of capecitabine, oxaliplatin plus bevacizumab as perioperative treatment of patients with poor-risk colorectal liver-only metastases not selected for upfront resection. Annals of Oncology. 2011;**22**(9):2042–8. DOI: 10.1093/annonc/mdq714

[109] Ebos JM, Mastri M, Lee CR, et al. Neoadjuvant antiangiogenic therapy reveals contrasts in primary and metastatic tumor efficacy. EMBO Molecular Medicine. 2014;**6**(12):1561–76. DOI: 10.15252/emmm.201403989

[110] National Cancer Institute: FDA Approval for Ramucirumab [Internet]. 2015. Available from: http://www.cancer.gov/about-cancer/treatment/drugs/fda-ramucirumab [Accessed 2016-06-12].

[111] Fuchs, Charles S, et al. Ramucirumab monotherapy for previously treated advanced gastric or gastro-oesophageal junction adenocarcinoma (REGARD): an international, randomised, multicentre, placebo-controlled, phase 3 trial. The Lancet. 2014;**383**:31–9. DOI: 10.1016/S0140-6736(13)61719-5

[112] Garen, EB. Ramucirumab plus docetaxel versus placebo plus docetaxel for second-line treatment of stage IV non-small-cell lung cancer after disease progression on platinum-based therapy (REVEL): a multicentre, double-blind, randomised phase 3 trial. The Lancet 2014;**384**(9944):665–73. DOI: 10.1016/S0140-6736(14)60845-X

[113] Li J, et al. Randomized, double-blind, placebo-controlled phase III trial of apatinib in patients with chemotherapy-refractory advanced or metastatic adenocarcinoma of the stomach or gastroesophageal junction. Journal of Clinical Oncology. 2016;**34**(13):1448–54. DOI: 10.1200/JCO.2015.63.5995.

[114] Fontanella C, Ongaro E, Bolzonello S, Guardascione M, Fasola G, Aprile G. Clinical advances in the development of novel VEGFR2 inhibitors. Annals of Translational Medicine. 2014;**2**(12):123.

[115] U.S. Food and Drug Administration. Cabozantinib (CABOMETYX) [Internet]. 2016. Available from: http://www.fda.gov/Drugs/InformationOnDrugs/ApprovedDrugs/ucm497483.htm [Accessed 2016-06-09].

[116] Duong T, Koopman P, Francois M. Tumor lymphangiogenesis as a potential therapeutic target. Journal of Oncology. 2012, Article ID 204946, 2012, 23 p. DOI:10.1155/2012/204946

[117] Chen H-M, Tsai C-H, Hung W-C. Foretinib inhibits angiogenesis, lymphangiogenesis and tumor growth of pancreatic cancer in vivo by decreasing VEGFR-2/3 and TIE-2 signaling. Oncotarget. 2015;**6**(17):14940–52. DOI: 10.18632/oncotarget.3613

[118] Yoo K-H, Park J-H, Lee D-Y, et al. Corosolic acid exhibits anti-angiogenic and anti-lymphangiogenic effects on *in vitro* endothelial cells and on an *in vivo* CT-26 colon carcinoma animal model. Phytotherapy Research. 2015;**29**(5):714–23. DOI: 10.1002/ptr.5306

[119] Dewerchin M, Carmeliet P. Placental growth factor in cancer. Expert Opinion on Therapeutic Targets. 2014;**18**(11):1339–54. DOI: 10.1517/14728222.2014.948420

[120] Lou, K-J. PlGF point-counterpoint. Science–Business eXchange. [Internet]. 2010;**3**(16). DOI: 10.1038/scibx.2010.484

[121] Bessho H, et al. Inhibition of placental growth factor in renal cell carcinoma. Anticancer Research. 2015;**35**(1):531–41.

[122] Jayson G, Kerbel R, et al. Antiangiogenic therapy in oncology: current status and future directions. The Lancet. 2016;388 (10046):518-529. DOI: 10.1016/S0140-6736(15)01088-0

[123] Morserle L, Jimenez-Valerio G, Casanovas O. Antiangiogenic therapies: going beyond their limits. Cancer Discovery. 2014;**4**(1):31–41. DOI: 10.1158/2159-8290.CD-13-0199

[124] Ma J, Waxman D. Combination of anti-angiogenesis with chemotherapy for more effective cancer treatment. Molecular Cancer Therapeutics. 2008;**7**(12):3670–84. DOI: 10.1158/1535-7163.MCT-08-0715

[125] National Cancer Institute: FDA Approval for Bevacizumab [Internet]. 2014. Available from: http://www.cancer.gov/about-cancer/treatment/drugs/fda-bevacizumab [Accessed 2016-04-14].

[126] National Cancer Institute: FDA Approval for Pazopanib [Internet]. 2013. Available from: http://www.cancer.gov/about-cancer/treatment/drugs/fda-pazopanibhydrochloride [Accessed 2016-04-14].

[127] National Cancer Institute: FDA Approval for Ziv-Aflibercept [Internet]. 2013. Available from: update. http://www.cancer.gov/about-cancer/treatment/drugs/fda-ziv-aflibercept [Accessed 2016-04-14].

Chapter 20

Antiangiogenic Therapy for Hepatocellular Carcinoma

Kosuke Kaji and Hitoshi Yoshiji

Additional information is available at the end of the chapter

http://dx.doi.org/10.5772/66503

Abstract

Angiogenesis plays a pivotal role in many pathological processes, including hepatocellular carcinoma (HCC). This indicates that antiangiogenic agents could be promising candidates for chemoprevention against HCC. Several inhibitors targeting receptor tyrosine kinases (RTKs) for the regulation of tumoral vascularization have been developed and employed in clinical practice, including sorafenib. However, there seem to be several issues for the long-term use of this agent as some patients have experienced adverse effects while taking sorafenib. Therefore, it is desirable for patients with chronic liver diseases to be administered sorafenib as little as possible by combining other safe-to-use antiangiogenic compounds. Various factors, such as renin-angiotensin-aldosterone system (RAAS) and insulin resistance (IR), reciprocally contribute to the promotion of angiogenesis. A blockade of RAAS with an angiotensin-converting enzyme inhibitor (ACE-I) or angiotensin-II (AT-II) receptor blocker (ARB) markedly attenuates HCC in conjunction with the suppression of angiogenesis. Moreover, the IR status has demonstrated direct acceleration in the progression of HCC via the augmentation of tumoral neovascularization. These findings suggest that a combination therapy involving a lower dose of sorafenib with other clinically used agents [e.g., RAAS blockers, insulin sensitizer agents, and branched-chain amino acids (BCAA)] may reduce the adverse effects of sorafenib without attenuating the inhibitory effect against HCC in comparison to a high-dose administration.

Keywords: hepatocellular carcinoma, fibrosis, renin-angiotensin system

1. Introduction

Angiogenesis is the development of new vasculature from preexisting blood vessels or circulating endothelial cell (EC) stem cells. Emerging evidence indicates that angiogenesis develops in many organs and under multiple pathologic situations, as well as during conditions of tissue growth and regeneration. Abnormal pathological angiogenesis is observed in patients with rheumatoid arthritis, psoriasis, diabetic retinopathy, fibrogenesis, and tumor growth [1]. Although early studies were conducted to determine the molecular processes associated with carcinogenesis and angiogenesis that were performed independently, more recent studies have revealed that both biological phenomena emerge synergistically [2].

Hepatocellular carcinoma (HCC) is the sixth most common cancer and the second leading cause of cancer-related mortality worldwide, accounting for more than 600,000 new cases annually. The greatest risk factors for developing HCC include liver cirrhosis induced by hepatitis B virus (HBV) or hepatitis C virus (HCV) infections, excessive alcohol intake, and metabolic syndrome. Regardless of the etiology, since HCC commonly develops in patients with a chronic liver disease (e.g., liver cirrhosis) only approximately one-third of the patients diagnosed with HCC are eligible for curative treatments (e.g., surgical resection) [3]. Consequently, several alternative therapies have been employed, including percutaneous radiofrequency ablation (RFA) and transarterial chemoembolization (TACE). However, no satisfactory improvement of HCC prognosis has been achieved to date. The notable characteristic of HCC that accounts for its poor prognosis is the risk of high frequency in recurrence attributed to intrahepatic metastasis or the multicentric development. The key feature of HCC progression is also hypervascularity formed by intratumoral angiogenesis as well as the frequent recurrence. Several studies have demonstrated that angiogenesis is implicated in the survival and growth of HCC. It has also been reported that angiogenesis can be induced during the early stages of tumor formation and the various carcinogenic mechanisms have been demonstrated in several different experimental models [4–7]. Therefore, several antiangiogenic agents (i.e., sorafenib) have been developed as novel treatment options for HCC.

In this chapter, mechanistic insights into angiogenesis and its contribution to hepatocarcinogenesis will initially be reviewed. In addition, newly developed antiangiogenic agents will be described in detail.

2. Angiogenesis in HCC

In HCC, tumor angiogenesis leads to a pathologic vascularization pattern, of which intratumoral vascularization is critical for the diagnosis and treatment of HCC, as well as for pathogenesis and patient prognosis [1, 8, 9]. In general, HCC is supplied with blood flow primarily via the hepatic arteries, while noncancerous lesions and the normal liver parenchyma are supplied predominantly by the portal vein. This distinct vascularization is clinically utilized to diagnose HCC radiographically by emphasizing the tumor lesions. Any tumor mass more than 1–2 mm^3 depends entirely on the formation of a vascular network that provides the growing tumor with oxygen and essential nutrients [10].

Of the various proangiogenic factors, vascular endothelial growth factor (VEGF) is one of the most potent and required for both physiological and pathological angiogenesis [11]. VEGF induces EC proliferation, promotes migration and differentiation as well as stimulates permeabilization of blood vessels and vasculogenesis. The several forms of VEGF bind to two tyrosine kinase receptors, *fms*-like tyrosine kinase (flt-1: VEGFR-1) and the kinase insert domain-containing receptor/murine homolog, fetal liver kinase-1 (KDR/Flk-1: VEGFR-2) [11, 12]. Recent reports have demonstrated that upregulated VEGF expression is more frequently observed in the tumor lesions of HCC than noncancerous lesions [13–15]. Moreover, the marked increase of VEGF expression is shown during both hepatocarcinogenesis and HCC growth in accordance with the augmented neovascularization. Our basic studies elucidated that monoclonal antibodies (mAb) against both VEGFR-1 and VEGFR-2 ameliorated the HCC development with antiangiogenic activity in rodents [16]. These findings indicate that a blockade of the VEGF-VEGFR axis contributes to the suppressive effect on HCC development.

In tumor neovascularization, VEGF often coordinates with other angiogenic pathways. The angiopoietins (Ang) bind with receptor tyrosine kinases (RTKs) with immunoglobulin-like and EGF-like domains (Tie1 and Tie2). Increased levels of Ang2 promote tumor angiogenesis, metastasis, and inflammation with augmentation of VEGF activity. VEGF-A is also upregulated by interaction with multiple growth factors, including fibroblast growth factor (FGF), insulin-like growth factor-1 (IGF-1), platelet-derived growth factor (PDGF), and the transforming growth factors (TGF) [17]. Tissue hypoxia also stimulates VEGF-A upregulation via the hypoxia-inducible factors (HIF)-1α and HIF-2α [17].

3. Molecular targeted therapy

Several small-molecule, orally available RTK inhibitors exhibit an antiangiogenic effect of inhibiting VEGF and other kinases. They are expected to have high clinical utility and are currently being tested in clinical trials of varying stages for the treatment of advanced HCC (**Table 1**).

Agent	Target
Sorafenib	A-RAF, B-RAF, C-RAF/Raf-1VEGFR-2, VEGFR-3, PDGFR-β, Flt-3, c-Kit
Sunitinib	VEGFR-1, 2, and 3, PDGFR-α, β, c-Kit, Flt3
Brivanib	VEGFR-1, 2, and 3, FGFR-1, 2, and 3
Lenvatinib	VEGFR-1, 2, and 3, FGFR-1, 2, 3, and 4,PDGFR-α, c-Kit, RET
Cabozantinib	VEGFR-2, MET, RET

Table 1. Molecularly targeted antiangiogenic agents for advanced HCC.

3.1. Sorafenib

Sorafenib (Nexavar®) was developed in 1995 and is the only chemotherapeutic drug that has demonstrated to improve the survival rate in patients with HCC [18, 19]. Sorafenib acts by inhibiting the RAF serine/threonine kinases that play a key role in the transduction of mitogenic and oncogenic pathways through the Raf/mitogen-activated protein kinase (MEK)/

extracellular signal-regulated kinase (ERK)/mitogen-activated protein kinase (MAPK) signaling pathway [20]. Such signaling results in a lower cyclin D1 expression as well as cell cycle arrest. Sorafenib also potently inhibits VEGFR-2, VEGFR-3, PDGFR-β, Flt-3, and c-Kit, which promote angiogenesis [19, 20]. The repression blocks a broad spectrum of different processes involved in proliferation, angiogenesis, or apoptosis, causing a reduction in the blood vessel regions of the tumor and the starving of cancerous cells. Furthermore, sorafenib enhances tumor necrosis factor (TNF)-related apoptosis-inducing ligand (TRAIL)-induced cell death through an SH2 domain, which causes a tyrosine phosphatase (SHP-1)-dependent reduction of signal transducers and activators of transcription type 3 (STAT3) phosphorylation and the related protein myeloid cell leukemia 1 (Mcl-1) (i.e., survivin and cyclin D1) in HCC cells [21]. Sorafenib is also able to repress Mcl-1 activity through an MAPK-independent mechanism, which increases the intrinsic apoptosis pathway in tumor cells. Moreover, recent studies have claimed that the eukaryotic translation initiation factor 4E (eIF4E) might be implicated in sorafenib-dependent Mcl-1 inhibition [22]. Clinically, sorafenib can extend the mean patient survival from 7.9 to 10.7 months [19]. Representative adverse events caused by the treatment of sorafenib consist of diarrhea, weight loss, hand-foot skin reaction, and hypophosphatemia. Currently, sorafenib is the first and only agent to demonstrate a beneficial overall survival (OS) and be approved by regulators globally in patients with advanced HCC [19].

3.2. Sunitinib

Sunitinib (Sutent®) is an oral multi-RTK inhibitor targeting VEGFR-1, 2, and 3, PDGFRs, c-Kit, and other RTKs associated with angiogenesis [23]. Several phase II clinical trials have shown favorable results regarding the antitumor activity of this drug against advanced HCC. In one phase III trial, the median OS was 7.9 and 10.2 in the sunitinib and sorafenib groups, respectively [24]. This indicates that sunitinib had no benefit over sorafenib as a first-line therapy for advanced HCC.

3.3. Brivanib

Brivanib, a dual tyrosine kinase inhibitor, shows potent and selective inhibition of VEGFR and FGFR [25]. Brivanib has exerted an anticancerous effect in xenograft human HCC models expressing FGF receptors [26]. Two phase III trials have been performed: (1) the BRISK-FL study, in which brivanib vs. sorafenib as first-line therapy was evaluated in patients with advanced HCC and (2) the BRISK-PS study, in which brivanib was administered to patients with advanced HCC who were resistant to sorafenib [27, 28]. However, both trials failed to meet the primary endpoint of statistically improving the OS rate.

3.4. Lenvatinib

Lenvatinib (Lenvima®) is an oral multityrosine kinase inhibitor with potent antiangiogenic effects that has recently been approved for use in differentiated thyroid cancer [29]. The drug was established in patient-derived xenograft models that reliably recapitulated the genetic and phenotypic features of HCC [30]. Moreover, in models expressing high levels of FGF receptor

1, lenvatinib exhibited a greater efficacy than sorafenib. Lenvatinib has also shown highly promising data in phase I/II clinical trials involving patients with advanced HCC [31].

3.5. Cabozantinib

Cabozantinib (Cometriq®) was approved in 2012 by the FDA and is a small-molecule RTK inhibitor with potent activity toward VEGFR-2, MET, and RET (rearranged during transfection), leading to the inhibition of tumor angiogenesis [32]. In a phase II study, the observed disease control rate following 12 weeks of treatment with cabozantinib was found to be 68 or 78% of the patients with or without prior sorafenib treatment exhibited tumor regression. A phase III randomized double-blind, controlled trial is ongoing to compare the efficacy of cabozantinib with a placebo as the second-line treatment modality for advanced HCC patients who have previously received sorafenib.

4. Alternative therapy

Sorafenib is the standard therapeutic agent administered for the treatment of advanced stages of HCC and it is likely that other RTK inhibitors will also become commonly utilized drugs. However, chronic liver damage usually lowers the capacity of drug metabolism in patients, and the long-term administration of sorafenib may induce excessive adverse effects. Therefore, to reduce dosage of sorafenib, an alternative approach may be required to identify a clinically available compound targeting tumor angiogenesis. Among the various factors to affect angiogenic activities, many researchers have focused their attention on the mechanisms of angiotensin-II (AT-II) and insulin resistance (IR). These factors have been shown to affect angiogenesis in the liver via close interactions [33]. Moreover, since these factors could also be involved in the HCC, the regulation of these factors might contribute to suppressing the progression of the chronic liver disease.

4.1. RAAS blockers

The renin-angiotensin-aldosterone system (RAAS) is a hormone system that is involved in the regulation of the plasma sodium concentration and arterial blood pressure to maintain body fluid homeostasis [34]. Recent reports have demonstrated that RAAS is locally expressed in a number of tissues, including the kidneys, adrenal glands, heart, vasculature and nervous system, and liver. Actually, RAAS is frequently activated in patients with chronic liver diseases, such as liver cirrhosis [35, 36]. AT-II is an octapeptide derived from its precursor, AT-I, after AT-I converting enzyme (ACE) acts AT-I, proteolytically cleaving the C-terminal dipeptide. During the progression of chronic liver diseases, AT-II is considered to be a potential mediator of portal hypertension. It has been reported that AT-II plasma levels are clinically increased in patients with cirrhosis, and an animal study has shown the elevation of the portal pressure by AT-II administration [37, 38].

AT-II plays a crucial role in the development of several cancers, including HCC. Lever et al. has previously shown the outcome of a retrospective cohort study consisting of 5207 patients with treatment of either an ACE inhibitor (ACE-I) or other antihypertensive agents such as calcium channel blockers, diuretics, and β-blockers with a 10-year follow-up (Glasgow study). Interestingly, in their study, the incidence of cancer and fetal cancer was decreased in the patients with ACE-I treatment as compared with those with other drugs [39]. A recent cohort study has also demonstrated a lower incidence of cancer in patients using ACE-I or an AT-II receptor blocker (ARB) than nonusers [40]. Furthermore, it has been reported that the addition of ACE-I or ARB provided the prolonged survival for the patients with advanced non–small cell lung cancer undergoing platinum-based chemotherapy [41]. Additionally, inhibition of RAAS possibly exerted the beneficial effects on the prognosis of patients with advanced hormone-refractory prostate cancer and pancreatic cancer receiving gemcitabine [42, 43]. In regard to liver cancer, ACE-I showed the suppressive effect on the tumor growth in a murine HCC experimental model [44].

The RAAS, especially AT-II, is potently involved in the regulation of both rarefaction and expansion of the vascular network. Circulating AT-II leads to drive a variety of signaling cascades leading to VEGF, FGF, IGF, and TGF-β expression through mainly binding to the AT1R on ECs [45–47]. AT-II/AT1-R axis plays a key role in the regulation of angiogenic activity in various pathological events, including tumor neovascularization. Actually, inhibition of AT-II by ACE-I and ARB reportedly attenuates **intratumoral neovascularization with down-regulation of** VEGF expression in several cancers [48–50]. These findings indicate that ACE-I and ARB can be candidates for novel antiangiogenic agents against HCC. However, previous report has suggested that monotherapy with only antiangiogenic agent does not exert the sufficient effect on the prognosis in patients with advanced cancer [51]. Therefore, the combination treatment of antiangiogenic agents has been approached to show a synergistic inhibitory effect on cancer progression [51, 52]. For example, the combination of ACE-I and interferon (IFN) suppressed HCC growth more potently than monotherapy with ACE-I [53]. Our report demonstrated that the antitumoral effect of 5-fluorouracil (5-FU) is also enhanced by combination with ACE-I [54].

As well as tumor growth and metastasis, the early stages of carcinogenesis are also regulated by RAAS-mediated angiogenesis [5, 55]. Our animal study has shown that ACE-I significantly suppressed hepatocarcinogenesis at a clinically comparable low dose together with an attenuated neovascularization [56]. Additionally, a combination of ACE-I with supplementation of vitamin K (VK), which is often administered to the patients with osteoporosis, showed a more potent inhibitory effect on rat hepatocarcinogenesis than ACE-I monotherapy [57]. This combination regimen consisting of ACE-I and VK also exhibited the beneficial effect on ameliorating hepatocarcinogenesis in our clinical study [58]. A 48-month follow-up study revealed that a combined ACE-I with VK significantly suppressed the cumulative recurrence of HCC with reduced serum VEGF levels. The serum level of lectin-reactive α-fetoprotein (AFP-L3), known as one of the HCC tumor markers, was also decreased in parallel with VEGF. Accordingly, this combination regimen may represent a new strategy for chemoprevention against HCC.

Aldosterone (Ald), a downstream component of AT-II in RAAS, also affects in the regulation of angiogenesis. **Endocrinologically**, Ald is a mineralocorticoid hormone regulating the plasma sodium (Na^+), the extracellular potassium (K^+) and arterial blood pressure, blood pressure, and electrolyte balance via mineralocorticoid receptors (MR) [59]. Recent data have suggested that Ald plays a key role in endothelial dysfunction, as well as a suggested involvement in the pathogenesis of hypertension [60]. Moreover, the possible involvement of Ald and the MR systems in pathological ocular neovascularization has been reported [61]. Ald was shown to stimulate the proliferation and tubulogenesis of EC, and exacerbated angiogenesis in oxygen-induced retinopathy. In addition, these events could be attenuated by spironolactone. Eplerenone, a selective Ald blocker (SAB), is clinically used as a novel option for the treatment of hypertension. SAB is a selective MR antagonist with higher affinity than spironolactone, contributing to lower side effect by binding the progesterone and androgen receptors. The animal study revealed that murine hepatocarcinogenesis was markedly suppressed by the treatment of SAB with attenuation of VEGF-mediated angiogenesis [62]. These results indicate that SAB is also a viable option for treatment of HCC.

4.2. Regulation of insulin resistance

Recent studies have revealed a close relationship between IR and the progression of liver disease, including HCC [63, 64]. In general, chronic liver diseases impair the metabolic homeostasis of glucose as a result of IR, glucose intolerance, and DM [65]. Several clinical studies have also identified the hyperinsulinemia in patients with chronic hepatitis C (CHC) [66–68]. Experimental evidence with the HCV-transgenic mouse model confirms the contribution of HCV in the development of IR and DM [69]. In this model, the overproduced TNF-α appears to play a pivotal role in the induction of IR and DM. TNF-α is a proinflammatory cytokine, dramatically elevated during inflammation-induced disease pathology. HCV itself induces the phosphorylation of the serine residues associated with the insulin receptor substrate (IRS)-1 and -2 and stimulates the overproduction of suppressor of cytokine-3 (SOC-3), inhibiting the phosphorylation of Akt/PI3K, leading to the blockade of transactivation of GLUT-4, which contributes to inhibit intracellular glucose uptake. Additionally, nonalcoholic fatty liver disease (NAFLD) is a common liver disorder associated with IR and DM [70]. Various factors participate in the progression of NAFLD, such as oxidative stress, endotoxemia, obesity, genetic factors, and IR. Several reports have suggested the association of IR and mitochondrial abnormalities [71].

Recently, a reciprocal relationship between diabetes and HCC has been noticed. A two to threefold increase in the risk of HCC has been observed in the patients with DM, regardless of the etiology of chronic liver diseases [72–74]. A large longitudinal study in the United States demonstrated the twofold higher incidence of HCC in the diabetic patients [74]. Moreover, a recent study has elucidated that the IR status directly facilitated hepatocarcinogenesis [64]. Hyperinsulinemia can generally induce the synthesis and activation of IGF-1, which has a potential to progress a variety of cancer [75]. The altered expression pattern of IGF-1 signaling has been found in human HCC as well as hepatocarcinogenesis in rodent models [76]. Furthermore, IR status may progress hepatocarcinogenesis through the augmentation of hepatic neovascularization and VEGF expression in a rat carcinogenesis model [64].

The diabetic patients with compensated liver diseases initially are treated by a lifestyle change. However, restrictive diets may be liable to aggravate malnutrition in some patients. Thus, the oral antidiabetic drugs are administered to treat the diabetic patients with advanced liver diseases such as cirrhosis [77, 78]. To avoid hyperinsulinemia affecting adversely HCC growth, the drugs exerting insulin-sensitizing effects are preferable such as metformin, pioglitazone, dipeptidyl peptidase 4 inhibitor, or sodium glucose cotransporter inhibitor. Another report has demonstrated that the use of statins, a class of lipid-lowering medications by inhibiting HMG-CoA reductase that plays a central role in the production of cholesterol, significantly lowered the risk of HCC in the patients with DM [79].

The branched-chain amino acid (BCAA), an amino acid having aliphatic side chains with a branch (a central carbon atom bound to three or more carbon atoms), comprises three essential amino acids: leucine, isoleucine, and valine. Several clinical studies have suggested the beneficial effect of the long-term supplementation with BCAA granules on hypoalbuminemia and event-free survival in the patients with cirrhosis [80, 81]. BCAAs have also been shown to induce glucose uptake and improve glucose metabolism in a rat cirrhotic model. Intriguingly, the animal study using obese diabetic rat showed a chemopreventive effect of BCAAs against HCC with the downregulation of VEGF and antiangiogenic activity [82, 83]. Multicenter study in Japan also revealed that BCAAs decreased the incidence of HCC in patients with HCV-related cirrhosis as well as the type 2 DM and obesity [84]. However, a monotherapy with BCAA did not inhibit the recurrence of HCC after curative treatment. Therefore, to utilize BCAAs with sufficient effect against HCC, it is strongly recommended to combine them with other drugs. From previous research, AT-II also plays a key role in the development of IR. Actually, mice genetically lacking ACE exhibited the improvement of glucose tolerance through the reduced fat mass [85]. Moreover, additional administration of ACE-I or ARB to BCAAs is also shown to improve the IR status [33, 86]. Our randomized control trial study demonstrated that the combined BCAAs with ACE-I suppresses the cumulative recurrence of HCC in the patients with IR [87].

Taken together, these findings indicate that the combination of BCAAs supplementation and RAAS blockade may represent a potentially novel therapeutic strategy against HCC in the patients with IR.

5. Conclusions and future perspectives

Angiogenesis plays a crucial role in hepatocarcinogenesis and HCC progression, indicating the requirement of an antiangiogenic therapy as a tool for suppressing HCC. Sorafenib has become a breakthrough drug in the field of HCC, with an improvement in the median survival of almost 3 months. This represents a reduction of greater than 30% for the probability of death during the follow-up period.

However, when using RTK inhibitors, including sorafenib for patients with chronic liver diseases, many patients exhibit adverse effects, and several symptoms are very severe. Since the adverse effects induced by RTK inhibitors emerge in a dose-dependent manner, it is desirable for patients with chronic liver diseases to avoid these drugs as much as possible. Therefore, to lower the dose of such treatments, a clinically available compound to use in combination with RTK inhibitors may be required.

ACE-I, ARB, and SAB are extensively employed as antihypertensive agents in clinical practice without serious adverse effects. Thus, these RAAS blocking agents may provide a novel strategy targeting HCC. However, several reports also suggest that there is a close relationship between AT-II polymorphisms and the progression of chronic liver diseases and cancers. In certain types of cancers, the elevated ACE genetic polymorphisms are significantly involved in their poor prognosis [88, 89]. Additionally, AT-II type I receptor polymorphism reportedly contributes to the occurrence of nonalcoholic steatohepatitis (NASH) [90]. These evidences suggest that the efficacy of RAAS inhibition may vary in each case. Since combination treatment of ACE-I and VK exerted substantially more potent inhibitory effects, a combination treatment involving these agents may be preferable for future clinical applications. Furthermore, under IR conditions, the combination treatment of BCAA and ACE-I would be a promising approach against HCC via the suppression of VEGF-mediated angiogenesis. Since these agents are widely used in clinical practice, the combination of these agents with RTK inhibitors such as sorafenib represents a potential alternative approach against HCC.

Author details

Kosuke Kaji* and Hitoshi Yoshiji

*Address all correspondence to: kajik@naramed-u.ac.jp

Third Department of Internal Medicine, Nara Medical University, Shijo-cho, Kashihara, Nara, Japan

References

[1] Carmeliet P. Angiogenesis in life, disease and medicine. Nature. 2005;438(7070):932–6.

[2] Kalluri R, Sukhatme VP. Fibrosis and angiogenesis. Current Opinion in Nephrology and Hypertension. 2000;9(4):413–8.

[3] Llovet JM, Schwartz M, Mazzaferro V. Resection and liver transplantation for hepatocellular carcinoma. Seminars in Liver Disease. 2005;25(2):181–200.

[4] Li CY, Shan S, Huang Q, Braun RD, Lanzen J, Hu K, et al. Initial stages of tumor cell-induced angiogenesis: evaluation via skin window chambers in rodent models. Journal of the National Cancer Institute. 2000;92(2):143–7.

[5] Bergers G, Benjamin LE. Tumorigenesis and the angiogenic switch. Nature Reviews Cancer. 2003;3(6):401–10.

[6] Bergers G, Javaherian K, Lo KM, Folkman J, Hanahan D. Effects of angiogenesis inhibitors on multistage carcinogenesis in mice. Science. 1999;284(5415):808–12.

[7] Brandvold KA, Neiman P, Ruddell A. Angiogenesis is an early event in the generation of myc-induced lymphomas. Oncogene. 2000;19(23):2780–5.

[8] Carr BI. Hepatocellular carcinoma: current management and future trends. Gastroenterology. 2004;127(5 Suppl 1):S218–24.

[9] Kerbel RS. Tumor angiogenesis. The New England Journal of Medicine. 2008;358(19): 2039–49.

[10] Carmeliet P. VEGF as a key mediator of angiogenesis in cancer. Oncology. 2005;69(Suppl 3):4–10.

[11] Shibuya M. Structure and function of VEGF/VEGF-receptor system involved in angiogenesis. Cell Structure and Function. 2001;26(1):25–35.

[12] Karkkainen MJ, Petrova TV. Vascular endothelial growth factor receptors in the regulation of angiogenesis and lymphangiogenesis. Oncogene. 2000;19(49):5598–605.

[13] Miura H, Miyazaki T, Kuroda M, Oka T, Machinami R, Kodama T, et al. Increased expression of vascular endothelial growth factor in human hepatocellular carcinoma. Journal of Hepatology. 1997;27(5):854–61.

[14] Yamaguchi R, Yano H, Iemura A, Ogasawara S, Haramaki M, Kojiro M. Expression of vascular endothelial growth factor in human hepatocellular carcinoma. Hepatology. 1998;28(1):68–77.

[15] Yamaguchi R, Yano H, Nakashima Y, Ogasawara S, Higaki K, Akiba J, et al. Expression and localization of vascular endothelial growth factor receptors in human hepatocellular carcinoma and non-HCC tissues. Oncology Reports. 2000;7(4):725–9.

[16] Yoshiji H, Kuriyama S, Yoshii J, Ikenaka Y, Noguchi R, Hicklin DJ, et al. Halting the interaction between vascular endothelial growth factor and its receptors attenuates liver carcinogenesis in mice. Hepatology. 2004;39(6):1517–24.

[17] Cook KM, Figg WD. Angiogenesis inhibitors: current strategies and future prospects. CA: Cancer Journal for Clinicians. 2010;60(4):222–43.

[18] Forner A, Llovet JM, Bruix J. Hepatocellular carcinoma. Lancet. 2012;379(9822):1245–55.

[19] Llovet JM, Ricci S, Mazzaferro V, Hilgard P, Gane E, Blanc JF, et al. Sorafenib in advanced hepatocellular carcinoma. The New England Journal of Medicine. 2008;359(4):378–90.

[20] Wilhelm S, Carter C, Lynch M, Lowinger T, Dumas J, Smith RA, et al. Discovery and development of sorafenib: a multikinase inhibitor for treating cancer. Nature Reviews Drug Discovery. 2006;5(10):835–44.

[21] Chen KF, Tai WT, Liu TH, Huang HP, Lin YC, Shiau CW, et al. Sorafenib overcomes TRAIL resistance of hepatocellular carcinoma cells through the inhibition of STAT-Clinical Cancer Research: An Official Journal of the American Association for Cancer Research. 2010;16(21):5189–99.

[22] Rosato RR, Almenara JA, Coe S, Grant S. The multikinase inhibitor sorafenib potentiates TRAIL lethality in human leukemia cells in association with Mcl-1 and cFLIPL down-regulation. Cancer Research. 2007;67(19):9490–500.

[23] Zhu AX, Raymond E. Early development of sunitinib in hepatocellular carcinoma. Expert Review of Anticancer Therapy. 2009;9(1):143–50.

[24] Cheng AL, Kang YK, Lin DY, Park JW, Kudo M, Qin S, et al. Sunitinib versus sorafenib in advanced hepatocellular cancer: results of a randomized phase III trial. Journal of Clinical Oncology: Official Journal of the American Society of Clinical Oncology. 2013;31(32):4067–75.

[25] Bhide RS, Cai ZW, Zhang YZ, Qian L, Wei D, Barbosa S, et al. Discovery and preclinical studies of (R)-1-(4-(4-fluoro-2-methyl-1H-indol-5-yloxy)-5- methylpyrrolo[2,1-f][1,2,4]triazin-6-yloxy)propan-2-ol (BMS-540215), an in vivo active potent VEGFR-2 inhibitor. Journal of Medicinal Chemistry. 2006;49(7):2143–6.

[26] Huynh H, Ngo VC, Fargnoli J, Ayers M, Soo KC, Koong HN, et al. Brivanib alaninate, a dual inhibitor of vascular endothelial growth factor receptor and fibroblast growth factor receptor tyrosine kinases, induces growth inhibition in mouse models of human hepatocellular carcinoma. Clinical Cancer Research: An Official Journal of the American Association for Cancer Research. 2008;14(19):6146–53.

[27] Johnson PJ, Qin S, Park JW, Poon RT, Raoul JL, Philip PA, et al. Brivanib versus sorafenib as first-line therapy in patients with unresectable, advanced hepatocellular carcinoma: results from the randomized phase III BRISK-FL study. Journal of Clinical Oncology: Official Journal of the American Society of Clinical Oncology. 2013;31(28):3517–24.

[28] Llovet JM, Decaens T, Raoul JL, Boucher E, Kudo M, Chang C, et al. Brivanib in patients with advanced hepatocellular carcinoma who were intolerant to sorafenib or for whom sorafenib failed: results from the randomized phase III BRISK-PS study. Journal of Clinical Oncology: Official Journal of the American Society of Clinical Oncology. 2013;31(28):3509–16.

[29] Yeung KT, Cohen EE. Lenvatinib in advanced, radioactive iodine-refractory, differentiated thyroid carcinoma. Clinical Cancer Research: An Official Journal of the American Association for Cancer Research. 2015;21(24):5420–6.

[30] Gu Q, Zhang B, Sun H, Xu Q, Tan Y, Wang G, et al. Genomic characterization of a large panel of patient-derived hepatocellular carcinoma xenograft tumor models for preclinical development. Oncotarget. 2015;6(24):20160–76.

[31] Oikonomopoulos G, Aravind P, Sarker D. Lenvatinib: a potential breakthrough in advanced hepatocellular carcinoma? Future Oncology. 2016;12(4):465–76.

[32] Xiang Q, Chen W, Ren M, Wang J, Zhang H, Deng DY, et al. Cabozantinib suppresses tumor growth and metastasis in hepatocellular carcinoma by a dual blockade of VEGFR2 and MET. Clinical Cancer Research: An Official Journal of the American Association for Cancer Research. 2014;20(11):2959–70.

[33] de Kloet AD, Krause EG, Woods SC. The renin angiotensin system and the metabolic syndrome. Physiology & Behavior. 2010;100(5):525–34.

[34] Ardaillou R. Angiotensin II receptors. Journal of the American Society of Nephrology: JASN. 1999;10(Suppl 11):S30–9.

[35] Helmy A, Jalan R, Newby DE, Hayes PC, Webb DJ. Role of angiotensin II in regulation of basal and sympathetically stimulated vascular tone in early and advanced cirrhosis. Gastroenterology. 2000;118(3):565–72.

[36] Munshi MK, Uddin MN, Glaser SS. The role of the renin-angiotensin system in liver fibrosis. Experimental Biology and Medicine. 2011;236(5):557–66.

[37] Beyazit Y, Ibis M, Purnak T, Turhan T, Kekilli M, Kurt M, et al. Elevated levels of circulating angiotensin converting enzyme in patients with hepatoportal sclerosis. Digestive Diseases and Sciences. 2011;56(7):2160–5.

[38] Lugo-Baruqui A, Munoz-Valle JF, Arevalo-Gallegos S, Armendariz-Borunda J. Role of angiotensin II in liver fibrosis-induced portal hypertension and therapeutic implications. Hepatology Research: the Official Journal of the Japan Society of Hepatology. 2010;40(1):95–104.

[39] Lever AF, Hole DJ, Gillis CR, McCallum IR, McInnes GT, MacKinnon PL, et al. Do inhibitors of angiotensin-I-converting enzyme protect against risk of cancer? Lancet. 1998;352(9123):179–84.

[40] Christian JB, Lapane KL, Hume AL, Eaton CB, Weinstock MA, Trial V. Association of ACE inhibitors and angiotensin receptor blockers with keratinocyte cancer prevention in the randomized VATTC trial. Journal of the National Cancer Institute. 2008;100(17): 1223–32.

[41] Wilop S, von Hobe S, Crysandt M, Esser A, Osieka R, Jost E. Impact of angiotensin I converting enzyme inhibitors and angiotensin II type 1 receptor blockers on survival in patients with advanced non-small-cell lung cancer undergoing first-line platinum-based chemotherapy. Journal of Cancer Research and Clinical Oncology. 2009;135(10): 1429–35.

[42] Uemura H, Hasumi H, Kawahara T, Sugiura S, Miyoshi Y, Nakaigawa N, et al. Pilot study of angiotensin II receptor blocker in advanced hormone-refractory prostate cancer. International Journal of Clinical Oncology. 2005;10(6):405–10.

[43] Nakai Y, Isayama H, Ijichi H, Sasaki T, Sasahira N, Hirano K, et al. Inhibition of renin-angiotensin system affects prognosis of advanced pancreatic cancer receiving gemcitabine. British Journal of Cancer. 2010;103(11):1644–8.

[44] Yoshiji H, Kuriyama S, Kawata M, Yoshii J, Ikenaka Y, Noguchi R, et al. The angiotensin-I-converting enzyme inhibitor perindopril suppresses tumor growth and angiogenesis: possible role of the vascular endothelial growth factor. Clinical cancer Research: An Official Journal of the American Association for Cancer Research. 2001;7(4):1073–8.

[45] Miura S, Saku K. Regulation of angiogenesis and angiogenic factors by cardiovascular medications. Current Pharmaceutical Design. 2007;13(20):2113–7.

[46] Heffelfinger SC. The renin angiotensin system in the regulation of angiogenesis. Current Pharmaceutical Design. 2007;13(12):1215–29.

[47] Greene AS, Amaral SL. Microvascular angiogenesis and the renin-angiotensin system. Current Hypertension Reports. 2002;4(1):56–62.

[48] Huang W, Wu YL, Zhong J, Jiang FX, Tian XL, Yu LF. Angiotensin II type 1 receptor antagonist suppress angiogenesis and growth of gastric cancer xenografts. Digestive Diseases and Sciences. 2008;53(5):1206–10.

[49] Kosaka T, Miyajima A, Takayama E, Kikuchi E, Nakashima J, Ohigashi T, et al. Angiotensin II type 1 receptor antagonist as an angiogenic inhibitor in prostate cancer. The Prostate. 2007;67(1):41–9.

[50] Noguchi R, Yoshiji H, Ikenaka Y, Namisaki T, Kitade M, Kaji K, et al. Synergistic inhibitory effect of gemcitabine and angiotensin type-1 receptor blocker, losartan, on murine pancreatic tumor growth via antiangiogenic activities. Oncology Reports. 2009;22(2):355–60.

[51] Kerbel RS. Clinical trials of antiangiogenic drugs: opportunities, problems, and assessment of initial results. Journal of Clinical Oncology: Official Journal of the American Society of Clinical Oncology. 2001;19(18 Suppl):45S–51S.

[52] Scappaticci FA. Mechanisms and future directions for angiogenesis-based cancer therapies. Journal of Clinical Oncology: Official Journal of the American Society of Clinical Oncology. 2002;20(18):3906–27.

[53] Noguchi R, Yoshiji H, Kuriyama S, Yoshii J, Ikenaka Y, Yanase K, et al. Combination of interferon-beta and the angiotensin-converting enzyme inhibitor, perindopril, attenuates murine hepatocellular carcinoma development and angiogenesis. Clinical Cancer Research: An Official Journal of the American Association for Cancer Research. 2003;9(16 Pt 1):6038–45.

[54] Yanase K, Yoshiji H, Ikenaka Y, Noguchi R, Kitade M, Kaji K, et al. Synergistic inhibition of hepatocellular carcinoma growth and hepatocarcinogenesis by combination of 5-fluorouracil and angiotensin-converting enzyme inhibitor via anti-angiogenic activities. Oncology Reports. 2007;17(2):441–6.

[55] Staton CA, Chetwood AS, Cameron IC, Cross SS, Brown NJ, Reed MW. The angiogenic switch occurs at the adenoma stage of the adenoma carcinoma sequence in colorectal cancer. Gut. 2007;56(10):1426–32.

[56] Yoshiji H, Yoshii J, Ikenaka Y, Noguchi R, Yanase K, Tsujinoue H, et al. Suppression of the renin-angiotensin system attenuates vascular endothelial growth factor-mediated tumor development and angiogenesis in murine hepatocellular carcinoma cells. International Journal of Oncology. 2002;20(6):1227–31.

[57] Yoshiji H, Kuriyama S, Noguchi R, Yoshii J, Ikenaka Y, Yanase K, et al. Combination of vitamin K2 and the angiotensin-converting enzyme inhibitor, perindopril, attenuates the liver enzyme-altered preneoplastic lesions in rats via angiogenesis suppression. Journal of Hepatology. 2005;42(5):687–93.

[58] Yoshiji H, Noguchi R, Toyohara M, Ikenaka Y, Kitade M, Kaji K, et al. Combination of vitamin K2 and angiotensin-converting enzyme inhibitor ameliorates cumulative recurrence of hepatocellular carcinoma. Journal of Hepatology. 2009;51(2):315–21.

[59] Williams GH. Aldosterone biosynthesis, regulation, and classical mechanism of action. Heart Failure Reviews. 2005;10(1):7–13.

[60] Funder JW. Minireview: Aldosterone and mineralocorticoid receptors: past, present, and future. Endocrinology. 2010;151(11):5098–102.

[61] Wilkinson-Berka JL, Tan G, Jaworski K, Miller AG. Identification of a retinal aldosterone system and the protective effects of mineralocorticoid receptor antagonism on retinal vascular pathology. Circulation Research. 2009;104(1):124–33.

[62] Kaji K, Yoshiji H, Kitade M, Ikenaka Y, Noguchi R, Shirai Y, et al. Selective aldosterone blocker, eplerenone, attenuates hepatocellular carcinoma growth and angiogenesis in mice. Hepatology Research: The Official Journal of the Japan Society of Hepatology. 2010;40(5):540–9.

[63] Llovet JM, Bruix J. Novel advancements in the management of hepatocellular carcinoma in Journal of Hepatology. 2008;48 Suppl 1:S20–37.

[64] Kaji K, Yoshiji H, Kitade M, Ikenaka Y, Noguchi R, Yoshii J, et al. Impact of insulin resistance on the progression of chronic liver diseases. International Journal of Molecular Medicine. 2008;22(6):801–8.

[65] Nielsen MF, Caumo A, Aagaard NK, Chandramouli V, Schumann WC, Landau BR, et al. Contribution of defects in glucose uptake to carbohydrate intolerance in liver cirrhosis: assessment during physiological glucose and insulin concentrations. American journal of physiology Gastrointestinal and Liver Physiology. 2005;288(6):G1135–43.

[66] Kawaguchi T, Yoshida T, Harada M, Hisamoto T, Nagao Y, Ide T, et al. Hepatitis C virus down-regulates insulin receptor substrates 1 and 2 through up-regulation of suppressor of cytokine signaling The American Journal of Pathology. 2004;165(5):1499–508.

[67] Hui JM, Sud A, Farrell GC, Bandara P, Byth K, Kench JG, et al. Insulin resistance is associated with chronic hepatitis C virus infection and fibrosis progression [corrected]. Gastroenterology. 2003;125(6):1695–704.

[68] Petit JM, Bour JB, Galland-Jos C, Minello A, Verges B, Guiguet M, et al. Risk factors for diabetes mellitus and early insulin resistance in chronic hepatitis C. Journal of Hepatology. 2001;35(2):279–83.

[69] Shintani Y, Fujie H, Miyoshi H, Tsutsumi T, Tsukamoto K, Kimura S, et al. Hepatitis C virus infection and diabetes: direct involvement of the virus in the development of insulin resistance. Gastroenterology. 2004;126(3):840–8.

[70] Bugianesi E, McCullough AJ, Marchesini G. Insulin resistance: a metabolic pathway to chronic liver disease. Hepatology. 2005;42(5):987–1000.

[71] Sanyal AJ, Campbell-Sargent C, Mirshahi F, Rizzo WB, Contos MJ, Sterling RK, et al. Nonalcoholic steatohepatitis: association of insulin resistance and mitochondrial abnormalities. Gastroenterology. 2001;120(5):1183–92.

[72] Davila JA, Morgan RO, Shaib Y, McGlynn KA, El-Serag HB. Diabetes increases the risk of hepatocellular carcinoma in the United States: a population based case control study. Gut. 2005;54(4):533–9.

[73] El-Serag HB, Tran T, Everhart JE. Diabetes increases the risk of chronic liver disease and hepatocellular carcinoma. Gastroenterology. 2004;126(2):460–8.

[74] El-Serag HB, Richardson PA, Everhart JE. The role of diabetes in hepatocellular carcinoma: a case-control study among United States Veterans. The American Journal of Gastroenterology. 2001;96(8):2462–7.

[75] Siddique A, Kowdley KV. Insulin resistance and other metabolic risk factors in the pathogenesis of hepatocellular carcinoma. Clinics in Liver Disease. 2011;15(2):281–96, vii-x.

[76] Alexia C, Fallot G, Lasfer M, Schweizer-Groyer G, Groyer A. An evaluation of the role of insulin-like growth factors (IGF) and of type-I IGF receptor signalling in hepatocarcinogenesis and in the resistance of hepatocarcinoma cells against drug-induced apoptosis. Biochemical Pharmacology. 2004;68(6):1003–15.

[77] Donadon V, Balbi M, Mas MD, Casarin P, Zanette G. Metformin and reduced risk of hepatocellular carcinoma in diabetic patients with chronic liver disease. Liver International: Official Journal of the International Association for the Study of the Liver. 2010;30(5):750–8.

[78] Khattab M, Emad M, Abdelaleem A, Eslam M, Atef R, Shaker Y, et al. Pioglitazone improves virological response to peginterferon alpha-2b/ribavirin combination therapy in hepatitis C genotype 4 patients with insulin resistance. Liver International: Official Journal of the International Association for the Study of the Liver. 2010;30(3): 447–54.

[79] El-Serag HB, Johnson ML, Hachem C, Morgana RO. Statins are associated with a reduced risk of hepatocellular carcinoma in a large cohort of patients with diabetes. Gastroenterology. 2009;136(5):1601–8.

[80] Marchesini G, Bianchi G, Merli M, Amodio P, Panella C, Loguercio C, et al. Nutritional supplementation with branched-chain amino acids in advanced cirrhosis: a double-blind, randomized trial. Gastroenterology. 2003;124(7):1792–801.

[81] Muto Y, Sato S, Watanabe A, Moriwaki H, Suzuki K, Kato A, et al. Effects of oral branched-chain amino acid granules on event-free survival in patients with liver cirrhosis. Clinical Gastroenterology and Hepatology: The Official Clinical Practice Journal of the American Gastroenterological Association. 2005;3(7):705–13.

[82] Yoshiji H, Noguchi R, Kaji K, Ikenaka Y, Shirai Y, Namisaki T, et al. Attenuation of insulin-resistance-based hepatocarcinogenesis and angiogenesis by combined treatment with branched-chain amino acids and angiotensin-converting enzyme inhibitor in obese diabetic rats. Journal of Gastroenterology. 2010;45(4):443–50.

[83] Yoshiji H, Noguchi R, Kitade M, Kaji K, Ikenaka Y, Namisaki T, et al. Branched-chain amino acids suppress insulin-resistance-based hepatocarcinogenesis in obese diabetic rats. Journal of Gastroenterology. 2009;44(5):483–91.

[84] Muto Y, Sato S, Watanabe A, Moriwaki H, Suzuki K, Kato A, et al. Overweight and obesity increase the risk for liver cancer in patients with liver cirrhosis and long-term oral supplementation with branched-chain amino acid granules inhibits liver carcinogenesis in heavier patients with liver cirrhosis. Hepatology Research: The Official Journal of the Japan Society of Hepatology. 2006;35(3):204–14.

[85] Jayasooriya AP, Mathai ML, Walker LL, Begg DP, Denton DA, Cameron-Smith D, et al. Mice lacking angiotensin-converting enzyme have increased energy expenditure, with reduced fat mass and improved glucose clearance. Proceedings of the National Academy of Sciences of the United States of America. 2008;105(18):6531–6.

[86] Manrique C, Lastra G, Gardner M, Sowers JR. The renin angiotensin aldosterone system in hypertension: roles of insulin resistance and oxidative stress. The Medical Clinics of North America. 2009;93(3):569–82.

[87] Yoshiji H, Noguchi R, Ikenaka Y, Kaji K, Aihara Y, Yamazaki M, et al. Combination of branched-chain amino acids and angiotensin-converting enzyme inhibitor suppresses the cumulative recurrence of hepatocellular carcinoma: a randomized control trial. Oncology Reports. 2011;26(6):1547–53.

[88] Fabris C, Smirne C, Fangazio S, Toniutto P, Burlone M, Minisini R, et al. Influence of angiotensin-converting enzyme I/D gene polymorphism on clinical and histological correlates of chronic hepatitis C. Hepatology Research: The Official Journal of the Japan Society of Hepatology. 2009;39(8):795–804.

[89] Medeiros R, Vasconcelos A, Costa S, Pinto D, Lobo F, Morais A, et al. Linkage of angiotensin I-converting enzyme gene insertion/deletion polymorphism to the progression of human prostate cancer. The Journal of Pathology. 2004;202(3):330–5.

[90] Yoneda M, Hotta K, Nozaki Y, Endo H, Uchiyama T, Mawatari H, et al. Association between angiotensin II type 1 receptor polymorphisms and the occurrence of nonalcoholic fatty liver disease. Liver International: Official Journal of the International Association for the Study of the Liver. 2009;29(7):1078–85.

Chapter 21

MCAM and its Isoforms as Novel Targets in Angiogenesis Research and Therapy

Jimmy Stalin, Lucie Vivancos, Nathalie Bardin, Françoise Dignat-George and Marcel Blot-Chabaud

Additional information is available at the end of the chapter

http://dx.doi.org/10.5772/66765

Abstract

Melanoma cell adhesion molecule (MCAM) (CD146) is a membrane glycoprotein of the mucin family. It is one of the numerous proteins composing the junction of the vascular endothelium, and it is expressed in other cell types such as cancer cells, smooth muscle cells, and pericytes. Some recent works were designed to highlight its structural features, its location in the endothelium, and its role in angiogenesis, vascular permeability, and monocyte transmigration, but also in the maintenance of endothelial junctions and tumor development. MCAM exists in different splice variants and is shedded from the vascular membrane by metalloproteases. Studies about MCAM spliced and cleaved variant on human angiogenic physiological and pathological models permit a better understanding on the roles initially described for this protein. Furthermore, this knowledge will help in the future to develop therapeutic and diagnostic tools targeting specifically the different MCAM variant. Recent advances in research on angiogenesis and in the implication of MCAM in this process are discussed in this chapter.

Keywords: angiogenesis, MCAM (CD146), melanoma, physiology, pathology

1. Introduction

Angiogenesis is the process of new blood vessel formation from preexisting vessels. It contributes to physiological processes such as development and wound healing, but also to pathological processes, such as tumor angiogenesis. The identification of new targets involved in angiogenesis remains an important challenge to fully understand the involved mechanisms and to generate new therapeutic tools. Recent studies have highlighted CD146, an endothelial junctional molecule, as a key factor in angiogenesis. This molecule that displays different isoforms and that is present on different cell types could hence constitute a novel target for therapy. Different reviews have underlined its structural features, localization, and functions in the endothelium. This chapter thus mainly addresses the differences in CD146 isoforms with a special focus on their role in angiogenesis and the therapeutic tools targeting the molecule.

Historically, CD146 was discovered in 1987 by Professor J.P. Jonhson for the first time. It was identified as a marker of melanoma progression. These data were obtained by using an antibody generated by mouse immunization with a cell lysate of metastasizing melanoma. This antibody (MUC18) allowed the identification of a 113 kDa transmembrane protein. MCAM (melanoma cell adhesion molecule) described as a marker of metastasizing melanoma [1].

In 1991, the team of Professor. F. Dignat-George identified Sendo-1 antigen as a marker of circulating endothelial cells in the blood by flow cytometry. This was made possible through the generation of a mouse monoclonal antibody named Sendo -1 [2] obtained by mice immunization with a HUVEC cell lysate. Sendo-1 was able to stain the human endothelium whatever the vessel size and its anatomical location within the vascular tree [3, 4]. Gicerin and HEMCAM refer both to the avian homologues of the molecule [5].

As reported in Kobé in 1997, CD146 (cluster of differentiation 146) is now the official name grouping Sendo-1/MUC18/MCAM/gicerin/HEMCAM (Sendo-MUC18 preCD, Workshop Report).

2. Structure and characteristics of CD146

2.1. Genomic description

The specific location of the CD146 gene is on the arm q23.3 of the chromosome 11 in humans and on the chromosome 9 in mice (www.ensembl.org). The gene encoding the CD146 protein extends over 14 kb. It consists of five immunoglobulin-like domains, two variable domains, and three constant domains of C2 type, as well as a transmembrane domain and an intracytoplasmic portion [6]. The extracellular part of the molecule, including the five immunoglobulin domains, is encoded by 13 exons; the transmembrane domain and the intracellular domain are encoded by three exons.

The promoter of CD146 presents different putative binding sites and motifs including AP1, AP-2, CRE, SP1, CArG, and c-myb. Analysis of this DNA segments suggests that the four SP-1 sites, the two AP-2 domains, and one response element to AMPc-(CRE) form the minimal promotor of CD146 [7]. Specific sites play a role in CD146 expression. The AP-2 sites, which are located at −131 and −302 by relative to the initial ATG, inhibit the expression of CD146 by 70 and 44%, respectively. Moreover, when mutated, the CRE site inhibits by 70% the transcription of the genes. Therefore, AP-2 [8] and CRE sites [9] have been described to modulate CD146 expression in melanoma cells, leading to an increase in tumor growth and metastatic potential in these cancers. In fact, the AP-2 binding site located in the promoter (located at −23 bp) is an inhibitor of the transcription of CD146 while the other AP-2 sites (located at −131 and −302, respectively) are transcription activators [8].

The size of CD146 mRNA is around 3.3 kb and has been first identified in human melanoma cancer cells [10]. Its encoding region is about 1940 bp. A large homology in the mRNA sequences exists between human and mouse, but differences can be noted. Thus, in humans, there is a lengthening of the 3′ and 5′ UTR region as wells as a loss of 6 pb in exon 2. The encoding regions and 5′UTR have a homology of about 80 and 72%, respectively, between the murine and human genes and there is only 31% of homology for the 3'UTR fragment. Finally, the protein sequence shares about 76% of homology between these two species [1, 10, 11].

2.2. Proteic structure and isoforms

The proteic structure of CD146 is composed of a signal peptide of 28 amino acids (AA), five immunoglobulin domains (including two variable domains and three constant domains), a hydrophobic transmembrane region (AA 561–585), and an intracellular region. The protein sequence derived from the coding region of CD146 has a theoretical molecular weight of about 72 kDa. However, CD146 has a molecular weight of about 113 kDa. This difference is due to the glycosylation sites present on the protein sequence. Indeed, glycosylations represent about 35% of the total molecular weight of CD146 with mainly N-glycosylations. The presence of sialylation has also been shown [12].

CD146 has many similarities with other immunoglobulin family members such as BCAM (B-cell adhesion molecule) and ALCAM (activated leukocyte cell adhesion molecule), including the same number of immunoglobulin-like domains, similarity of functions and expression on tumor and endothelial cells. Thus, the ALCAM protein plays a role in CD4+ T lymphocytes and in tumor invasion [13, 14].

A short and a long isoform generated by alternative splicing have been identified as the two isoforms of membrane CD146. They have not been identified simultaneously. The long isoform was the first discovered in human melanocytes in 1987 and the short isoform was identified as a complementary DNA from chicken more recently [15]. In addition, a soluble form of CD146 was also identified in endothelial cell culture supernatant (HUVEC) and in bloodstream in patient [16].

Concerning the extracellular sequence, it is common to both isoforms. The difference is located in the intracytoplasmic portion [15]. The two isoforms are the result of an alternative splicing on exon 15 causing a reading frame shift. The short isoform displays a shorter intracytoplasmic domain containing a phosphorylation site for protein kinase C (PKC) and an interaction site for the protein with PDZ domain while the long isoform displays two domains for phosphorylation by PKC and an endocytosis signal sequence [15].

The intracytoplasmic domain sequence is similar to mice and human at 95 and 93% for the short isoform and long isoform, respectively. This conservation across species is in accordance with the important functions carried by the intracytoplasmic domain of CD146.

Finally, a soluble CD146 isoform with a molecular mass around 100 kDa, was identified for the first time in 1998 [16]. This isoform is detectable in human plasma and serum [17] and is generated by a metalloprotease-dependant shedding of the extracellular domain of CD146. The use of nonspecific inhibitors of metalloproteinase (GM6001) inhibits the formation of soluble CD146 [18].

3. CD146 localization

All the data concerning the expression of the different isoforms of CD146 and their functions are summarized in **Figures 1** and **2**.

3.1. Localization in cancer cells

CD146 has been identified for the first time in melanoma where it plays an important role in disease progression. Thereafter, CD146 has been shown to be expressed in various cancers, such as pancreatic/breast/prostate/ovarian/lung/kidney cancers, osteosarcoma, Kaposi sarcoma, angiosarcoma, Schwann cell tumors, or leiomyosarcoma (**Figure 1**). The mechanism of this neo-expression is still largely unknown but, in prostate cancer, it was reported that high expression of CD146 resulted from hypermethylation at the promoter of the CD146 gene [19].

However, almost nothing is known on the differential expressions and localizations of the different isoforms of CD146 in these cells. A recent study has shown that many cancer cells expressing CD146 were able to secrete soluble CD146 through a metalloprotease-dependant shedding [20].

Tissue/Organs/Cell lines	CD146 isoform expression	Effects/roles	Pathology	References
Human endothelial cell and cell lines HUVEC/EPC	CD146	Interaction endothelial-stromal cells / angiogenesis	Tumor angiogenesis	22, 33, 37, 59, 64
	short CD146	Angiogenesis	*nd*	23, 39
	long CD146	Stabilization of new vascular structure	*nd*	23
	soluble CD146	Pro-angiogenic factor-chemotactic properties	*nd*	16,17, 33, 39, 41
Zebrafish endothelial cells	CD146	Involved in VEGF-a signalization / regulate blood flow rate and vessel lumen size	*nd*	33, 34
Central Nervous System	CD146	Increases neurite extension / involved in optic tectum process extension	*nd*	30, 31, 32, 55
Bone marrow stroma	CD146	Able to generate bone tissue and hematopoietic environment	*nd*	29
Mesenchymal cells	CD146	Increases differenciation capacity	*nd*	28
Intermediate trophoblast	CD146	Regulates embryon implantation	Obstetric complication	70, 71
	soluble CD146	Decreases EVT migration	Obstetric complication	72
Human B lymphocyte	CD146	Increases adhesion	Rheumatoid arthritis	25
Human T lymphocyte	CD146	Increases adhesion	Rheumatoid arthritis	25, 26, 34,36
	long CD146	Increases adhesion	*nd*	26
Human Natural Killer cells	CD146	Increases adhesion	Rheumatoid arthritis	25
Mesengial/tubular cells	CD146	Endocapillary proliferation/proteinuria/inflammatory syndrome	Nephropathy	73
	soluble CD146	Increased in blood patient with chronic renal failure	Type 2 diabetic nephropathy patient	74
Non Small Cell Lung Cancer	soluble CD146	Increases in plasma	Poor prognosis factor	51
Gastric cancer	CD146	Increases metastasis/EMT inducer	Cancer development	49
	soluble CD146	*nd*	*nd*	74
Breast cancer	CD146	Increased cell motility	Poor prognosis factor	46, 47, 48, 50
Osteosarcoma	CD146	Increases metastatic dissemination	Cancer development	44, 45
Ovarian cancer	CD146	Increases metastatic dissemination and cancer cell survival	Cancer development	43
Prostate cancer	CD146	Increases invasiveness and metastatic potential	Cancer development/poor prognosis marker	19, 42
	soluble CD146	*nd*	*nd*	74
Human melanoma cancer	CD146	Increases metastatic dissemination	Poor prognosis marker	8, 9, 10, 61, 62, 63
	soluble CD146	Increases tumor angiogenesis and cancer cell survival	*nd*	20
Murin melanoma cell line	CD146	Increases metastatic dissemination	*nd*	11
Suprabasal Keratinocyte	CD146	*nd*	Kaposi's sarcoma/acute chronic dermatitis	75

Figure 1. Summary table for the different isoforms of CD146 expressed in several organs and cells related to their functions, pathologies, and references associated.

http://dx.doi.org/10.5772/66765

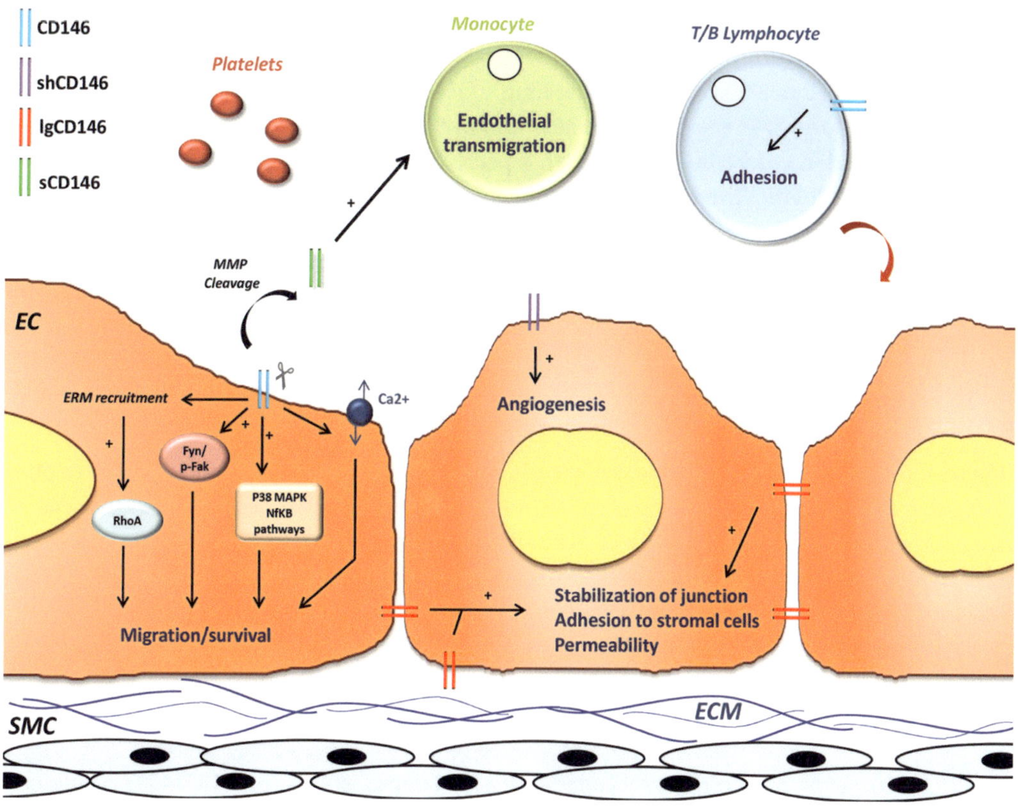

Figure 2. Expression, cell localization, and functions of the different isoforms of CD146 by endothelial cells (EC) and blood circulating cells.

3.2. Vascular localization

CD146 is expressed on the whole vascular tree whatever the vessel anatomical location and caliber. The localization of the long and short isoforms of CD146 is different. The induction of long CD146 expression in the CHO cell line (which does not constitutively express CD146) results in the expression of the protein at the intercellular junctions. Costaining of CD146 with VE-cadherin, focal adhesion kinase (FAK), PECAM, and the complex catenin/cadherin shows no colocalization, suggesting that CD146 is not located in the adherent junctions, tight junctions, or focal adhesions sites [21, 22].

Overexpression of the long form of CD146 in the MDCK cell line (Madin-Darby canine kidney) leads to a basolateral localization of the protein. A dileucine motif on its intracytoplasmic peptide sequence is necessary for this localization [21]. An immunohistochemical staining of long CD146 in endothelial colony-forming cells (ECFC) confirmed this junctional localization of the protein. In addition, the presence of a cytoplasmic pool of long CD146 that can be redistributed to the cell membrane was also described in Ref. [23].

The short isoform of CD146 does not share the same cellular localization. Transfection shows an apical localization of the protein in MDCK cells [21] that was confirmed in ECFC in a culture with a specific antibody generated against this isoform [23].

The confluence state of endothelial cells appears to regulate the spatial distribution of the two isoforms. Indeed, the long CD146 isoform was not detected at the junction in nonconfluent endothelial cells. Under this condition, the long CD146 isoform was intracytoplasmic and the short CD146 isoform was essentially nuclear and at the migration front [23]. In other experiments performed in chickens, it was shown a preferential localization of the long isoform of CD146 in the microvilli where the protein plays a role in their formation. Overexpression of CD146 increased the size of these microvilli [24].

3.3. Localization on immune cells

On peripheral blood of healthy patients approximately 1% of blood mononuclear cells express CD146. An analysis by flow cytometry of different lymphocyte populations showed an expression of CD146 on B and T lymphocytes in humans [25].

Research has shown that about 1% of B lymphocytes cells express CD146 and its expression is upregulated by a factor 5 following stimulation with IL-4 and CD40. Moreover, CD146 can be neo-expressed on some cell populations after stimulation [25]. The generation of two antibodies by rat immunization using cells from the T lymphocytic cell line HUT102 deepened these studies and shown that 2% of CD3+, CD3+/CD4+, and CD3+/CD8+ lymphocytes express CD146.

Moreover, stimulations with IL-2 [25] and PHA (phytohemagglutinin) [26] increases the amount of CD146+ T lymphocytes. The cells are also found *in vivo* in the synovial fluid of patients with rheumatoid arthritis [26].

In mice, a leucocytes screening was carried out which demonstrated that CD146 is not detectable on T/B lymphocyte populations, monocytes, and dendritic cells while 30% of neutrophils and 60% of NK cells express CD146. CD146 expression was correlated with an increased expression of CD11b and CD27 reflecting the maturity of NK. These CD146+ NK cells have a decreased cytotoxicity and produce gamma interferon in smaller quantities [27].

3.4. Bone marrow environment

In adults, hematopoiesis takes place in the bone marrow located in long bones of the human body. It is composed of a dense network of discontinuous capillaries allowing easy passage of cells produced in the bone marrow into the blood. A vascular sinus network which is mainly composed of stromal cells (reticular, endothelial, adipocyte, and osteoblast) serves to support the hematopoiesis process.

In one particular study, a subpopulation of bone marrow stroma cells was shown to express CD146 and to display characteristics of mural cells. They were characterized as a subpopulation of advential reticular cells which are abundant in the bone marrow and are able to generate bone tissue and a hematopoietic environment after isolation and implantation into an immunodeficient mouse [28].

Furthermore, angiopoietin -1 is regulated by CD146+ stromal cells. A decrease in the expression of CD146 by siRNA or FGF-2 (CD146 and Ang-1 regulator) reduces the capacity of these cells to participate in the remodeling and the assembly of pseudovascular structures *in vitro*

http://dx.doi.org/10.5772/66765

and to form hematopoietic microenvironment *in vivo*. From data on the spatial location of adventitial reticular cells and the expression of Tie-2 (the angiopoietin-1 receptor), it was suggested that CD146 and angiopoietin-1 are involved in the interaction between endothelial and stromal cells [29].

3.5. Localization in the central nervous system (CNS)

CD146 is found in the central nervous system (CNS). It is expressed during fetal development of the embryo but decreases after birth. Studies performed in chickens and rats have shown an expression of CD146 in the cerebellum, hippocampus, Purkinje cells, and sensorimotor cells of the spinal cord [30]. In chickens, CD146 binds NOF (neurite outgrowth factor), causing neurite extension [31], and increases the extension of the optic tectum process [32].

4. The different functions of CD146

CD146 was reported to be involved in many physiological processes. It has been described to play a role during the vascular development but also during the angiogenic process. As others junction molecules, it was described to be an actor during inflammation by modulating the migration of leucocytes through vascular endothelium.

4.1. CD146 during the vascular development

The role of CD146 was studied during vascular development. To this end, a model of CD146 inactivation by antisense morpholino-oligonucleotides was developed in zebrafish. Authors observed a decrease in intersomitic vessels followed by a decrease in blood flow and a reduction in vessel lumen observed by microangiography after CD146 inactivation [33]. It was also shown an inhibition of the VEGF-dependent angiogenesis [34].

4.2. Permeability and leucocytes migration

CD146 has been shown to be involved in endothelial permeability [33]. Using both a monocyte cell line, THP-1, and freshly isolated monocytes, it was also showed that it modulates monocytes transmigration. Junctional CD146 was shown to bind monocytes through a heterophilic interaction to increase their transmigration. In addition, an increased transmigration was observed following the binding of soluble CD146 on monocytes [33]. Another study showed that neo-expression of CD146 on lymphocytes induced new cellular properties. Indeed, an increase in the adhesion of CD146+ T lymphocytes effectors was observed after stimulation with IL-1 beta. This effect was blocked by the addition of anti-CD146 blocking antibodies [34]. An increase in the adhesion of CD4+/CD146+ T lymphocytes on endothelium was also observed after an inflammatory stimulus. In this study, *in vitro* transfection of the long isoform of CD146 in NKL.1 cell line induced a reduction of rolling cells and an increased adhesion to the endothelial monolayer. Moreover, these phenomena were accompanied by an increase in microvilli in T lymphocyte cell membrane. Another study showed an increased permeability of HMVEC (human microvascular endothelial cells) following incubation with an anti-CD146 antibody (P1H12) [35]. Finally, CD146 is coexpressed with CCR6 on a population of TH17 lymphocytic cells [36].

4.3. Angiogenesis

Angiogenesis is an important mechanism, both in fetal life and at adulthood. Endothelial cells with angiogenic capacities are able to proliferate, migrate, adhere, and generate new capillaries from a preexisting one.

The injection of an anti-CD146 antibody (AA98) led to a decrease of 70% in the number of vessels in a membrane model, chorioallantoic membrane model, in chicken. Furthermore, in mice, this antibody reduced the number of vessels in different models of xenografted tumors (hepatocellular carcinoma, pancreatic, and leiomyosarcoma) [37], demonstrating a role of CD146 in tumor angiogenesis.

The recent discovery of the existence of two isoforms of CD146 and the description of a soluble form of CD146 led to study their implications in the angiogenic process. Specific siRNA directed against these two isoforms has shown that the absence of the short CD146 decreased the proliferation, migration, and adhesion of endothelial cells, whereas its overexpression led to the reverse phenomena. These experiments showed that the long CD146 was also necessary to generate pseudocapillaries in Matrigel *in vitro* by stabilizing the junctions of neovessels. It thus appears that both the short and long isoforms of CD146 display complementary effects to generate neovessels. The effects of the short CD146 were confirmed *in vivo* by the transplantation of endothelial colony-forming cells (ECFC) overexpressing this isoform in a mouse model of hind limb ischemia. Indeed, it increased the incorporation of ECFC in ischemic muscle and favored the generation of neovessels [23]. A study of the mechanism showed that the short CD146 is associated with VEGF-R2 [38], but also angiomotin and VEGF-R1 at the endothelial cell surface [39, 40]. This association is essential for these different pathways. Indeed, the absence of the short CD146 isoform decreases the phosphorylation of VEGF-R2 in endothelial cells and prevents the proangiogenic effect of vascular endothelial growth factor (VEGF).

Soluble CD146 is also able to increase the formation of pseudocapillaries *in vitro* and to induce neovascularization in a rat model of hindlimb ischemia. In addition, subcutaneous injection of Matrigel containing soluble CD146 in mice increased the recruitment of both mature and immature endothelial cells, as well as smooth muscle cells, resulting in the formation of capillary-like structures [41]. Of interest, it was reported that soluble CD146 stimulates the short CD146 isoform through its binding on angiomotin [39] and that the angiogenic properties of soluble CD146 are additive to those of VEGF [41]. The roles of the different forms of CD146 are summarized in **Figure 2**.

4.4. Cancer cell growth and dissemination

CD146, which is neo-expressed on cancer cells, modulates their growth and dissemination. In prostate cancer, CD146 expression was observed in different cell lines. CD146 overexpression increased their invasiveness and metastatic potential [42]. CD146 overexpression was also observed in biopsies of patients. Its expression was correlated with a poor prognosis. In ovarian carcinomas, CD146 expression was also correlated with the increase of the metastatic potential. In addition, inhibition of CD146 protein expression in ovarian cancer cell lines led to inhibition of invasiveness, tumor spread and induced cancer cell apoptosis. This was explained by the fact that a lack of CD146 induced a decreased activity of Rho GTPase [43] involved in the invasion, proliferation, and metastatic spread of cancer cells.

It was also demonstrated that CD146 expression is increased in osteosarcomas as compared to nonpathological osteoblasts [44]. Injection of antibodies against CD146 decreased the amount of lung metastases in an immunodeficient mouse model injected with cells derived from human osteosarcoma [45].

In breast cancer, it was reported that CD146 would act as a tumor suppressor [46] while other studies have described CD146 as a poor prognosis marker [47]. Indeed, CD146 overexpression in a breast cancer cell line induced an increased motility and tumorigenicity [48]. Recent studies have also shown that CD146 induces the epithelial-mesenchymal transition (EMT) in so far as its expression is correlated with markers of EMT in gastric cancer [49]. Moreover, in triple negative breast cancers, an increase of CD146 expression in epithelial cells correlates with a loss of epithelial markers in favor of mesenchymal markers, increasing their invasiveness, migration, and the number of mammospheres. In addition CD44 expression increases and CD24 expression decreases on the cell surface suggesting that cells acquire phenotypic characteristics of cancer stem cells [50].

At present, there is no data on the differential expression and roles of the two membrane isoforms of CD146 on cancer cells. However, recent studies have shown an important role of soluble CD146 in tumor development. First, an increase of soluble CD146 concentration was described in blood of cancer patients with nonsmall cell lung cancer as compared to patients with respiratory inflammatory disease and healthy subjects [51]. In this chapter, we showed that association between an increased soluble CD146 concentration and an increased number of circulating endothelial cells (CEC) constitute a poor prognostic factor [51].

Recently, a study showed that human cancer cells that express membrane CD146 on their surface have also the ability to secrete the soluble form of CD146 [20]. This was described in melanoma, colorectal and pancreatic cancer cell lines. The authors demonstrated that soluble CD146 secreted by cancer cells could display autocrine effects on cancer cells and paracrine effects on vascular endothelial cells. Indeed, *in vitro* stimulation of cancer cells with recombinant soluble CD146 increased their proliferation and the production of protumorigenic factor such as VEGF. They also demonstrated that this stimulation protected cancer cells from apoptosis induced by H_2O_2 and decreased cancer cell senescence. In particular, the c-myc signaling pathway appeared to be upregulated by soluble CD146. Soluble CD146 secreted by cancer cells also increased the proliferation of surrounding endothelial cells, stimulating tumor angiogenesis. These effects were confirmed *in vivo* in different models of xenografted mice and an antisoluble CD146 antibody was able to block these effects. Thus, soluble CD146 was described as a proangiogenic factor and seems to have a major role in tumor development.

5. Ligand and cell signalization

Historically, the first molecule interacting with the extracellular portion of CD146 is NOF (neurite outgrowth factor). A stable transfection of complementary DNA encoding for CD146 induces an adhesion of neuronal cells on a NOF matrix [32]. More recently, laminin-8 has been identified as a new vascular ligand of CD146 expressed by TH17 lymphocytes. In this study, it has been demonstrated that the laminin-411/CD146 interaction favor adhesion and tissue transmigration of these lymphocytes, leading to an increased inflammation [52]. Furthermore, one study showed that CD146 DNA transfection in the CD146-deficient melanoma cell line Mel-888 induced an increased aggregation between these cells and cells which do not express CD146 suggesting that there are other still unidentified partners [53].

The existence of a homophilic interaction for CD146 is controversial. One study showed that CD146 transfection in neuronal cells induced their aggregation, suggesting that CD146 could create homophilic bonds [32]. Another *in vitro* study demonstrated that the neurite growth of PC12 cells is increased when cells are in a chimeric CD146 protein substrate. In addition, under these conditions, the use of an anti-CD146 antibody blocks neurite growth. This inhibition would be associated with an inhibition of CD146-CD146 homophilic interaction [54]. CD146 dimerization at the cell membrane following stimulation with an activating CD146 antibody (clone AA98) was also demonstrated using fluorescence resonance energy transfer (FRET) and pull-down. The use of an NFkB signaling pathway inhibitor reduced this dimerization [55]. Finally, a recent study highlighted dimerization after stimulation with VEGF [56].

Conversely, other studies could not replicate the homophilic interaction, in particular, between soluble CD146 and CD146-Fc [33].

Recently, new ligands for CD146 were identified. A direct and strong interaction between CD146 and VEGFR-2 was demonstrated in endothelial cells and this association was important for VEGFR-2 phosphorylation by VEGF. These results were confirmed in a CD146 KO mouse model where the absence of CD146 inhibited vessel formation induced by VEGF. Experiments in mouse models of pancreas and melanoma cancer cell xenograft have shown that the combined use of anti-VEGF antibody (bevacizumab) and anti-CD146 antibody (AA98) displayed a synergistic effect on tumor development [57].

Another work identified galectin 1 as a new CD146 ligand on the endothelium [58]. This protein induced apoptosis of endothelial cells and specifically bound to CD146 via extracellular glycosylations. This interaction is specific for galectin 1 since it is not found with galectin 2. Using siRNA or antibodies able to block CD146 resulted in an increased cell apoptosis, suggesting a protective role of CD146 against apoptosis.

Different factors have been shown to modulate CD146 expression:

- A stimulation with TNF-alpha increases the amount of CD146 present at the endothelial cell surface [33].

http://dx.doi.org/10.5772/66765

- TGF-beta administered to hepatocyte cells pretreated with an inducer of acute hepatitis (tetrachloride carbonate) increases the amount of CD146 mRNA and the regenerative capacity of these cells [59].
- HSP27 (heat shock protein 27), a chaperone molecule involved mainly in tumor differentiation and tumorigenesis, inhibits the migration and invasion of melanoma cells and thus acts on the tumor phenotype [60]. Overexpression of HSP27 has been shown to decrease the expression of CD146 and increase the expression of E-cadherin in melanoma cell lines. These variations in protein expression determine, among other, malignant phenotype of melanoma cells [61].
- AKT activation by PD98059 and Wortmannin increases CD146 expression at the cell membrane in melanoma cell lines. Conversely in these cell lines, overexpression of CD146 increases AKT which inhibits BAD (Bcl-2-associated death promoter), increasing cell survival [62].

Membrane CD146 activates multiple signaling pathways, leading to the activation of the NFkB pathway. CD146 dimerization has been described in the membrane of endothelial cells following the addition of culture medium of tumor cells (A375 cell line). Inhibition of the NFkB pathway (by BAY11-7082 compound) causes a reduction of the nuclear translocation of NFKB but also inhibits the dimerization of CD146 [63, 64]. The junctional molecules involved in adhesion such as VE-cadherin or claudins are also involved in a phenomenon of actin cytoskeleton reorganization. CD146 is also connected to the actin cytoskeleton.

Indeed, CD146 targeting with the S-ENDO1 antibody led to FAK phosphorylation and an increase in the release of intracellular calcium and extracellular calcium entry. This mechanism of action of calcium flux was mediated by the recruitment and activation of Fyn leading to the phosphorylation of PLC gamma. Calcium entry also caused the recruitment of PYK2 and p130. On the other hand, FAK activation led to signaling pathways involved in the reorganization of the actin cytoskeleton and also modulated transcription factors involved in cells survival and migration. In these studies, there was no evidence of direct interaction between CD146, paxillin, and FAK. It seems therefore important to identify the intermediate partners [65, 66].

Recently, a study confirmed the role of CD146 in the migration and induction of signals related to the actin cytoskeleton. Indeed, CD146 displays direct physical interaction with the ezrin-radixin-moesin (ERM) proteins, allowing the recruitment of ERM at the protrusions of melanoma cells. This phenomenon induces the elongation and expansion of microvilli at these protrusions [67].

Recruitment by CD146 allows the sequestration of a RhoA inhibitor (Rho guanine nucleotide dissociation inhibitory factor 1) leading to RhoA activation and an increased cell motility. Another study showed that CD146 is redistributed in a polarized structure named W-RAMP (Wnt5a-mediated actin-myosin receptor-polarity) in subconfluent melanoma cells stimulated with Wnt5a. W-RAMP is involved in membrane retraction and the direction of cell migration with an intervention of Rho-A [68].

In another study that focused on the priming of ECFC with soluble CD146 in order to improve the therapeutic potential of these cells *in vivo*, the authors showed that a priming of these cells

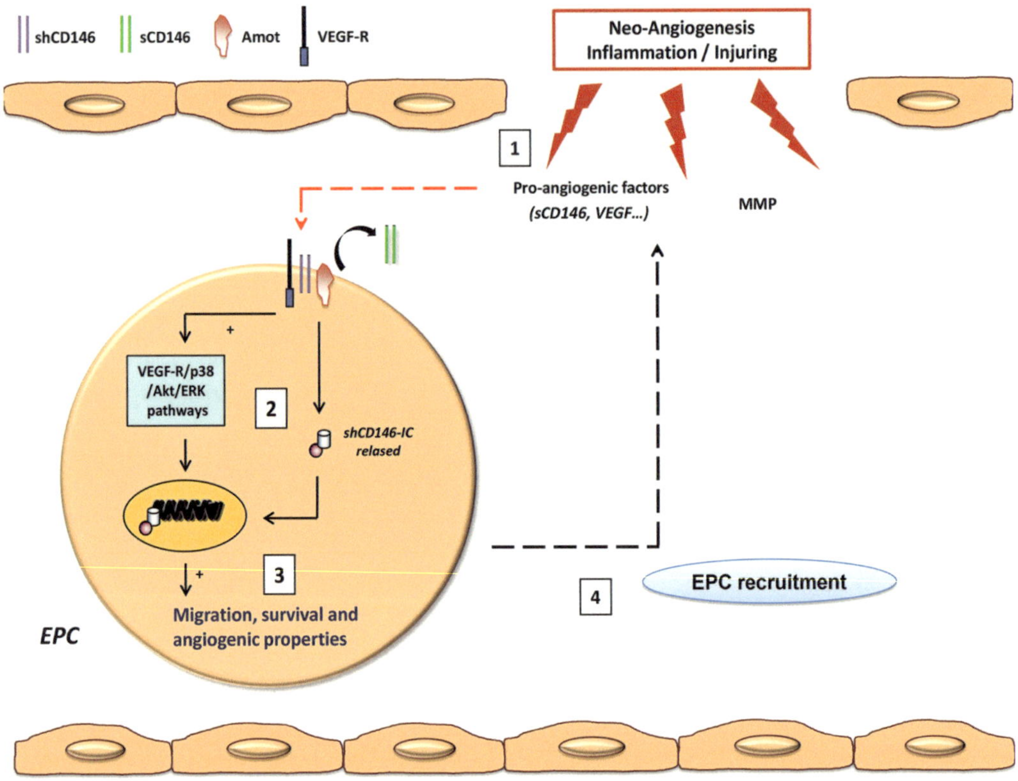

Figure 3. Mechanism of actions of endothelial progenitor cells (EPC) activation leads to their recruitment after inflammatory or angiogenic stimulation.

with soluble CD146 did not modify the number of engrafted ECFC in the ischemic muscle but improved their survival capacity leading to an enhanced revascularization [39]. They showed that in ECFC, it exists a signalosome that is located in a particular region of cell membrane called lipid rafts. This signalosome contains soluble CD146, the short isoform of CD146 (shCD146), presenilin-1 but also the two VEGF receptor called flt1 and flk1. The mechanism of action is characterized by a sequential proteolytic cleavage, induced by soluble CD146, with an extracellular shedding of the short CD146 followed by an intramembrane cleavage which is mediated by both the ADAM/matrix metalloproteases (MMP) and the gamma-secretase protein. The consequences of this shedding involved a nuclear translocation of the new intracellular peptide of shCD146 which binds to the transcription factor CSL and is associated with a modulation of gene transcription leading to angiogenesis (eNOS) and cell survival (FADD, Bcl-xl). The association between CD146 and VEGFR2 was described in a previous paper and based on these results the authors showed that the effect of soluble CD146 on EFCF is dependent on VEGFR2 but also VEGFR1 which are phosphorylated by soluble CD146. All these findings show that the stimulation of this cell by soluble CD146 and the proteolytic cleavage of shCD146 is a promising pathway to increase the regenerative properties of endothelial progenitor cells for the treatment of cardiovascular diseases (**Figure 3**).

http://dx.doi.org/10.5772/66765

6. CD146 in pathology

6.1. Obstetrical pathologies

About 2% of fertile women are affected by spontaneous fetal loss. The mechanism of this fetal loss is not yet understood.

One study showed that CD146 is highly expressed during the implantation window. During the following steps, the level of CD146 decreased rapidly and CD146 blocking with an antibody caused abortion [69]. CD146 is expressed by the intermediate trophoblasts (or extravillous) in humans but is not detected on the syncytiotrophoblasts and cytotrophoblasts [70].

After this work, soluble CD146 was described as a novel physiological factor with angiogenic properties involved in the regulation of placenta vascular development by acting on extravillous trophoblast (EVT). Using placenta explants, soluble CD146 was demonstrated to inhibit the growth of extravillous trophoblasts and the ability of EVT to migrate and form pseudocapillary tubes on Matrigel. A clinical study on the role of soluble CD146 in 50 pregnant women was also conducted. A physiological decrease of plasmatic soluble CD146 was observed in pregnant women as compared to nongestational women. These results inspired the authors to study the effects of prolonged administration of soluble CD146 in a pregnant rat model. Repeated systemic injection of soluble CD146 after mating caused a significant decrease in the pregnancy rate and the number of embryos. Histological studies of placenta showed a decreased migration of glycogen cells (cells that are similar to the EVT in rat) in female rat treated with soluble CD146.

In mice the use of a specific antibody blocking CD146 (AA98) caused a decrease in the blastocysts adhesion on a uterine epithelium cell monolayer and a decrease in the growth of trophoblastic cells. In addition, injection of this antibody in the uterine horn of the mouse at 3.5 dpc (days post coitum) resulted in a decrease of embryo implantation at 7.5 dpc. Histological analysis showed that the embryos were present but smaller and in poor condition [69]. Two clinical studies were in line with these observations. A first clinical study showed that the rate of membrane CD146 expression was lower on intermediate trophoblasts in the placenta of preeclamptic patients when compared to patients with nonpathological pregnancies [70]. In a second study, two populations of women have been used to compare the blood level of soluble CD146. In this study, the authors used 100 blood samples which were taken 2 months after the last obstetrical events between women with no pregnancy lost which have at least one living child and 100 blood samples from women with at least two consecutive losses at/ or before 21 weeks of gestation. They found an increase in the level of soluble CD146 in the second population compared to the first control population [71]. In this study, the two populations used are age matched.

Thus, in view of these results soluble CD146 may represent an attractive biomarker of vascular placental development as well as a therapeutic target in obstetric complications.

6.2. Inflammatory diseases

Endothelial functions are altered in inflammatory diseases.

In inflammatory kidney disease, biopsies of patients with nephropathy show an increased expression of membrane CD146 on endothelial cells, but also on the mesangial cells and a neo-expression of CD146 on tubular cells [72]. In addition, there is a correlation between CD146 expression and proteinuria, endocapillary proliferation and inflammatory syndrome. The serum level of soluble CD146 is also modulated. Thus, an increase in CD146 secretion was observed in chronic renal failure which was correlated with the severity of this disease in type 2 diabetic nephropathy patients [73].

In a second type of inflammatory disease, CD146 has also been identified in primary cultures of keratinocytes while its expression was not observed on healthy skin. An increase in the expression of CD146 has been observed in various skin diseases. For example, CD146 is expressed in suprabasals keratinocytes of psoriasis patients [74]. CD146 is also detected in Kaposi's sarcoma, lichen planus, on the skin overlying skin neoplasms or in chronic and acute chronic dermatitis [74]. On the other hand, the expression of CD146 is not increased in other skin diseases such as lupus erythematosus.

6.3. Tumor pathologies

CD146 is expressed in many cancers, such as melanoma, prostate cancer, breast cancer, pancreatic cancer, lung cancer, Kaposi sarcoma, angiosarcoma, Schwann cells tumors, or leiomyosarcoma.

The role of tumor CD146 was first studied in melanoma. A direct correlation has been demonstrated between the increase in metastasizing capacities and the increased expression of CD146 [75]. The level of expression of CD146 by human melanoma cell lines has been shown to correlate with their ability to form tumors and metastasis in a mouse xenograft model in immunodeficient nude or SCID mice [76]. In addition, CD146 increases the number of lung metastases following intravenous injection of melanoma cells in nude mice *in vivo* [77]. These observations were confirmed through the use of interfering RNA directed against CD146 leading to a decrease in migration, proliferation, and invasion *in vitro* [78].

CD146 immunohistochemistry staining was performed on human primary melanoma tissue, showing a CD146 expression on tumor-associated endothelium and on smooth muscle cells [79]. The role of CD146 in tumor angiogenesis has been described in particular thanks to the use of the AA98 antibody [37, 64] that is able to block tumor angiogenesis and decrease tumor growth of human melanoma xenograft model in immunodeficient mice.

Currently, mechanisms involved in melanoma progression are unclear. A study showed that a particular population of B lymphocyte cells, the B1 lymphocytes, has a prometastatic potential. Indeed, depletion of this population caused a decrease of tumor growth and metastasis dissemination in mice in an experimental metastasis model, following a B16 cell line injection. The decrease in metastases dissemination involved homophilic interactions between B1 and B16 cells thanks to CD146 [80]. In addition, coculture of B1 cells with melanoma cells increased the expression of CD146 at the cell membrane of cancer cells, increasing the number of metastases *in vivo*.

A clinical study was conducted on a cohort of patients with skin cancer. Patients were divided into two groups: early and late stage melanoma, in order to analyze the presence of different commonly used cancer markers including CD146. Analysis in the blood of patients showed that CD146 was the only protein correlated with the advanced stages of the disease [81]. Another study confirmed this finding by demonstrating that CD146 is a marker of poor prognosis and survival in melanoma patients. CD146 constitutes a better marker than biopsies analysis of sentinel lymph node [82].

6.4. Angiogenesis-related diseases and therapeutic approaches

Recent studies revealed that both isoforms of CD146 are involved in angiogenesis with a promigratory and a proproliferative role of the short CD146 and a vessel stabilization role of long CD146, which is also described in this chapter. Soluble CD146 secreted by both endothelial and cancer cells is also able to stimulate angiogenesis. These different forms are involved in physiological angiogenesis but also in pathological angiogenesis, in particular in tumor angiogenesis.

Therefore, different antibodies have been generated to block its functions. The first one was ABX-MA1, an antibody recognizing the human form of this molecule. This antibody was able to inhibit the formation of spheroids containing melanoma cells, reducing metastasis, tumorigenicity, and vascularization of the tumor *in vivo*. This reduction was related to the inhibition of MMP-2 expression which is heavily involved in metastasis formation [83].

Another team-generated monoclonal antibody specifically directed against the vascular endothelium of tumors. During the screening of these antibodies, the authors focused on the AA98 antibody. This antibody recognizes CD146 localized in the intratumoral vasculature but not recognizes CD146 expressed on blood vessels in healthy tissues [37]. This antibody inhibits both *in vitro* and *in vivo* angiogenic properties of CD146 in human tumors xenografted in immunodeficient mice. In addition, it was demonstrated that the AA98 antibody is a potential diagnostic and therapeutic agent in vascular and cancer diseases. Following this work, it was shown that AA98 antibody inhibits phosphorylation of p38/MAPK, suppresses NFkB activation, and inhibits MMP-9 and ICAM-1 expression. This suggests that deleting NFkB is a pivotal point of the inhibitory effects of the antibody on endothelial cell migration, angiogenesis, and development of tumor metastases [64].

Of interest, this antibody displays additive inhibitory effects when used in combination with the anti-VEGF antibody bevacizumab in xenografted models of human pancreatic tumors and melanoma [57]. In addition, it reduces significantly the chronic inflammation in the colon in a mouse model and prevents the development of cancer associated with this chronic inflammation [38].

Recently, a novel antibody was generated against the soluble form of CD146 [20]. The authors demonstrated that this antibody was able to decrease tumor angiogenesis and growth but to also induce apoptosis of human melanoma and pancreatic tumors xenografted in immunodeficient mice. Of interest, this antibody cannot bind membrane CD146, a property that should limit the side effects that could be observed with antibodies targeting the membrane form.

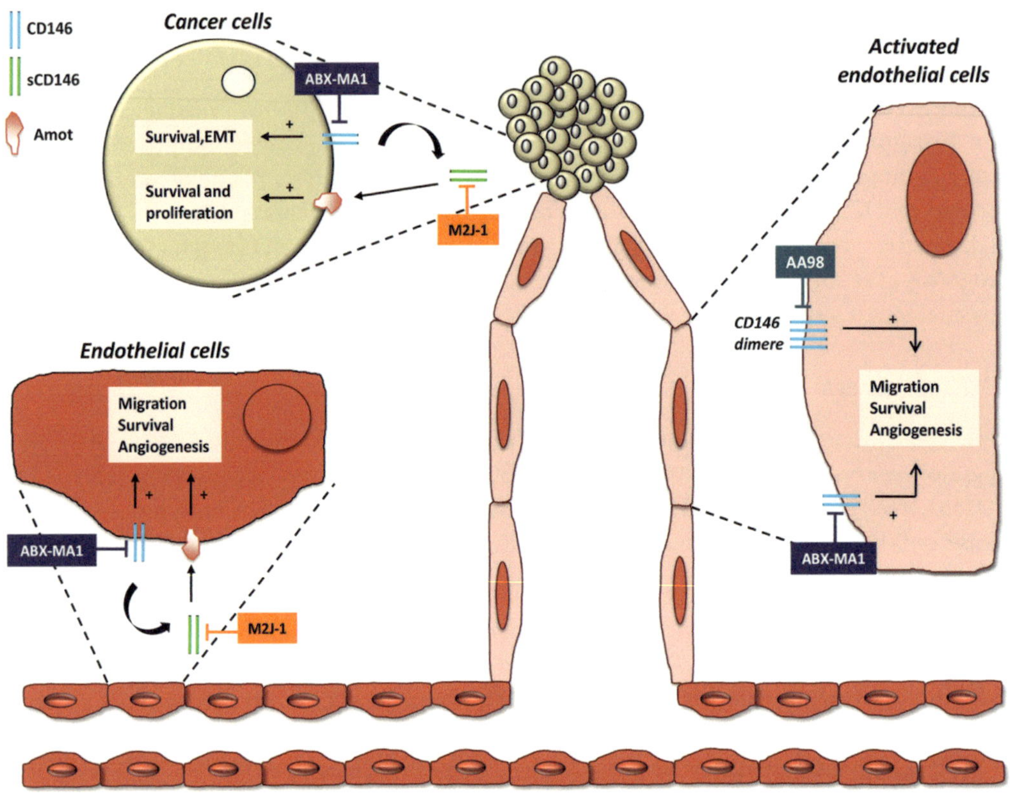

Figure 4. Functions of the different isoforms of CD146 and the inhibitory antibodies associated during tumor growth and angiogenesis.

Functions of the different CD146 isoforms and the inhibitory antibodies associated are summarized in **Figure 4**.

Author details

Jimmy Stalin[1]*, Lucie Vivancos[2], Nathalie Bardin[3], Françoise Dignat-George[3] and Marcel Blot-Chabaud[3]

*Address all correspondence to: jimmy.stalin@unige.ch

1 Department of Pathology and Immunology, University Medical Center, Geneva University, Switzerland

2 Pediatric Hematology-Oncology Research Laboratory, Pediatric Division, University Hospital CHUV, Lausanne, Switzerland

3 INSERM UMR-S 1076, Aix-Marseille University, UFR Pharmacy, Marseille, France

References

[1] Lehmann JM, Holzmann B, Breitbart EW, Schmiegelow P, Riethmüller G, Johnson JP. Discrimination between benign and malignant cells of melanocytic lineage by two novel antigens, a glycoprotein with a molecular weight of 113,000 and a protein with a molecular weight of 76,000. Cancer Res. 1987 Feb 1;47(3):841–845.

[2] George F, Poncelet P, Laurent JC, Massot O, Arnoux D, Lequeux N, Ambrosi P, Chicheportiche C, Sampol J. Cytofluorometric detection of human endothelial cells in whole blood using S-Endo 1 monoclonal antibody. J Immunol Methods. 1991 May 17;139(1):65–75.

[3] Bardin N, George F, Mutin M, Brisson C, Horschowski N, Francés V, Lesaule G, Sampol J. S-Endo 1, a pan-endothelial monoclonal antibody recognizing a novel human endothelial antigen. Tissue Antigens. 1996 Nov;48(5):531–539.

[4] Bardin N, Francès V, Lesaule G, Horschowski N, George F, Sampol J. Identification of the S-Endo 1 endothelial-associated antigen. Biochem Biophys Res Commun. 1996 Jan 5;218(1):210–216.

[5] Vainio O, Dunon D, Aïssi F, Dangy JP, McNagny KM, Imhof BA. HEMCAM, an adhesion molecule expressed by c-kit+ hemopoietic progenitors. J Cell Biol. 1996 Dec;135(6 Pt 1):1655–1668.

[6] Sers C, Kirsch K, Rothbächer U, Riethmüller G, Johnson JP. Genomic organization of the melanoma-associated glycoprotein MUC18: implications for the evolution of the immunoglobulin domains. Proc Natl Acad Sci U S A. 1993 Sep 15;90(18):8514–8518.

[7] Mintz-Weber CS, Johnson JP. Identification of the elements regulating the expression of the cell adhesion molecule MCAM/MUC18. Loss of AP-2 is not required for MCAM expression in melanoma cell lines. J Biol Chem. 2000 Nov 3;275(44):34672–34680.

[8] Jean D, Gershenwald JE, Huang S, Luca M, Hudson MJ, Tainsky MA, Bar-Eli M. Loss of AP-2 results in up-regulation of MCAM/MUC18 and an increase in tumor growth and metastasis of human melanoma cells. J Biol Chem. 1998 Jun 26;273(26):16501–16508.

[9] Xie S, Price JE, Luca M, Jean D, Ronai Z, Bar-Eli M. Dominant-negative CREB inhibits tumor growth and metastasis of human melanoma cells. Oncogene. 1997 Oct 23;15(17):2069–2075.

[10] Lehmann JM, Riethmüller G, Johnson JP. MUC18, a marker of tumor progression in human melanoma, shows sequence similarity to the neural cell adhesion molecules of the immunoglobulin superfamily. Proc Natl Acad Sci U S A. 1989 Dec;86(24):9891–9895.

[11] Yang H, Wang S, Liu Z, Wu MH, McAlpine B, Ansel J, Armstrong C, Wu G. Isolation and characterization of mouse MUC18 cDNA gene, and correlation of MUC18 expression in mouse melanoma cell lines with metastatic ability. Gene. 2001 Mar 7;265(1–2):133–145.

[12] Schön M1, Kähne T, Gollnick H, Schön MP. Expression of gp130 in tumors and inflammatory disorders of the skin: formal proof of its identity as CD146 (MUC18, Mel-CAM). J Invest Dermatol. 2005 Aug;125(2):353–363.

[13] Ihnen M, Kilic E, Köhler N, Löning T, Witzel I, Hagel C, Höller S, Kersten JF, Müller V, Jänicke F, Milde-Langosch K. Protein expression analysis of ALCAM and CEACAM6 in breast cancer metastases reveals significantly increased ALCAM expression in metastases of the skin. J Clin Pathol. 2011 Feb;64(2):146–152. doi: 10.1136/jcp.2010.082602.

[14] Kijima N, Hosen N, Kagawa N, Hashimoto N, Nakano A, Fujimoto Y, Kinoshita M, Sugiyama H, Yoshimine T. CD166/activated leukocyte cell adhesion molecule is expressed on glioblastoma progenitor cells and involved in the regulation of tumor cell invasion. Neuro Oncol. 2012 Oct;14(10):1254–1264.

[15] Taira E, Nagino T, Taniura H, Takaha N, Kim CH, Kuo CH, Li BS, Higuchi H, Miki N. Expression and functional analysis of a novel isoform of gicerin, an immunoglobulin superfamily cell adhesion molecule. J Biol Chem. 1995 Dec 1;270(48):28681–28687.

[16] Bardin N, Francès V, Combes V, Sampol J, Dignat-George F. CD146: biosynthesis and production of a soluble form in human cultured endothelial cells. FEBS Lett. 1998 Jan 2;421(1):12–14.

[17] Bardin N1, Moal V, Anfosso F, Daniel L, Brunet P, Sampol J, Dignat George F. Soluble CD146, a novel endothelial marker, is increased in physiopathological settings linked to endothelial junctional alteration. Thromb Haemost. 2003 Nov;90(5):915–920.

[18] Boneberg EM, Illges H, Legler DF, Fürstenberger G. Soluble CD146 is generated by ectodomain shedding of membrane CD146 in a calcium-induced, matrix metalloprotease-dependent process. Microvasc Res. 2009 Dec;78(3):325–331. doi: 10.1016/j.mvr.2009.06.012.

[19] Liu JW, Nagpal JK, Jeronimo C, Lee JE, Henrique R, Kim MS, Ostrow KL, Yamashita K, van Criekinge V, Wu G, Moon CS, Trink B, Sidransky D. Hypermethylation of MCAM gene is associated with advanced tumor stage in prostate cancer. Prostate. 2008 Mar 1;68(4):418–426. doi: 10.1002/pros.20709.

[20] Stalin J, Nollet M, Garigue P, Fernandez S, Vivancos L, Essaadi A, Muller A, Bachelier R, Foucault-Bertaud A, Fugazza L, Leroyer AS, Bardin N, Guillet B, Dignat-George F, Blot-Chabaud M. Targeting soluble CD146 with a neutralizing antibody inhibits vascularization, growth and survival of CD146-positive tumors. Oncogene. 2016 Apr 11. doi: 10.1038/onc.2016.83.

[21] Guezguez B1, Vigneron P, Alais S, Jaffredo T, Gavard J, Mège RM, Dunon D. A dileucine motif targets MCAM-l cell adhesion molecule to the basolateral membrane in MDCK cells. FEBS Lett. 2006 Jun 26;580(15):3649–3656. Epub 2006 Jun 2.

[22] Bardin N1, Anfosso F, Massé JM, Cramer E, Sabatier F, Le Bivic A, Sampol J, Dignat-George F. Identification of CD146 as a component of the endothelial junction involved in the control of cell-cell cohesion. Blood. 2001 Dec 15;98(13):3677–3684.

[23] Kebir A, Harhouri K, Guillet B, Liu JW, Foucault-Bertaud A, Lamy E, Kaspi E, Elganfoud N, Vely F, Sabatier F, Sampol J, Pisano P, Kruithof EK, Bardin N, Dignat-George F, Blot-Chabaud M. CD146 short isoform increases the proangiogenic potential of endothelial progenitor cells *in vitro* and *in vivo*. Circ Res. 2010 Jul 9;107(1):66–75. doi: 10.1161/CIRCRESAHA.109.213827.

[24] Okumura S, Muraoka O, Tsukamoto Y, Tanaka H, Kohama K, Miki N, Taira E. Involvement of gicerin in the extension of microvilli. Exp Cell Res. 2001 Dec 10;271(2):269–276.

[25] Elshal MF, Khan SS, Takahashi Y, Solomon MA, McCoy JP Jr. CD146 (Mel-CAM), an adhesion marker of endothelial cells, is a novel marker of lymphocyte subset activation in normal peripheral blood. Blood. 2005 Oct 15;106(8):2923–2924.

[26] Pickl WF1, Majdic O, Fischer GF, Petzelbauer P, Faé I, Waclavicek M, Stöckl J, Scheinecker C, Vidicki T, Aschauer H, Johnson JP, Knapp W. MUC18/MCAM (CD146), an activation antigen of human T lymphocytes. J Immunol. 1997 Mar 1;158(5):2107–2115.

[27] Despoix N1, Walzer T, Jouve N, Blot-Chabaud M, Bardin N, Paul P, Lyonnet L, Vivier E, Dignat-George F, Vély F. Mouse CD146/MCAM is a marker of natural killer cell maturation. Eur J Immunol. 2008 Oct;38(10):2855–2864. doi: 10.1002/eji.200838469.

[28] Sorrentino A, Ferracin M, Castelli G, Biffoni M, Tomaselli G, Baiocchi M, Fatica A, Negrini M, Peschle C, Valtieri M. Isolation and characterization of CD146+ multipotent mesenchymal stromal cells. Exp Hematol. 2008 Aug;36(8):1035–1046. doi: 10.1016/j.exphem.2008.03.004.

[29] Sacchetti B1, Funari A, Michienzi S, Di Cesare S, Piersanti S, Saggio I, Tagliafico E, Ferrari S, Robey PG, Riminucci M, Bianco P. Self-renewing osteoprogenitors in bone marrow sinusoids can organize a hematopoietic microenvironment. Cell. 2007 Oct 19;131(2):324–336.

[30] Taira E1, Kohama K, Tsukamoto Y, Okumura S, Miki N. Characterization of Gicerin/MUC18/CD146 in the rat nervous system. J Cell Physiol. 2004 Mar;198(3):377–387.

[31] Taira E1, Takaha N, Taniura H, Kim CH, Miki N. Molecular cloning and functional expression of gicerin, a novel cell adhesion molecule that binds to neurite outgrowth factor. Neuron. 1994 Apr;12(4):861–872.

[32] Taira E1, Tsukamoto Y, Kohama K, Maeda M, Kiyama H, Miki N. Expression and involvement of gicerin, a cell adhesion molecule, in the development of chick optic tectum. J Neurochem. 2004 Feb;88(4):891–899.

[33] Bardin N1, Blot-Chabaud M, Despoix N, Kebir A, Harhouri K, Arsanto JP, Espinosa L, Perrin P, Robert S, Vely F, Sabatier F, Le Bivic A, Kaplanski G, Sampol J, Dignat-George F. CD146 and its soluble form regulate monocyte transendothelial migration. Arterioscler Thromb Vasc Biol. 2009 May;29(5):746–753. doi: 10.1161/ATVBAHA.108.183251.

[34] Elshal MF1, Khan SS, Raghavachari N, Takahashi Y, Barb J, Bailey JJ, Munson PJ, Solomon MA, Danner RL, McCoy JP Jr. A unique population of effector memory lymphocytes

identified by CD146 having a distinct immunophenotypic and genomic profile. BMC Immunol. 2007 Nov 13;8:29.

[35] Solovey AN1, Gui L, Chang L, Enenstein J, Browne PV, Hebbel RP. Identification and functional assessment of endothelial P1H12. J Lab Clin Med. 2001 Nov;138(5):322–331.

[36] Kamiyama T1, Watanabe H, Iijima M, Miyazaki A, Iwamoto S. Coexpression of CCR6 and CD146 (MCAM) is a marker of effector memory T-helper 17 cells. J Dermatol. 2012 Oct;39(10):838–842. doi: 10.1111/j.1346-8138.2012.01544.x.

[37] Yan X1, Lin Y, Yang D, Shen Y, Yuan M, Zhang Z, Li P, Xia H, Li L, Luo D, Liu Q, Mann K, Bader BL. A novel anti-CD146 monoclonal antibody, AA98, inhibits angiogenesis and tumor growth. Blood. 2003 Jul 1;102(1):184–191.

[38] Wellbrock J1, Fiedler W. CD146: a new partner for VEGFR2. Blood. 2012 Sep 13;120(11):2164–2165. doi: 10.1182/blood-2012-07-439646.

[39] Stalin J1, Harhouri K1, Hubert L1, Garrigue P2, Nollet M1, Essaadi A1, Muller A1, Foucault-Bertaud A1, Bachelier R1, Sabatier F3, Pisano P1, Peiretti F4, Leroyer AS1, Guillet B2, Bardin N1, Dignat-George F1, Blot-Chabaud M5. Soluble CD146 boosts therapeutic effect of endothelial progenitors through proteolytic processing of short CD146 isoform. Cardiovasc Res. 2016 Aug 1;111(3):240–251. doi: 10.1093/cvr/cvw096.

[40] Stalin J1, Harhouri K, Hubert L, Subrini C, Lafitte D, Lissitzky JC, Elganfoud N, Robert S, Foucault-Bertaud A, Kaspi E, Sabatier F, Aurrand-Lions M, Bardin N, Holmgren L, Dignat-George F, Blot-Chabaud M. Soluble melanoma cell adhesion molecule (sMCAM/sCD146) promotes angiogenic effects on endothelial progenitor cells through angiomotin. J Biol Chem. 2013 Mar 29;288(13):8991–9000. doi: 10.1074/jbc.M112.446518.

[41] Harhouri K1, Kebir A, Guillet B, Foucault-Bertaud A, Voytenko S, Piercecchi-Marti MD, Berenguer C, Lamy E, Vely F, Pisano P, Ouafik L, Sabatier F, Sampol J, Bardin N, Dignat-George F, Blot-Chabaud M. Soluble CD146 displays angiogenic properties and promotes neovascularization in experimental hind-limb ischemia. Blood. 2010 May 6;115(18):3843–3851. doi: 10.1182/blood-2009-06-229591.

[42] Wu GJ1, Peng Q, Fu P, Wang SW, Chiang CF, Dillehay DL, Wu MW. Ectopical expression of human MUC18 increases metastasis of human prostate cancer cells. Gene. 2004 Mar 3;327(2):201–213.

[43] Wu Z1, Wu Z, Li J, Yang X, Wang Y, Yu Y, Ye J, Xu C, Qin W, Zhang Z. MCAM is a novel metastasis marker and regulates spreading, apoptosis and invasion of ovarian cancer cells. Tumour Biol. 2012 Oct;33(5):1619–1628. doi: 10.1007/s13277-012-0417-0.

[44] Schiano C1, Grimaldi V, Casamassimi A, Infante T, Esposito A, Giovane A, Napoli C. Different expression of CD146 in human normal and osteosarcoma cell lines. Med Oncol. 2012 Dec;29(4):2998–3002. doi: 10.1007/s12032-012-0158-3.

[45] McGary EC1, Heimberger A, Mills L, Weber K, Thomas GW, Shtivelband M, Lev DC, Bar-Eli M. A fully human antimelanoma cellular adhesion molecule/MUC18 antibody

inhibits spontaneous pulmonary metastasis of osteosarcoma cells in vivo. Clin Cancer Res. 2003 Dec 15;9(17):6560–6566.

[46] Shih LM1, Hsu MY, Palazzo JP, Herlyn M. The cell-cell adhesion receptor Mel-CAM acts as a tumor suppressor in breast carcinoma. Am J Pathol. 1997 Sep;151(3):745–751.

[47] Zabouo G, Imbert AM, Jacquemier J, Finetti P, Moreau T, Esterni B, Birnbaum D, Bertucci F, Chabannon C. CD146 expression is associated with a poor prognosis in human breast tumors and with enhanced motility in breast cancer cell lines. Breast Cancer Res. 2009;11(1):R1. doi: 10.1186/bcr2215.

[48] Zeng G1, Cai S, Liu Y, Wu GJ. METCAM/MUC18 augments migration, invasion, and tumorigenicity of human breast cancer SK-BR-3 cells. Gene. 2012 Jan 15;492(1):229–238. doi: 10.1016/j.gene.2011.10.024.

[49] Liu WF1, Ji SR, Sun JJ, Zhang Y, Liu ZY, Liang AB, Zeng HZ. CD146 expression correlates with epithelial-mesenchymal transition markers and a poor prognosis in gastric cancer. Int J Mol Sci. 2012;13(5):6399–6406. doi: 10.3390/ijms13056399.

[50] Zeng Q, Li W, Lu D, Wu Z, Duan H, Luo Y, Feng J, Yang D, Fu L, Yan X. CD146, an epithelial-mesenchymal transition inducer, is associated with triple-negative breast cancer. Proc Natl Acad Sci U S A. 2012 Jan 24;109(4):1127–1132. doi: 10.1073/pnas.1111053108.

[51] Ilie M1, Long E1, Hofman V2, Selva E3, Bonnetaud C3, Boyer J4, Vénissac N5, Sanfiorenzo C6, Ferrua B7, Marquette CH6, Mouroux J5, Hofman P2. Clinical value of circulating endothelial cells and of soluble CD146 levels in patients undergoing surgery for non-small cell lung cancer. Br J Cancer. 2014 Mar 4;110(5):1236–1243. doi: 10.1038/bjc.2014.11.

[52] Flanagan K1, Fitzgerald K, Baker J, Regnstrom K, Gardai S, Bard F, Mocci S, Seto P, You M, Larochelle C, Prat A, Chow S, Li L, Vandevert C, Zago W, Lorenzana C, Nishioka C, Hoffman J, Botelho R, Willits C, Tanaka K, Johnston J, Yednock T. Laminin-411 is a vascular ligand for MCAM and facilitates TH17 cell entry into the CNS. PLoS One. 2012;7(7):e40443. doi: 10.1371/journal.pone.0040443.

[53] Johnson JP1, Bar-Eli M, Jansen B, Markhof E. Melanoma progression-associated glycoprotein MUC18/MCAM mediates homotypic cell adhesion through interaction with a heterophilic ligand. Int J Cancer. 1997 Nov 27;73(5):769–774.

[54] Taira E1, Kohama K, Tsukamoto Y, Okumura S, Miki N. Gicerin/CD146 is involved in neurite extension of NGF-treated PC12 cells. J Cell Physiol. 2005 Aug;204(2):632–637.

[55] Bu P1, Zhuang J, Feng J, Yang D, Shen X, Yan X. Visualization of CD146 dimerization and its regulation in living cells. Biochim Biophys Acta. 2007 Apr;1773(4):513–520.

[56] Zhuang J1, Jiang T, Lu D, Luo Y, Zheng C, Feng J, Yang D, Chen C, Yan X. NADPH oxidase 4 mediates reactive oxygen species induction of CD146 dimerization in VEGF signal transduction. Free Radic Biol Med. 2010 Jul 15;49(2):227–236. doi: 10.1016/j.freeradbiomed.2010.04.007.

[57] Jiang T1, Zhuang J, Duan H, Luo Y, Zeng Q, Fan K, Yan H, Lu D, Ye Z, Hao J, Feng J, Yang D, Yan X. CD146 is a coreceptor for VEGFR-2 in tumor angiogenesis. Blood. 2012 Sep 13;120(11):2330–2339. doi: 10.1182/blood-2012-01-406108.

[58] Jouve N1, Despoix N, Espeli M, Gauthier L, Cypowyj S, Fallague K, Schiff C, Dignat-George F, Vély F, Leroyer AS. The involvement of CD146 and its novel ligand Galectin-1 in apoptotic regulation of endothelial cells. J Biol Chem. 2013 Jan 25;288(4):2571–2579. doi: 10.1074/jbc.M112.418848.

[59] Tsuchiya S1, Tsukamoto Y, Taira E, LaMarre J. Involvement of transforming growth factor-beta in the expression of gicerin, a cell adhesion molecule, in the regeneration of hepatocytes. Int J Mol Med. 2007 Mar;19(3):381–386.

[60] Aldrian S1, Trautinger F, Fröhlich I, Berger W, Micksche M, Kindas-Mügge I. Overexpression of Hsp27 affects the metastatic phenotype of human melanoma cells in vitro. Cell Stress Chaperones. 2002 Apr;7(2):177–185.

[61] Aldrian S1, Kindas-Mügge I, Trautinger F, Fröhlich I, Gsur A, Herbacek I, Berger W, Micksche M. Overexpression of Hsp27 in a human melanoma cell line: regulation of E-cadherin, MUC18/MCAM, and plasminogen activator (PA) system. Cell Stress Chaperones. 2003 Fall;8(3):249–257.

[62] Li G1, Kalabis J, Xu X, Meier F, Oka M, Bogenrieder T, Herlyn M.Reciprocal regulation of MelCAM and AKT in human melanoma. Oncogene. 2003 Oct 9;22(44):6891–6899.

[63] Zheng C1, Qiu Y, Zeng Q, Zhang Y, Lu D, Yang D, Feng J, Yan X. Endothelial CD146 is required for in vitro tumor-induced angiogenesis: the role of a disulfide bond in signaling and dimerization. Int J Biochem Cell Biol. 2009 Nov;41(11):2163–2172. doi: 10.1016/j.biocel.2009.03.014.

[64] Bu P1, Gao L, Zhuang J, Feng J, Yang D, Yan X. Anti-CD146 monoclonal antibody AA98 inhibits angiogenesis via suppression of nuclear factor-kappaB activation. Mol Cancer Ther. 2006 Nov;5(11):2872–2878.

[65] Anfosso F1, Bardin N, Francès V, Vivier E, Camoin-Jau L, Sampol J, Dignat-George F. Activation of human endothelial cells via S-endo-1 antigen (CD146) stimulates the tyrosine phosphorylation of focal adhesion kinase p125(FAK). J Biol Chem. 1998 Oct 9;273(41):26852–26856.

[66] Anfosso F1, Bardin N, Vivier E, Sabatier F, Sampol J, Dignat-George F. Outside-in signaling pathway linked to CD146 engagement in human endothelial cells. J Biol Chem. 2001 Jan 12;276(2):1564–1569.

[67] Luo Y1, Zheng C, Zhang J, Lu D, Zhuang J, Xing S, Feng J, Yang D, Yan X. Recognition of CD146 as an ERM-binding protein offers novel mechanisms for melanoma cell migration. Oncogene. 2012 Jan 19;31(3):306–321. doi: 10.1038/onc.2011.244.

[68] Witze ES1, Litman ES, Argast GM, Moon RT, Ahn NG. Wnt5a control of cell polarity and directional movement by polarized redistribution of adhesion receptors. Science. 2008 Apr 18;320(5874):365–369. doi: 10.1126/science.1151250.

[69] Liu Q1, Zhang B, Zhao X, Zhang Y, Liu Y, Yan X. Blockade of adhesion molecule CD146 causes pregnancy failure in mice. J Cell Physiol. 2008 Jun;215(3):621–626. doi: 10.1002/jcp.21341.

[70] Shih IM, Kurman RJ. Expression of melanoma cell adhesion molecule in intermediate trophoblast. Lab Invest. 1996 Sep;75(3):377–388.

[71] Pasquier E1, Bardin N, De Saint Martin L, Le Martelot MT, Bohec C, Roche S, Mottier D, Dignat-George F. The first assessment of soluble CD146 in women with unexplained pregnancy loss. A new insight? Thromb Haemost. 2005 Dec;94(6):1280–1284.

[72] Daniel L1, Bardin N, Moal V, Dignat-George F, Berland Y, Figarella-Branger D. Tubular CD146 expression in nephropathies is related to chronic renal failure. Nephron Exp Nephrol. 2005;99(4):e105–111.

[73] Wang F1, Xing T, Wang N, Liu L. Clinical significance of plasma CD146 and P-selectin in patients with type 2 diabetic nephropathy. Cytokine. 2012 Jan;57(1):127–129. doi: 10.1016/j.cyto.2011.10.010.

[74] Weninger W1, Rendl M, Mildner M, Mayer C, Ban J, Geusau A, Bayer G, Tanew A, Majdic O, Tschachler E. Keratinocytes express the CD146 (Muc18/S-endo) antigen in tissue culture and during inflammatory skin diseases. J Invest Dermatol. 2000 Aug;115(2):219–224.

[75] Luca M1, Hunt B, Bucana CD, Johnson JP, Fidler IJ, Bar-Eli M. Direct correlation between MUC18 expression and metastatic potential of human melanoma cells. Melanoma Res. 1993 Feb;3(1):35–41.

[76] Schlagbauer-Wadl H1, Jansen B, Müller M, Polterauer P, Wolff K, Eichler HG, Pehamberger H, Konak E, Johnson JP. Influence of MUC18/MCAM/CD146 expression on human melanoma growth and metastasis in SCID mice. Int J Cancer. 1999 Jun 11;81(6):951–955.

[77] Xie S, Luca M, Huang S, Gutman M, Reich R, Johnson JP, Bar-Eli M. Expression of MCAM/MUC18 by human melanoma cells leads to increased tumor growth and metastasis. Cancer Res. 1997 Jun 1;57(11):2295–2303.

[78] Watson-Hurst K1, Becker D. The role of N-cadherin, MCAM and beta3 integrin in melanoma progression, proliferation, migration and invasion. Cancer Biol Ther. 2006 Oct;5(10):1375–1382.

[79] Sers C1, Riethmüller G, Johnson JP. MUC18, a melanoma-progression associated molecule, and its potential role in tumor vascularization and hematogenous spread. Cancer Res. 1994 Nov 1;54(21):5689–5694.

[80] Staquicini FI1, Tandle A, Libutti SK, Sun J, Zigler M, Bar-Eli M, Aliperti F, Pérez EC, Gershenwald JE, Mariano M, Pasqualini R, Arap W, Lopes JD. A subset of host B lymphocytes controls melanoma metastasis through a melanoma cell adhesion molecule/

MUC18-dependent interaction: evidence from mice and humans. Cancer Res. 2008 Oct 15;68(20):8419–8428. doi: 10.1158/0008-5472.CAN-08-1242.

[81] Rapanotti MC1, Bianchi L, Ricozzi I, Campione E, Pierantozzi A, Orlandi A, Chimenti S, Federici G, Bernardini S. Melanoma-associated markers expression in blood: MUC-18 is associated with advanced stages in melanoma patients. Br J Dermatol. 2009 Feb;160(2):338–344. doi: 10.1111/j.1365-2133.2008.08929.x.

[82] Pearl RA1, Pacifico MD, Richman PI, Wilson GD, Grover R. Stratification of patients by melanoma cell adhesion molecule (MCAM) expression on the basis of risk: implications for sentinel lymph node biopsy. J Plast Reconstr Aesthet Surg. 2008;61(3):265–271.

[83] Mills L1, Tellez C, Huang S, Baker C, McCarty M, Green L, Gudas JM, Feng X, Bar-Eli M. Fully human antibodies to MCAM/MUC18 inhibit tumor growth and metastasis of human melanoma. Cancer Res. 2002 Sep 1;62(17):5106–5114.